GASTROINTESTINAL PATHOLOGY

Parakrama Chandrasoma, MD, MRCP (UK)
Professor of Pathology
University of Southern California
Los Angeles

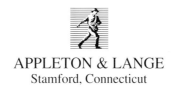

APPLETON & LANGE
Stamford, Connecticut

99 00 01 02 03/ 10 9 8 7 6 5 4 3 2 1

Prentice Hall International (UK) Limited, *London*
Prentice Hall of Australia Pty. Limited, *Sydney*
Prentice Hall Canada, Inc., *Toronto*
Prentice Hall Hispanoamericana, S.A., *Mexico*
Prentice Hall of India Private Limited, *New Delhi*
Prentice Hall of Japan, Inc., *Tokyo*
Simon & Schuster Asia Pte. Ltd., *Singapore*
Editora Prentice Hall do Brasil Ltda., *Rio de Janeiro*
Prentice Hall, *Upper Saddle River, New Jersey*

Library of Congress Cataloging-in-Publication Data

Chandrasoma, Para.
   Gastrointestinal pathology / Parakrama Chandrasoma.
      p.   cm.
   Includes index.
   ISBN 0-8385-3093-1 (case : alk. paper)
   1. Gastrointestinal system—Diseases.   2. Gastrointestinal system—
Histopathology.   3. Gastrointestinal system—Diseases—Diagnosis.
I. Title
   [DNLM: 1. Gastrointestinal System—pathology.   2. Gastrointestinal
Diseases—diagnosis.   WI   141C456g   1999]
RC802.9.C47   199
616.3′3—dc21
DNLM/DLC   98-25826
for Library of Congress   CIP

Acquisitions Editor: Michael P. Medina
Production Service: York Production Services
Designer: Janice Barsevich Bielawa
Cover Design: Aimee Nordin
PRINTED IN HONG KONG

ISBN 0-8385-3093-1

To my parents
for life, genes, love, and education

Parakrama Chandrasoma, MD

PREFACE

Learning to make pathologic diagnoses is a complex process. Rarely is a disease diagnosed using one overriding diagnostic criterion; rather, diagnosis often uses a combination of criteria. Although it is easy to list these criteria, each specimen expresses these features to different degrees. Although each criterion has a different amount of diagnostic value, criteria are rarely weighted according to their importance. When different examples of the same pathologic process are evaluated, it is not uncommon that different diagnostic criteria dominate. This is very confusing to the trainee pathologist, and even more intimidating for the clinician who looks at slides in a more superficial manner.

Diagnostic criteria are important; however, most pathologic diagnoses are made instantly by recognizing and analyzing a constellation of criteria simultaneously. It is a matter of considerable frustration when a pathology resident brings a slide to me and I make an instant diagnosis. In my early teaching years, I thought this process unfair and attempted to backtrack my chain of reasoning so as to enumerate all the criteria I had used subconsciously. I no longer believe this to be appropriate. My function as a teacher is to be totally honest with my students and to let them know the thought processes that I am conscious of when I look at a slide. If these do not involve criteria, so be it.

When asked the perennial question, "Dr. Chandrasoma, does this specimen demonstrate high-grade dysplasia?" by junior residents, I tell them that my overall experience tells me that this is so. I then tell them that they can have total trust in the fact that I am correct and encourage them to carefully study the slide, comparing it with other similar epithelial proliferations and develop their own diagnostic criteria. Truth is not what anyone says; it is to be found in the slide itself. My most important function as a teacher is to be honest. When I make a diagnosis, I must be correct. When I am uncertain, I must say so. My greatest thrill as a teacher is when a resident examines the slide carefully and challenges what I have said. Those cases where they prove me wrong provide me with my ultimate learning experiences.

The process of making a pathologic diagnosis is akin to the value system of the Jedi Knights in the movie *Star Wars*. Luke Skywalker, piloting his X-wing fighter through a treacherous trench of the Death Star, squints his eyes, scanning the intricate surface of the space station for his miniscule target. All his predecessors have failed to see and hit the target. Luke readies his computerized aiming device, locking on to the ventilation shaft he must hit to destroy the Death Star. His ears prick up suddenly as the voice of his trainer, Jedi Master Obi-Wan Kenobi, echoes in his brain: "Let go, Luke; use the Force." A brief internal debate flickers in Luke's eyes, and to the astonishment of all, he shuts down the computer, switching to manual aim. His finger tenses on the trigger and two ellipses of energy rocket from his fighter, slipping right down the vent to the center of the Death Star, initiating a chain reaction that destroys the space station and saves the galaxy.

I tell the residents that the secret to learning to make pathologic diagnoses is equivalent to acquiring the Force. The Force is acquired by analyzing large numbers of slides, and entering data into one's brain that involves not only criteria but the different weights that are ascribed to each criterion in each different case. When a pathologist has acquired the Force, diagnoses will be made instantly and instinctively; not by evaluating criteria. The Force is superior to all other diagnostic methods.

What is the role of books in this learning process, and specifically what do I hope to achieve by this book? The usefulness of this book will vary depending on who is using it. Practicing pathologists will find it useful because it provides a review of pathologic technique and diagnostic methods. This book may even slightly improve the way they approach specimens and make diagnoses ("fine-tuning the Force"). Pathology trainees will find it useful because it provides basic diagnostic criteria of most diseases. They will be able to use the text and photographs as they study slides and develop the experience ("developing the Force") they need to become adept at microscopic diagnosis. They will also find a rational basis for what they do at gross examination that will help them develop good techniques.

To function well as a pathologist, diagnostic ability alone is not sufficient. All pathologists must have a knowledge of the clinical practice of gastroenterology to allow them to understand the clinical relevance of their reports; without this, they function in a vacuum. This book provides what I believe is the relevant clinical information critical to pathologists to work in the same universe as their clinical colleagues. Communication is 80% of a successful pathologist.

Gastroenterologists will find this book useful because it provides a liaison for the meaning of different terms and diagnoses. The text attempts to discuss the clinical relevance of pathologic diagnosis in the hope that gastroenterologists will increase their accuracy in interpreting surgical pathology re-

ports. Gastroenterology trainees will find a clinically oriented presentation of pathology that makes sense as they review slides with pathologists. No one expects the gastroenterologist to develop the ability to make diagnoses, but the closer a clinician is to the "Force" the better he or she can communicate with and understand the pathologist. The microscopic photographs should provide the basic knowledge required of pathology residents at their Board examination.

Although this book is not a substitute for long and arduous study of microscopic slides, I do hope that it will facilitate many pathologists to develop and fine-tune their diagnostic skills. I trust that the clinicopathologic correlates emphasized throughout this text will enable pathologist and clinician to understand each other, ultimately to the benefit of the patients they care for.

"May the Force be with you"
Obi-Wan Kenobi, Jedi master: *Star Wars*

CONTENTS

CONTRIBUTORS

Joel Chan, MD
Clinical Assistant Professor
University of Southern California School of Medicine
Physician Resident
Department of Pathology
Los Angeles County-University of Southern California
    Medical Center
Los Angeles, California

Jennifer Cho Sartorelli, MD
Physician Resident
Department of Pathology
University of Southern California
Los Angeles, California

Evelyn Choo, MD
Fellow in Cytopathology
Los Angeles County-University of California-Los Angeles
    Medical Center
Los Angeles, California

Patricia Dalton, MD
Clinical Assistant Professor
University of Southern California School of Medicine
Physician Resident
Department of Pathology
Los Angeles County-University of Southern California
    Medical Center
Los Angeles, California

Roger Der, MD
Clinical Assistant Professor
University of Southern California School of Medicine
Physician Resident
Department of Pathology
Los Angeles County-University of Southern California
    Medical Center
Los Angeles, California

Milton Kiyabu, MD
Assistant Professor of Clinical Pathology
University of Southern California School of Medicine
Associate Director, Surgical Pathology
Los Angeles County-University of Southern California
    Medical Center
Los Angeles, California

Greg Kobayashi, MD
Resident in Pathology
Department of Pathology
University of Southern California
Los Angeles, California

Yanling Ma, MD
Clinical Assistant Professor
University of Southern California School of Medicine
Physician Resident
Department of Pathology
Los Angeles County-University of Southern California
    Medical Center
Los Angeles, California

Wesley Naritoku, MD, PhD
Clinical Assistant Professor
University of Southern California School of Medicine
Attending Staff Pathologist
Los Angeles County-University of Southern California
    Medical Center
Los Angeles, California

Anwar Sultana Raza, MD
Assistant Professor of Clinical Pathology
Department of Cytopathology
Los Angeles County-University of Southern California
Los Angeles, California

Rashida Soni, MD
Clinical Assistant Professor
University of Southern California School of Medicine
Physician Resident
Department of Pathology
Los Angeles County-University of Southern California
    Medical Center
Los Angeles, California

Pamela B. Sylvestre, MD
Clinical Assistant Professor of Pathology
University of Southern California School of Medicine
Los Angeles, California

Mark T. Taira, MD
Associate Deputy Medical Examiner
Los Angeles County Department of Coroner
Los Angeles, California

Gail Wehrli, MD
Clinical Assistant Instructor
University of Southern California School of Medicine
Los Angeles, California

Helen Yen, MD
Clinical Assistant Professor
University of Southern California School of Medicine
Physician Resident
Department of Pathology
Los Angeles County-University of Southern California
    Medical Center
Los Angeles, California

1

BASIC PRECEPTS

Parakrama Chandrasoma

RULES OF CLINICAL INTERACTION

The importance of gastrointestinal (GI) pathology in the daily workload of the pathologist has both increased and changed with the increasing use of endoscopy. Although the number of large resection specimens from surgery has remained fairly constant, in the past 20 years endoscopic GI biopsies have proliferated. This proliferation has shifted the clinical focus in GI pathology from surgical to medical pathology. Dividing this discussion into medical and surgical gastrointestinal pathology is useful, because the gastroenterologist and surgeon need different things from the pathologist.

Medical GI Pathology

The endoscopic biopsy represents the end-point of an interaction between a patient with symptoms related to the gastrointestinal tract and a gastroenterologist. In most cases, the gastroenterologist is seeking a diagnosis to direct the patient's care. Most biopsy specimens are diagnostic by virtue of their histologic features; in these cases, very little clinical information is necessary. Some GI biopsies, however, do not have features diagnostic of a specific disease; in these cases, the surgical pathologist's success correlates directly with the degree of interaction between gastroenterologist and pathologist. Unfortunately, such interaction appears to be decreasing. In general medical practice, the vast majority of endoscopic biopsies are read by the pathologist, who is given scanty clinical data, resulting in a suboptimal pathology report that is of limited value to the gastroenterologist. Knowledge of the patient's symptoms, laboratory testing, radiologic and endoscopic findings, and the gastroenterologist's diagnostic thought process dramatically increases the usefulness of information that the surgical pathologist can provide. As managed care providers dictate to physicians the numbers of patients and specimens they are required to handle, this type of interaction falls by the wayside, and endoscopic procedures, although achieving a "satisfactory care outcome" often fail to provide optimum patient care.

It is important for both gastroenterologist and pathologist to attempt to optimize the endoscopic diagnostic process within the constraints of their medical practice. The following practical adjustments to the routine of endoscopy, biopsy, specimen transmittal (by gastroenterologist), specimen processing, microscopic examination, pathology report generation and transmittal (by pathologist), and pathology report interpretation (by gastroenterologist) are recommended.

Develop a Good Pathology Request Form

The pathologist should develop a request form that emphasizes clinical data. This is easy to achieve. Getting adequate clinical data on the request form from the clinician is more difficult. Because the vast majority of cases have information that the nurse can appropriately insert (eg, abdominal pain, colon polyp), this function is commonly delegated to the nurse. In complicated cases, however, it is crucial for the gastroenterologist to break this routine by including a brief statement on the nature of the problem. Just a short explanation can mean the difference between a useless and a helpful pathology report. One gastroenterologist I deal with provides, along with the biopsy specimen, a dictated report of the procedure, which includes the symptoms, indication for endoscopy, endoscopic findings, location of specimens taken, and the treatment plan after the procedure. Another gastroenterologist routinely provides a copy of all color photographs taken at endoscopy. Such information is invaluable and increases the accuracy of pathologic diagnosis dramatically.

Increase Communication Between Gastroenterologist and Pathologist

The patient who undergoes endoscopy and biopsy is really consulting two physicians. The patient only speaks with the gastroenterologist, but, in many cases, the pathologist provides the crucial information for deciding the patient's treatment. In the vast majority of cases, the pathologist can communicate all the necessary pathologic information in the surgical pathology report. Unfortunately, this has the effect of preventing communication between the pathologist and gastroenterologist. Communication is essential in the following situations:

1. *When the pathology report provides a diagnosis that does not fit with the gastroenterologist's impression.*

    One common example is minimal early gastric cancer in which a pathology report provides a diagnosis of adenocarcinoma (Fig. 1–1) that surprises the endoscopist who really did not see anything indicative of malignancy. Although most of these cases turn out to be correctly diagnosed as early gastric cancers, I have seen several examples in which the reparative reaction associated with a healing erosion was misdiagnosed as cancer (Fig. 1–2). The gastroenterologist's vigilance and request for a second opinion in these cases was the only thing that prevented an unnecessary gastrectomy.

2. *When the gastroenterologist has no clear idea of the patient diagnosis or how to proceed after reading the pathology report.*

    Discussing the problem with the pathologist who has examined the patient's sample under the microscope is frequently helpful. The pathologist may have some insights that were not expressed in the pathology report that may provide direction, or the gastroenterologist may provide information

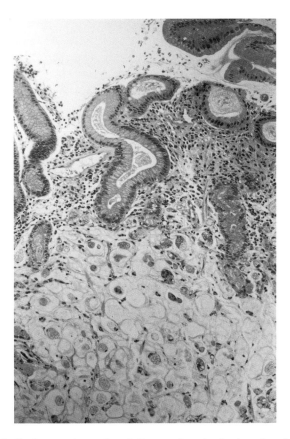

Figure 1–1. Gastric mucosa in an endoscopic biopsy specimen showing signet ring cell adenocarcinoma in the lamina propria. The gastroenterologist, who did not see a lesion indicative of malignancy, requested a second opinion, which confirmed the diagnosis of carcinoma.

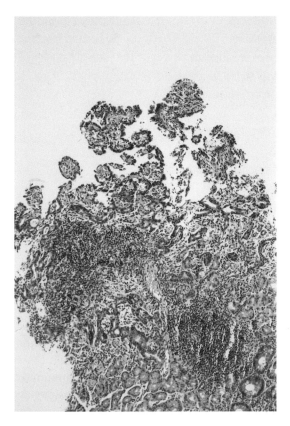

Figure 1–2. Healing gastric erosion with atypical regenerative changes. The surface has a papillary appearance with marked cytologic atypia of the epithelial cells. This was diagnosed as adenocarcinoma; request for a second opinion by the gastroenterologist led to the diagnosis of healing erosion. Patient had a negative repeat endoscopic examination 3 months later.

that precipitates further study of the specimen. A recent case will demonstrate the value of this type of interaction: A 42-year-old male with abdominal pain and iron deficiency anemia had a gastric biopsy that was reported as showing reactive gastropathy with congestion. The gastroenterologist called the pathologist to inquire about a possible etiology. Discussion of the clinical findings (patient with a history of chronic alcoholism and evidence of liver dysfunction) and biopsy findings resulted in a conclusion that the changes were most likely the result of portal hypertension affecting the gastric mucosa.

Communication between gastroenterologist and pathologist is best done in the pathologist's office over a double-headed microscope. The telephone is a reasonable substitute if dictated by time constraints. The effectiveness of communication is ultimately dependent on very personal factors. Pathologists who make the interaction positive by their enthusiastic participation in the diagnostic process and gastroenterologists who understand the value of pathology in patient care communicate the most effectively with one another. Unfortunately, it is often the case that the pathologists and gastroenterologists who most need to improve their communication skills so as to improve patient care are the least likely to believe in its importance and the least likely to seek it.

Surgical GI Pathology

The handling of surgical procedures related to the gastrointestinal tract requires skills that are very different from those needed for interpreting endoscopic biopsies. In most elective cases, the diagnosis has been established by prior endoscopic biopsy or radiologic imaging. In these cases, the pathologist may be called on intraoperatively to confirm the preoperative diagnosis and, in neoplastic diseases, to help establish surgical margin adequacy by gross and frozen section examination.

In emergency cases, usually the treatment of intestinal obstruction or perforation, the pathologist may have a greater intraoperative diagnostic role. The value of the pathologist here is based on his or her expertise in the diagnosis of gross specimens. Surgeons and pathologists have equivalent ability in diagnosis when the organs are in situ, but the pathologist has greater expertise once the specimen has been removed, and particularly when it has been opened. The frequency with which the pathologist is called in this type of situation is a function of the surgeon's belief that the pathologist will provide useful information, which in turn is a function of the pathologist's level of expertise and reputation.

For the most part, however, diagnosis is a function of how the specimen removed at surgery is handled by the pathologist. This procedure provides a definitive pathologic diagnosis, staging, and information regarding adequacy of the surgery in cases of neoplasms. Unlike endoscopic biopsies, surgically resected specimens must result in a definitive diagnosis, assuming that the pathologic tissue has been removed. The pathologist does not require a great deal of communication with the surgeon in most cases. When a pathologic diagnosis is not obvious, however, knowledge of the radiologic features (eg, colon removed for bleeding from angiodysplasia), operative findings (eg, a small bowel removed for obstruction secondary to adhesions), or previous history (eg, gastric cancer that has received preoperative chemotherapy) can be essential for correct diagnosis.

SOME BASIC RULES OF PATHOLOGY

Recognition of Normal Tissue

Most experienced surgical pathologists have learned most of their GI pathology by dealing with surgical specimens. When tissue is removed at surgery, a pathologic abnormality is usually present in the tissue that justifies the surgical procedure. The invariable need of a pathologic diagnosis in a surgical specimen inhibits pathologists from using the words "normal" or "no pathologic abnormality" in a final diagnosis. This has resulted in the creation of nonexistent pathologic entities, such as "chronic nonspecific colitis." The diagnostic criteria for chronic nonspecific colitis, when enumerated, cannot be clearly distinguished from normal colonic mucosa. When real chronic inflammation exists in the colon, it must satisfy criteria for some recognized type of colitis such as microscopic colitis, diversion colitis, or idiopathic inflammatory bowel disease.

In endoscopic biopsies, "normal" is a common diagnosis and provides information that is often as valuable to the gastroenterologist as a specific diagnosis. Unlike a surgical resection, which must remove pathologically abnormal tissue, endoscopic biopsies are frequently the result of exploring for possible pathology. In a patient with occult GI bleeding, for example, the first diagnostic procedure may be lower GI endoscopy. Biopsies of normal colonic mucosa, when reported as "chronic nonspecific colitis" may prevent further study in the patient and result in diagnostic failure if a significant cause of bleeding is present elsewhere in the GI tract. In a patient with diarrhea, the clinical diagnosis of irritable bowel syndrome requires that endoscopy and histologic examination of a mucosal biopsy specimen be normal. When the gastroenterologist receives a diagnosis of normal on a colonic biopsy, irritable bowel syndrome can be diagnosed clinically. A pathologic diagnosis of "chronic nonspecific colitis" creates a problem, however. Many well-informed gastroenterologists learn to equate "nonspecific chronic colitis" with normal and essentially ignore this as a diagnosis. It is to be hoped that no gastroenterologist believes that "chronic nonspecific colitis" is a disease that necessitates some treatment!

Speak the Same Language as Your Clinician

A recent study[1] tested the understanding of the meaning of dysplasia in ulcerative colitis and the effect of dysplasia in a biopsy on patient treatment among a group of senior gastroenterology trainees and two groups of academic and community gastroen-terologists in the western United States. The understanding of the process was not uniform or consistently accurate among the participants. The majority could not identify the correct definition of dysplasia. In particular, 50% of the gastroenterologists underestimated the cancer risk in high-grade dysplasia, and 30% did not recommend colectomy when high-grade dysplasia was diagnosed on the surveillance biopsy.

It is a mistake for pathologists to assume that their clinical colleagues understand their jargon, including such well-known concepts as dysplasia. I have had clinicians ask me whether metaplasia was a neoplastic process. There is no easy solution to this problem. Increasing surgical pathology training from the present level, which usually consists of intermittent clinico-pathologic conferences, is difficult to achieve in busy clinical residency programs. Increasing communication between pathologists and gastroenterologists would help, but this generally occurs most among those physicians who need it the least. Comments in the pathology report elaborating on the relevance of pathologic diagnoses are helpful, but they must be adjusted to the clinical setting and the personalities involved.

Know the Effect of the Pathologic Diagnosis

Pathologic diagnosis is sometimes not a black-and-white issue; in many conditions, gray areas exist. The best example of this is the grading of dysplasia. Dysplasia occurs in a spectrum from low grade to high grade, and pathologists draw artificial lines that separate no dysplasia from low-grade and low-grade dysplasia from high-grade. These lines can be adjusted to increase sensitivity or specificity of diagnosis (Fig. 1–3). Knowing the effect of a diagnosis is crucial to where the pathologist sets his or her lines. In Barrett's esophagus, a diagnosis of high-grade dys-

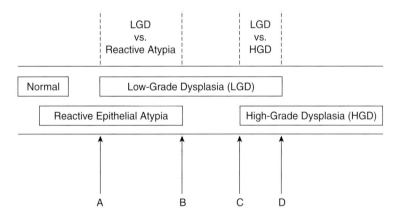

Figure 1–3. Spectrum of epithelial dysplasia ranging from normal to high-grade dysplasia. Note that the changes of reactive epithelial changes and low-grade dysplasia (LGD), and LGD and high-grade dysplasia (HGD) can overlap. The specificity and sensitivity of the diagnoses of LGD and HGD can be adjusted by changing the dividing line between these conditions. If LGD is diagnosed at point A, it will have a high sensitivity (all LGD will be called LGD) and low specificity (many cases called LGD will be reactive atypias). If LGD is diagnosed at point B, it will have low sensitivity but high specificity. Similarly, if HGD is diagnosed at point C, it will have high sensitivity but, by including some cases of LGD, the specificity will be lower. Diagnosing HGD at point D will make specificity 100%, but some cases of HGD will be missed (ie, lower sensitivity).

plasia must be made with 100% specificity (ie, at point D in Fig. 1–3) in a clinical setting in which this diagnosis is an indication for esophagectomy. In clinical situations in which high-grade dysplasia is handled with extremely careful follow-up, the diagnosis of high-grade dysplasia can have a greater degree of sensitivity and less than 100% specificity (ie, at point C in Fig. 1–3). There is sufficient data in the literature to justify both types of patient treatment after a diagnosis of high-grade dysplasia in Barrett's esophagus.

It is even more important for the pathologist to recognize that the consequences of pathologic diagnosis can suddenly change without their knowledge. For many years, the diagnosis of low-grade dysplasia in ulcerative colitis was an indication for increasing the frequency of surveillance. If this is true, a high sensitivity of diagnosis is desirable. Recently, evidence in the literature could indicate that low-grade dysplasia in ulcerative colitis is an indication for prophylactic colectomy. If this is true, the diagnosis of low-grade dysplasia must have a much higher specificity (ie, at point B in Fig. 1–3). A pathologist *must* know whether a diagnosis of low-grade dysplasia in a patient with ulcerative colitis will precipitate increased surveillance or colectomy. The pathologist needs to know this at the time of examination of the endoscopic biopsy, not when he or she receives the colon 3 weeks later. Ideally, gastroenterologists should communicate any such crucial change in their thinking to the pathologist. Such information is rarely provided, however, because most gastroenterologists believe that all pathologic diagnoses are based on definitive and unchangeable criteria.

Interobserver Variation of Pathologic Diagnosis

Significant variation exists among observers in pathologic diagnosis, even among experts.[2] Consultation between several pathologists within a group removes some of this interobserver variation. Consultation with a recognized expert in the field, particularly in difficult cases, permits community pathologists to fine-tune their diagnostic criteria, bringing these criteria into line with those of the expert. Although this process sounds good, experts may disagree in difficult cases, and interobserver variation cannot be completely removed.

Geographic variation also exists in diagnosis, and this may result in greatly different disease statistics. It has been known for many years that a high percentage of gastric cancer cases are detected at an intramucosal stage in Japan, and that the survival from gastric cancer is much higher in Japan than in the rest of the world. A recent study comparing the pathologic interpretation of gastric biopsies in Japan and other Western countries suggested that the diagnosis of intestinal-type adenocarcinoma was made more aggressively in Japan because it is based entirely on cytologic criteria.[3] In the West, a diagnosis of intramucosal carcinoma requires lamina propria invasion in addition to cytologic criteria. Cases that were diagnosed as high-grade dysplasia and even low-grade dysplasia in the West were called intramucosal carcinoma by Japanese pathologists. This study illustrates the importance of interobserver variability of pathologic diagnosis in assessing the medical literature.

Review Prior Pathologic Material

When a new patient is seen by a gastroenterologist, any prior pathologic material must be reviewed by the pathologist who usually interacts with that gastroenterologist. The only reason not to do this is cost: the reviewing pathologist charges a fee for this assessment. Disagreements between the original diagnosis and the review interpretation arise often enough to make this review imperative. All hospitals should have a policy that mandates such slide review, particularly in patients coming to surgery at that hospital. Unfortunately, many do not. Significant and justifiable malpractice risk is associated with failure to review outside pathologic material before instituting treatment, especially radical surgery for malignancy.

SPECIMEN HANDLING

Endoscopic Biopsies

The aim of handling endoscopic biopsy specimens is to ensure that all the material is appropriately evaluated by the pathologist. This requires establishment of a routine that is as free of error as possible. Although most cases are free of error, problems arise that the gastroenterologist and pathologist must take care to prevent and recognize when they occur.

Specimen Collection and Labeling

The pathologist has a responsibility to establish the correct procedure of specimen collection in the gastroenterologist's office. This can be done by means of a written manual generated by the pathologist, but an on-hands training session must also be conducted by the pathologist, gastroenterologist, or senior office nurse for any new employees.

Biopsy specimens must be lesion-specific and site-specific. It is not appropriate, for example, to place colon polyps from different locations into the same container. Even polyps that look absolutely benign may have cancer within them, resulting in obvious problems. Even when random biopsies are done on two different areas, the specimens must be placed in separate containers.

The labeling process must be rigidly adhered to to prevent mislabeling of specimens within different sites of the same patient and between patients. Such serious problems can arise as a result of mislabeling that only the most careful employees should be given this task.

The following steps are suggested for correctly labeling a specimen:

1. Have an adequate supply of prepared labels and the pathology request form that includes the patient's name and at least one other additional identifying feature (eg, medical record number, date of birth) at hand at the endoscopy.
2. When a biopsy is performed, place the specimen into the container, close the container, write the site of the biopsy on one label, affix the label onto the container, and record the site of the biopsy on the request form. It is essential to do this for each specimen before taking the next specimen. When multiple specimens are taken from one patient, label these using sequential letters (A, B, C, etc) or numbers (1, 2, 3, etc). *Do not place sequential biopsies into a series of bottles for later labeling of specimen site.* A distraction such as a medical emergency or a telephone call can result in change in the order of the bottles and faulty labeling. *Under no circumstances should a second endoscopy begin before labeling from the first patient is complete.* Eliminate every possibility of interpatient specimen mixing during the collection process.
3. Ensure that the labels on the containers match the specimen list on the request form.
4. Complete the request form. It is strongly recommended that the gastroenterologist fills in the clinical data section in the request form, including endoscopic findings and diagnostic possibilities.
5. Include endoscopic reports and endoscopic photographs whenever possible.

The samples may be placed into the formalin solution directly or on a piece of paper prior to placement in formalin. Small unbreakable plastic containers prefilled with adequate amounts of formalin are recommended. These can be transported by courier or even by mail.

Mislabeling can lead to significant diagnostic error. A biopsy from the gastroesophageal junction that is mislabeled "gastric antrum" can result in a patient with Barrett's esophagus and low-grade epithelial dysplasia being misdiagnosed as having chronic antral gastritis with intestinal metaplasia, diseases with different etiology, treatment, and surveillance programs. Interposed colonic polyp sites can lead to resection of the wrong colonic segment if one polyp is carcinomatous. Some instances of mislabeling can be detected, for example, interposed labels for antral and esophageal biopsies are apparent when the epithelial linings are antral and squamous. If any such mislabeling is detected, it should be taken as an indication that the routine of specimen labeling is faulty, and that in-service training of personnel is necessary.

Special Handling of Specimens

The vast majority of endoscopic specimens are immediately placed in formalin. Rarely, a need arises for special handling of specimens, including such instances as (1) specimens taken for cultures that must be placed in the appropriate microbiologic transport media; (2) specimens that may need electron microscopy (eg, for diagnosis or microsporidiosis or Whipple's disease), which must be placed in glutaraldehyde, a fixative required for electron microscopy; (3) specimens that may need special immunologic or genetic studies (eg, lymphoid neoplasms), which may need to be snap-frozen in liquid nitrogen; (4) specimens that may require cell culture, chemosensitivity, or enzymatic studies (eg, certain neoplastic lesions), which may require collection into tissue culture media. If special handling is necessary, ensure that the endoscopy is performed where facility exists for appropriate specimen collection.

Specimen Orientation

The majority of endoscopic biopsy specimens are collected and processed without orientation, which has the disadvantage of resulting in randomly sectioned pieces of mucosa without clear orientation of surface and mucosal base. This lack of orientation makes evaluation of mucosal thickness imperfect. In small-intestine biopsies, the relationship of the length of villi and crypts is crucial for the diagnosis of villous atrophy, which is impossible in unoriented specimens. In most cases, this disadvantage can be overcome by using multiple specimens cut at multiple levels. The probability of finding correctly oriented mucosa for appropriate evaluation when this is done is high, and accurate diagnosis is possible even in those specimens for which there was no attempt made to accurately orient the specimen.

In some academic centers, the personnel involved in collecting the specimen in the endoscopy suite are specially trained to orient the collected specimen. This requires teasing the biopsy so that it is laid flat on a piece of paper with the mucosal surface facing upward. Fixation of the specimen is then possible in an oriented position, resulting in oriented sections. Such specimens are easier to evaluate, particularly for mucosal thickness characteristics, than unoriented specimens. The advantages gained in diagnostic accuracy, however, have not been great enough to justify mandating this technique for general use. The required expertise in the endoscopy office setting, and the fact that the delicate mucosal biopsies can easily be destroyed by handling if orientation is attempted by someone not adept at it, has precluded widespread use of specimen orientation. Although encouraged, specimen orientation is not considered essential.

Specimen Processing

The routine in the laboratory must guarantee that the specimen slide contains a representative section of the material submitted that identifies the patient and the location of the biopsy. Again, the laboratory's routine should be rigidly adhered to, and laboratory personnel processing specimens must be those who act in a manner that prevents any error.

Accessioning is the system whereby a pathology number is assigned to a pathology request. This number is used throughout tissue processing and associates the slide that results from processing with the surgical pathology report developed by the clerical process. Each patient request should be assigned a unique number (eg, S99-0000) and each specimen for that patient given a unique letter or number (eg, A, B, C or 1, 2, 3). These pathology numbers must be placed on the request form and specimen containers prior to gross examination.

Gross examination of the specimen is performed by the pathologist. All biopsy samples must be picked out of the container and placed into a tea bag or other device to ensure that small specimens are not lost. The tissue is then placed in a cassette labeled with the surgical pathology number (eg, S99-0000A), and the labeled cassettes are placed in formalin for transport to the tissue processor with all the other specimens for the day.

The gross description of the specimen should accurately detail the number of specimens present and the size of the largest specimen. The use of disposable cassettes has become almost universal in the United States. This method is preferable to the use of older reusable metal cassettes. Where metal cassettes are still used, however, care should be taken to ensure that specimens are completely removed before the cassettes are reused; otherwise, interpatient contamination can occur.

After processing, the tissue is embedded in paraffin blocks, and sections are cut in the microtome. The cut sections are placed in a water bath before being transferred onto a glass slide that has been prelabeled with the surgical pathology number. Precise routine is necessary here as well, because of the potential for both specimen mix up and carryover of tissue from one specimen to another. Errors in this process are rare, but they can be devastating as the following example illustrates. The slide from a specimen stated to be a rectal polyp in a 64-year-old female showed anal mucosa from the anorectal junction with carcinoma in situ of the squamous epithelium. To ensure lack of invasive carcinoma, deeper sections were ordered. When the deeper sections were examined the next day, they showed a hyperplastic polyp, completely unlike the original section. All the blocks and slides from the day were reviewed and showed that the numbers on slides from two blocks had been interposed. The 64-year-old woman's block of hyperplastic polyp had been interposed with a specimen from a 46-year-old HIV-positive man who really had the squamous carcinoma in situ of the anal canal. Repeat examination and biopsies in both patients in addition to DNA fingerprinting of both patients and both tissue blocks were required to prove this. This egregious error could have led to an unnecessary abdomino-perineal resection in the 64-year-old female and a delay or complete lack of proper treatment of the carcinoma in the man. Such errors were avoided purely by the chance ordering of a deeper cut on a mislabeled slide. Such cases are shocking because they call into question the fundamental processes on which the entire practice of pathology depends. The pathologist must continually ensure the highest standards of practice in even the simplest laboratory procedures.

There is no standard method for cutting sections from the paraffin block. In most centers, the block is cut at one level to produce a strip of sections that fills one slide. In other centers, the block is cut at three levels, producing three slides. The latter method provides a more exhaustive examination of the biopsy sample. If only one level is examined, deeper sections should be liberally used whenever examination of the slide suggests that this may provide additional information.

Microscopic Examination

The pathologist examines the slide in conjunction with the demographic information, a specimen key, any available clinical information, and the gross description. The number and size of pieces of tissue on the slide must correspond with the information in the gross description. Any discrepancy should alert the pathologist to possible problems in labeling, and deeper sections should be requested because the sections may have been cut too superficially in the paraffin block.

Surgical Specimens

General Handling

Specimens resulting from surgery are usually large. They should be handled in one of two ways, depending on the need for intraoperative consultation.

The pathologist is usually involved in intraoperative consultation for either diagnosis or margin evaluation. The pathologist is either called to the operating room, or the fresh specimen is transported to the surgical pathology frozen section area. The first alternative is generally preferable because it guarantees communication between the pathologist and surgeon. Intraoperative specimen handling is also essential when fresh specimens are needed for culture, immunologic and genetic studies, electron microscopy, and other special techniques that are precluded by fixation. Photography of specimens for documentation of lesions and teaching conferences is also best done with the sample in the fresh state prior to fixation.

Large solid specimens, such as liver, spleen, large segments of intestine, and large tumors, do not fix well in formalin unless cut, and such specimens are also best transported immediately to the surgical pathology department for processing and appropriate fixation. Smaller specimens (eg, appendix or small pieces of nontumorous intestine) that do not require intraoperative consultation can be placed in formalin for transport to the laboratory. It is important to use enough formalin to completely immerse the specimen.

The pathologist examines these large surgical specimens, describes gross findings, and takes appropriate samples. Examination and sampling of different specimens is described in the appropriate chapters later in the book.

Margin Evaluation in Neoplasms

In neoplasms treated by radical surgical procedures, the surgical pathologist must ensure complete removal of the neoplasm. This requires careful evaluation of the surgical margin. The surgical margin is defined as that part of the surface of the specimen that has been actively separated by surgical dissection from tissue still in the patient.

Evaluation of the margin requires the following steps: (1) The margin is marked with indelible ink that persists through tissue processing. Inks of different colors can be used to designate different margins. (2) Sections are submitted to include all margins that need to be examined. (3) When the slides are examined, the ink indicates where the margin is. In cases where the entire inked margin does not appear on the slide, deeper sections may be needed to ensure complete evaluation.

The Surgical Pathology Report

The surgical pathology report must contain three sections: (1) demographic information and labeling information, (2) a gross description, and (3) a pathologic diagnosis. A microscopic description and comments are also commonly present, but not required.

The gross description is probably the most important part of the surgical pathology report from the standpoint of documentation. This element of the report converts the specimen received in the laboratory to a description that represents the only permanent record of the specimen. Specimens that are not completely submitted for microscopy (eg, most large surgical specimens) are usually discarded within a few weeks after the report is generated.

A microscopic description is not as necessary because the microscopic slide is stored in the laboratory for several years, and its features can be studied at any time by reviewing the slide. Any microscopic description that is provided, however, must accurately describe the features seen on the slide that led to the diagnosis. A pathologist rarely functions in this orderly manner. In most cases, the pathologist makes a microscopic diagnosis instantly, using pattern recognition and his or her collective experience, rather than a deliberate examination of all the individual microscopic features. If a microscopic description is generated in such a case, it is important for the pathologist to reexamine the slide carefully after the diagnosis has been made and verify all the microscopic features being described. The microscopic description should not describe the diagnosis that has been made.

The diagnosis should be precise and succinct. A long descriptive sentence in a diagnosis usually indicates lack of certainty. The use of "hedge" words, such as "suggestive of," "suspicious for," "most likely," and "possibly representing," should be avoided. Such common hedge phrases represent the avoidance of responsibility on the part of pathologists and have the long-term effect of undermining the trust of their clinical colleagues. The pathologist must take final responsibility for interpreting the specimen, as the following example illustrates. A biopsy of the esophagus shows a squamous epithelial proliferation associated with ulceration. The pathologist thinks this is squamous carcinoma, but has a slight uncertainty about the possibility of regenerative squamous epithelium at an ulcer edge. It is a mistake to report this case as: "squamous epithelial proliferation highly suggestive of (or any of the other hedge phrases) squamous carcinoma" without any other comment. Although an accurate statement, this diagnosis does not provide the clinician with sufficient information to allow for an informed decision on treatment. Because the pathologist has the most critical information about the presence or absence of malignancy, he or she must make the diagnosis. To pass that responsibility back to the clinician, who has less information, is unfair to the patient and the clinician. The most appropriate way to handle such cases is by direct conversation with the clinician. The pathologist should describe the problem, and together both physicians can arrive at the most appropriate solution. If consultation is impossible, the diagnosis can read: "atypical squamous epithelial proliferation; criteria for malignancy not present in this biopsy" with a comment that describes the problem, the difficulty in excluding malignancy, and possibly a suggestion that the biopsy be repeated after the ulcer has been treated. The difference between these two reports is subtle, but crucial because in the second report the pathologist takes responsibility for determining that the patient should not be treated for esophageal cancer at this time. The only alternative to this diagnosis is "squamous carcinoma, invasive," which should be made only when the diagnosis is absolutely certain and the patient can be treated accordingly.

The only hedge phrase that has value is "consistent with." This term can be used to indicate a most likely pathologic diagnosis in a biopsy specimen with nonspecific features when clinical features are used to assist in the diagnosis. "Consistent with" must never be used for the diagnosis of a malignant neoplasm; a diagnosis of malignant neoplasm must be made on the basis of definitive pathologic criteria and should never be predicated on clinical suspicion. In a patient with cirrhosis who presents with upper GI bleeding, however, the diagnosis "reactive gastropathy with vascular ectasia, consistent with portal hypertensive gastropathy" is perfectly appropriate.

A request that a biopsy be repeated should not be made lightly by the pathologist. Repeat biopsy entails a second procedure for the patient and sometimes creates more problems than it solves. Repeat biopsy is clearly indicated (1) if thorough pathologic examination of a sample from an endoscopically or radiologically defined lesion shows that the biopsy is inadequate for diagnosis and (2) when additional studies that cannot be performed on the submitted specimen are necessary for diagnosis, such as when gene rearrangement studies are indicated for diagnosis of a lymphoid mass. Repeat biopsy is less helpful in the following situations: (1) when the pathologic findings of concern are from a poorly defined endoscopic lesion. Here, a negative repeat biopsy does not remove the concern caused by the first biopsy because the sampling in the second biopsy cannot be guaranteed to come from the area of concern. (2) When the pathologic interpretation is difficult, but not on account of sample inadequacy. In such cases, repeat biopsy will likely provide a sample with the same difficulty.

The use of comments in a surgical pathology report is encouraged. Comments represent a method of clarifying the pathologic diagnosis or providing direction to patient treatment. The need for such clarification and direction varies in different situations. For example, when intramucosal carcinoma is found in a pedunculated colonic adenoma, it is wise to include the comment that this has no risk of metastasis and that the polypectomy is adequate treatment. Although such a comment can be misunderstood by the clinician as unnecessary and insulting, it forestalls the pursuit of inappropriate treatment.

References

1. Bernstein CN, Weinstein WM, Levine DS, et al. Physicians' perceptions of dysplasia and approaches to surveillance colonoscopy in ulcerative colitis. *Am J Gastroenterol.* 1995;90:2106–2114.
2. Riddell RH, Goldman H, Ranschoff DF, et al. Dysplasia in inflammatory bowel disease: Standardized classification with provisional clinical applications. *Hum Pathol.* 1983; 14:931–966.
3. Schlemper RJ, Itabashi M, Kato Y, et al. Differences in diagnostic criteria for gastric carcinoma between Japanese and Western pathologists. *Lancet.* 1997;349:1725–1729.

2

NON-NEOPLASTIC DISEASES OF THE ESOPHAGUS

Parakrama Chandrasoma

ANATOMY AND PHYSIOLOGY

The esophagus is a muscular tube lined by squamous epithelium that has a tonically contracted sphincter at each end. The upper esophageal, or cricopharyngeal, sphincter (UES) is made up of the cricopharyngeus muscle and the inferior constrictor muscle of the pharynx. The lower esophageal sphincter (LES) is not clearly defined anatomically. Both sphincters are recognized at manometry as zones with high resting pressure.

The upper end of the esophagus is at the C5–C6 vertebral level and 16–20 cm from the incisors at endoscopy. The esophagus passes posteriorly in the thorax and passes through the diaphragm to join the stomach immediately below the diaphragmatic hiatus. The gastroesophageal junction is the anatomic junction between esophagus and stomach recognized by external examination.

The muscle wall of the esophagus has an inner circular and outer longitudinal layer. The upper third of the esophagus is composed of striated muscle and the lower two thirds of smooth muscle. A ganglionated myenteric and submucosal plexus of nerves, innervated mainly by the vagus nerve, controls esophageal peristalsis. The muscularis mucosae of the esophagus is a well-defined layer of smooth muscle separated by a highly vascularized submucosa from the underlying muscularis externa. A layer of lamina propria connective tissue separates the squamous epithelium from the muscularis mucosae. This

TABLE 2–1. CRITERIA FOR DEFINING THE DIFFERENT TYPES OF EPITHELIA FOUND IN THE GASTROESOPHAGEAL REGION

Type of Epithelium	Definition
Squamous epithelium	Stratified squamous epithelium
Cardiac (= junctional*) mucosa	Mucosa lined by gastric-type surface and foveolar cells with glands containing only mucous cells
Oxyntocardiac (= fundic*) mucosa	Mucosa lined by gastric-type surface and foveolar cells with glands containing a mixture of mucous, oxyntic, and chief cells
Gastric fundic mucosa†	Mucosa lined by gastric-type surface and foveolar cells with glands containing only oxyntic and chief cells
Intestinal (= specialized*) epithelium	Mucosa with surface, foveolae, or glands containing a mixture of mucous cells and goblet cells

*The terms in parentheses were those originally used by Paull and colleagues[30] for the three types of epithelia seen in Barrett's esophagus. Junctional mucosa is also identical to that described by Hayward[6] as being present normally between squamous epithelium of the esophagus and oxyntic mucosa of the gastric fundus.

†Gastric fundic mucosa occurs in the stomach; all other epithelial types in this table occur in the esophagus or junctional region.

lamina propria can develop smooth muscle fibers in reactive conditions, particularly Barrett's esophagus.

The LES, which was first discovered in 1956,[1] is defined manometrically,[2] and its limits cannot be recognized accurately at surgery, pathologic examination, or endoscopy.[3] At manome-

try, the LES is recognized as a high-pressure zone 3–5 cm long that has thoracic and abdominal components. Minimum requirements for adequate function of the LES have been defined[4] as (1) an overall length greater than 2 cm, (2) an abdominal length greater than 1 cm, and (3) a resting pressure of more than 6 Hg-mm. If any one of these elements is below these values, the sphincter is defective. Combined lesser defects of these elements, however, may also result in a defective sphincter.

The LES's function, to prevent gastroesophageal reflux, is assessed by ambulatory 24-h pH monitoring, in which the patient has a pH electrode placed 5 cm above the LES during the day. The electrode is attached to a measuring device that monitors the pH continuously.[5] Acid reflux is identified by a drop in esophageal pH below 4. Because nearly all asymptomatic people have a low level of reflux, abnormal reflux is defined quantitatively as the percentage of time the pH is below 4. If pH is below this level for more than 4.5% of the 24-h period, the patient is likely to have clinical reflux disease. Correlation between symptoms and pH scores is not exact.

Much confusion exists about the various epithelia that line the gastroesophageal region (as defined in Table 2–1 and Figures 2–1 through 2–7.) The esophagus is lined by stratified squamous epithelium throughout its extent. The lining of the LES is also squamous, at least in its upper part. The normal squamous epithelium is flat and nonkeratinized, with a basal cell layer that is less than 20% of the mucosal thickness and lamina propria papillae that extend upward less than 70% of the mucosal thickness (Figs. 2–1 and 2–2). There are normally no

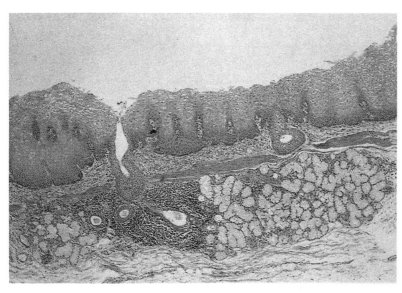
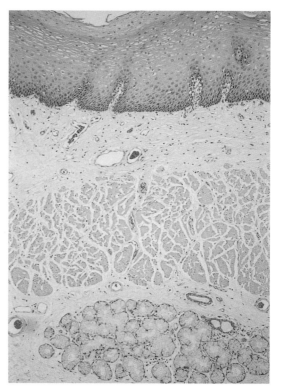

A **B**

Figure 2–1. A: Normal esophagus showing flat stratified squamous epithelium with normal maturation, muscularis mucosa, and submucosal glands draining to the surface through squamous-lined ducts. B: Normal esophagus. The muscularis mucosae is thicker and the submucosal glands are deeper than in part A.

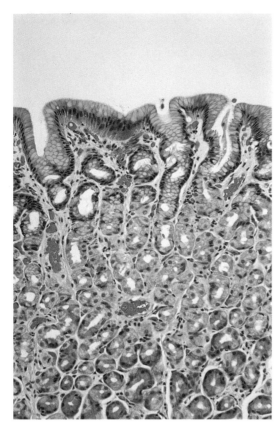

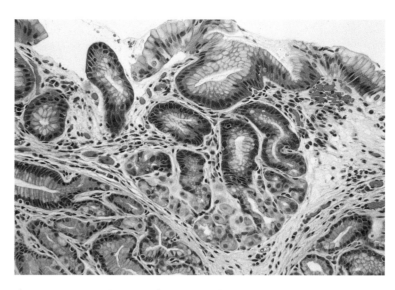

Figure 2–4. Oxyntocardiac mucosa showing scattered parietal cells in the mucous cardiac glands. The glands are better formed and less distorted than pure cardiac mucosa. Inflammation is present.

Figure 2–2. Normal oxyntic mucosa of the gastric fundus. This shows a short pit lined by foveolar mucous cells and gastric glands containing parietal and chief cells only. No significant inflammation is apparent.

intraepithelial inflammatory cells. In some patients, intraepithelial lymphocytes are present (Fig. 2–8); these have no specific pathologic significance. The esophagus is also characterized by the presence of submucosal mucous glands, which drain to the surface via ducts that are frequently squamous-lined (Fig. 2–1). These glands can sometimes be seen in biopsy specimens and provide evidence that the location of the biopsy is esopha-

gus, because ducts such as these are not present in the stomach (Fig. 2–9).

In 1961, Hayward[6] postulated that a junctional mucous-producing mucosa must exist between the squamous epithelium of the esophagus and the oxyntic mucosa of the gastric fundus. He suggested that this epithelium lined the lower 1–2 cm of the esophagus and also extended a little way into the stomach. This assertion was not based on any published studies or personal observations. It has, however, become the basis of the confusion that exists regarding the normal histology of this region. This junctional mucosa is identical to cardiac mucosa (see Fig. 2–4) that is believed to normally line the most proximal stomach. It is also the reason that the presence of junctional (cardiac) mucosa in the lower 1–2 cm of the tubular esophagus is regarded by most endoscopists as a normal finding.

The squamocolumnar junction can be recognized at en-

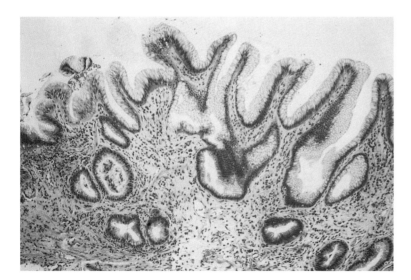

Figure 2–3. Cardiac mucosa in a biopsy sample, showing a mucosa composed of a foveolar region and mucous glands devoid of parietal cells. Note the inflammation and distorted appearance of glands, which is usual for cardiac mucosa.

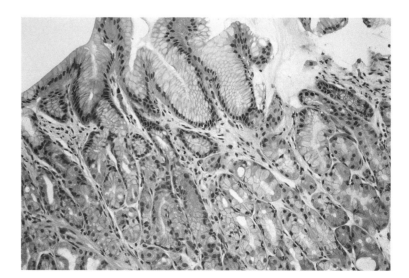

Figure 2–5. Oxyntocardiac mucosa with more straight glands resembling oxyntic mucosa, but containing a mixture of parietal and mucous cells. Only minimal foveolar elongation and chronic inflammation are evident.

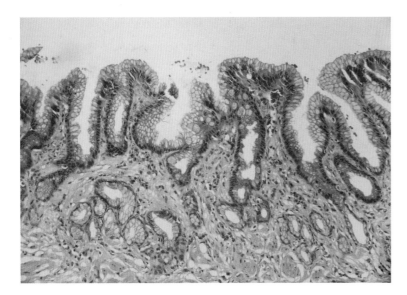

Figure 2–6. Cardiac mucosa with a villous surface resulting from hyperplasia of the foveolar region. A small area in the center shows goblet cells, indicating early intestinal metaplasia occurring in the cardiac mucosa.

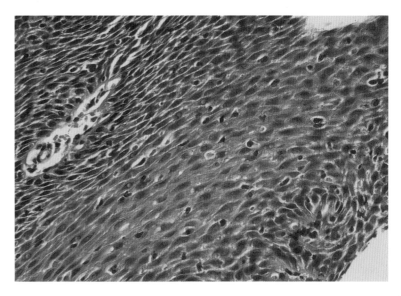

Figure 2–8. Unoriented biopsy specimen showing squamous epithelium with scattered intraepithelial lymphocytes. Although not normally present, intraepithelial lymphocytes have no specific diagnostic significance.

doscopy and is called the Z-line. The Z-line is normally approximately 40 cm from the incisors and is commonly irregular. The relationship of the Z-line to the anatomic gastroesophageal junction and the manometrically defined LES is uncertain. Because of the existing belief that the lower 1–2 cm of the tubular esophagus can be lined by junctional (cardiac) mucosa, most endoscopists do not consider the Z-line to be situated abnormally unless it is above this level in the tubular esophagus.[7]

An autopsy study of the gastroesophageal junctional region at the University of Southern California (USC) (unpublished data) showed that in the majority of normal children, the squamous epithelium transitions directly to oxyntic mucosa. With increasing age, a junctional or cardiac mucosa develops between the oxyntic and squamous epithelium in the majority

of people. In approximately 30% of our autopsy population, however, no cardiac mucosa occurred. This study suggests to us that cardiac mucosa is not a normal part of the stomach; later we will present evidence that cardiac mucosa is generated by transformation of esophageal squamous epithelium by gastroesophageal reflux (See Fig. 2–9).

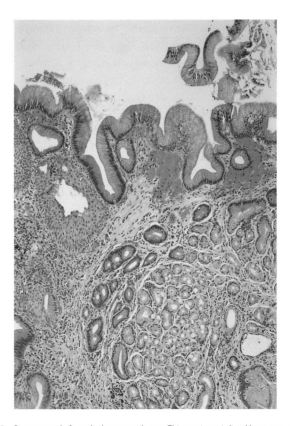

Figure 2–9. Biopsy sample from the lower esophagus. This specimen is lined by oxynto-cardiac mucosa with inflammation and contains a squamous-lined duct in the lamina propria. The presence of squamous-lined ducts indicates that this specimen is from the esophagus, where such ducts are normally found (see Fig. 2–1).

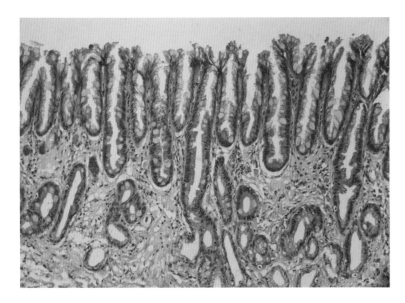

Figure 2–7. Mucosa with a villous surface showing extensive intestinal metaplasia characterized by the presence of numerous goblet cells. Note the inflammation and gland distortion under the foveolar region, which is similar to that seen in cardiac mucosa.

ANATOMIC ABNORMALITIES

A large number of anatomic abnormalities occur in the esophagus (Table 2–2). Although these are clinically important, they rarely produce pathologic specimens and are therefore rarely encountered by the surgical pathologist.

Gastric heterotopia in the esophagus is present in 3–5% of otherwise normal esophagi,[8] occurring in the upper third of the esophagus as a pink patch of variable size in the white squamous epithelium ("inlet patch"). They are usually composed of either oxyntic gastric mucosa or mixed oxyntic–cardiac mucosa. Rarely, inflammation is present; intestinal metaplasia is exceptional, and adenocarcinoma associated within this mucosa has been reported very rarely.[8] Heterotopic gastric mucosa in the esophagus may secrete acid.

Two clinicopathologic abnormalities may be encountered in relation to the squamous epithelium in esophageal biopsies: (1) Glycogen acanthosis, in which glycogen accumulates in the superficial squamous epithelial cells, which become enlarged. In routine sections, the glycogen is dissolved during processing, and the cytoplasm appears clear or vacuolated. Glycogen acanthosis is commonly patchy, resulting in slightly raised white plaques that may endoscopically resemble *Candida* esophagitis. (2) Melanosis esophagii, in which black pigment-containing macrophages are found scattered in the lamina propria (Fig. 2–10). The pigment is black and finely granular, resembling

---

TABLE 2–2. ANATOMIC ABNORMALITIES OF THE ESOPHAGUS

Congenital Tracheoesophageal Fistula

Type A	8%	Atresia of esophagus without TE fistula
Type B	1%	Atresia with fistula between blind upper segment and trachea
Type C	85%	Atresia with fistula between lower segment and trachea
Type D	1%	Atresia with tracheal fistulae to both upper and lower segments
Type E	5%	No atresia; fistula between normal esophagus and trachea

Acquired Tracheoesophageal Fistula

Secondary to malignant neoplasms of the mediastinum that simultaneously erode trachea and esophagus; commonly bronchogenic or esophageal carcinoma; rarely secondary to benign diseases like tuberculosis and Crohn's disease.

Esophageal Webs

Mucosal folds that extend into the lumen as a crescentic fold. Associated with Plummer-Vinson syndrome (dysphagia, koilonychia, atrophic glossitis associated with severe iron deficiency anemia). Rare.

Schatzki Ring

Concentric mucosal fold in the distal esophagus; a concentric fold of thickened mucosa lined by squamous and cardiac mucosa. Associated with sliding hiatal hernia and gastroesophageal reflux. Causes dysphagia when luminal narrowing is severe.

Zenker's Diverticulum

Pulsion diverticulum of the posterior pharynx immediately above the cricopharyngeal sphincter. Associated with cricopharyngeal sphincter dysfunction. May be large enough to produce a neck mass or cause external compression of the cervical esophagus.

Epiphrenic Diverticulum

Pulsion diverticulum of the lower esophagus. Associated with achalasia and hiatal hernia. Common, usually found incidentally. Rarely symptomatic.

Midbody Esophageal Diverticulum

Traction diverticulum associated with adherent tuberculous lymph nodes in the mediastinum. Rare.

Sliding Hiatal Hernia

Common (90% of hiatal hernias). Upward displacement of the esophagus causes the stomach to slide into the thorax through the diaphragmatic hiatus. Displacement of the LES into the thorax commonly results in dysfunction, and gastroesophageal reflux is common. Asymptomatic if LES function is normal.

Paraesophageal (Rolling) Hiatal Hernia

The fundus of the stomach herniates into the diaphragmatic hiatus alongside the lower esophagus, causing part of the stomach to become intrathoracic. Not associated with reflux because the LES is not altered. The intrathoracic stomach is liable to complications such as ischemic mucosal necrosis and bleeding.

Esophageal Varices

Dilated tortuous veins in the mucosa and submucosa of the esophagus occurring in portal hypertension. Common cause of upper GI hemorrhage in patients with cirrhosis of the liver.

Mallory-Weiss Syndrome

Linear, longitudinal mucosal lacerations in the lower esophagus and upper stomach resulting from severe vomiting. Rupture of mucosal vessels can lead to hemorrhage.

Esophageal Perforation

May complicate endoscopy and particularly balloon dilatation. Also occurs in severe vomiting (Boerhaave's syndrome). Produces severe chest pain associated with air in the mediastinum (mediastinal emphysema). Emergent treatment is necessary to prevent secondary infection of the mediastinum.

Abbreviations: TE = tracheoesophageal; LES = lower esophageal sphincter.

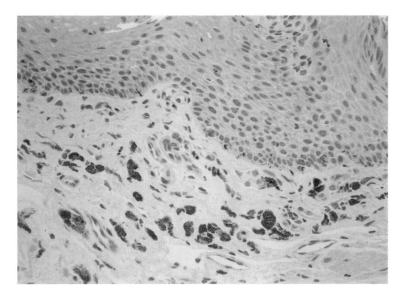

Figure 2–10. Melanosis of the esophagus. Numerous macrophages containing black pigment are present in the lamina propria.

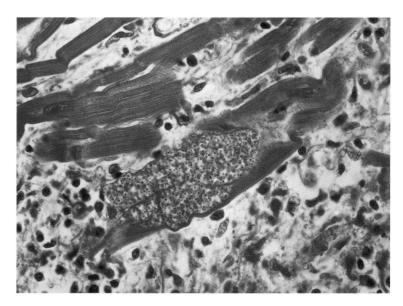

Figure 2–11. *Trypanosoma cruzi* infection of a muscle fiber. *Note:* This is from myocardium in acute *T. cruzi* infection causing death from myocardial failure. In the chronic phase of infection in which esophageal motility dysfunction occurs, organisms are scarce.

melanin, but there is controversy as to whether it represents true melanin or lipofuscin.

MOTOR DYSFUNCTION

Motor disorders of the esophagus present with dysphagia for liquids as well as solids and chest pain that commonly mimics cardiac pain ("noncardiac chest pain"). These disorders are assessed by manometry, and treatment generally consists of drugs that influence motility, endoscopic dilatation, and surgical myotomy. Because myotomy does not generate a pathologic specimen, the surgical pathologist has little role to play in the diagnosis of these diseases.

Achalasia of the Cardia

Achalasia is defined by a failure of relaxation of the LES during swallowing. This is usually associated with a failure of peristalsis in the body of the esophagus. Achalasia is the result of an abnormality of the neural plexuses in the esophagus, and aganglionosis has been reported. A clinical syndrome similar to achalasia occurs in chronic Chagas' disease in which, aganglionosis results from infection by *Trypanosoma cruzi* (Fig. 2–11).

Patients commonly present with dysphagia. Heartburn occurs occasionally and is believed to be caused by irritation from the food collecting in the esophagus rather than gastroesophageal reflux. The obstruction results in dilatation of the esophagus due to food accumulation in it. The dilated esophagus with the beak-like narrowing of the distal end produces a classical radiologic appearance (Fig. 2–12). Patients commonly maintain good nutrition because the hydrostatic pressure of the accumulated food column in the esophagus intermittently overcomes the LES pressure, resulting in entry of food into the

stomach. Rarely, the clinical, radiologic, and manometric features of achalasia are mimicked by malignancy (secondary achalasia).[9]

Complications of achalasia include regurgitation of food into the pharynx and aspiration pneumonia. The squamous epithelium of the esophagus is reported to become thickened, but no specific histologic changes occur. A slightly increased incidence of squamous carcinoma is reported.

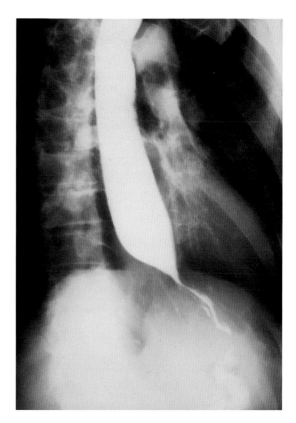

Figure 2–12. Barium swallow in achalasia of the cardia, showing the dilated esophagus and the typical distal narrowing.

Medical treatment of achalasia is by a combination of balloon dilatation and the use of intrasphincteric botulinum toxin injection. Surgical myotomy, done as an open procedure, by thoracoscopy or laparoscopy, is highly effective, but is commonly (except in the thoracoscopic procedure) combined with some anti-reflux procedure to prevent gastroesophageal reflux. Very rarely, esophagectomy is necessary. The esophagus shows a greatly increased circumference (Fig. 2–13), and the mucosa may show thickening. Most cases that require surgical removal of the esophagus have evidence of reflux disease due to prior myotomy or dilatations.

Progressive Systemic Sclerosis (Scleroderma)

Esophageal involvement occurs in over 80% of patients with progressive systemic sclerosis[10] and much less commonly in other collagen diseases. CREST syndrome is a limited variant of progressive systemic sclerosis characterized by calcinosis cutis, Raynaud's phenomenon, esophageal dysmotility, sclerodactyly, and telangiectasia. Progressive systemic sclerosis results in smooth muscle atrophy and fibrous replacement of the esophageal wall. It is manometrically defined by (1) Diminution of peristalsis in the lower two thirds of the esophagus. The UES and the upper striated muscle part of the esophagus generates normal peristaltic waves. (2) Hypotensive LES, which results in reflux and heartburn. Symptoms of reflux commonly dominate over dysphagia (Fig. 2–14). Complicated reflux with stricture is common in scleroderma.[11]

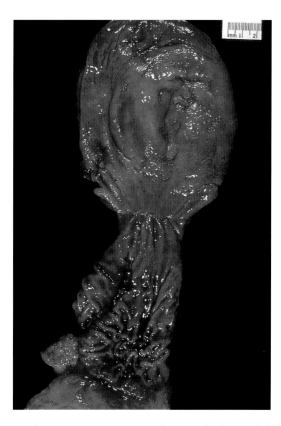

Figure 2–14. Esophagogastrectomy in a patient with severe scleroderma with failure of gastric motility and marked reflux disease of the lower esophagus. Note the marked erythema and dilatation of the lower third of the esophagus.

Other Motility Disorders

Several motility disorders have been defined by abnormalities detected at manometry and radiologic examination (Table 2–3). The relationship of these manometric abnormalities to symptoms must be evaluated with caution because similar abnormalities occur in asymptomatic people. In patients being evaluated by manometry for noncardiac chest pain, the common abnormalities are nutcracker esophagus (50%), ineffective esophageal motility (35%), and diffuse esophageal spasm (also called "corkscrew esophagus"; 10%). In patients undergoing manometric testing for dysphagia, the commonly encountered conditions are achalasia of the cardia (35%), ineffective esophageal motility (35%), diffuse esophageal spasm (15%), and

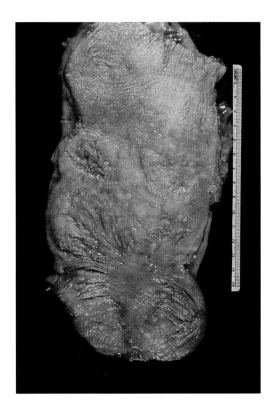

Figure 2–13. Esophagectomy specimen in a patient with achalasia of the cardia, showing the opened esophagus, which has a markedly increased circumference and thickening of the squamous epithelium.

TABLE 2–3. MOTOR DISORDERS OF THE ESOPHAGUS: MANOMETRIC FEATURES

Cricopharyngeal achalasia	Failure of relaxation of UES; associated with pharyngeal bar
Achalasia of the cardia	Absent peristalsis in body of esophagus; failure of LES relaxation
Progressive systemic sclerosis	Absent peristalsis in lower esophagus; hypotensive LES
Diffuse esophageal spasm	Simultaneous nonperistaltic contractions; normal LES
Nutcracker esophagus	High pressure, prolonged contractions; normal LES
Hypertensive LES	Normal esophageal peristalsis; high LES resting pressure with incomplete relaxation; >30% hypotensive or nontransmitted contractions

Abbreviations: UES = upper esophageal sphincter; LES = lower esophageal sphincter.

nutcracker esophagus (10%). Hypertensive LES is extremely uncommon.

GASTROESOPHAGEAL REFLUX DISEASE

Definition

Ambulatory 24-h pH studies clearly show that most asymptomatic people have infrequent reflux episodes associated with a drop in esophageal pH to below 4. These episodes are usually of short duration, and the refluxed material rapidly clears from the lower esophagus. Most such reflux episodes are asymptomatic. Acid reflux is quantitated by the percentage of time the pH is below 4 during the 24-h period of the test.[12] Alkaline reflux is the result of the presence of duodenal contents in gastric juice. It is quantitated by the percentage of time the esophageal pH is above 7, and the presence of duodenal contents can be identified by placing a bilirubin-detecting probe (Bilitec) in the esophagus. Patients who have abnormal acid reflux (pH < 4, for longer than 4.5% of the time) and a positive Bilitec test are classified as having mixed acid–alkaline reflux.[13,14]

Because reflux is almost universal, the definition of abnormal reflux must be established by correlation of the degree of pH abnormality with a recognizable end-point. This method is similar to defining abnormal blood pressure as the level associated with increased mortality from vascular complications. Unfortunately, recognizing a clinical or pathologic end-point to define reflux disease is difficult.

Comparison of pH studies of asymptomatic and symptomatic patients established the upper limit of normal as a pH below 4 less than 4.5% of the time.[12] If the pH is less than 4 less than 4.5% of the time, the likelihood is high that the patient does not have symptomatic reflux disease. Although ambulatory pH studies are considered the gold standard for the diagnosis of reflux disease, their specificity and sensitivity are 96–98%. Patients with abnormal pH scores may be asymptomatic, and those who are symptomatic rarely have scores within the normal range. Despite its less than 100% diagnostic accuracy, no better established test presently exists for diagnosing reflux disease than pH testing.

A major problem regarding the use of reflux symptoms as an end-point for defining reflux disease is the fact that some patients who develop Barrett's esophagus and adenocarcinoma have never been symptomatic prior to the occurrence of malignancy. Because adenocarcinoma is the most serious end-result of reflux disease, it would be preferable to use a criterion to define reflux disease that is more sensitive to adenocarcinoma than symptoms.

Manometric Abnormalities

A defective LES is demonstrable in 60% of patients with reflux disease,[15] increasing to 100% when severe mucosal disease is present.[16] In patients who have reflux disease with no LES ab-

normality at manometry, it is believed that transient dysfunction of the LES may be responsible for reflux episodes. In some reflux patients, abnormal peristalsis in the body of the esophagus suggests the possibility that decreased esophageal clearing may be responsible for prolonged exposure of the esophagus to refluxed gastric contents.

Accepted Morphologic Changes

Mild (grade 1) esophagitis may produce no recognizable endoscopic change or the presence of mild erythema of the squamous epithelium. In more severe cases, the mucosa shows increasing erythema associated with red streaks, edema, and increased friability. In these nonerosive cases, the histologic criteria for gastroesophageal reflux are the following changes in the squamous epithelium: (1) Maturation abnormality characterized by hyperplasia of the basal cell region greater than 20% of mucosal thickness associated with papillary elongation greater than 70% of mucosal thickness (Fig. 2–15). This maturation abnormality resembles the changes of psoriasis in the skin and probably results from an increased rate of surface cell loss due to reflux injury. (2) The presence of intraepithelial eosinophils (Figs. 2–15B and 2–16). This criterion is controversial. According to some authorities, a few eosinophils can be found in the lowest 2 cm of the normal esophagus, and more than a "few" eosinophils or eosinophils at a level more than 2 cm above the squamocolumnar junction are required for a diagnosis of disease. The literature that questions the diagnostic specificity of eosinophils is flawed in that "normal" is defined by absence of symptoms rather than pH abnormality. At USC, the presence of eosinophils in squamous epithelium is considered diagnostic of reflux disease, irrespective of their number or the location of the biopsy sample.

Intraepithelial eosinophils are commonly associated with spongiosis (intraepithelial edema), characterized by separation of squamous cells from one another (see Fig. 2–16), papillary tip congestion, intraepithelial neutrophils, and intraepithelial lymphocytes. None of these "soft" criteria are diagnostic of reflux disease in the absence of eosinophils. The presence of intraepithelial neutrophils without eosinophils is abnormal and signifies acute esophagitis; although most commonly caused by reflux disease, neutrophils are not specific for it; they can be seen with any cause of esophagitis (Fig. 2–17). The occurrence of intraepithelial lymphocytes alone is a not uncommonly encountered histologic change (see Fig. 2–8); this is not considered diagnostic for reflux disease or any other esophageal disease.

More severe (grade 2) reflux esophagitis is characterized by erosion of the squamous epithelium, commonly seen endoscopically as linear streaks of yellow necrotic debris in the mucosa (Fig. 2–18). Grade 3 esophagitis is demonstrated by more extensive erosion or ulceration. Erosion and ulceration are commonly associated with severe erythema and friability of the intervening squamous epithelium. An erosion involves full thickness of the squamous epithelium; an ulcer involves the full thickness of the mucosa down to the muscularis mucosae. Deep ulcers may involve the muscularis externa (Fig. 2–19), poten-

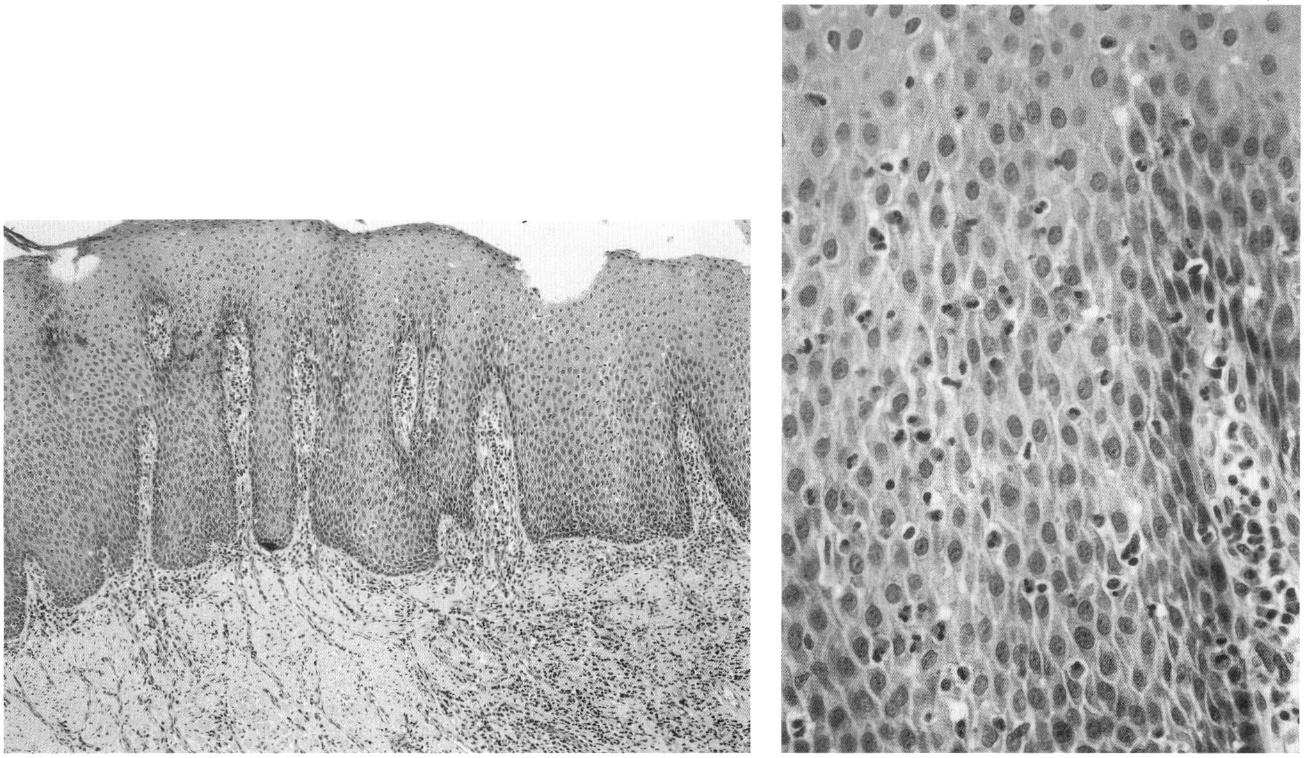

Figure 2–15. A: Reflux esophagitis. The squamous epithelium shows acanthosis, basal cell hyperplasia, and papillary elongation to a degree that is sufficient for a diagnosis of reflux disease. B: Higher power of part A, showing intraepithelial eosinophils, the presence of which makes diagnosis of reflux disease definite.

tially causing strictures and motility dysfunction. Biopsies of an erosion show acutely inflamed necrotic debris; in a deeper ulcer, the necrotic debris of the ulcer base is associated with inflamed granulation tissue. Biopsy evidence of erosion and ulceration are diagnostic of reflux disease only when associated with histologic criteria of reflux in the adjacent squamous epithelium. When erosion and ulceration are present but the squamous ep-

ithelium is either normal or shows only neutrophils and non-specific regenerative features at the ulcer's edge, other causes of esophageal ulcer must be excluded by history before erosive or ulcerative reflux esophagitis is diagnosed.

Complicated reflux is a term used for reflux disease associated with strictures of the lower esophagus that are characterized by extensive mural fibrosis and for the presence of Barrett's

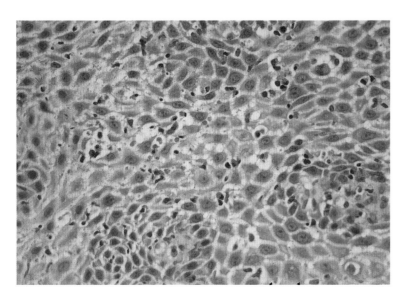

Figure 2–16. Reflux esophagitis. Unoriented biopsy specimen of squamous epithelium showing spongiosis and numerous intraepithelial eosinophils, the presence of which are diagnostic of reflux esophagitis.

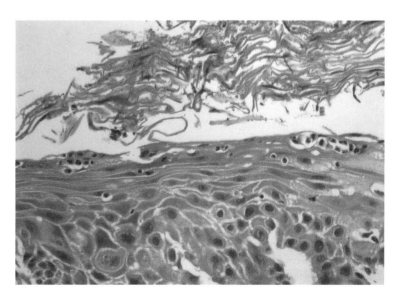

Figure 2–17. Esophageal squamous mucosa showing neutrophils in the superficial region of the epithelium. This biopsy specimen shows pseudohyphae of *Candida* species in the parakeratotic debris overlying the squamous epithelium.

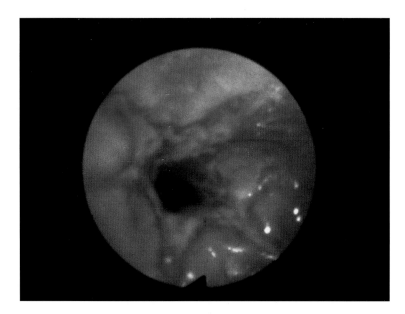

Figure 2–18. Reflux esophagitis with erosions at endoscopy.

TABLE 2–4. CAUSES OF ESOPHAGEAL STRICTURES

Disease	Incidence	Comments
Gastroesophageal reflux disease	30%	Higher incidence of impaired LES, hiatal hernia, esophageal dysmotility, and alkaline reflux than uncomplicated GERD
Carcinoma of the esophagus	30%	Both squamous and adenocarcinoma; rarely other neoplasms like malignant lymphoma
Rings and webs	15%	Schatzki ring commonest
Postoperative (anastomotic)	7%	Most commonly after transhiatal esophagectomy with a cervical anastomosis
Postradiation	5%	
Drug-induced ("pill esophagitis")	3%	Potassium chloride, iron (ferrous sulfate), antibiotics (doxycycline), salicylates, NSAIDs, ascorbic acid, oral contraceptives, quinidine, alendronate
Caustic esophagitis	2%	
Inflammatory diseases	5%	Tuberculosis, Crohn's disease, eosinophilic esophagitis
Nasogastric tube related	1%	Commonly cause long complicated strictures
Ischemic	Rare	Follows severe hypotensive and septic shock
Epidermolysis bullosa	Rare	

Abbreviations: GERD = gastroesophageal reflux disease; LES = lower esophageal sphincter; NSAIDs = nonsteroidal antiinflammatory drugs.

esophagus. Strictures due to reflux disease must be distinguished from other strictures that occur in the esophagus (Table 2–4). Reflux strictures, which occur at the squamocolumnar junction, are usually short and are commonly associated with Barrett's esophagus. Nonreflux strictures such as those resulting from caustic ingestion and nasogastric tubes tend to be more commonly complicated, long strictures and occur proximal to the squamocolumnar junction.

Evaluation of biopsy samples by presently used criteria in the squamous epithelium are of very little practical value in the diagnosis of reflux disease. Biopsy evidence of reflux esophagitis has a sensitivity of around 60% when measured against pH proven reflux, and the presence of maturation changes in the epithelium have been shown to be unreliable when they are not associated with eosinophils (Fig. 2–20).[17] The severity of the changes in the squamous epithelium has little correlation with the degree of reflux by pH studies. For this reason, many gastroenterologists consider the diagnosis of reflux esophagitis to

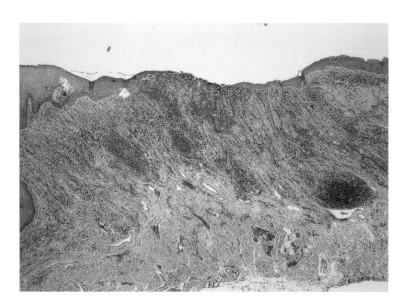

Figure 2–19. Low-power appearance of a reflux-associated esophageal stricture showing ulceration, with involvement of the deep muscle wall in the fibrosing, inflammatory process.

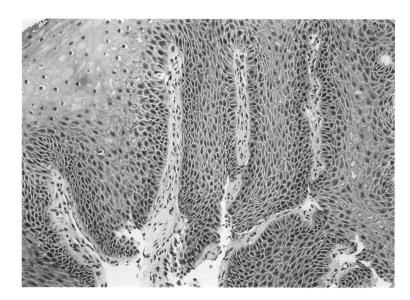

Figure 2–20. Esophageal mucosa with basal cell hyperplasia and papillary elongation without intraepithelial eosinophils. Although satisfying presently accepted criteria for reflux, this finding is not reliable for diagnosis.

TABLE 2–5. INTERPRETATION OF CHANGES IN BIOPSIES TAKEN IMMEDIATELY DISTAL TO THE SQUAMOCOLUMNAR JUNCTION, IRRESPECTIVE OF ANY ENDOSCOPIC OR CLINICAL DATA*

Finding	Reflux	pH Study Abnormality	Risk of Intestinal Metaplasia	Risk of Adenocarcinoma
Fundic mucosa only	0	0	0	0
Oxyntocardiac mucosa only	+	+/–	0	0
Cardiac mucosa < 1 cm long; no IM	+	+/–	+	0
Cardiac mucosa < 1 cm long; IM +	+	+/–	N/A	+
Reflux Carditis	++	+	+	0
Cardiac mucosa 1–2 cm long; No IM	++	+	+	0
Cardiac mucosa 1–2 cm long; IM +	++	+	N/A	+
Cardiac mucosa > 2 cm long; no IM	+++	++	++	0
Cardiac mucosa > 2 cm long; IM +	+++	++	N/A	++

Abbreviations: IM = intestinal metaplasia.
*Note that when a segment of abnormal glandular mucosa is observed at endoscopy, multiple specimens should be taken at 1–2-cm measured intervals.

be a clinical rather than a pathologic diagnosis, and many cases receive no biopsy at endoscopy. It is difficult to argue against this in the light of presently accepted criteria. Reflux esophagitis is the only significant mucosal disease in which histologic examination does not presently form the basis for diagnosis.

Criteria Used at USC for Diagnosis

At the University of Southern California, we have successfully developed a system of evaluation of biopsy samples[18] that permits accurate diagnosis of reflux and assessment of the severity of the disease (Table 2–5). This evaluation depends on recognizing the normal histology of this region. Understand, however, that the USC criteria presented here are not yet widely accepted.

In an autopsy study, we examined 69 patients who had an evaluable section across the squamocolumnar junction. Thirty percent of all cases, including 9 of 11 patients younger than age 20, did not have any cardiac mucosa; instead, the squamous epithelium transitioned directly to the oxyntic mucosa of the gastric fundus (Fig. 2–21). Despite postmortem changes, the flat, organized oxyntic mucosa was easy to distinguish from the disorganized cardiac mucosa, which showed large mucous cells (Figs. 2–22 and 2–23). In those that had cardiac mucosa, the length of this mucosa was small, being less than 1 cm in all but two cases (Fig. 2–23). In a study of the squamocolumnar junction in patients who had esophageal resection for squamous carcinoma of the esophagus, the length of cardiac mucosa was also commonly less than 1 cm (Fig. 2–24).

We contrasted this autopsy population with a series of 71 patients with reflux disease who had multiple biopsies, permitting evaluation of the extent of cardiac mucosa. All 71 patients had cardiac mucosa, and 30% had cardiac mucosal lengths of over 2 cm. The results of this comparison strongly suggest that cardiac mucosa is not a normal structure; rather, it is an abnormal mucosa that results from transformation of the squamous epithelium of the esophagus that is damaged by reflux (Table 2–6).

We also evaluated endoscopic biopsies taken from the squamocolumnar junctional region in 334 patients who had no endoscopic evidence of a columnar-lined esophagus.[19] The 246 patients in whom cardiac mucosa was present had significantly higher esophageal acid exposure and defective LES than the 88 patients who did not have evidence of cardiac mucosa on biopsy. This also suggests a relationship between the presence of cardiac mucosa and reflux disease. Csendes and colleagues[20] in an endoscopic study of healthy controls and patients with reflux disease showed that a proximal migration of the squamocolumnar junction occurred with increasing severity of disease. In other words, as the severity of reflux increases, the length of cardiac transformation of squamous epithelium increases.

If squamous epithelium normally transitions directly to oxyntic mucosa of the gastric fundus (Fig. 2–25A), the changes in reflux are easy to understand. Gastric oxyntic mucosa is not damaged by gastric juice. Reflux damages only squamous ep-

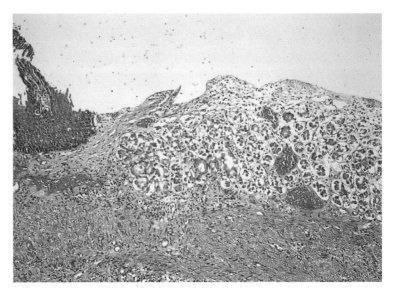

Figure 2–21. Section across the squamocolumnar junction in normal autopsy showing squamous epithelium transitioning directly to oxyntic fundic mucosa.

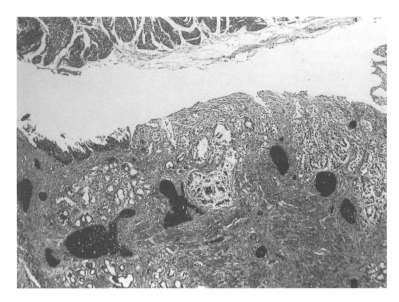

Figure 2–22. Section across squamocolumnar junction in normal autopsy showing squamous epithelium transitioning to oxynto-cardiac mucosa. Although cytologic features are difficult to recognize because of postmortem changes, the difference between cardiac and oxyntic mucosae (see Fig. 2–21) are apparent.

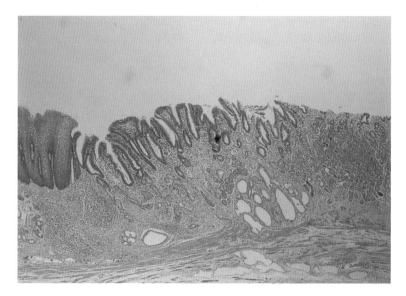

Figure 2–24. Section across the squamocolumnar junction in a patient with resection for squamous carcinoma of the esophagus. Note the short (<0.5 cm) length of cardiac mucosa between squamous epithelium and oxyntic mucosa.

ithelium, causing (1) changes in the squamous epithelium that are presently recognized as criteria of reflux disease and (2) cardiac transformation of the squamous epithelium. The length of cardiac mucosa increases as reflux severity increases[20] (Fig. 2–25B, C).

We consider the presence of cardiac mucosa a highly sensitive morphologic indicator of reflux disease, and we consider its presence as being morphologically definitional of reflux disease. Based on this hypothesis, the 30% of patients in our autopsy study and 88/334 patients in our biopsy study[19] who had

no evidence of cardiac mucosa had no morphologic evidence of reflux disease. The 70% in the autopsy study and 246/334 patients in our biopsy study[19] who had cardiac mucosa had morphologic evidence of reflux. Although it may seem that a 70% incidence of reflux disease in the population by this criterion is unreasonable, there is much evidence to support this. The increasing incidence of cardiac mucosa with patient age, as suggested by our autopsy study, suggests that cardiac mucosa is an acquired change. Evidence that reflux disease is involved is supported by the fact that on careful questioning over 30% of the

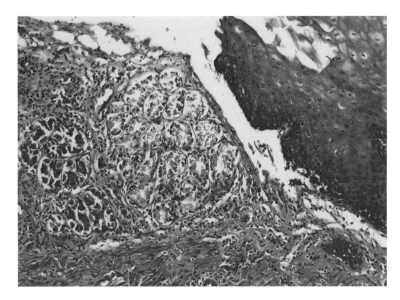

Figure 2–23. Normal autopsy in a child showing one focus of cardiac-type mucous glands (0.03 cm long) between squamous and oxyntic mucosa. Cell preservation is better, permitting parietal cells to be clearly identified in the oxyntic mucosa.

TABLE 2–6. MUCOSAL CHANGES IN GASTROESOPHAGEAL REFLUX DISEASE

Acid-induced (nonmutational; reversible)	
Ulceration and erosion	Diagnostic if other causes of ulceration or erosion are excluded.*
Squamous epithelial changes:	Basal cell hyperplasia > 20% of mucosal thickness + increased papillary height > 70% of mucosal height
	Intercellular edema, papillary congestion
	Intraepithelial eosinophils*
	Intraepithelial neutrophils, lymphocytes
Cardiac mucosal changes	Presence of cardiac mucosa†
	Increasing length of cardiac mucosa†
	Reflux carditis: foveolar hyperplasia, inflammation with prominent eosinophils†
Mutational (etiology unknown; irreversible)	
Intestinal metaplasia*	Always in cardiac mucosa; risk increases with increasing amounts of cardiac mucosa and reflux carditis
Dysplasia and adenocarcinoma	Always in intestinal metaplasia; possibility of increased risk with increasing amounts of intestinal metaplasia

*Generally accepted as diagnostic criteria for reflux disease.
†Used at USC as diagnostic criteria for reflux disease; not yet generally accepted.

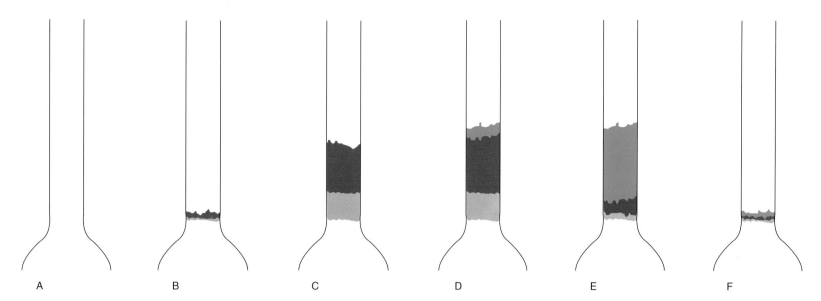

A   B   C   D   E   F

Figure 2–25. Changes in reflux esophagitis. **A.** Normal squamous–oxyntic fundic mucosal junction. **B.** Mild reflux disease showing a short segment of cardiac mucosa between squamous and fundic mucosa derived from transformation of damaged squamous epithelium. **C.** Severe reflux disease. The length of cardiac mucosa is longer. **D.** Intestinal metaplasia occurring in cardiac mucosa at the squamocardiac junction. Overall amount of intestinal metaplasia is small. **E.** Intestinal metaplasia has progressed caudally and involved a large area of the cardiac mucosa. **F.** Intestinal metaplasia occurring in mild reflux disease with a short segment of cardiac mucosa.

population report frequent episodes of heartburn.[21] The massive sales of over-the-counter acid suppressants in the United States also suggests a high incidence of reflux disease in the population.[22]

Cardiac mucosa is lined by gastric-type surface epithelium and has mucosal glands containing only mucous cells (see Fig. 2–4). This is the simplest epithelium that can result from glandular transformation of the squamous epithelium. In fact, transitional stages between squamous and glandular epithelium are frequently seen in biopsy samples (Fig. 2–26). Squamous-lined ducts are present in some samples lined by cardiac mucosa (see Fig. 2–9). Because squamous-lined ducts are seen only in the esophagus, this provides strong evidence that cardiac mucosa has replaced esophageal squamous epithelium in these specimens.

Cardiac mucosa, when found in the gastroesophageal region, almost always shows reactive changes and inflammation.[19] Because of the highly significant association of this change in cardiac mucosa with abnormalities on 24-h pH monitoring, we call these changes "reflux carditis" (see Table 2–6). An equivalent, less confusing, and preferable term is "reflux esophagitis, cardiac type," because cardiac mucosa represents the esophagus and not the stomach. The cardiac reactive changes are similar to those seen in reactive gastropathy in the stomach, and include villous-like surface (Fig. 2–27A) foveolar elongation (Fig. 2–27B) and serration (Fig. 2–27C), gland distortion (Fig. 2–27D) and smooth muscle proliferation in the lamina propria (Fig. 2–27D), which can sometimes be very prominent. The epithelial cells lining the foveolae of cardiac mucosa commonly show enlargement and distention of the cytoplasm

with mucin, which can appear as vacuoles ("pseudo-goblet cell change") (Fig. 2–27E). Mild reactive changes are commonly present in the cardiac epithelium, but true epithelial dysplasia does not occur in the absence of intestinal metaplasia. The inflammatory cells are a mixture of lymphocytes, plasma cells, and eosinophils (Fig. 2–27F). Eosinophils are frequently prominent. Neutrophils are not common. When present in significant numbers, they commonly signify erosion (Fig. 2–28) or *Helicobacter pylori* infection (Fig. 2–29). *Helicobacter pylori* infec-

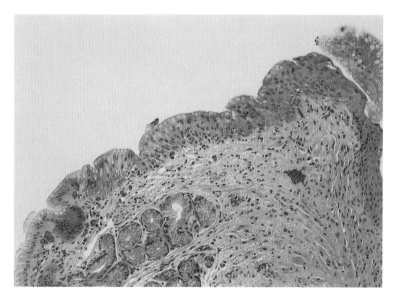

Figure 2–26. Cardiac mucosa at the junction. Note the stratified appearance of surface epithelium, which resembles reserve cell hyperplasia in other epithelia such as endocervical undergoing metaplasia.

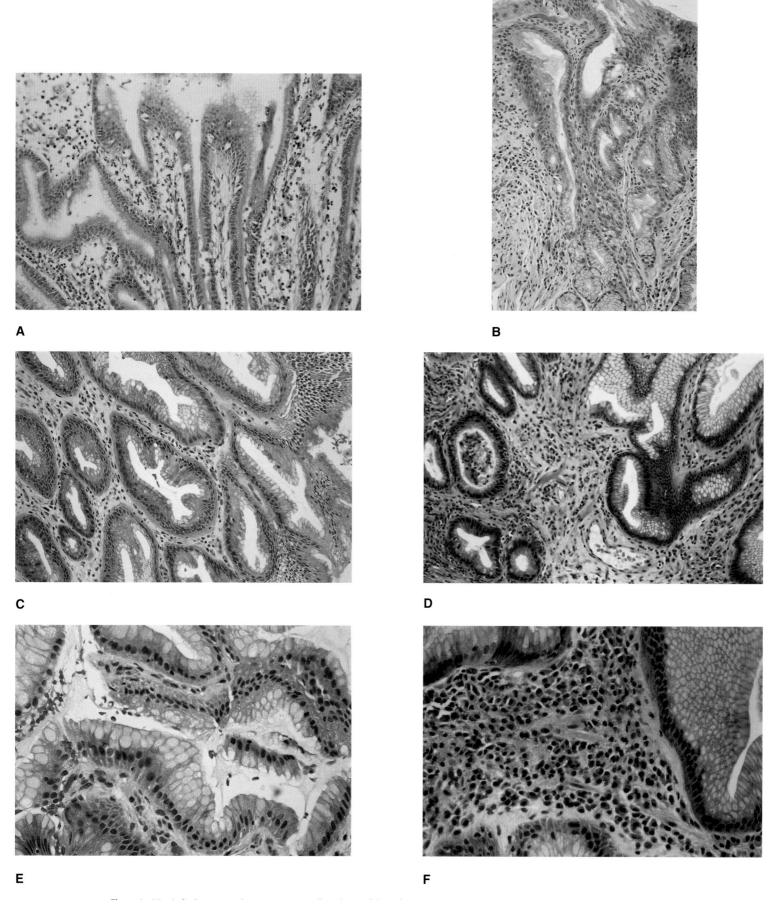

Figure 2–27. A: Cardiac mucosa showing prominent villous change of the surface due to marked foveolar elongation (reflux carditis). B: Cardiac mucosa showing marked chronic inflammation, foveolar elongation, and distortion (reflux carditis). C: Cardiac mucosa cut in tangential section, showing luminal serration of foveolar region, indicative of foveolar hyperplasia (reflux carditis). D: Cardiac mucosa showing chronic inflammation, gland distortion, and smooth muscle fibers in the lamina propria (reflux carditis). E: Cardiac mucosa showing enlargement of the cells due to mucin distention. The cytoplasm shows vacuolation due to the mucin (pseudo-goblet cell change). There are no definitive goblet cells. F: Cardiac mucosa, showing lamina propria inflammatory cells, which consist of lymphocytes, eosinophils, and plasma cells (reflux carditis).

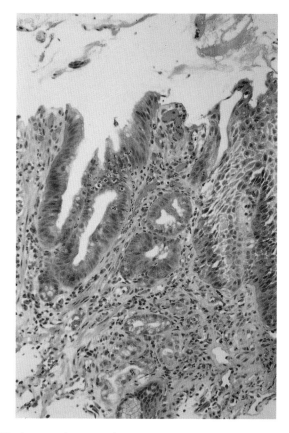

Figure 2–28. Squamocardiac junction showing reactive change and active inflammation associated with a healing erosion.

tion of cardiac mucosa occurs in patients with diffuse *H. pylori* gastritis when cardiac mucosa is present.

The incidence of *H. pylori* infection of cardiac mucosa varies among different populations. In the Los Angeles County Hospital, which caters to a predominantly nonwhite indigent population, the incidence is high, whereas at the private USC University Hospital, where the population is predominantly affluent and white, the incidence is low. Cardiac mucosal changes

in reflux disease, except for the higher incidence of active inflammation with neutrophils in patients positive for *H. pylori*, are identical in patients with and without *H. pylori* infection. In our studies, *H. pylori* infection of the stomach and cardiac mucosa do not correlate with the presence of reflux disease by pH studies.

Based on the preceding findings, we recommend the following protocol for biopsy during upper GI endoscopy: (1) In patients who have normal endoscopy, biopsies are recommended from the antrum, the gastric side of the squamocolumnar junction by a retroflex biopsy, and an antegrade biopsy of the squamocolumnar junction, which includes the lowest part of the squamous epithelium. (b) In patients who have a recognizable columnar-lined esophagus, specimens should be taken at intervals of 2 cm beginning at the gastric fundus (recognized by the typical rugal folds) up to the lowest part of the squamous epithelium. These biopsies permit estimation of the length of cardiac mucosa that is present in the patient, which provides reliable information regarding the severity of reflux disease (see Table 2–5). The squamous epithelium is relevant in this system only in that it permits the delineation of the upper limit of cardiac mucosa. Criteria of reflux disease in the squamous epithelium correlate poorly with pH scores; in fact, patients with the most severe disease and the longest lengths of cardiac mucosa commonly have no evidence of reflux disease in the squamous epithelium.

Metaplastic cardiac mucosa in the lower esophagus is exposed to the various components of refluxed gastric contents and is affected by numerous drugs used in the treatment of reflux. The simple mucous glands in the cardiac mucosa frequently develop specialized cells that become admixed with the mucous cells. Three specialized cell types are recognized.

1. Oxyntic cells. These convert the cardiac mucosa to a mixed oxyntocardiac mucosa (see Figs. 2–5 and 2–6). Oxyntic transformation tends to occur in the most distal part of the cardiac mucosa, adjacent to gastric fundic mucosa. Extensive

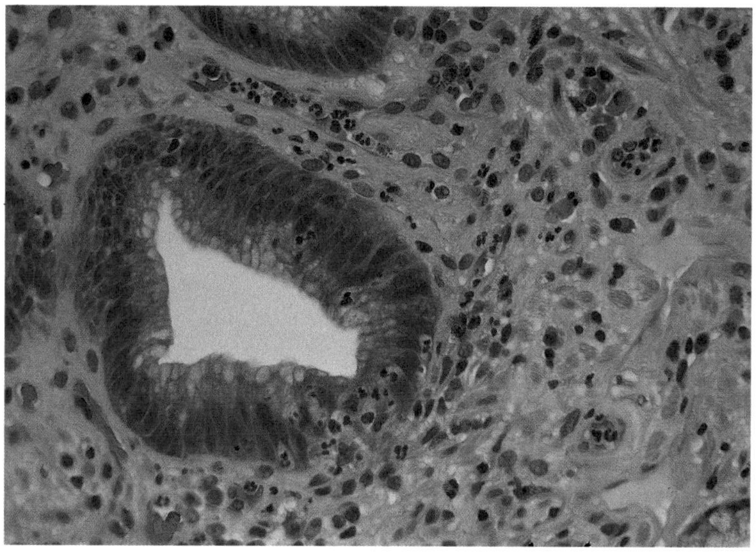

Figure 2–29. Cardiac mucosa with neutrophils in lamina propria and gland. *Helicobacter pylori* was present in this biopsy.

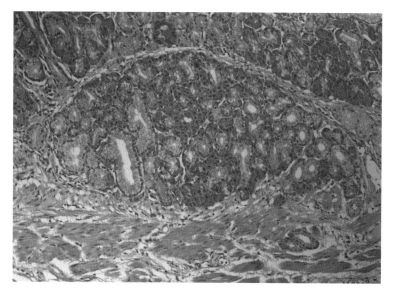

Figure 2–30. Cardiac mucosa with serous cells. Some of these show evidence of zymogenic granules, indicative of pancreatic differentiation.

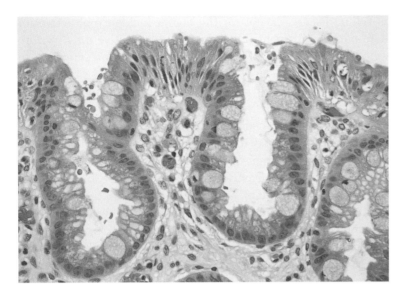

Figure 2–31. Intestinal metaplasia, characterized by goblet cells. The cytoplasm is denser, and the mucin vacuole is better defined, larger, and has a basophilic tinge, permitting differentiation from pseudo-goblet cells (see Fig. 2–27). This finding defines Barrett's esophagus.

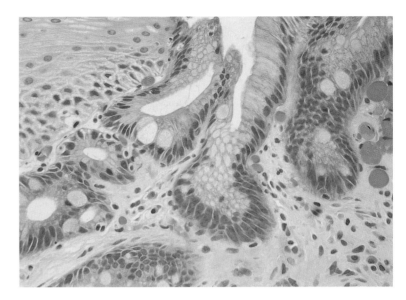

Figure 2–33. Intestinal metaplasia arising in cardiac mucosa adjacent to squamous epithelium.

oxyntic transformation of cardiac mucosa produces a mucosa that closely resembles gastric fundic mucosa (see Fig. 2–6). Oxyntic transformation of cardiac mucosa is associated with a lesser degree of inflammation and foveolar hyperplasia, suggesting that it is more resistant to the action of refluxed gastric juice than cardiac mucosa is. Intestinal metaplasia does not develop in oxyntocardiac mucosa. Complete transformation of all metaplastic cardiac mucosa into oxyntocardiac mucosa results in a junction between squamous epithelium and oxyntocardiac mucosa; this correlates with low levels of reflux disease and is a common finding in the asymptomatic autopsy population.

2. Serous cells. These resemble pancreatic acinar cells[23] or Paneth cells and are seen less frequently (Fig. 2–30).
3. Intestinal goblet cells. These (Fig. 2–31) result in the specialized Barrett's epithelium. Intestinal metaplasia invariably de-

velops in cardiac mucosa with reactive changes (Fig. 2–32) and first occurs at the junction between cardiac and squamous epithelium (Fig. 2–33).

The first phase of gastroesophageal reflux disease, which includes squamous epithelial maturation abnormalities, squamous inflammation, cardiac transformation, and reflux carditis, correlates with the amount of acid exposure of the lower esophagus and a defective lower esophageal sphincter.[19] The most reliable factor enabling histologic prediction of the severity of acid exposure is the length of cardiac mucosa[18] (see Table 2–6).

BARRETT'S ESOPHAGUS

Definition

Barrett's esophagus is presently defined as the presence of intestinal metaplasia in the esophagus. It is also accepted that Barrett's esophagus is a complication of gastroesophageal reflux disease. Rare cases of caustic ingestion have shown intestinal metaplasia unrelated to reflux disease; however, these cases would correctly be excluded from the definition of Barrett's esophagus if the definition included an etiologic reference to reflux. The noneponymous designation of this entity is therefore "reflux-associated intestinal metaplasia of the esophagus." It is highly recommended that this designation replace the term "Barrett's esophagus."

The term "Barrett's esophagus" has gone through numerous definitional changes (Table 2–7). Until the mid-1980s, Barrett's esophagus was an endoscopic diagnosis made when a length of columnar-lined esophagus greater than 3 cm was recognized. When the definition of Barrett's esophagus was restricted to include only the specialized (intestinal) type of ep-

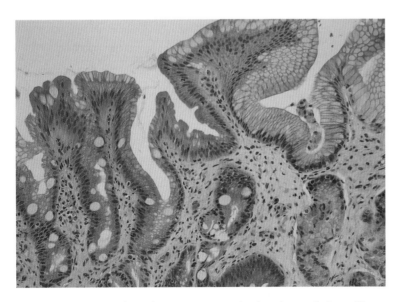

Figure 2–32. Intestinal metaplasia, arising in mucosa that shows features of reflux carditis.

TABLE 2–7. HISTORICAL DEFINITIONS OF BARRETT'S ESOPHAGUS

Year	Development
1950	Barrett declared that the columnar lining in the lower esophagus was in reality a tubular stomach associated with a congenitally shortened esophagus. He used the presence of a squamous lining to define esophagus.
1957	Barrett changed his mind on the basis of prevailing evidence presented and coined the term "columnar-lined lower esophagus"; this entity became synonymous with Barrett's esophagus. Barrett's opinion was that this was a congenital heterotopia of gastric mucosa in the esophagus.
1963	It became generally accepted that Barrett's esophagus was an acquired abnormality that was caused by gastroesophageal reflux.
1971	Paull and colleagues[30] classified the histologic types of glandular epithelia found in the lower esophagus. From this, three types of Barrett's esophagus were recognized: junctional (=cardiac), fundic(=oxyntocardiac), and specialized (=intestinal).
1980s	Adenocarcinoma arising in Barrett's esophagus was recognized as arising only in the specialized (intestinal) type of Barrett's. The definition of Barrett's was therefore restricted to only the specialized (intestinal) type of columnar epithelium.

ithelium, the diagnostic criterion changed from endoscopic to histologic because it is not possible to differentiate intestinal from other glandular epithelia at endoscopy (Fig. 2–34).

Endoscopic features associated with the greatest chance of finding intestinal metaplasia are[24] (1) long segments of esophageal columnar lining, which is strongly associated with intestinal metaplasia; (2) a jagged, irregular squamocolumnar junction; (3) a prominent squamocolumnar junction; and (4) discrete patches of columnar epithelium in the distal esophagus. Presence of features (2)–(4) are predictive of finding short-segment Barrett's esophagus only in 35–50% of cases. Absence of all of these features does not exclude the presence of intestinal metaplasia. Five to 15% of patients who have none of these features and who essentially have a normal junction have intestinal metaplasia at biopsy.[25] Vital staining of the columnar epithelium with methylene blue during endoscopy has been reported to selectively stain intestinal metaplastic mucosa.[26] This technique has not yet been accepted and is not widely used. These findings support the broad statement that the endoscopist cannot reliably differentiate intestinal metaplasia from cardiac and oxyntocardiac mucosa except by histologic sampling. The fact that a significant number of patients with reflux disease have intestinal metaplasia in the glandular mucosa immediately distal to the squamous epithelium even when endoscopic features are normal should mandate biopsy of this region in all patients who have endoscopy.

Intestinal metaplasia is most accurately diagnosed when clear-cut goblet cells are identified in a routine hematoxylin and eosin (H&E) stained section (see Figs. 2–31, 2–32, and 2–33). Goblet cells have a perfectly round cytoplasmic vacuole that has a faint basophilic tinge (see Fig. 2–31). Goblet cells show strongly positive staining with Alcian blue (AB) at pH 2.5 (Fig. 2–35), indicating their acid mucin content. Alcian blue staining is not necessary for the diagnosis of intestinal metaplasia in most cases in which goblet cells are obviously present.

In reflux disease, goblet cells invariably occur in cardiac

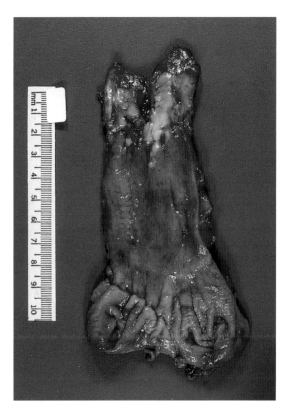

A

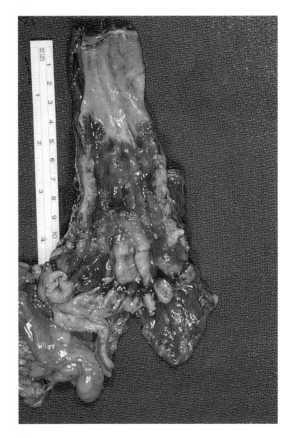

B

Figure 2–34. A: Long-segment glandular metaplasia of the esophagus showing a smooth glandular segment between the gastric mucosal folds and squamous epithelium. B: Long-segment glandular metaplasia of the esophagus showing surface irregularity. Only histologic examination can reliably differentiate between cardiac mucosa (reflux carditis) and intestinal metaplasia (Barrett's esophagus).

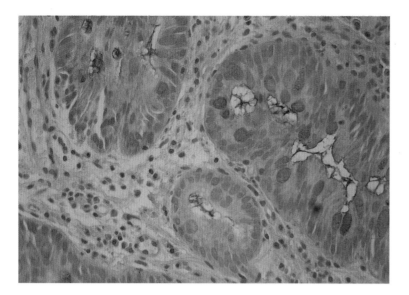

Figure 2–35. Alcian blue stain at pH 2.5, showing blue staining of goblet cells.

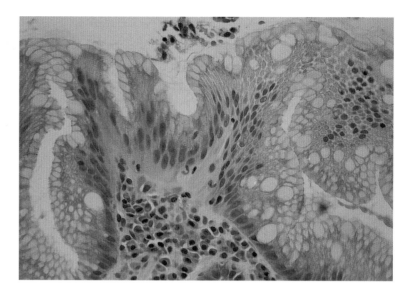

A

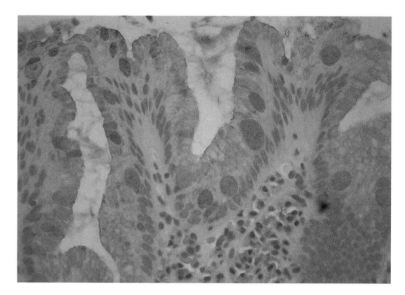

B

Figure 2–36. A: Cardiac mucosa containing both pseudo-goblet cells and definitive goblet cells. B: Alcian blue stain at pH 2.5. This shows varying degrees of Alcian blue positivity. Alcian blue stains are much more difficult to evaluate for goblet cells than hematoxylin and eosin (H&E) stain and have a high risk of false-positive diagnosis of Barrett's esophagus.

mucosa that shows reflux carditis (see Figs. 2–7 and 2–32). The occurrence of goblet cells in cardiac mucosa is preceded by two types of cytologic changes in cardiac mucosa: (1) The mucous cells lining the surface and foveolar region become enlarged and distended with mucin, frequently producing cytoplasmic vacuolation ("pseudo-goblet cells") (Fig. 2–36A, see Fig. 2–27C, E). On staining with Alcian blue at pH 2.5, the cardiac cells, which contain alcian blue-negative neutral mucin, show progressively increasing positivity without having the typical features of goblet cells. These cells, called "columnar blue cells," are commonly seen with (Fig. 2–36B) and without goblet cells (Fig. 2–37).[27] Similar columnar blue cells have been reported in the gastric mucosal foveolar region as a reactive phenomenon.[28] It is unclear at present whether pseudo-goblet cells and columnar blue cells represent intermediate stages in the development of goblet cells from mucous cells of the cardiac mucosa. As such, their presence does not warrant a diagnosis of intestinal metaplasia. There is a risk of false-positive diagnosis of Barrett's esophagus when Alcian blue-stained sections are used because Alcian blue-positive pseudo-goblet cells can easily be mistaken for intestinal metaplasia. For this reason, we have discontinued the use of routine Alcian blue staining for the diagnosis of Barrett's esophagus; we only use it to confirm that a goblet cell identified in an H&E-stained section actually contains acid mucin; a negative stain indicates negativity for intestinal metaplasia.

Presently Accepted Classification

Long-Segment Barrett's Esophagus

Long-segment Barrett's esophagus is defined as the presence of intestinal metaplasia in a columnar-lined esophagus greater than 2 cm in length (see Figs. 2–25D, E and 2–34). The diagnosis uses endoscopic (>2 cm of glandular mucosa in the esophagus) and histologic (presence of intestinal metaplasia) criteria and therefore needs clinicopathologic correlation. Long-segment Barrett's esophagus is the only entity universally accepted as being defini-

tively Barrett's esophagus. It is clearly associated with adenocarcinoma, and patients diagnosed as having long-segment Barrett's esophagus are entered into endoscopic surveillance programs.[24]

It is useful to consider the situation when no intestinal metaplasia is found in a patient with a greater than 2 cm length of columnar-lined esophagus (see Fig. 2–25C). In the 1970s, these patients would have been classified as having Barrett's esophagus, cardiac or fundic type, a condition that was associated with reflux disease. By diagnostic criteria accepted today, however, this condition is called "columnar lined esophagus without intestinal metaplasia," an entity whose significance is said to be uncertain.[24] According to the USC criteria, these patients, having a greater than 2 cm length of cardiac mucosa, are classified as having severe reflux disease; this finding correlates strongly with abnormal pH tests in our studies (Table 2–8).

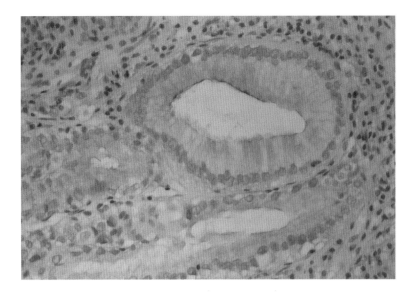

Figure 2–37. Faint blue staining (with Alcian blue) of gastric-type columnar cells. Blue staining with Alcian blue is not the diagnostic criterion for Barrett's esophagus.

Short-Segment Barrett's Esophagus

Short-segment Barrett's esophagus is the presence of intestinal metaplasia in a segment shorter than 2 cm of glandular mucosa in the lower esophagus (Figs. 2–38 and 2–39, see Fig. 2–25F). This differs from "intestinal metaplasia of the gastric cardia" only in the fact that, in the latter condition, the endoscopist has not perceived any abnormal columnar lining in the esophagus, and the intestinal metaplasia occurs in cardiac mucosa. Intestinal metaplasia has been reported to occur in 5–15% of patients with no perceived abnormal glandular mucosa in the esophagus at endoscopy, suggesting that this is a very common condition.[25] According to presently accepted thinking, these diagnoses must therefore be made using combined endoscopic and histologic criteria. The significance of these two conditions is uncertain, although the consensus is that at least short-segment Barrett's esophagus is associated with an increased risk of adenocarcinoma of the gastroesophageal junctional region. Surveillance is not generally recommended in either of these conditions at present.

USC Classification

In the USC scheme of biopsy evaluation, abnormal mucosa is defined histologically, not endoscopically. The presence of cardiac mucosa anywhere in this region is regarded as being derived from squamous epithelium as a consequence of reflux disease. Intestinal metaplasia occurring in cardiac mucosa therefore represents reflux-associated intestinal metaplasia, which is our preferred term for Barrett's esophagus. In the USC scheme, intestinal metaplasia of the gastric cardia does not exist, because cardiac mucosa is not part of the stomach.

One major difference between using presently accepted criteria and the USC criteria in the diagnosis of reflux disease and Barrett's esophagus is that in the USC system, all diagnostic decisions are based on histologic criteria without any need for endoscopic correlations. The pathologist can accurately identify tissue from the normal stomach (lined by gastric oxyntic mucosa), abnormal reflux-associated columnar esophagus (lined by cardiac mucosa and its various specializations), and normal esophagus (lined by squamous epithelium). The lack of dependence on endoscopic findings increases accuracy because identification of landmarks at endoscopy is notoriously unreliable.[29]

The second difference between the two classifications of Barrett's esophagus is that USC does not use the designations of long- and short-segment Barrett's esophagus. We presently quantitate the amount of intestinal metaplasia present in each patient by multiple biopsies (see Fig. 2–25D, E, F). It is logical, though unproven, that the risk of adenocarcinoma is related to the amount of intestinal metaplasia; it is possible that this will quantitate risk better than the present classification into long- and short-segment Barrett's esophagus.

Differential Diagnosis of Intestinal Metaplasia in the Junctional Region

Intestinal metaplasia may occur in gastric fundic oxyntic mucosa in patients with diffuse atrophic gastritis resulting from autoimmune gastritis, *Helicobacter pylori* gastritis, or omeprazole-induced atrophic gastritis (Fig. 2–40A). Atrophic gastritis is associated with atrophy of the oxyntic glands and replace-

TABLE 2–8. ANALYSIS OF SOME SITUATIONS BY PRESENTLY ACCEPTED CRITERIA AND BY USC CRITERIA

	Endoscopic Findings	Histologic Findings	Diagnosis by Present Criteria	Diagnosis by USC Criteria
Case 1	Normal	Normal squamous; cardiac mucosa	Normal	Mild reflux disease
Case 2	Normal	Normal squamous; IM in cardiac mucosa	IM of gastric cardia	Reflux-associated IM*
Case 3	< 2 cm CLE	Normal squamous; cardiac mucosa	Normal	Moderate reflux disease
Case 4	< 2 cm CLE	Normal squamous; IM in cardiac mucosa	Short-segment BE	Reflux-associated IM*
Case 5	> 2 cm CLE	Normal squamous; cardiac mucosa	?Normal ?CLE with no IM	Severe reflux disease
Case 6	> 2 cm CLE	Normal squamous; IM in cardiac mucosa	Long-segment BE	Reflux-associated IM*

Abbreviations: IM = intestinal metaplasia; CLE = columnar-lined esophagus; BE = Barrett's esophagus. NOTE: Reflux-associated IM is a term that is equivalent to Barrett's esophagus.
*The intestinal metaplasia is quantitated by serial biopsies in all cases.

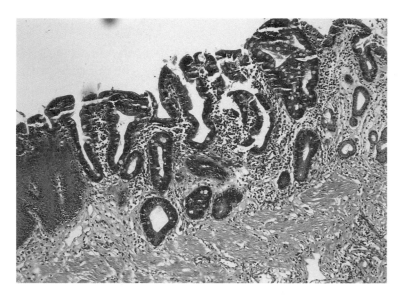

Figure 2–38. Short-segment Barrett's esophagus in resection specimen for esophageal squamous carcinoma. Note the typical zonation of epithelia—squamous to intestinal to cardiac—and the short length (<0.5 cm) of Barrett's epithelium.

ment with mucous cell-containing glands (pseudo-pyloric metaplasia); this resembles oxynto-cardiac mucosa and, in severe cases with complete parietal cell atrophy, cardiac mucosa. Intestinal metaplasia of the gastric fundus in chronic atrophic gastritis can be distinguished from reflux-associated intestinal metaplasia of cardiac mucosa by: (1) The presence of diffuse gastritis in the distal stomach. Atrophic gastritis almost never occurs as a condition restricted to the gastric side of the junctional region. (2) Occurrence in a flat mucosa without foveolar hyperplasia (Fig. 2–40B). This is quite different from reflux carditis, in which foveolar hyperplasia is marked and villiform change is frequent. Cases exist in which differentiating between the two is difficult from a single biopsy specimen, but the problem is resolved easily when multiple samples of distal stomach and esophagus are available.

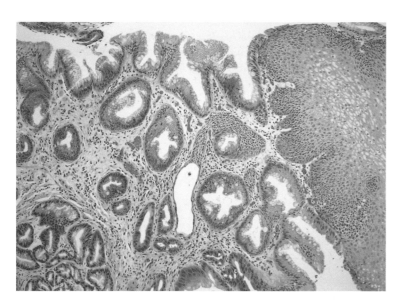

Figure 2–39. Squamocolumnar junction in a resection specimen for esophageal squamous carcinoma. There is a short segment of cardiac mucosa with rare goblet cells adjacent to the squamous epithelium. This represents ultrashort-segment Barrett's esophagus.

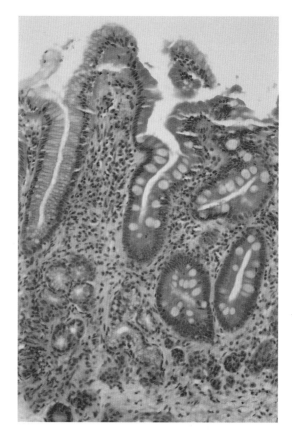

A

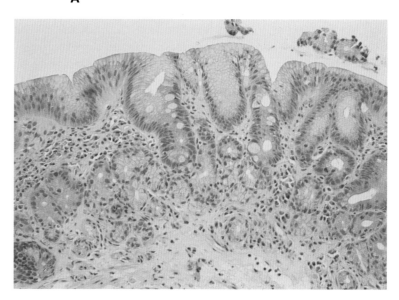

B

Figure 2–40. A: Chronic atrophic gastritis with intestinal metaplasia in a patient with autoimmune chronic atrophic gastritis. Note the relatively flat appearance of the mucosa that distinguishes this lesion from reflux carditis with intestinal metaplasia. Endocrine cell hyperplasia is also evident. B: Chronic atrophic gastritis with intestinal metaplasia in a flat mucosa.

Epithelial Zonation in Reflux Disease and Barrett's Esophagus

Paull and colleagues,[30] in 1971, described a regular zonation of the different types of epithelia that occur in Barrett's esophagus. Our observations confirm the zonation described by these researchers (see Figs. 2–25D, E, F, and 2–38). In all cases of significant reflux disease, three epithelial types occur: squamous (with or without criteria of reflux disease), metaplastic cardiac (with or without specialized cells), and normal gastric fundic oxyntic mucosa below the zone of reflux-induced cardiac mucosa. With increasing severity of reflux disease, the length of cardiac mucosa increases at the expense of the squamous epithelium, resulting in a cephalad migration of the squamocolumnar junction.[20] Two changes occurring in the cardiac mucosa are responsible for the epithelial zonation: (1) oxyntic transformation of the cardia occurring at the caudad end of the cardiac mucosa, and (2) intestinal metaplasia at the cephalad end of the cardiac mucosa. This leads to the following zones, starting cephalad and moving caudad: (1) squamous epithelium, with or without criteria of reflux, (2) intestinal metaplasia (in those patients who develop this change), (3) cardiac mucosa with reflux carditis, (4) oxyntocardiac mucosa, and (5) normal gastric fundic oxyntic mucosa.

Because intestinal metaplasia always occurs in cardiac mucosa immediately distal to the squamous epithelium (see Figs. 2–33 and 2–38), thorough sampling of the glandular mucosa immediately distal to the squamous epithelium will permit confident diagnosis or exclusion of intestinal metaplasia. If intestinal metaplasia is not found in this biopsy specimen, its presence elsewhere can be confidently excluded.

The incidence of intestinal metaplasia is directly related to the length of cardiac mucosa in the esophagus, ranging from 5–15% when no definite columnar lining is recognized in the esophagus at endoscopy to 93% when the columnar lining is longer than 3 cm.[31]

Intestinal metaplasia represents the only premalignant epithelium in reflux. Once it begins at the squamocardiac junction, intestinal metaplasia progresses caudally by progressive replacement of cardiac mucosa. The progression is contiguous without skip areas, but in any given area, intestinal metaplasia may coexist with carditis without the presence of goblet cells. Serial measured biopsy samples from the squamous epithelium to the lowest involved level permit accurate calculation of the extent of intestinal metaplasia. This quantitative assessment of intestinal metaplasia is presently being studied at USC as a cancer risk determinant.

Molecular and Histochemical Abnormalities in Barrett's Esophagus

Many histochemical and molecular abnormalities have been reported in Barrett's esophagus[32,33] (Table 2–9). Aneuploidy and genetic changes are present in nondysplastic Barrett's mucosa, increasing in frequency with increasing grades of dysplasia and malignancy. The presence of genetic changes in the nondysplastic Barrett's mucosa strongly indicates that intestinal metaplasia results from a genetic mutational change.

Changes in mucin content in the columnar epithelium in the esophagus has received much study. Cardiac and oxynto-cardiac surface and foveolar cells contain neutral mucin, which

TABLE 2–9. NONHISTOLOGIC MARKERS IN BARRETT'S ESOPHAGUS

Abnormal Finding	Significance
Sulfomucins	Expression of sulfomucin in sections stained with high iron diamine–Alcian blue pH 2.5 is negative in cardiac and fundic mucosa; positive in 50% of cases of intestinal metaplasia without cancer; and positive in 100% of cases of intestinal metaplasia with cancer.
Aberrant Lewis (a) antigen	Expression of aberrant Lea antigen among Lewis (a-b+) patients is negative in cardiac and fundic mucosa; positive in 35% of cases of intestinal metaplasia without cancer; and positive in 100% of cases of intestinal metaplasia with cancer.
Overexpression of p53 protein and 17p allelic deletion	Reported to occur early in the carcinogenesis of reflux-associated intestinal metaplasia, as indicated by their rare presence in nondysplastic and low-grade dysplastic epithelia. The frequency of p53 and 17p abnormalities increase with increasing grades of dysplasia and carcinoma.
Aneuploidy by flow cytometry	When aneuploidy was present in the initial biopsy of intestinal metaplastic epithelium, it was predictive of progression to high-grade dysplasia and adenocarcinoma in a subsequent biopsy. When flow cytometric abnormalities were absent, there was no progression to high-grade dysplasia and malignancy.

stains positively with periodic acid–Schiff (PAS) stain and negatively with Alcian blue stain at pH 2.5. Goblet cells in intestinal metaplasia stain a deep blue color with Alcian blue at pH 2.5. "Columnar blue cells" stain more faintly blue than goblet cells with AB, and with the combined PAS–AB stain at pH 2.5, they have a magenta color because of their mixed neutral and acid mucin content (Fig. 2–41). The acid mucin in intestinal metaplasia can be further classified by means of the combined high amine diamine (HID)–PAS stain at pH 2.5 into sialomucins (blue

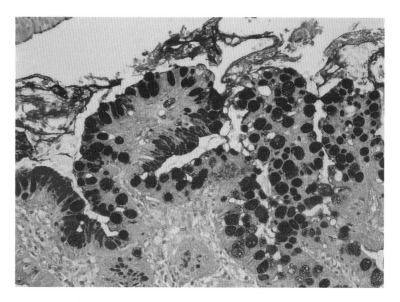

Figure 2–41. Barrett's esophagus, stained with PAS–Alcian blue at pH 2.5. The acid mucin of the goblet cells stains blue, but the neutral mucin stains pink with PAS.

cytoplasmic staining with HID–PAS) and sulfomucins (brown black cytoplasm on HID–PAS).[34] Sulfomucin indicates colonic-type intestinal metaplasia, and its presence is associated with an increased risk of adenocarcinoma, although the findings are not sufficiently specific or sensitive for routine clinical application.

Etiology

The etiologic relationship of Barrett's esophagus to gastro-esophageal reflux is certain. In other words, intestinal metaplasia always occurs in reflux-induced metaplastic cardiac mucosa. However, although cardiac mucosal length has a quantitative relationship with the severity of acid reflux (ie, the more acid reflux there is, the greater the length of metaplastic cardiac mucosa), the occurrence of intestinal metaplasia has no such quantitative relationship. The lack of quantitative association between acid exposure and intestinal metaplasia is indicated by the fact that intestinal metaplasia occurs in patients with low-level asymptomatic acid reflux and in 5–15% of patients who have no perceived abnormal columnar mucosa in the esophagus at endoscopy.[25] Abnormal pH scores correlate better with cardiac mucosal length than with the presence or absence of intestinal metaplasia (see Table 2–5). These findings, we believe, provide strong evidence that the occurrence of intestinal metaplasia in reflux-induced cardiac mucosa is independent of acid levels in the gastroesophageal refluxate.

Intestinal mucosa is very likely to result from genetic mutation in metaplastic cardiac mucosal cells, as indicated by the presence of aneuploidy and genetic changes in nondysplastic Barrett's esophagus.[32,33] This would explain the correlation between reflux carditis and intestinal metaplasia. Reflux carditis is a reactive mucosa associated with increased proliferation of the cardiac foveolar cells, and increased cellular proliferation is associated with an increased risk of genetic mutation.

Three possible etiologic factors in the initiation of intestinal metaplasia are considered.

1. Genetic Factors: Reflux-associated adenocarcinomas do not have a strong familial tendency. Evidence of a minor genetic susceptibility is suggested by a positive association of reflux-associated esophageal adenocarcinoma with Lewis(a+b–), nonsecretor and blood group A phenotypes.[35]
2. *Helicobacter pylori* Infection: Recently, evidence has been produced to suggest that *Helicobacter pylori* is involved in the etiology of Barrett's esophagus and adenocarcinoma in a manner similar to its association with gastric adenocarcinoma.[35,36] This suggestion has not been borne out in other studies,[37] including our own. Firstly, the epidemiologic features of reflux-associated adenocarcinoma are very different from both distal gastric carcinoma and *Helicobacter pylori* infection. The former is essentially a disease of affluent white males, whereas the latter has a high incidence in the less affluent nonwhite population. Secondly, the vast majority of our cases of reflux disease, Barrett's esophagus, and reflux-associated adenocarcinoma have occurred in patients with

no evidence of *Helicobacter pylori* gastritis as documented by distal gastric biopsies routinely performed in every case. Although it is possible that *H. pylori* contributes to carcinogenesis in those cases in which it is associated, it cannot be the universal or even main etiology for this cancer.

Care must be exercised in establishing a relationship between *Helicobacter pylori* infection and diseases of the stomach and esophagus. In institutions where *H. pylori* infection is common (eg, the Los Angeles County Hospital, which serves a nonwhite indigent population), *H. pylori* is associated with all diseases in this region. At the County Hospital, the majority of cases of reflux and Barrett's esophagus have associated *H. pylori* infection, simply because the majority of gastric biopsies are positive for the organism. The incidence of Barrett's esophagus and adenocarcinoma, however, is higher in the USC University Hospital, which serves an affluent white population, in which the incidence of *H. pylori* infection is much lower. Studies at the Los Angeles County Hospital may suggest a relationship between *H. pylori* and Barrett's esophagus; studies at the USC University Hospital, however, are much more meaningful in studying this relationship because incidence of *H. pylori* is low and permits more accurate evaluation of etiologic factors. All data presented here as "USC data" are derived from patients at the USC University Hospital.
3. Gastroduodenal Reflux: Duodenal contents have been shown to be a common component of gastroesophageal refluxate by pH studies ("alkaline reflux"), esophageal probes that detect bilirubin in the refluxate, and chemical testing of aspirated refluxate.[13] Levels of duodenal contents in refluxate have also been shown to correlate with the severity of reflux disease and particularly with the occurrence of strictures and intestinal (Barrett's) metaplasia in reflux disease.[13] The activity of duodenal components, particularly bile salts, is greatly influenced by pH.[38] Alteration of gastric pH with acid-suppressing drugs has been cited as a potential reason for the increasing incidence of Barrett's esophagus and adenocarcinoma associated with it. According to this thesis, acid suppressive drugs, although controlling reflux symptoms related to acid, may alter the bile salts and potentiate carcinogenesis because patients continue to reflux even though their symptoms are controlled. This hypothesis raises the disturbing possibility that the mutagenic phase of reflux disease, which includes intestinal metaplasia, dysplasia, and adenocarcinoma, may be iatrogenic.

Surveillance

At present, surveillance is recommended for patients with long-segment Barrett's esophagus. This consists of annual endoscopic examinations with multiple biopsies. Four-quadrant specimens are taken at 2-cm intervals along the abnormal glandular mucosa in the esophagus. Additional samples are taken from any abnormal appearing area.

Patients developing low-grade dysplasia during surveillance are entered into a 3-month course of intensive acid suppression with adequate dosages of omeprazole. Endoscopy is repeated after this with careful examination of multiple biopsy specimens. If low-grade dysplasia persists, the patient's surveillance interval is shortened or antireflux surgery or ablation therapy is performed.

The finding of high-grade dysplasia during surveillance is generally, but not universally, an indication for esophagectomy.

Dysplasia

Reflux-associated intestinal metaplasia (Barrett's esophagus) is the only premalignant epithelium in reflux disease. Intestinal metaplasia progresses through low-grade dysplasia and high-grade dysplasia to invasive carcinoma in those patients who progress along the cancer sequence.

The diagnosis of low-grade dysplasia in reflux-associated intestinal metaplasia lacks clearly definable criteria and is therefore associated with considerable interobserver variation. The cytologic changes of low-grade dysplasia include gland crowding with the lining epithelial cells showing mucin depletion, nuclear enlargement, hyperchromasia, and irregularity (Figs. 2–42, 2–43, 2–44). Mitotic figures may be present but are not numerous or atypical. The glands are simple. The cells retain at least a semblance of nuclear polarity, with nuclei being perpendicular to the basement membrane. These changes are difficult to distinguish from reactive changes that occur in the presence of healing erosions and acute inflammation (Fig. 2–45). For this reason, it is probably wise not to make a diagnosis of low-grade dysplasia in an area of ulcerated or actively inflamed mucosa. A category of "indefinite for dysplasia" is recommended when a decision between reactive atypia and low-grade dysplasia cannot be made. This diagnosis should be used sparingly.

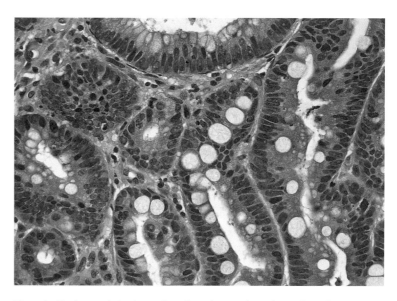

Figure 2–43. Low-grade dysplasia in Barrett's esophagus with significant cell stratification, nuclear enlargement, and irregularity in the absence of active inflammation and ulceration.

High-grade dysplasia, on the other hand, is a diagnosis for which clear criteria exist and the interobserver variation is less. Criteria for high-grade dysplasia are the presence of a severe cytologic abnormality characterized by almost complete mucin depletion and marked nuclear enlargement, pleomorphism, hyperchromasia, irregularity, and the presence of mitoses including atypical mitotic figures (Figs. 2–46 through 2–49). In addition to this severe cytologic abnormality, complete loss of nuclear polarity (Figs. 2–46 and 2–47) or gland complexity characterized by luminal bridging and cribriform change must occur (Fig. 2–48). The presence of these changes in the surface epithelium has a greater degree of diagnostic certainty than when they are restricted to the deeper glands (Fig. 2–49). Criteria for high-grade dysplasia do not occur in inflammatory and

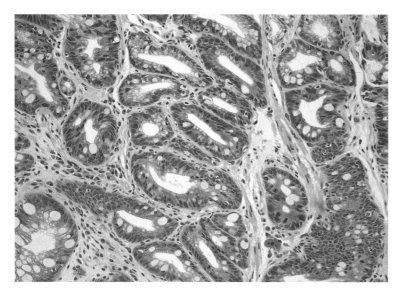

Figure 2–42. Barrett's esophagus with mild crowding of glands and mild cell stratification and nuclear hyperchromasia of lining cells in the absence of active ulceration or inflammation. This degree of change is in the indeterminate area between reactive atypia and low-grade dysplasia.

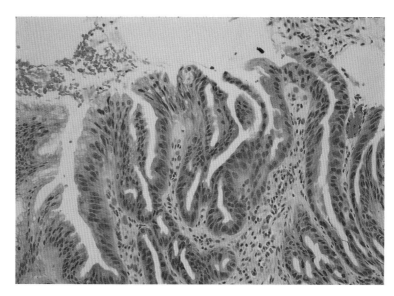

Figure 2–44. Low-grade dysplasia in Barrett's esophagus involving surface epithelium with significant cellular abnormalities in the absence of ulceration and acute inflammation.

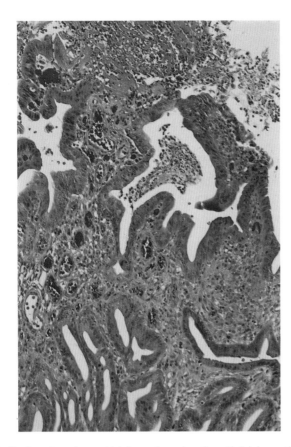

Figure 2–45. Barrett's esophagus with inflammation and reactive epithelial changes that are difficult to distinguish from low-grade dysplasia.

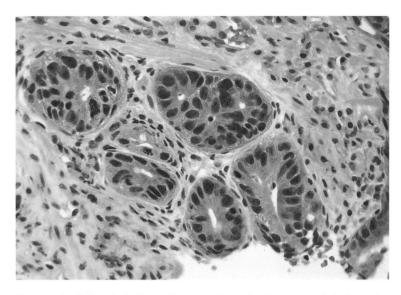

Figure 2–47. High-grade dysplasia in Barrett's esophagus showing severe cytologic abnormality, loss of nuclear polarity, and early gland complexity.

regenerative atypia; therefore high-grade dysplasia can be diagnosed in the presence of inflammation and erosion.

Although low- and high-grade dysplasia are recognized, it must be realized that dysplasia is a continuum of increasing abnormality, and borderline cases occur in which diagnostic uncertainty arises between low- and high-grade dysplasia (Figs. 2–50 and 2–51, see also Chapter 1–Fig. 1–3). In such cases, the

diagnosis should always be low-grade dysplasia. It has been recommended that the diagnosis of high-grade dysplasia be confirmed by an expert pathologist before patients are subject to esophagectomy.

The distinction between high-grade dysplasia and intramucosal adenocarcinoma can sometimes be difficult and subjective (Figs. 2–52, 2–53, and 2–54). Irregularity of glands showing features of high-grade dysplasia and the presence of small nests and individual malignant cells in the lamina propria are definitive criteria for intramucosal carcinoma (see Fig. 2–54). Use of a multiple-biopsy protocol with extensive sampling has been reported to be effective in excluding the presence of early adenocarcinoma in cases of high-grade dysplasia.[39] When marked irregularity of malignant glands, single malignant cells, and desmoplasia are present, the specimen should be diagnosed

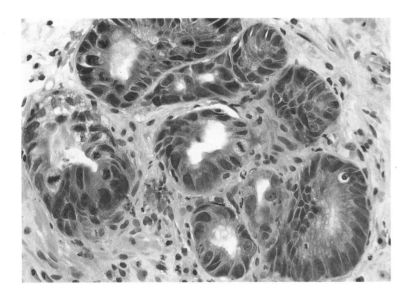

Figure 2–46. Focus of dysplastic glands in Barrett's esophagus showing transition of low-grade to high-grade dysplasia. The gland at right lower corner has retained nuclear polarity; the remainder show loss of nuclear polarity. Note that goblet cells are commonly absent in high-grade dysplasia.

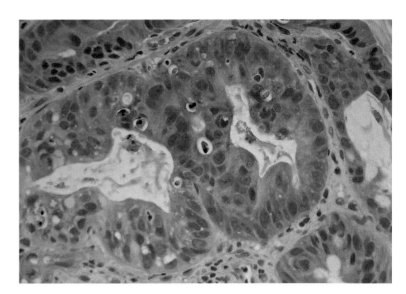

Figure 2–48. High-grade dysplasia in Barrett's esophagus showing severe cytologic abnormality, loss of nuclear polarity, and gland complexity with cribriform spaces.

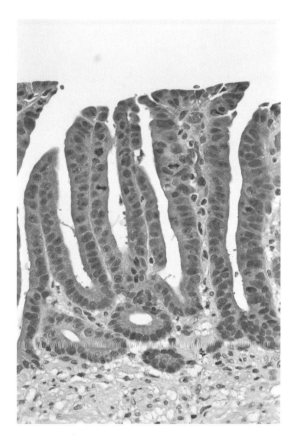

Figure 2–49. High-grade dysplasia in Barrett's esophagus involving villous surface epithelium showing severe cytologic abnormality and loss of nuclear polarity.

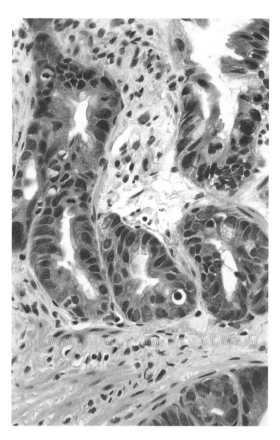

Figure 2–51. Dysplasia in Barrett's esophagus. Severe cytologic abnormality is present, and there is loss of nuclear polarity. This was called high-grade dysplasia, but it has potential for interobserver variation.

as invasive adenocarcinoma (Fig. 2–55). The presence of demoplasia in a mucosal biopsy is predictive of invasion deeper than the mucosa.

The progression of low-grade dysplasia to high-grade dysplasia to adenocarcinoma is uncertain both in terms of frequency and time frame. Although it is generally held that high-

grade dysplasia progresses to adenocarcinoma often and rapidly,[40] some studies show no progression of high-grade dysplasia during several years of follow-up.[41] On the other hand, other studies show that if esophagectomy is performed on a diagnosis of high-grade dysplasia, invasive carcinoma is found in the resection specimen in 30% of cases.[42]

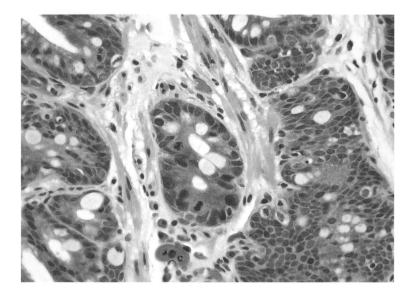

Figure 2–50. Dysplasia in Barrett's esophagus. This was classified as low-grade dysplasia, but the single gland in the center shows features consistent with high-grade dysplasia. This case is one with significant potential for interobserver variation.

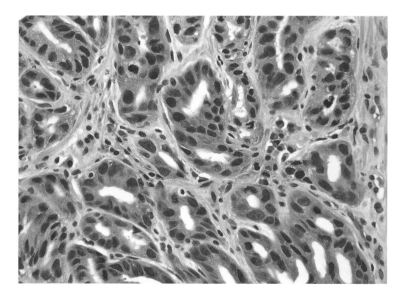

Figure 2–52. Irregular small glands with severe cytologic abnormality and loss of nuclear polarity. This was called high-grade dysplasia with the possibility of early intramucosal carcinoma. This also has potential for significant interobserver variation.

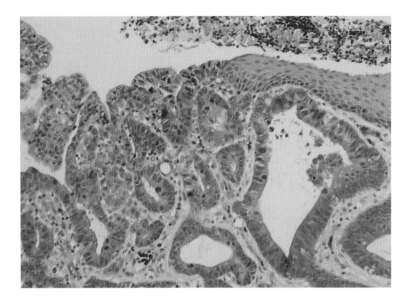

Figure 2–53. More definitive example of intramucosal carcinoma, characterized by small glands without clear basement membranes.

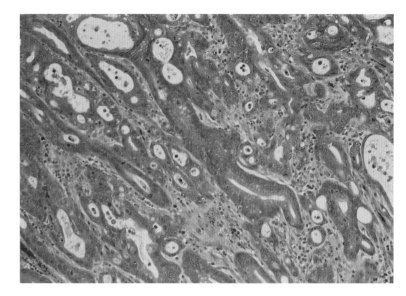

Figure 2–55. Moderately differentiated adenocarcinoma in Barrett's esophagus. The presence of desmoplasia in a mucosal biopsy is predictive for invasion below the muscularis mucosae.

As a pathologist, it is important to be aware of the consequences of different diagnoses. In some centers, low-grade dysplasia is an indication for shortening the surveillance intervals; in others, it is an indication for antireflux surgery or ablation therapy. In some centers, high-grade dysplasia is an indication for careful, multibiopsy surveillance; in others, it is an indication for esophagectomy. Diagnoses of intramucosal and invasive carcinoma precipitates cancer surgery unless there is a contraindication.

Reflux–Adenocarcinoma Sequence

Gastroesophageal reflux causes adenocarcinoma of the lower esophagus and, very likely, adenocarcinoma of the gastroesophageal junctional region. According to the USC scheme, the

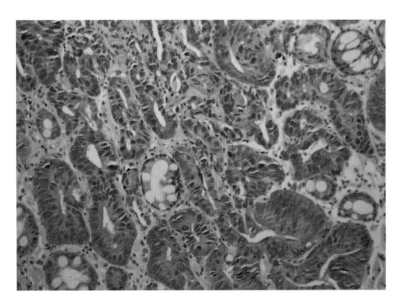

Figure 2–54. Intramucosal adenocarcinoma in Barrett's esophagus characterized by small infiltrative glands. The absence of deeper invasion cannot be excluded in a mucosal biopsy.

sequence of morphologic change whereby this happens is as follows: (1) acid reflux causes cardiac transformation of squamous epithelium; (2) acid reflux injures the cardiac mucosa, causing reflux carditis with increased cell turnover; (3) intestinal metaplasia occurs in the cardiac mucosa (reflux-associated intestinal metaplasia or Barrett's esophagus), a change that is very likely associated with genetic mutation; and (4) further genetic mutational events occur in the intestinal epithelium leading to low-grade dysplasia, high-grade dysplasia, and invasive carcinoma.

By this sequence, any adenocarcinoma arising in cardiac mucosa is reflux-induced; this includes all carcinomas of the gastroesophageal junctional region, which have epidemiologic characteristics that are identical to adenocarcinoma of the lower esophagus.

Reflux disease in children results in long segments of cardiac or fundic mucosa without intestinal metaplasia, which is rare in children.[43] In large studies of adults, there is 10-year difference in the median age of occurrence of specialized intestinal mucosa, high-grade dysplasia, and adenocarcinoma. These findings suggest a progression from reflux-induced cardiac metaplasia to intestinal metaplasia to high-grade dysplasia in the sequence set out previously. This is the only malignant sequence in reflux disease.

Changes in Barrett's Esophagus with Treatment

Medical treatment with acid-suppressing drugs are highly effective in controlling reflux symptoms. They do not control reflux, however, and the abnormal glandular mucosa in the esophagus remains exposed to all the components of the refluxate except the acid. Antireflux surgical procedures such as Nissen fundoplication, when successful, stop the reflux. There is evidence that progression of Barrett's esophagus to dysplasia is less in surgically treated patients than in medically treated patients.[44]

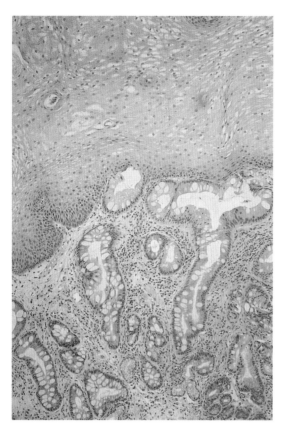

Figure 2–56. Overgrowth of squamous epithelium over Barrett's type glands with intestinal metaplasia.

Pathologic specimens from the esophagus in patients who have had successful antireflux surgery show the following changes:

1. Changes in Cardiac Mucosa: The amount of inflammation and foveolar hyperplasia (reflux carditis) is decreased. The frequency of oxyntocardiac mucosa increases, suggesting that reduction in acid exposure promotes oxyntic transformation of cardiac mucosa (see Fig. 2–6). Complete oxyntic transformation of cardiac mucosa results in a mucosa that is

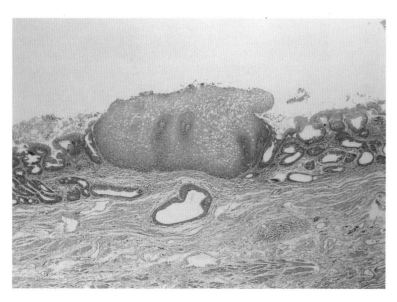

Figure 2–57. Squamous island in columnar-lined esophagus.

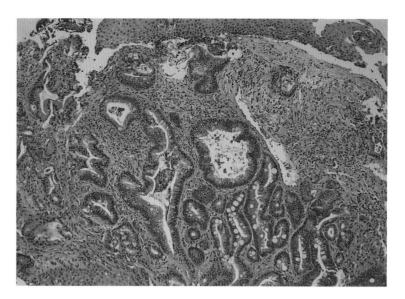

Figure 2–58. Low-grade dysplasia in Barrett's glands underlying squamous overgrowth. A high-power micrograph of these glands is shown in Figure 2–43.

essentially identical to normal fundic mucosa. Both these changes protect against the progression of disease to intestinal metaplasia. The decline in the cellular proliferation associated with reflux theoretically decreases the likelihood of mutational change, and intestinal metaplasia almost never occurs in oxyntocardiac mucosa.

2. Squamous "Overgrowth": This probably represents a reversion of differentiation of surface epithelium from glandular to squamous and occurs over both cardiac mucosa and in-

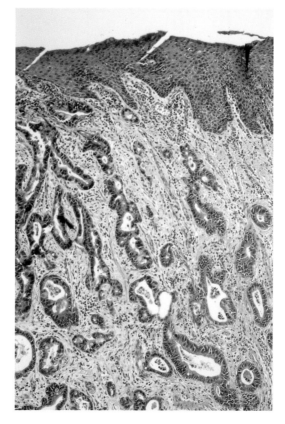

Figure 2–59. Adenocarcinoma of Barrett's esophagus in glands under squamous surface epithelium.

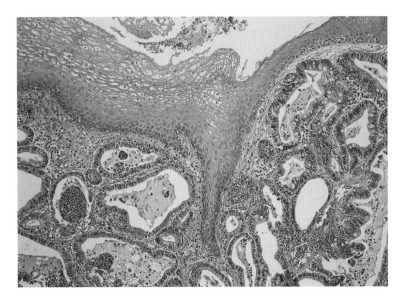

Figure 2–60. Adenocarcinoma of Barrett's esophagus with malignant glands under squamous epithelium.

testinal mucosa (Fig. 2–56). Overgrowth occurs in patients after ablation therapy, surgical antireflux procedures without mucosal ablation, and effective medical therapy with omeprazole. Overgrowth of squamous epithelium results in squamous islands in the columnar epithelium (Fig. 2–57) followed by a decrease in the area lined by columnar epithelium.[45] The fate of the residual glands under the squamous epithelium is unknown; they may progressively disappear or remain and become potential sites for dysplasia (Fig. 2–58) and malignant transformation under the squamous epithelium. It is not uncommon to see Barrett's adenocarcinoma in mucosa lined by squamous epithelium on the surface (Figs. 2–59 and 2–60); whether this represents occurrence of adenocarcinoma in lamina propria in cases with squamous overgrowth over Barrett's epithelium or undermining of squamous epithelium by adenocarcinoma is unknown.

NONREFLUX ESOPHAGITIS

Drug-Induced ("Pill") Esophagitis

Since it was first reported in 1970 by Pemberton,[46] over 250 cases of drug-induced esophagitis have been reported. Tablets and capsules have been shown to take more than 5 min to pass down the esophagus when a small volume of fluid is used and when the person lies down immediately after ingestion. Large size of the pill and its chemical composition are important factors in how long it can remain in the esophagus. In most cases, the pill becomes obstructed at the point of physiologic narrowing at aortic arch level. When pathologic narrowing or dysmotility exists, pills can become held up at the site of abnormality. In patients with reflux disease, pills can exacerbate mucosal injury and contribute to stricture formation.

The most commonly implicated drugs are potassium chlo-

ride tablets (particularly Slow-K), doxycycline, tetracycline, quinidine gluconate, ferrous sulfate, vitamin C, NSAIDs, aspirin, oral contraceptives, and alendronate (Fosamax). Drug impaction leads to acute mucosal injury. With drugs such as ferrous sulfate and doxycycline, the injury reverses rapidly when the drug is withdrawn. With potassium chloride, quinidine gluconate, and alendronate, the acute injury is followed by fibrosis and stricture formation. Potassium chloride, which is the most lethal, has been reported to cause severe ulceration with hemorrhage and perforation.

Pill-induced ulcers of the esophagus are recognized at endoscopy by their focal nature and occurrence at an atypical location. Rarely, long segments of ulceration and stricture formation occur and resemble malignant strictures.[47] Biopsy specimens are nonspecific. For the pathologist, lack of clinical information may result in the samples with ulceration being misinterpreted as representing reflux disease.

Corrosive Esophagitis

Severe acute injury of the esophagus results from ingestion of concentrated acid or concentrated alkali. These caustic materials are present in household cleaners such as toilet bowl cleaners and drain cleaners. Lye is a caustic alkali used in cleaners and several industrial chemicals. Accidental ingestion of caustic household chemicals by young children is the most common cause of caustic injury. Lye ingestion in suicide attempts is less common.

Caustic ingestion produces mucosal injury from the pharynx to the stomach[48] (Fig. 2–61). Severe injury is associ-

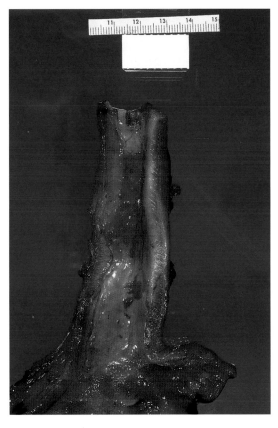

Figure 2–61. Caustic ingestion, chronic phase with complicated strictures in the midesophagus.

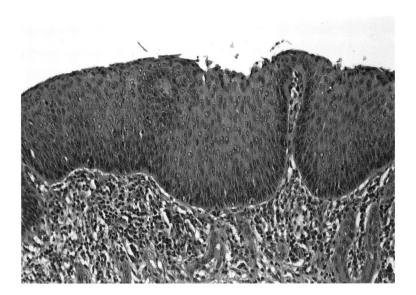

Figure 2–62. Regenerative squamous epithelium after lye injury.

atcd with extensive ulceration, transmural necrosis, and perforation, requiring emergency surgery. Resected cases show ulceration and healing with fibrosis and squamous epithelial regeneration (Fig. 2–62). We have encountered an unusual combination of goblet cells within squamous epithelium in a case of resected lye ingestion (Fig. 2–63). Less severe cases heal with fibrous stricture formation and require repeated dilatations throughout life. The incidence of squamous carcinoma in patients with chronic caustic strictures of the esophagus is greatly increased.

Esophagitis Associated with Dermatologic Diseases

Pemphigus vulgaris may involve the esophagus. In most cases, this occurs in patients who have an established diagnosis of cutaneous pemphigus vulgaris. Rarely, mucosal and esophageal lesions are the first manifestation of the disease. When dysphagia is the presenting symptom and esophagoscopy shows irregular ulcerations from which biopsy specimens are provided, the diagnosis can be difficult. In one case, a cytologic specimen of a brushing from an ulcer showed the acantholytic cells as markedly atypical cells that were initially misdiagnosed as malignant cells (Fig. 2–64A), until histologic examination showed the typical denuded suprabasal vesicles with the basal cells appearing as a "row of tombstones" (Fig. 2–64B). It should be noted that poor fixation (resulting most commonly when the biopsy sample is placed in saline prior to transfer into formalin) can result in artefactual suprabasal separation that bears a superficial resemblance to pemphigus vulgaris. The absence of basal villi, lack of acantholytic cells, and lack of separation of the lateral borders of the basal cells should permit differentiation of this artefact from pemphigus vulgaris (Fig. 2–65).

The recessive dystrophic form of epidermolysis bullosa is commonly associated with esophageal involvement. Vesicles, ulcers, fibrous strictures are most commonly seen in the upper esophagus.[49]

The esophagus can also be involved in severe cases of Stevens-Johnson syndrome. The changes in the esophageal squamous epithelium resemble erythema multiforme, with in-

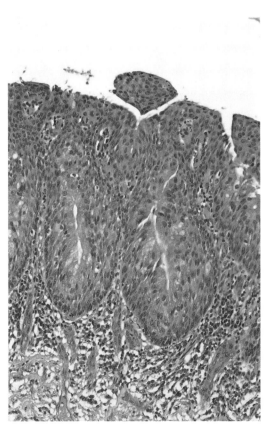

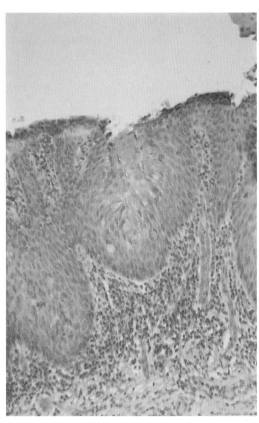

Figure 2–63. A: Epithelial reaction after lye injury showing goblet cells in regenerating squamous epithelium. B: Alcian blue stain at pH 2.5 in lye injury, showing acid mucin positivity in goblet cells. This does not represent Barrett's esophagus, which is defined as intestinal metaplasia complicating reflux disease.

A

B

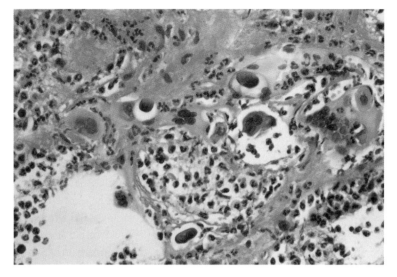

A

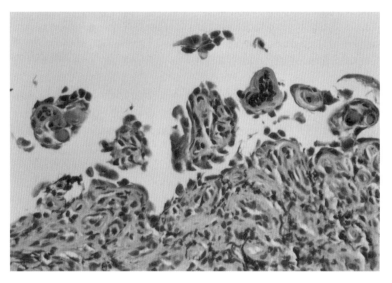

B

Figure 2–64. A: Pemphigus vulgaris. Cell block from esophageal cytology specimen showing markedly atypical cells that were called squamous carcinoma at the original read-out. B: Pemphigus vulgaris of the esophagus showing deroofed vesicle with its base composed of villous structures lined by the typical "row of tombstones" appearance of the nonacantholytic basal cells. The acantholytic cells are represented in the cytologic sample and show marked atypia.

dividual necrotic keratinocytes being the most typical feature.[50] Ulceration is common. The histologic changes seen in Stevens-Johnson syndrome resemble those seen in esophageal involvement in graft-versus-host disease. The latter occurs in patients who have had bone marrow transplantation.

Infectious and Inflammatory Esophagitis

In the Immunocompetent Host

Esophageal infections are extremely uncommon in the immunocompetent host. Sometimes, esophageal ulcers in patients with reflux disease show overgrowth of *Candida* species in the ulcer base, but this does not constitute *Candida* esophagitis.

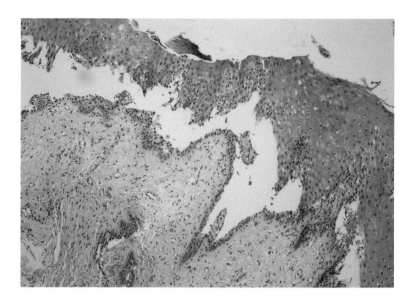

Figure 2–65. Poorly fixed esophageal biopsy specimen showing artefactual suprabasal separation of the epithelium. This can be differentiated from pemphigus vulgaris by the absence of acantholytic cells and the lack of the "row of tombstones" appearance.

Bacterial infections are rare. In the past, β-hemolytic streptococcal infections were reported in patients severely ill from other causes.[51] These resulted in a diffuse acute inflammation involving the full thickness of the esophagus (esophagitis dissecans). Tuberculosis rarely affects the esophagus.

Generalized inflammatory diseases of the gastrointestinal tract such as Crohn's disease[52] and eosinophilic gastroenteritis rarely involve the esophagus.

In the Immunocompromised Host

Esophageal infections are common in the immunocompromised host, particularly in patients with acquired immunodeficiency syndrome (AIDS). Patients with all types of infections present with dysphagia and odynophagia. Upper GI bleeding occurs in cases associated with ulceration, particularly cytomegalovirus infection and idiopathic human immunodeficiency virus (HIV)-related ulcers. Esophageal symptoms occur in 40% of patients with AIDS.[53]

Infection with *Candida* species is the most common infection, and is frequently an AIDS-defining infection in HIV-positive patients. It has been recommended that antifungal therapy effective against *Candida* be tried empirically in all AIDS patients with odynophagia, and endoscopy performed only in those in whom symptoms persist after 2 weeks.[53] *Candida* infects the surface layers of the squamous epithelium, which undergoes hyperkeratosis and parakeratosis in the areas of infection. Neutrophil infiltration of the involved area is common. The neutrophils tend to aggregate in the superficial region of the epithelium (see Fig. 2–17). The affected area appears endoscopically as a white plaque; in severe infections, plaques become confluent and may cover large areas of the mucosa. The diagnosis is usually obvious endoscopically. It can be confirmed by biopsy of the white plaques or brush cytology, both of which show the typical budding yeasts and pseudohyphae of *Candida* species (Fig. 2–66A). Staining with fungal stains such as methenamine silver and PAS are helpful in cases in which yeasts are not obvious on H&E (Fig. 2–66B).

Herpes simplex esophagitis commonly accompanies lesions in the oropharynx. The virus infects the squamous epithelial cells, resulting in blisters, which rapidly turn into multiple superficial apthous ulcers surrounded by erythema (Fig. 2–67). Biopsies show mucosal ulceration. Biopsies from the edge of the ulcer are the most diagnostic. The diagnosis is made by the finding of typical infected epithelial cells, which show multinucleation and viral inclusions in biopsies (Fig. 2–68A) and brushings (Fig. 2–68B). Viral inclusions commonly appear as a glassy basophilia of the nucleus; typical Cowdry A inclusions also

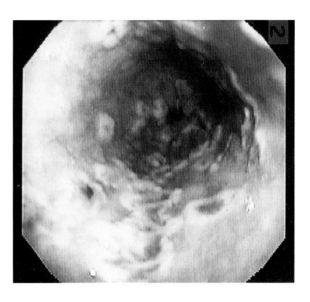

Figure 2–67. Endoscopy in an AIDS patient presenting with dysphagia, showing inflammation and multiple ulcers in the lower esophagus. This appearance can represent herpes simplex virus infection, cytomegalovirus infection, or idiopathic esophageal ulceration. This particular case was HSV esophagitis.

occur. In cases in which the inclusions are not definitive histologically, immunoperoxidase staining is helpful in confirming the diagnosis.

Cytomegalovirus (CMV) esophagitis is common in AIDS patients, but it also occurs in transplant patients and patients on cancer chemotherapy.[54] Endoscopy shows ulcers in the mid and distal esophagus; the ulcers are surrounded by normal mucosa. Ulcers are multiple in half the cases, and giant (larger than 1 cm) in 25%.[55] Clinical and endoscopic features are not specific. Multiple biopsy specimens should be taken from the center and edge of the ulcer; the samples must be large enough to contain sufficient lamina propria, which contains the diagnostic cells. CMV does not infect squamous cells; it infects endothelial cells in the lamina propria (Fig. 2–69). Biopsies show ulcer debris, reactive squamous epithelium, and lamina propria inflammation. CMV-infected endothelial cells are present in the endothelial cells of the lamina propria, appearing as enlarged cells with large intranuclear inclusions or granular basophilic cytoplasmic inclusions (or both). Enlarged cells with smudged nuclei may be seen. These could represent either reactive fibroblasts or CMV-infected cells; in cases with such histologically nondiagnostic cells, immunoperoxidase staining for CMV is helpful. Treatment with ganciclovir and foscarnet induces healing, but prolonged treatment is often necessary.

HIV-associated idiopathic esophageal ulcer (IEU) cannot be distinguished clinically or endoscopically from CMV and herpes simplex virus esophagitis.[56] Ulcers usually occur in the middle and distal esophagus, are frequently multiple, and larger than 1 cm in more than a third of patients. The diagnosis of IEU is made when biopsies and brushings are negative for CMV and herpes simplex virus. Histologic exclusion of these viruses in multiple levels of the specimens is usually adequate. Some cen-

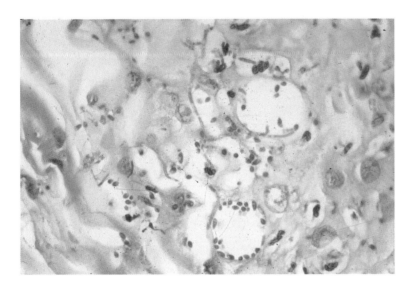

A

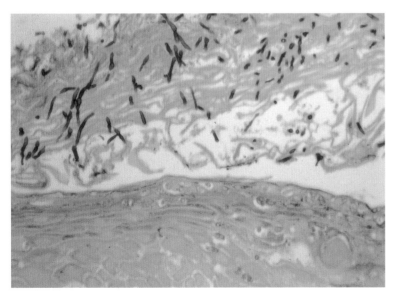

B

Figure 2–66. A: Surface region of the squamous epithelium tangentially cut showing yeast and pseudohyphal forms of *Candida*. B: Methenamine silver stain showing *Candida* species in esophageal biopsy.

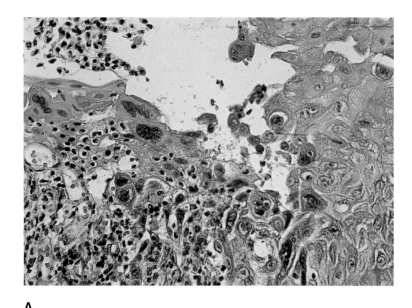

A

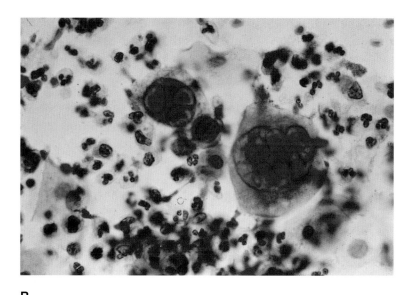

B

Figure 2–68. A: Herpes simplex virus infection showing multinucleated giant cells with glassy intranuclear appearance. B: Esophageal brushings in herpes simplex virus esophagitis showing multinucleation and intranuclear inclusions with both glassy and typical Cowdry A appearance.

ters also require negative culture of brushings and negative immunoperoxidase staining or negative in situ hybridization of tissue sections before a viral etiology is excluded. HIV has been demonstrated in biopsies from IEU by polymerase chain reaction,[57] but HIV is not thought to be the cause of IEU. HIV-associated IEU responds to steroid therapy.

Figure 2–69. Cytomegalovirus esophagitis showing enlarged cells with glassy inclusions in the nuclei of lamina propria stromal cells. Atypical viral features such as this are common with CMV esophagitis and require confirmation with immunohistochemistry.

References

1. Fyke FE, Code CF, Schlegel JF. The gastroesophageal sphincter in healthy human beings. *Gastroenterologia.* 1956;86:135–150.
2. Stein HJ, Liebermann-Meffert D, DeMeester TR, et al. Three-dimensional pressure image and muscular structure of the human lower esophageal sphincter. *Surgery.* 1995;117:692–698.
3. Kim SL, Waring PJ, Spechler SL, et al. Diagnostic inconsistencies in Barrett's esophagus. *Gastroenterology.* 1994;107:945–949.
4. Zaninotto G, DeMeester TR, Schwizer W, et al. *Am J Surg.* 1988;155:104–111.
5. Jamieson JR, Stein HJ, DeMeester TR, et al. Ambulatory 24-h esophageal pH monitoring: Normal values, optimal thresholds, specificity, sensitivity, and reproducibility. *Am J Gastroenterol.* 1992;87:1102–1111.
6. Hayward J. The lower end of the esophagus. *Thorax.* 1961;16:36–41.
7. Spechler SJ. Esophageal columnar metaplasia (Barrett's esophagus). *Gastrointest Endosc Clin North Am.* 1997;7:1–18.
8. Christensen WN, Sternberg SS. Adenocarcinoma of the upper esophagus arising in ectopic gastric mucosa. *Am J Surg Pathol.* 1987;11:397–402.
9. Tucker HJ, Snape WJ, Cohen S. Achalasia secondary to carcinoma: Manometric and clinical features. *Ann Intern Med.* 1978;89:315.
10. Cohen S. Laufer I, Snape WJ, et al. The gastrointestinal manifestations of scleroderma. *Gastroenterology.* 1980;79:155.
11. Zamost BJ, Hirschberg J, Ippoliti AF, et al. Esophagitis in scleroderma. *Gastroenterology.* 1987;92:421.
12. Jamieson JR, Stein HJ, DeMeester TR, et al. Ambulatory 24-h esophageal pH monitoring: Normal values, optimal thresh-

olds, specificity, sensitivity, and reproducibility. *Am J Gastroenterol.* 1992;87:1102–1111.

13. Kauer WKH, Peters JH, DeMeester TR, et al. Mixed reflux of gastric and duodenal juices is more harmful to the esophagus than gastric juice alone. *Ann Surg.* 1995;222:525–533.

14. Liron R, Parrilla P, de Haro LFM, et al. Quantification of duodenogastric reflux in Barrett's esophagus. *Am J Gastroenterol.* 1997;92:32.

15. Zaninotto G, DeMeester TR, Schwitzer W, et al. The lower esophageal sphincter in health and disease. *Am J Surg.* 1988;155:104–111.

16. Stein HJ, DeMeester TR, Naspetti R, et al. Three-dimensional imaging of the lower esophageal sphincter in gastroesophageal reflux disease. *Ann Surg.* 1991;214:364–384.

17. Schindlbeck NE, Wiebecke B, Klauser AG, et al. Diagnostic value of histology in non-erosive gastro-oesophageal reflux disease. *Gut.* 1996;39:151–154.

18. Chandrasoma P. Pathophysiology of Barrett's esophagus. *Semin Thorac Cardiovasc Surg.* 1997;9:270–278.

19. Oberg S, Peters JH, DeMeester TR, et al. Inflammation and specialized intestinal metaplasia of cardiac mucosa is a manifestation of gastroesophageal reflux disease. *Ann Surg.* 1997;226:522–532.

20. Csendes A, Maluenda F, Braghetto I, et al. Location of the lower oesophageal sphincter and the squamous columnar mucosa junction in 109 healthy controls and 778 patients with different degrees of endoscopic oesophagitis. *Gut.* 1993;34:21–27.

21. Nebel OT, Fornes MF, Castell DO. Symptomatic gastroesophageal reflux. Incidence and precipitating factors. *Dig Dis Sci.* 1976;21:955.

22. Graham DY, Smith JL, Patterson DJ. Why do apparently healthy people use antacid tablets. *Am J Gastroenterol.* 1983;78:257.

23. Krishnamurthy S, Dayal Y. Pancreatic metaplasia in Barrett's esophagus. An immunohistochemical study. *Am J Surg Pathol.* 1995;19:1172–1180.

24. Spechler SJ. Esophageal columnar metaplasia (Barrett's esophagus). *Gastrointest Endosc Clin North Am.* 1997;7:1–18.

25. Spechler SJ, Zeroogian JM, Antonioli DA, et al. Prevalence of metaplasia at the gastroesophageal junction. *Lancet.* 1994;344:1533–1536.

26. Canto MIF, Setrakian S, Petras RE, et al. Methylene blue selectively stains intestinal metaplasia in Barrett's esophagus. *Gastrointest Endosc.* 1996;44:1–7.

27. Weinstein WM. Precursor lesions for cancer of the cardia. *Gastrointest Endosc Clin North Am.* 1997;7:19–28.

28. Haggitt RC. Barrett's esophagus, dysplasia, and adenocarcinoma. *Hum Pathol.* 1994;25:982–993.

29. Kim SL, Waring PJ, Spechler SJ, et al. Diagnostic inconsistencies in Barrett's esophagus. *Gastroenterology.* 1994;107:945–949.

30. Paull A, Trier JS, Dalton MD, et al. The histologic spectrum of Barrett's esophagus. *N Engl J Med.* 1976;295:476–480.

31. Spechler SJ, Zeroogian JM, Wang HH, et al. The frequency of specialized intestinal metaplasia at the squamocolumnar junction varies with the extent of columnar epithelium lining the esophagus. *Gastroenterology.* 1995;108:A224.

32. Blount PL, Ramel S, Raskind WH, et al. 17p allelic deletions and p53 protein overexpression in Barrett's adenocarcinomas. *Cancer Res.* 1991;51:5482–5486.

33. Reid BJ, Blount PL, Rubin CE, et al. Flow cytometric and histologic progression to malignancy in Barrett's esophagus: Prospective endoscopic surveillance of a cohort. *Gastroenterology.* 1992;102:1212–1219.

34. Antonioli DA, Esophagus. *In* Henson DE, Albers-Saavedra J (eds.): *Pathology of Incipient Neoplasia,* ed 2, Philadelphia, WB Saunders, 1993. pp. 64–84.

35. Torrado J, Ruiz B, Garay J, et al. Blood-group phenotypes, sulfomucins, and *Helicobacter pylori* in Barrett's esophagus. *Am J Surg Pathol.* 1997;21:1023–1029.

36. Loffeld RJLF, Tiji BJT, Arends JW. Prevalence and significance of *Helicobacter pylori* in patients with Barrett's esophagus. *Am J Gastroenterol.* 1992;87:598–600.

37. Quddus MR, Henley JD, Sulaiman RA, et al. *Helicobacter pylori* infection and adenocarcinoma arising in Barrett's esophagus. *Hum Pathol.* 1997;28:1007–1009.

38. Barthlen W, Liebermann-Meffert D, Feussner H, et al. Influence of pH on bile acid concentration in human, pig and commercial bile: Implications for "alkaline" gastro-esophageal reflux. *Dis Esophagus.* 1994;7:127–130.

39. Levin DS, Haggitt RC, Blount RL, et al. An endoscopy biopsy protocol can differentiate high grade dysplasia from early adenocarcinoma in Barrett's esophagus. *Gastroenterology.* 1993;107:40–50.

40. Hameeteman W, Tytgat GNJ, Houthoff HJ, et al. Barrett's esophagus: Development of dysplasia and adenocarcinoma. *Gastroenterology.* 1989;96:1249–1256.

41. Lee RG. Dysplasia in Barrett's esophagus. A clinicopathologic study of six patients. *Am J Surg Pathol.* 1985;9:845–852.

42. Altorki NK, Sunagawa M, Little AG, et al. High grade dysplasia in the columnar lined esophagus. *Am J Surg.* 1991;161:97–100.

43. Qualman SJ, Murray RD, McClung J, et al. Intestinal metaplasia is age related in Barrett's esophagus. *Arch Pathol Lab Med.* 1990;114:1236–1240.

44. Peters JH. The surgical management of Barrett's esophagus. *Gastroenterol Clin North Am.* 1997;26:647–668.

45. Hassall E, Weinstein WM. Partial regression of childhood Barrett's esophagus after fundoplication. *Am J Gastroenterol.* 1992;87:1506–1512.

46. Pemberton J. Esophageal obstruction and ulceration caused by oral potassium therapy. *Br Heart J.* 1970;32:267–268.

47. Bonavina L, DeMeester TR, McChesney L, et al. Drug-induced esophageal strictures. *Ann Surg.* 1987;206:173–183.

48. Zargor SA, Kochlar R, Mehta S, et al. The role of fiberoptic endoscopy in the management of corrosive ingestion and modified endoscopic classification of burns. *Gastrointest Endosc.* 1991;37:165–169.

49. Travis SPL, Eady RAJ, Thompson RPH. Esophageal complications in epidermolysis bullosa. *Gut.* 1991;32:1569–1570.

50. Zweiban B, Cohen H, Chandrasoma P. Gastrointestinal involvement complicating Stevens-Johnson's syndrome. *Gastroenterology.* 1986;91:469–474.

51. Walsh TJ, Belitsos NJ, Hamilton SR. Bacterial esophagitis in immunocompromised patients. *Arch Intern Med.* 1986;146:1345–1348.

52. D'Haens G, Rutgeerts P, Geboes K, et al. The natural history of esophageal Crohn's disease: Three patterns of evolution. *Gastrointest Endosc.* 1994;40:296–300.

53. Laine L, Bonacini M. Esophageal disease in human immunodeficiency virus infection. *Arch Intern Med.* 1994;154:1577–1582.

54. Buckner FS, Pomeroy C. Cytomegalovirus disease of the gastroin-

testinal tract in patients without AIDS. *Clin Infect Dis.* 1993;17: 644–656.

55. Wilcox CM, Straub RF, Dietrich DA. Prospective endoscopic characterization of cytomegalovirus esophagitis in AIDS. *Gastrointest Endosc.* 1994;40:481–484.

56. Wilcox CM, Schwartz DA. Endoscopic characterization of idiopathic esophageal ulceration associated with human im-munodeficiency virus infection. *J Clin Gastroenterol.* 1993;16: 251–256.

57. Wilcox CM, Zaki SR, Coffield LM, et al. Evaluation of idiopathic esophageal ulceration for human immunodeficiency virus. *Modern Pathol.* 1995;8:568–572.

3

ESOPHAGEAL NEOPLASMS

Roger Der and Parakrama Chandrasoma

Esophageal carcinoma is one of the most lethal types of cancer, with an overall 5-year survival of less than 10%.[1] In 1996, 12,300 persons developed esophageal carcinoma, and 11,200 persons died of this disease.[2]

Prior to 1975, squamous carcinoma accounted for 95% of all cases of esophageal cancer. Since 1975, there has been a marked increase in the percentage of adenocarcinomas among cancers of the esophagus. This has resulted mainly from an increase in the incidence of adenocarcinoma, but a decreased incidence of squamous carcinoma during this period has also contributed.[3] Comparison of the incidence of squamous carcinomas seen between 1988–1990 and 1976–1978 showed a decline of 28% during this period. In contrast, the incidence of

adenocarcinoma of the lower esophagus in the United States was three times higher in the same period.[4]

The overall relative incidence between squamous carcinoma and adenocarcinoma of the esophagus at the present time is about equal in the United States.[4] The relative incidence depends on the patient population served. At the Los Angeles County—University of Southern California (USC) Medical Center, which serves a predominantly nonwhite population, squamous carcinoma still accounts for more than 70% of the esophageal carcinomas. At the USC University Hospital, which serves an affluent white population, over 80% of the cancers are adenocarcinomas. Overall, in the United States, the rate of adenocarcinoma exceeded that of squamous carcinoma in white males under the age of 55 years in the 1984–1987 period.[5] This trend of increasing adenocarcinoma prevalence continues.

Malignant neoplasms of the esophagus other than squamous carcinoma and adenocarcinoma account for less than 3% of esophageal cancers (Table 3–1).

SQUAMOUS CARCINOMA

Epidemiology

Squamous carcinoma of the esophagus has an incidence of 2.5–5 for males and 1.5–2.5 for females per 100,000 population[1] in the United States and other areas of the world where the incidence is "normal." In some areas of the world, however, the incidence is much higher, in the range of 50–200/100,000 population. These include a large Asian belt stretching from the Caspian Sea to Northern China, including parts of Iran,

TABLE 3–1. MALIGNANT NEOPLASMS OF THE ESOPHAGUS

Squamous carcinoma

Adenocarcinoma arising in Barrett's esophagus

Rare types of malignancies (less than 3% of all malignancies)

    Variants of squamous carcinoma

        Spindle cell squamous carcinoma

        Verrucous squamous carcinoma

        Basaloid squamous carcinoma

        EBV-associated lymphoepithelioma-like squamous carcinoma

    Variants of adenocarcinoma

        Mucoepidermoid carcinoma

        Adenoid cystic carcinoma

        Carcinoma arising in ectopic gastric mucosa

        Adenocarcinoma with germ cell elements (choriocarcinoma and yolk sac carcinoma)

    Neuroendocrine neoplasms

        Carcinoid tumor

        Small-cell undifferentiated neuroendocrine carcinoma

    Primary malignant melanoma

    Malignant lymphoma (see Chapter 15).

    Malignant stromal neoplasm (leiomyosarcoma) (See Chapter 14)

Abbreviation: EBV = Epstein-Barr virus

Afghanistan, Northern India, Southern Russia, Mongolia, and China.[6] In the United States, the highest incidence of esophageal squamous carcinoma occurs in South Carolina, Washington D.C., and Alaska.

In the United States, squamous carcinoma of the esophagus is a disease affecting mainly nonwhite males in lower socioeconomic groups. It is rare under the age of 40 years, but increases progressively after this. Men are affected two to three times more frequently than women, except in Northern Iran and in cases of esophageal carcinoma that complicates Plummer-Vinson syndrome, in which there is a higher female incidence. In the United States, African-Americans are affected five times more frequently than Caucasians.

Etiology

The cause of esophageal squamous carcinoma is unknown. The reason for the high incidence in certain parts of the world is believed to be environmental rather than genetic. There is no significant familial tendency for the development of esophageal carcinoma. Gastroesophageal reflux is not etiologically related to squamous carcinoma.

In North China, where the incidence of esophageal cancer is 160/100,000 population and accounts for 50% of all cancers, there is a strong correlation between esophageal cancer and intake of pickled vegetables. This is believed to be the result of contamination of the food with a white moldy fungus, *Geotrichum candidum.*[7] Human papillomavirus infection is also believed to be important in these cancers.[7] Smoking of opiates and ingestion of hot tea and hot rice have also been suggested as contributing to esophageal cancer in China.

Cigarette smoking and alcohol ingestion are strongly associated with esophageal squamous carcinoma; together, they have a synergistic effect. Drinking "moonshine" whiskey is believed to be responsible for a high risk of esophageal carcinoma in coastal South Carolina.[8] Esophageal cancer is associated with other cancer types that are strongly associated with smoking, such as cancers of the lung, larynx, and oropharynx.

Most esophageal squamous carcinomas occur de novo, although it is likely that the epithelium progresses through increasing degrees of dysplasia before invasive carcinoma develops (Fig. 3–1). Premalignant conditions, which are associated with only a small number of squamous carcinomas of the esophagus are:

1. Caustic lye strictures: Patients with strictures induced by lye ingestion have a 1000-fold increase in the incidence of squamous carcinoma. Carcinoma develops in 5–10% of patients,

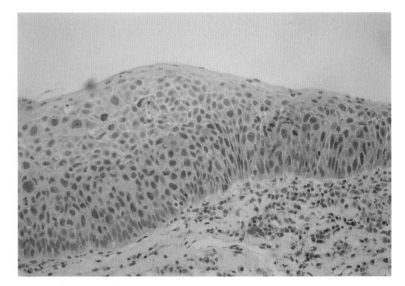

A

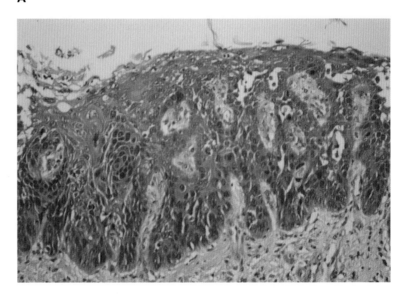

B

Figure 3–1. A: Squamous dysplasia of the esophagus. This occurred in an esophagus removed for early squamous carcinoma. The dysplasia is low grade on the left and high grade on the right of the figure. B: High-grade squamous dysplasia (carcinoma in situ) of the esophagus, showing failure of maturation, marked cytologic abnormality, and mitotic activity in the midlevel of the epithelium.

usually more than 40 years after the initial injury.[9] Lye strictures are an indication for surveillance, but most of these patients need regular evaluation and dilatation for their strictures in any case.

2. Tylosis palmaris: A congenital disease characterized by hyperkeratosis and pitting of the palms and soles, has a high incidence of esophageal squamous carcinoma.[10] The incidence is so high as to justify regular surveillance and consideration of prophylactic esophagectomy.

3. Plummer-Vinson syndrome: A disease caused by severe iron deficiency anemia associated with glossitis, koilonychia, dysphagia, and esophageal mucosal webs, has a high incidence of squamous carcinoma of the upper third of the esophagus. The disease was common among Northern Scandinavian females, but has declined greatly in incidence.

4. Achalasia of the cardia is associated with an incidence of esophageal carcinoma of 3.4/1000 patients, which represents a greater than 30-fold increase over the general population.[11] Annual radiologic or endoscopic surveillance has been suggested.

5. Squamous carcinoma of the esophagus has also been associated with human papillomavirus infection, celiac disease, prior gastric resection, and prior radiation. Patients who have squamous carcinomas of the oropharynx and larynx have an increased incidence of synchronous and metachronous esophageal squamous carcinoma. Esophageal endoscopy is indicated in all patients diagnosed with head and neck squamous carcinoma.

Molecular Biology

Although a large number of molecular abnormalities have been identified[12] (Table 3–2), with many showing a negative correlation with survival, the biology of squamous carcinoma of the esophagus is highly complex and poorly understood.[13] There is no defined sequence of genetic abnormalities in the pathogenesis of squamous carcinoma. None of these abnormalities is useful for routine use in diagnosis or predicting prognosis.

Clinical Presentation

In a nonscreened population, which represents almost all squamous carcinomas of the esophagus, symptoms occur at a late stage of the disease. Dysphagia, which is the commonest presenting symptom, occurs when the lumen is reduced by at least half its normal caliber. Dysphagia is first for solid foods, followed by inability to swallow liquids at a late stage of the disease. Patients make changes in their diet with increasing dysphagia, frequently avoiding hard meats. The time they take to complete a meal also commonly increases. Sialorrhea occurs when there is severe luminal obstruction. Weight loss is almost always present and is frequently severe. Persistent pain, persistent hiccups, pleural effusion, chylothorax, and pneumonia due either to aspiration or tracheoesophageal fistula are late features that indicate involvement of mediastinal structures. Hematemesis is common and may be severe when it is caused by erosion into a large vessel; aortic erosion causes rapidly fatal hemorrhage. Patients with advanced symptoms have a median survival of less than 1 year.

Surveillance for squamous carcinoma of the esophagus is justified in high-incidence areas and in high-risk patients such as those with lye strictures, tylosis, Plummer-Vinson syndrome, and achalasia. In developed countries, endoscopic surveillance is indicated in all patients with high-risk premalignant lesions, but is not cost-effective in the general population. In developing countries the use of balloon abrasion cytologic screening is a more viable option than endoscopic screening because of the resources available.[14]

Diagnosis

Distribution

Approximately half of the esophageal squamous carcinomas occur in the middle third of the esophagus, 25–32 cm from the incisors at endoscopy. One third occur in the lower esophagus; the rest are in the upper third. Squamous carcinomas very rarely extend into the stomach.

Endoscopic and Gross Features

Advanced tumors are fungating masses (Figs. 3–2 and 3–3) (60%), malignant ulcers (Figs. 3–4, 3–5, and 3–6) (25%), or diffusely infiltrative lesions (Fig. 3–7). These features are obvious at endoscopy. Prospective evaluation of the number of specimens needed for pathologic diagnosis showed that one biopsy specimen was diagnostic in 93% of cases, increasing to 100% when seven samples were obtained from the edge and base of the tumor.[15] Biopsy diagnosis is easiest and most accurate when an obvious lesion is seen and the lumen is not obstructed.

TABLE 3–2. MOLECULAR BIOLOGIC ABNORMALITIES IN SQUAMOUS CARCINOMA OF THE ESOPHAGUS

Abnormality	Significance
Epidermal growth factor	Amplified; overexpression of mRNA and the protein product appears to decrease survival.
EGF receptor gene	Overexpression correlates with higher stage.
Transforming growth factor α	Overexpression correlates with decreased survival.
hst-1 and int-2 oncogenes	Coamplification correlates with worse prognosis.
Cyclin A	Overexpression correlates with poor prognosis.
ras oncogenes	Overexpression frequently present.
p53 mutation (17p)	Present in one third.
Retinoblastoma gene (13q)	Loss of heterozygosity seen in half.
APC gene (5p)	Loss of heterozygosity present in majority.
DCC gene (18q)	Loss more common in poorly differentiated carcinomas.
bcl-2	Reactivity in poorly differentiated carcinomas.

Abbreviations: EGF = epidermal growth factor; APC = adenomatous polyposis coli; DCC = deleted in colon cancer

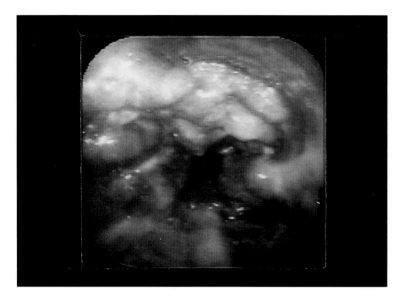

A

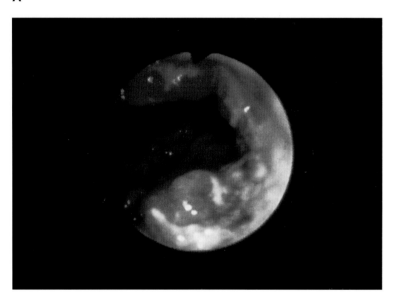

B

Figure 3–2. A: Esophageal carcinoma, endoscopic appearance, showing ulcerated large mass. B: Advanced squamous carcinoma of the esophagus, endoscopic appearance, showing a fungating tumor mass. (Figure A courtesy of Aslam Godil, MD, Dept. of Gastroenterology, Loma Linda University, CA)

When the lumen is obstructed or the tumor has an infiltrative growth pattern, multiple specimens are necessary. In cases where a tight stricture prevents passage of the endoscope, brush cytology is extremely useful.[16]

Early, asymptomatic esophageal carcinomas may be encountered at upper gastrointestinal (GI) endoscopy done for any reason. These lesions are often subtle, appearing as slight changes in color, small protuberances, depressions, or erosions of the mucosa (Fig. 3–8). They can easily be missed if the endoscopist traverses the "normal-appearing" esophagus too rapidly. Performance of upper GI endoscopy for any reason must be regarded as an opportunity to screen the esophagus carefully, particularly in patients older than 40 years. Early esophageal cancers are defined as tumors restricted to the mucosa and submucosa; they are classified by their macroscopic features in

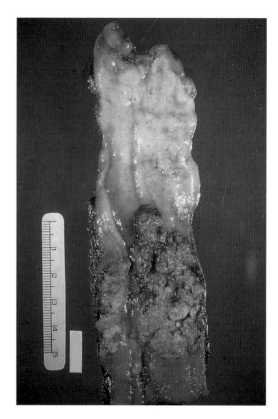

Figure 3–3. Squamous carcinoma of the midesophagus, showing a fungating mass.

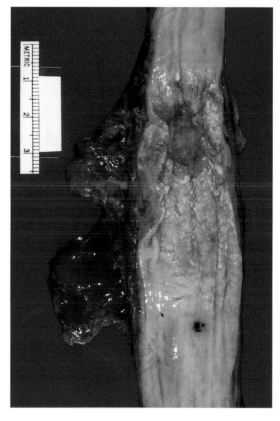

Figure 3–4. Squamous carcinoma of the midesophagus, showing a malignant ulcer with slightly elevated edges and a necrotic base.

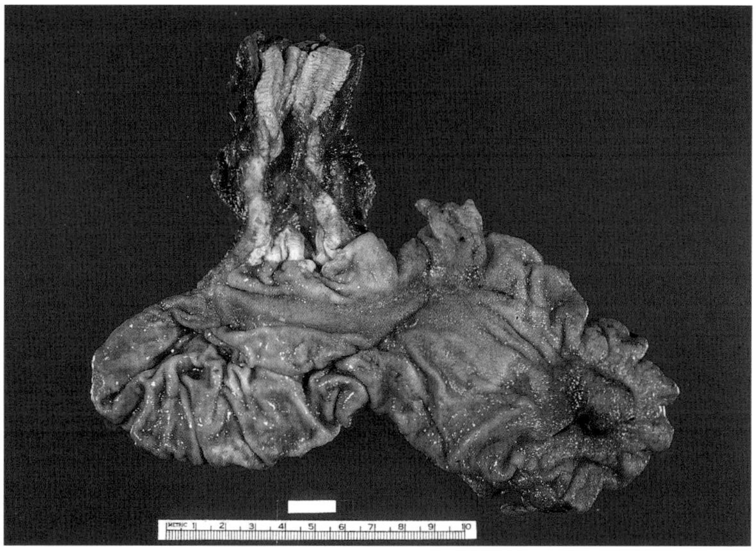

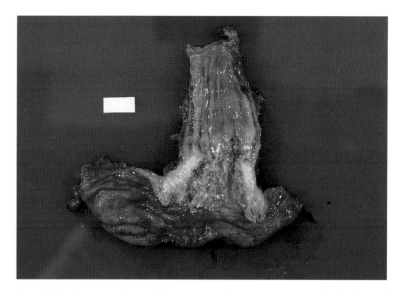

Figure 3–5. Squamous carcinoma of the lower esophagus, showing a large malignant ulcer. Note the white squamous epithelium at the lower edge of the tumor, indicating that the tumor is entirely in squamous-lined mucosa.

Figure 3–7. Squamous carcinoma of the esophagus, infiltrative type, showing marked thickening of the wall with relatively mild mucosal changes.

a manner similar to that for early gastric cancers[17] (Table 3–3) and by the depth of invasion.[18] They have 5-year survival rates of approximately 90% after surgical resection.[19] Early tumors are not commonly detected in the United States; they are much more commonly found in Japan, where endoscopic screening for gastric cancer permits concomitant screening of the esophagus.

Pathologic Diagnosis

The majority of squamous carcinomas are obvious on histologic examination of endoscopic biopsies. The presence of irregular infiltrating nests of squamous epithelial cells with malignant cytologic features, surrounded by desmoplasia and inflammation, are easy to recognize (Fig. 3–9). Focal keratinization and

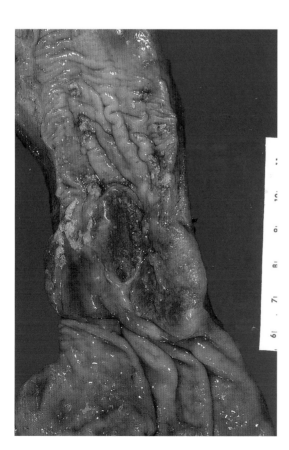

Figure 3–6. Squamous carcinoma of the esophagus, showing a malignant ulcer in the lower esophagus.

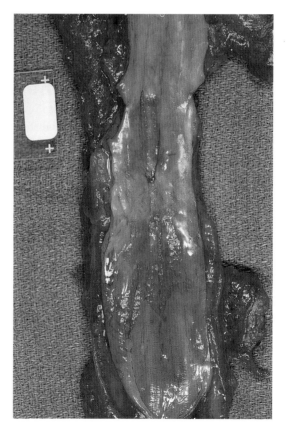

Figure 3–8. Early squamous carcinoma of the esophagus, showing mucosal discoloration and a small, elevated area.

TABLE 3–3. CLASSIFICATION OF EARLY CANCERS OF THE ESOPHAGUS.*

Macroscopic/Endoscopic Classification

Type I	Protruded type	Presents as a small polyp or nodule less than 3 mm in height.
Type II	Flat type	
Type IIa	Elevated	Presents as an elevated plaque that is raised < 3 mm from the mucosal surface.
Type IIb	Flat	Recognized only by changes in the color and vascular pattern of the mucosa.
Type IIc	Depressed	Depressed slightly from the surface but has an intact surface or shallow erosion.
Type III	Excavated type	A deeper ulcer with tumor restricted microscopically to mucosa and submucosa.

Pathologic Classification

Intraepithelial	ep-cancer	High-grade dysplasia (carcinoma in situ).
Intramucosal	mm-cancer	Invasion confined to mucosa, ie, no invasion deeper than muscularis mucosae.
Submucosal	sm-cancer	Invasion beyond muscularis mucosae, but not involving muscularis externa.

*This classification was developed for squamous carcinoma, but can be equally applied to adenocarcinomas.

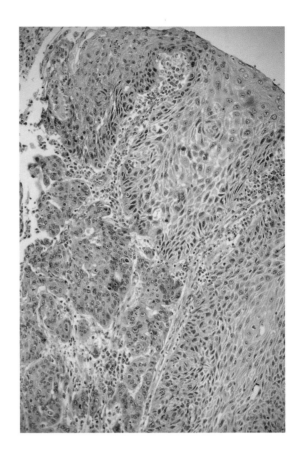

A

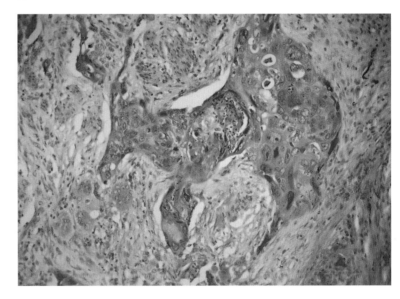

B

Figure 3–9. A: Esophageal biopsy specimen showing invasive squamous carcinoma, consisting of nests of malignant cells arising from the squamous epithelium and infiltrating the lamina propria. The contrast in the cytologic features between the malignant tumor and the overlying epithelium is striking. B: Esophageal biopsy sample showing invasive squamous carcinoma, characterized by malignant squamous cells surrounded by a desmoplastic stroma and smooth muscle of the muscularis mucosae.

the presence of intercellular bridges (Fig. 3–10A). and well-formed squamous epithelial pearls (Fig. 3–10B) permit classification of the tumor as squamous carcinoma.

Poorly differentiated squamous carcinomas without any intercellular bridges or keratinization (Fig. 3–11) must be distinguished from poorly differentiated adenocarcinoma. This can be difficult on purely cytologic grounds because no totally reliable cytologic features exist that permit differentiation of undifferentiated squamous and adenocarcinoma. Eosinophilic cytoplasm, giving a "squamoid" appearance, and large nucleoli can be seen in both, and cytoplasmic vacuolation is not reliable. Stains for mucin (mucicarmine, diastase-digested periodic acid–Schiff (PAS) stain) are helpful; if they are positive, a diagnosis of adenocarcinoma or adenosquamous carcinoma can be made. In cases of undifferentiated carcinoma that are negative for mucin, the biopsy diagnosis should be "undifferentiated carcinoma." Immunoperoxidase staining for cytokeratins of different molecular weights are unreliable in an individual case for distinguishing squamous from adenocarcinoma. The final classification of these tumors is usually possible when a larger specimen is available after the tumor is resected. In unresectable tumors, the lack of an accurate classification is not of great practical significance.

More rarely, the biopsy shows a tumor that is so undifferentiated that there is doubt as to whether it represents carcinoma or some other malignant neoplasm. In these cases, immunoperoxidase staining is extremely useful in distinguishing undifferentiated carcinoma (cytokeratin+ CD45− CD34− S100 protein and HMB45−) from malignant lymphoma (cytokeratin− CD45+ CD34− S100 protein and HMB45−), malignant melanoma (cytokeratin± CD45− CD34− S100 protein and HMB45+), and malignant GI stromal neoplasm (cytokeratin± CD45− CD34+ S100 protein± HMB45−).

False-negative pathologic diagnosis is very unusual in esophageal carcinoma. Even a single biopsy specimen is diagnostic in over 90% of cases.[15] In only very rare cases of

A

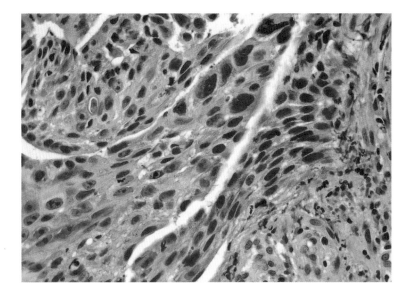

A

B

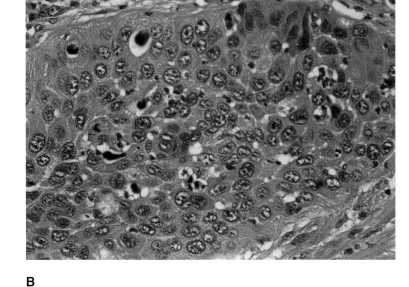

B

Figure 3–10. A: Squamous carcinoma of the esophagus, showing evidence of focal keratinization of malignant cells and intercellular bridges. B: A typical malignant squamous epithelial "pearl" in a well-differentiated squamous carcinoma showing an irregular nest of malignant cells with a central mass of parakeratotic cells.

Figure 3–11. A: Squamous carcinoma of the esophagus, poorly differentiated, but with "squamoid" appearance. B: Poorly differentiated squamous carcinoma of the esophagus showing poorly differentiated malignant cells without evidence of keratinization. The tumor cells show a "squamoid" appearance resulting from diffuse cytoplasmic eosinophilia.

esophageal carcinoma is the pathologic diagnosis difficult. When the pathologist has any difficulty, therefore, the likelihood is that no esophageal carcinoma exists. In cases of real difficulty, conversing with the endoscopist is helpful because the only cases in which real diagnostic difficulty may be encountered and in which repeat biopsy may be necessary is in infiltrative tumors with tight strictures in which accessing the tumor may be difficult. It is important, however, never to let an endoscopist's impression that "there was an obvious malignant tumor" convince a pathologist that a doubtful biopsy represents carcinoma. An obvious tumor should always be obvious at histologic examination, and the diagnosis of cancer must be made on the presence of definitive morphologic criteria.

False-positive pathologic diagnosis, on the other hand, is a

real danger in esophageal biopsies. Ulceration from any cause can induce regenerative changes in the squamous epithelium and cytologically atypical granulation tissue that can mimic squamous carcinoma. Regenerating squamous epithelium may show nuclear enlargement, hyperchromasia, nuclear irregularity, prominent nucleoli, and mitotic activity that closely mimic malignancy (Fig. 3–12A). Irregularity of the epithelial proliferation in regeneration and tangential sectioning of biopsies can make the resemblance to carcinoma very close, and careful attention to cytologic changes is necessary to avoid false-positive diagnosis (Fig. 3–12B). Association of these changes with ulceration and the fact that regenerating epithelium usually is disposed horizontally at the surface without much vertical extent are helpful features, features which are easier to assess in larger

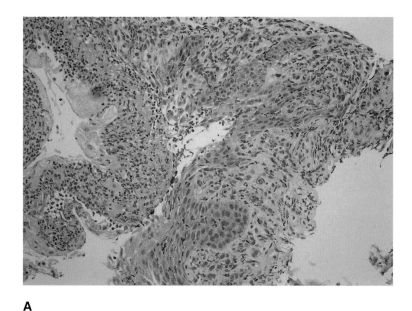

A

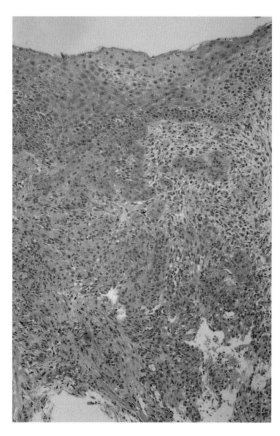

B

Figure 3–12. A: Regenerating squamous epithelium at the edge of an ulcer in reflux disease, showing regenerative cytologic atypia. B: Regenerating epithelium at the edge of an ulcer, showing cytologic atypia and hyperplasia.

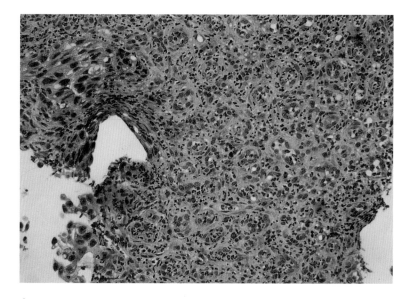

A

B

Figure 3–13. A: Granulation tissue in the base of a malignant ulcer showing acutely inflamed granulation tissue. There is a small focus of malignant epithelial cells at the upper edge. The size and degree of atypia of the malignant cells provides a sharp contrast to the active atypical endothelial cells. B: Active granulation tissue, higher power micrograph of part A, showing enlargement and atypia of endothelial cells. This appearance, which is commonly seen in all esophageal ulcers, must never be misinterpreted as carcinoma.

specimens. Atypical granulation tissue is usually easy to recognize (Fig. 3–13). In some cases, though, the proliferating endothelial cells in the new vessels show not only atypia, but appear as solid nests without apparent lumina, mimicking carcinoma (Fig. 3–13). In these cases, immunoperoxidase staining is very helpful in distinguishing carcinoma (cytokeratin+ CD34–) from granulation tissue (cytokeratin– CD34+).

Another situation that sometimes causes difficulty is the differentiation of reactive changes in ulcerative reflux disease from squamous carcinoma in situ (Fig. 3–14). The cytologic changes in the epithelium can be very difficult to interpret with absolute accuracy in these cases. The fact that reflux disease is not associated with squamous carcinoma does not preclude squamous carcinoma occurring in patients with reflux. In cases in which real difficulty exists, it is appropriate to describe the difficulty and recommend reexamination after aggressive treatment of the reflux disease; hopefully, the regenerative changes will have reversed by this time. This is not totally satisfactory as

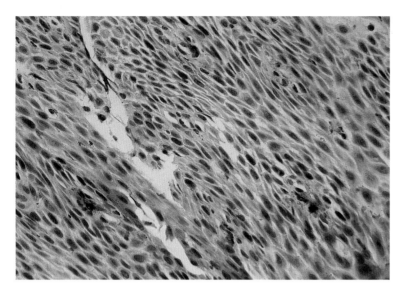

Figure 3–14. Reflux esophagitis, showing marked reactive atypia. Distinction from true dysplasia is difficult and may require repeat biopsy with extensive sampling after acute inflammation has subsided. Although squamous carcinoma has no etiologic association with reflux, the two diseases can coexist coincidentally.

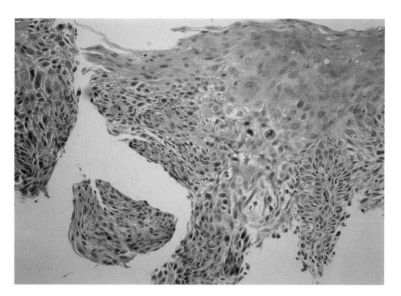

A

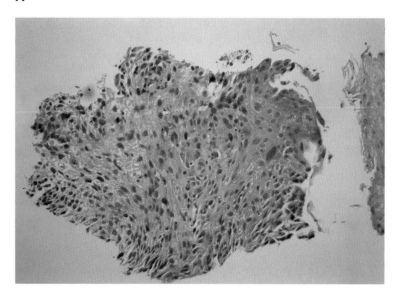

B

Figure 3–15. A and B: Esophageal biopsy sample, showing cytologically malignant squamous epithelium without underlying stroma. This was called high-grade dysplasia and on resection showed superficially invasive squamous carcinoma restricted to the mucosa.

a solution because the absence of a well-defined lesion leaves open the possibility that the area of concern is not accurately sampled at the second biopsy.

Another problem arises when the biopsy shows only detached small pieces of squamous epithelium with high-grade dysplasia without underlying stromal tissue (Fig. 3–15), even after deeper sections have been taken. When an obvious endoscopic mass lesion was present, a superficial biopsy most commonly represents poor biopsy technique, and if there is any doubt as to the nature of the process, a repeat biopsy should be requested. If, however, the endoscopic lesion was subtle, suggesting the possibility of an early lesion, and the cytologic criteria of malignancy are definitive, a diagnosis of carcinoma in situ can be made, with comments that the biopsy is superficial, invasion is not demonstrated in the specimen, but that the specimen is inadequate to evaluate for invasive carcinoma.

Brush cytology of the esophagus improves diagnostic yield in most studies.[16] Reactive changes, however, sometimes mimic malignancy to an extent that a false-positive diagnosis is possible even when expert cytologic interpretation is available (see Chapter 18). A positive cytologic diagnosis must always be confirmed by biopsy before treatment is undertaken. When cytology is positive but histology is negative, the case must be reexamined carefully with multiple biopsies if no lesion is visible to exclude a flat high-grade dysplasia or malignancy. We have experience with a case of pemphigus vulgaris of the esophagus that had a false-positive cytology (see Chapter 2).

The pathologist must be definitive in reporting a biopsy in a case suspected clinically or pathologically as being malignant. The diagnosis of esophageal carcinoma is one that should be made only when absolute histologic criteria for malignancy are present in the biopsy. In such cases, the diagnosis line should read: "Esophagus, biopsy: Squamous carcinoma, invasive." When the biopsy does not contain any features of malignancy,

it should be reported as some variant of "benign." In rare cases when the pathologist sees features that suggest carcinoma, but in which even the slightest possibility exists that the lesion is some reactive phenomenon mimicking carcinoma, the diagnosis should read: "Esophagus, biopsy: Atypical cellular proliferation; criteria for malignancy are not satisfied." The cytologic features of concern should be described, and a comment regarding the possibility that they may represent malignancy or that further study of this patient is indicated is desirable. Under no circumstances should the phrases "highly suspicious for carcinoma" or "consistent with carcinoma" be used in the diagnosis. These "hedge" phrases do not protect the pathologist; on the contrary, they are dangerous. It enables the clinician to interpret the lesion as being malignant if the clinical impression is one of cancer. If the resection specimen does not contain malignancy, the pathologist's diagnosis of "consistent with carcinoma" is regarded as a false-positive diagnosis. If, on the other hand, the clinician decides to follow the patient because of the absence of a definitive pathologic diagnosis, and the patient comes back a year later with advanced cancer, the pathologist's diagnosis of "suspicious for carcinoma" will be regarded as a false-negative diagnosis, because it did not persuade the clinician to take immediate action.

Pretreatment Staging

The majority of squamous carcinomas are unresectable for cure at the time of presentation. Preoperative staging includes assessment of degree of invasion of the wall, mediastinal involvement, lymph node involvement, involvement of adjacent structures, and evidence of metastatic disease. Accuracy of staging is highest with a combination of endoscopic ultrasound (which is most accurate for assessing depth of wall invasion and nodal involvement), and computed tomography (most accurate for distant metastases). The best studies have a 90% concordance between preoperative staging and the final pathologic stage.[16] Thoracoscopy, mediastinoscopy, and laparoscopy improve preoperative staging, particularly with regard to assessment of microscopic disease in the mediastinum and lymph nodes.

Treatment

Esophageal squamous carcinoma is usually detected at a stage that precludes curative resection in approximately 70–80% of patients because of the presence of metastatic disease or mediastinal involvement. In patients undergoing surgery, another 10–15% have evidence of mediastinal and lymph node involvement that precludes curative resections.

Many forms of palliation are used for unresectable cases, including external beam radiation and several endoscopically delivered methods of tumor control designed to maintain luminal patency. These latter include dilatation, stenting, and attempts at decreasing tumor load with tumor probes which deliver heat, neodymium-yttrium-aluminum-garnet (Nd. YAG) laser therapy, brachytherapy (intracavitary radiation), photodynamic therapy using ultraviolet light after administration of a photosensitizer such as protoporphyrin that is selectively taken up by the malignant cells, and chemotherapy.[16] Combined regimens, most commonly chemotherapy and external beam radiation, have been shown to slightly increase survival times; the median length of survival is increased to approximately 1 year.[20] In rare cases, radiation and chemotherapy produce a dramatic reduction in the tumor size, resulting in downstaging of the tumor and making a previously unresectable tumor amenable to surgery. In some of these cases, the resection specimen contains no or minimal evidence of carcinoma (Fig. 3–16). These specimens show marked hyalinization with vascular changes of radiation (Fig. 3–17A), cytologic changes of radiation in stromal cells (Fig. 3–17B), and necrosis of esophageal glands with squamous metaplasia of the glands

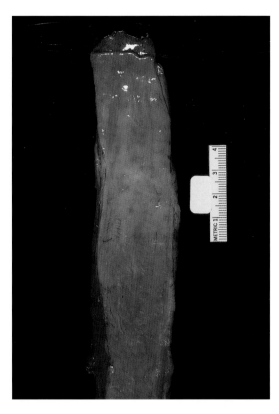

Figure 3–16. Esophagectomy performed after radiation therapy. No tumor is visible.

and ducts (Fig. 3–17C). These must not be mistaken for residual carcinoma.

Surgical resection is of two kinds: (1) En bloc esophagectomy, which involves a thoracotomy, removes the tumor with adequate margins, often including the proximal stomach, and all regional lymph nodes (Fig. 3–18). Lymph node groups that are removed include subcarinal, paraesophageal, hiatal, and abdominal nodes around the celiac axis. (2) Transhiatal esophagectomy, which does not involve a thoracotomy. Mediastinal lymph node dissection is incomplete with a transhiatal resection, which usually has a lesser curative intent than en bloc resection. Reconstruction requires gastric pull-up or interposition of a segment of small intestine or colon.

The overall operative mortality and morbidity rate is considerable with en bloc resection, and there is controversy over whether it should be used to manage a disease with such a poor final outcome. Surgery, however, represents the only possibility of cure for patients with esophageal carcinoma, and in specialized centers experienced in the performance of esophagectomy, morbidity and mortality rates are lower than in centers where the operation is performed sporadically.

Endoscopic mucosal resection and ablation therapy is feasible for early squamous carcinoma of the esophagus. These treatment modalities are more fully discussed under the section on adenocarcinoma because early esophageal carcinomas are most frequently encountered in the United States in the screened population with Barrett's esophagus. Paradoxically, though, the present literature on localized treatment for early cancers is more developed for early squamous carcinoma because of the Japanese experience.

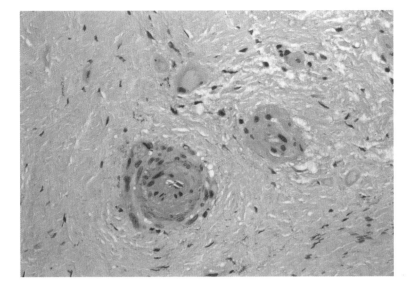

A

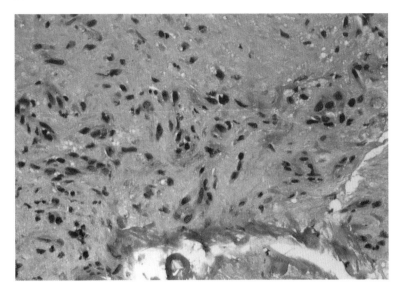

C

B

Figure 3–17. A: Radiation change in the esophagus, showing stromal fibrosis and hyalinization of blood vessels. B: Radiation change in stromal cells in the esophagus. C: Radiation-induced changes in the esophagus, showing squamous metaplasia of radiation-affected submucosal glands and ducts. The organization of the squamous proliferation and benign cytologic features argue against squamous carcinoma.

Pathologic Features

Examination of the Esophagectomy Specimen

The pathologist must know whether an esophagectomy is a transhiatal or en bloc resection because several lymph node groups need to be assessed in the latter procedure. Lymph node assessment for staging only requires evaluation of all the nodes in the specimen for evidence of metastases. However, involvement of nodes, specifically in the subcarinal and celiac regions, provide useful clinical information because they represent the highest and lowest nodes in the specimen.

In most cases, the mediastinal soft tissue around the esophagus is so irregular that complete assessment of the mediastinal margin of resection is difficult. Inking the external surface of the specimen must be done only when there is a reasonable amount of continuity of the mediastinal connective tissue.

The esophagus should be opened longitudinally. The size and gross characteristics of the tumor should be recorded. The distance of the proximal and distal edge of the tumor to the mucosal margins should be measured. The esophagus should then be sectioned serially in a transverse direction. The sections through the tumor should be evaluated for evidence of deepest wall invasion and sections taken accordingly (Fig. 3–19). When a definite soft tissue margin is present and has been inked, evaluation of this margin should be done with appropriate sections for microscopy.

Mucosal margin evaluation is of importance in esophageal carcinoma because of the tendency of these tumors to spread in the submucosal lymphatics (Fig. 3–20). Submucosal lymphatic invasion must be assessed in multiple random sections of the esophagus taken away from the tumor mass. Sometimes, satellite nodules are present in the submucosa due to lymphatic spread; these should be carefully searched for by palpating the entire mucosal surface. An adequate mucosal surgical margin

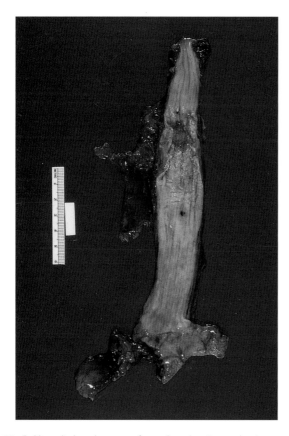

Figure 3–18. En bloc radical esophagectomy for esophageal carcinoma, showing tumor with wide mucosal margins and lymph node containing mediastinal soft tissue around the esophagus.

should have 10 cm between the margin and the nearest tumor edge.

The information required in a pathology report of a resected specimen for esophageal carcinoma are summarized in Table 3–4.

Pathologic Staging

Esophageal carcinoma is staged according to the tumor, nodes, and metastases (TNM) system recommended by the American Joint Committee on Cancer[21] (Table 3–5). Other staging systems exist that divide patients with positive lymph nodes into different stages based on the number of positive lymph nodes. The pathology report should therefore contain information regarding the number of nodes present and the number that are positive.

Prognosis

The overall 5-year survival rate for all patients with squamous carcinoma of the esophagus is less than 10%.[1] In the 10–20% of selected patients who undergo curative surgical resections, the 3-year survival rate is 58% if there is no nodal metastasis and 32% if nodes are positive; a survival rate of 75% is reported with en bloc resection in patients with T1 or T2 tumors with fewer than five positive lymph nodes.[22]

Pathologic staging represents the best indicator of progno-

TABLE 3–4. THE PATHOLOGY REPORT FOR ESOPHAGEAL CARCINOMA TREATED BY ESOPHAGECTOMY

Pathology Laboratory Information

Patient Demographic Information	Dates
Pathology Number	
Clinical Data (including physicians involved)	
Specimens Submitted	
Intraoperative Consultation Results (including frozen sections)	
Gross Description	

    Location of tumor

        Obligatory: Upper third/middle third/lower third/upper and middle third/middle and lower third

        Desirable: tumor size; gross characteristics; distance of proximal and distal margins from tumor edges

    Extent of Surgery

        Obligatory: (i) En bloc or transhiatal esophagectomy

               (ii) Length of removed esophagus and stomach

        Desirable: Extent of lymphadenectomy

Microscopic Description and Diagnosis

    Histomorphology

        Obligatory: (i) Type and degree of differentiation

               (ii) Lymphovascular invasion

    Staging/primary tumor

        Obligatory: Depth of infiltration (Tis–T4)

    Staging/lymph nodes

        Obligatory: TNM lymph node status (N0 or N1)

        Desirable: Number of nodes examined and number involved; topography of involved nodes

    Surgical Margin

        Obligatory: Microscopic margin status (clear or involved)

Other lesions in the specimen, if any

Abbreviation: TNM = tumor, node, metastasis (system)

sis in esophageal carcinoma. Histologic grade does not have significant predictive value, mainly because there are very few poorly differentiated carcinomas among tumors confined to the esophageal wall.

Unresectable tumors result in large mediastinal tumor masses, usually involving lymph nodes (Fig. 3–21). They commonly invade adjacent structures, resulting in a variety of problems. Thoracic duct involvement may cause chylous effusion, pleural and pericardial involvement may result in malignant effusions, involvement of the tracheobronchial tree may lead to tracheoesophageal fistula and pneumonia (Fig. 3–22), and involvement of the aorta may result in lethal hemorrhage.

Esophageal carcinoma can metastasize to lymph nodes even when it is restricted to the mucosa; in some studies, 30% of intramucosal carcinomas have been associated with minimal nodal disease.[23] The survival rate from intramucosal carcinoma after resection even with limited nodal metastases is good. The incidence of nodal involvement increases in submucosal tumors, and this is associated with a decline in survival rate.[24]

Molecular prognosis indicators are only of value in early-

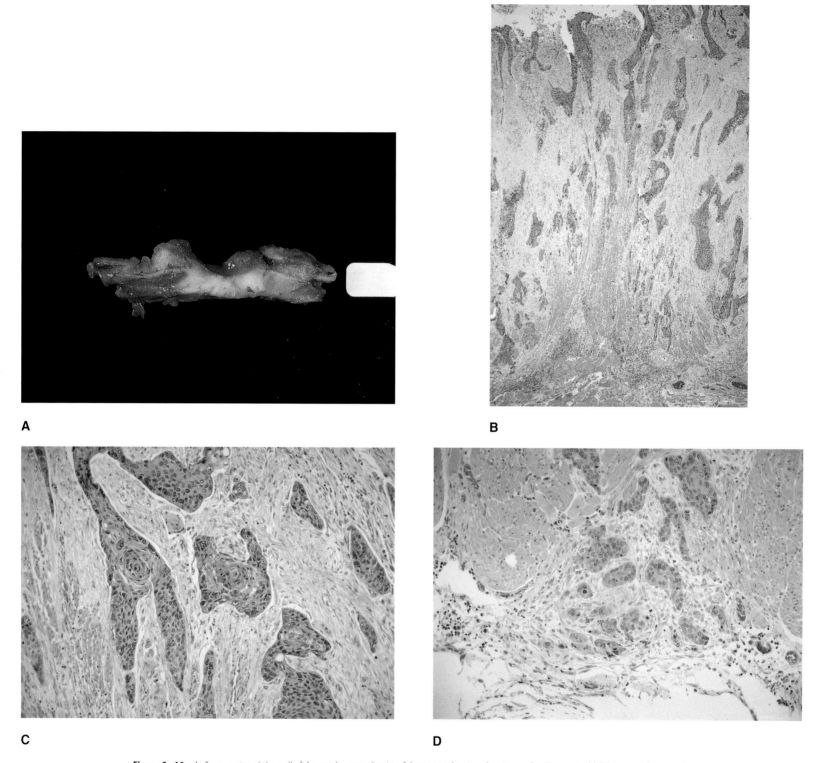

Figure 3–19. A: Cross section of the wall of the esophagus at the site of the tumor, showing ulceration and replacement of full thickness of the muscle wall by tumor. B: Diffuse infiltration of the esophageal wall by squamous carcinoma. The ulcerated mucosa is at the top. C: Higher power micrograph of part B, showing well-differentiated, keratinizing squamous carcinoma. D: Transmural extension of squamous carcinoma, seen here infiltrating beyond the outer limit of the muscle wall into the mediastinal connective tissue.

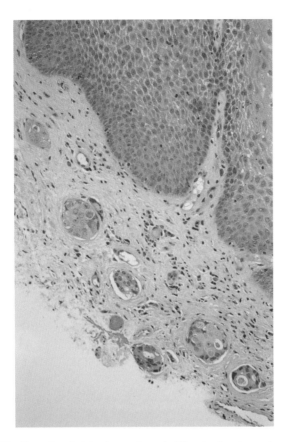

Figure 3–20. Mucosal lymphatic involvement by poorly differentiated carcinoma, showing tumor in an area covered by normal mucosa.

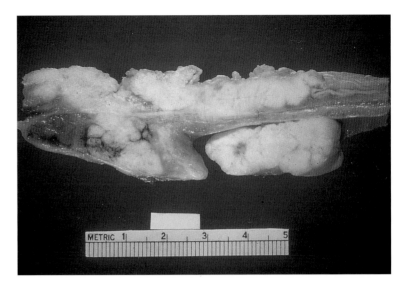

Figure 3–21. Advanced squamous carcinoma of the esophagus at autopsy, showing a cross section of the tumor that infiltrates the full thickness of the wall of the esophagus and has resulted in a large mediastinal mass.

stage disease with carcinoma restricted to the wall of the esophagus with negative nodes. Although many potential prognostic indicators have been identified in esophageal squamous carcinoma (see Table 3–2), none have proved of value in the practical assessment of prognosis.[25] Evaluation of lymph nodes for micrometastases using immunoperoxidase staining for cytokeratin has shown the presence of single tumor cells in previously negative lymph nodes (Fig. 3–23). When found in a node-negative patient, micrometastases are associated with a reduced expectation of cure.[26]

TABLE 3–5. TNM STAGING SYSTEM FOR ESOPHAGEAL CARCINOMA

Tumor (T)

Tis	Carcinoma in situ
T1	Tumor invades mucosa or submucosa
T2	Tumor invades muscularis externa
T3	Tumor invades through the muscle wall into mediastinal adventitia
T4	Tumor invades adjacent structures

Lymph Nodes (N)

N0	No regional node involvement
N1	Regional node metastases present*

Metastasis (M)

M0	No distant metastases
M1	Distant metastases present*

Stage Groupings of TNM Designations		5-Year Survival Rate† (%)
Stage 0	Tis N0 M0	100
Stage I	T1 N0 M0 or T2 N0 M0	75
Stage IIA	T3 N0 M0 or T1 N1 M0	37
Stage IIB	T2 N1 M0 or T3 N1 M0	27
Stage III	T4 any N M0	13
Stage IV	Any T any N M1	0

*Celiac node involvement is counted as regional nodal disease for adenocarcinoma; for squamous carcinoma, it represents distant metastasis.
†Survival figures are only for those patients undergoing surgical resection.
Abbreviation: TNM = tumor, node, metastasis.

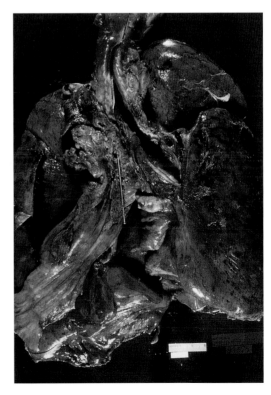

Figure 3–22. Large squamous carcinoma of the esophagus involving adjacent bronchus and resulting in a tracheoesophageal fistula (metal probe).

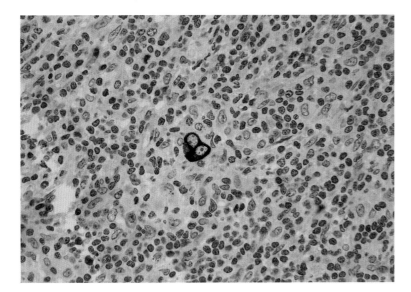

Figure 3–23. Lymph node in esophagectomy specimen showing a single malignant cell stained by immunoperoxidase for cytokeratin. This represents a micrometastasis not detected by routine stain microscopy.

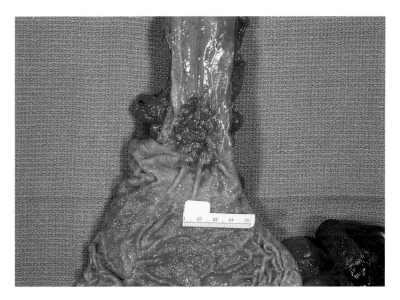

Figure 3–24. Tumor at the gastroesophageal junction with more than 50% in the tubular esophagus. This is classified as an adenocarcinoma of the esophagus. Note that the mucosa immediately below the tumor appears different from the gastric mucosa.

ADENOCARCINOMA

Epidemiology

The incidence of adenocarcinoma of the lower esophagus in the United States was three times higher in the 1988–1990 period compared with the 1976–1978 period,[4] according to data from the National Cancer Institute's Surveillance, Epidemiology, and End-Results Program. A parallel increase was seen in carcinomas of the gastroesophageal junction. This was accompanied by decreasing rates for squamous carcinoma of the esophagus and distal gastric cancers. According to these figures, adenocarcinoma of the lower esophagus and gastroesophageal junction have the most rapidly increasing incidence among all carcinomas in the United States.[4] In 1988–1990, the incidence rate for esophageal and gastroesophageal junction adenocarcinomas combined in white men in the United States was 5.9/100,000.[4]

Adenocarcinoma of the lower esophagus and gastroesophageal junction is a disease that predominantly affects affluent white males. Males are affected eight times more frequently than females. The incidence is four times higher in Caucasian men than in African-American men. Smoking and alcohol use are not strongly associated with esophageal adenocarcinoma. The epidemiologic factors for adenocarcinoma of the lower esophagus are exactly parallel to those for adenocarcinoma of the gastroesophageal junction and gastric cardia, strongly suggesting that they have a similar etiology.

The classification of adenocarcinoma in the junctional region is based on a convention that if more than half the tumor is in the esophagus, it is classified as an esophageal adenocarcinoma (Fig. 3–24), whereas if more than half is in the cardia, the tumor is classified as an adenocarcinoma of the gastric cardia (Fig. 3–25). Evidence is emerging that even tumors that are almost entirely in the gastric cardia (Fig. 3–26) have the same epi-

demiology and association with reflux disease as lower esophageal adenocarcinoma, very likely occurring in short-segment Barrett's esophagus. This suggests that present anatomic perceptions of the location of the true lower end of the esophagus may be incorrect. In fact, careful examination of resected specimens frequently show a transition from abnormal flat cardiac mucosa to gastric mucosa, which has normal rugal folds some distance below the tubular esophagus (see Fig. 3–24) (see also Figs. 3–32 and 3–33).

Because intestinal metaplasia was rarely reported prior to 1971[27,28] and is very commonly seen today, the increasing incidence of adenocarcinoma is likely the result of an increasing incidence of intestinal metaplasia. The possibility exists that the incidence of carcinogenesis in intestinal metaplasia is also increasing.

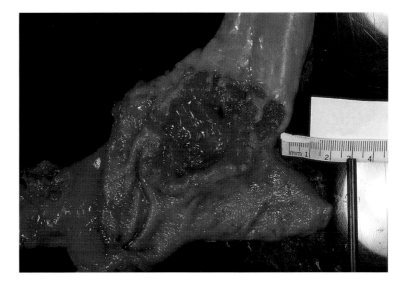

Figure 3–25. Tumor at the gastroesophageal junction with more than 50% in the gastric cardia. By convention, this is classified as a gastric cardiac adenocarcinoma. This is epidemiologically similar to lower esophageal adenocarcinoma.

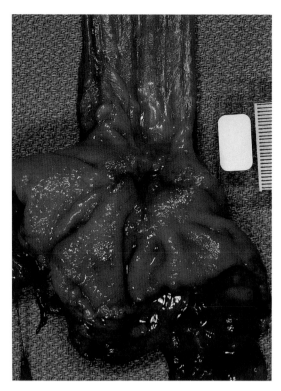

Figure 3–26. Tumor entirely in the gastric cardia. This patient had reflux disease, short-segment Barrett's esophagus, and a normal distal stomach.

Etiology

Most lower esophageal adenocarcinomas arise in Barrett's esophagus, which in turn is a complication of gastroesophageal reflux. The risk of adenocarcinoma in patients with Barrett's esophagus is about 1 cancer per 100 patient years of follow-up.[29] Evidence is accumulating that most adenocarcinomas of the gastroesophageal junction develop in short-segment Barrett's esophagus, though this is till debated. Residual intestinal metaplasia is found in only 42% of cases of adenocarcinomas at the junction,[30] but this may be due to the fact that the small area of intestinal metaplasia associated with short-segment Barrett's esophagus becomes quickly obliterated by the cancer.

The risk factors for adenocarcinoma in patients with Barrett's esophagus are unclear. At present, the risk is considered high enough in patients with a long segment of glandular mucosa in the lower esophagus with intestinal metaplasia (long-segment Barrett's esophagus) to be placed under regular surveillance. Long-segment Barrett's esophagus is relatively uncommon compared with intestinal metaplasia restricted to the gastroesophageal junctional region, which occurs in 18–20% of all patients.[31] The high prevalence of intestinal metaplasia in the junctional region could explain the frequency of adenocarcinomas in the junctional region, despite a lower risk of malignant transformation. Our studies provide strong evidence that intestinal metaplasia at the junction is caused by reflux disease.[32] At present, short-segment Barrett's esophagus is not a universally accepted indication for surveillance, though many individual patients are placed under some kind of surveillance.

Carcinogenesis in intestinal metaplasia results from progressive genetic changes induced in the cells by some compo-

nent of refluxed gastroesophageal contents. The fact that adenocarcinoma complicating Barrett's esophagus has continued to increase in frequency even as the ability to suppress acid secretion has improved suggests that this factor is not acid. Bile acids may be important etiologically, and it has been suggested that alteration of gastric pH by acid suppression therapy may result in the conversion of bile acids into promoters of carcinogenesis.[33] More study is needed in these areas.

The presently accepted sequence of adenocarcinoma in the lower esophagus is that reflux causes long-segment Barrett's esophagus (intestinal metaplasia), which progresses through increasing grades of dysplasia to adenocarcinoma. Recognition of this sequence provides the rationale for surveillance of patients with long-segment Barrett's esophagus. There is no evidence that any type of treatment causes reversal of intestinal metaplasia, most likely because it is associated with irreversible genetic abnormalities.[34]

At USC, we believe the reflux–adenocarcinoma sequence is as follows (Fig. 3–27):

1. Acid reflux causes cardiac transformation of the squamous epithelium, with reactive changes and inflammation in the metaplastic cardiac mucosa, which we call reflux carditis.
2. Unknown etiologic factors cause a genetic change that is manifested as intestinal metaplasia. This genetic change is favored by the increased cell proliferation that accompanies reflux carditis.
3. Progression of genetic abnormalities, also due to unknown etiologic factors, leads to increasing dysplasia, finally resulting in invasive adenocarcinoma.

Recognition of the earlier stages of this sequence such as cardiac metaplasia and reflux carditis, which are probably re-

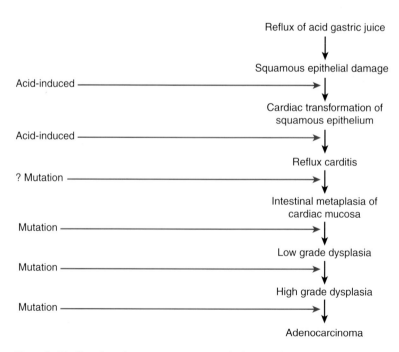

Figure 3–27. The reflux-adenocarcinoma sequence in the lower esophagus and lower esophageal sphincter region.

versible because they are not associated with genetic changes, permits prevention of Barrett's esophagus and entry into the irreversible phase of this sequence. Although the exact cause of intestinal metaplasia is unknown, there is good evidence that it is related to some component of refluxed gastric contents. As such, early antireflux surgery at the stage of reflux carditis represents a logical method of preventing Barrett's esophagus.[35] The large number of patients with reflux carditis (very likely 30–70% of the general population) makes this impractical. Identifying high-risk factors for developing intestinal metaplasia (eg, greater length of cardiac mucosa, persistence of reflux carditis after acid suppressive therapy) within this group may provide a rational basis in the future for selecting individuals for early antireflux surgery with the intent of preventing Barrett's esophagus.

Molecular Biology

Reid and colleagues[34] showed that aneuploidy was associated with nondysplastic Barrett's metaplasia, suggesting that the occurrence of intestinal metaplasia in cardiac mucosa represented an irreversible biologic change. Aneuploidy in intestinal metaplasia is associated with a large variety of chromosomal abnormalities.[36]

Loss of heterozygosity and mutation of the tumor suppressor *p53* gene is seen frequently in Barrett's esophagus. Although *p53* mutates with increasing frequency further along in the carcinogenic sequence, such mutations are present relatively early, sometimes even in nondysplastic, diploid intestinal metaplastic cells.[36] Studies to date suggest that DNA mismatch repair gene mutations and adenomatous polyposis coli (APC) gene mutations are found rarely in esophageal adenocarcinoma.

Among the oncogenes that are expressed, *c-erb* B-2 oncogene expression is present at all stages of Barrett's carcinogenesis, including the early nondysplastic stage. None of these molecular abnormalities are of sufficient specificity and sensitivity to be of routine diagnostic or prognostic value at this time.

Clinical Presentation

Many patients with adenocarcinoma complicating Barrett's esophagus present for the first time with symptoms of advanced cancer that are identical to those described for squamous carcinoma, including progressive dysphagia, loss of weight, and hemorrhage. These patients may never have had symptoms of reflux disease or they may give a long history of medically treated reflux. The treatment of these patients is identical to that for patients with advanced squamous carcinoma, and their prognosis is similarly dismal, with a median survival time of less than a year.

Patients with Barrett's esophagus who are under a screening protocol are usually detected at a much earlier stage in the disease. The presence of high-grade dysplasia in surveillance biopsies is an indication for esophagectomy in most centers.[37] Some of these patients have no invasive carcinoma at esophagectomy. A variable number, ranging from rare to 66% in different series, however, had invasive carcinoma in the esophagectomy specimen.[37] Most of these invasive cancers were intramucosal or submucosal.

Diagnosis

Distribution

Ninety percent of esophageal adenocarcinomas that complicate Barrett's esophagus occur in the lower third (Figs. 3–28, 3–29, and 3–30); the rest are in the middle third of the esophagus. When adenocarcinoma occurs above the gastroesophageal junction, the mucosa between the lower edge of the tumor and the stomach is lined by glandular mucosa of cardiac type with or without intestinal metaplasia (see Figs. 3–28 and 3–29). In cases of adenocarcinoma at the junction, residual Barrett's epithelium is found only in 42% of cases.[30]

Rare esophageal adenocarcinomas occur independent of Barrett's esophagus. These include adenocarcinomas arising in heterotopic gastric mucosa in the upper third of the esophagus ("inlet patch") and in esophageal glands. These tumors are discussed separately.

Macroscopic–Endoscopic Features

Advanced tumors present features identical to those in advanced squamous carcinomas. The only difference is the association of adenocarcinoma with glandular metaplasia of the lower esophagus. In screened patients with high-grade dysplasia and early cancers, the macroscopic and endoscopic appearance of the lesions correspond to the descriptions of early squamous carcinomas (Figs. 3–31, 3–32, and 3–33) (Table 3–3).

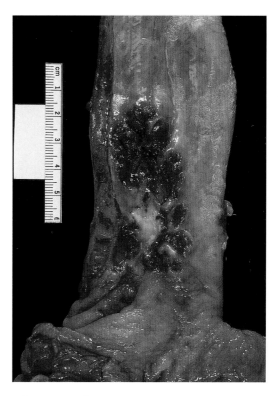

Figure 3–28. Adenocarcinoma of the lower esophagus, appearing as a flat ulcerated lesion. Note the glandular mucosa below the tumor.

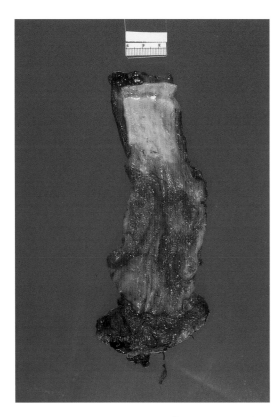

Figure 3–29. Carcinoma in the midesophagus with an infiltrative appearance. This can be differentiated from squamous carcinoma because of the presence of glandular mucosa in the esophagus below the tumor.

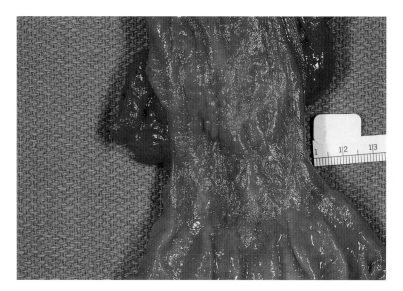

Figure 3–31. Early intramucosal adenocarcinoma of the esophagus occurring in a patient having esophagectomy, for a diagnosis of high-grade dysplasia during a surveillance protocol for Barrett's esophagus. The mucosa is slightly polypoid without any obviously visible lesions.

Pathologic Diagnosis

The pathologic diagnosis of high-grade dysplasia in Barrett's esophagus is discussed in Chapter 2.

When biopsies are performed on large tumors, the diagnosis of adenocarcinoma is usually obvious, with infiltrative malignant glands or cell nests surrounded by desmoplasia, often associated with high-grade dysplasia (Fig. 3–34). The histologic features of

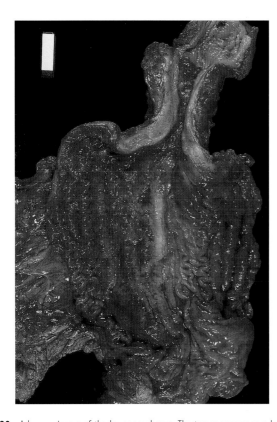

Figure 3–30. Adenocarcinoma of the lower esophagus. The tumor appears as a long malignant stricture. Note the reddened mucosal lining representing carcinoma and Barrett's esophagus.

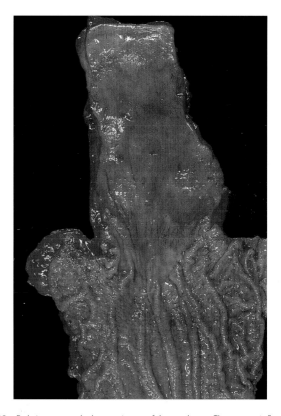

Figure 3–32. Early intramucosal adenocarcinoma of the esophagus. The mucosa is flat without any obviously visible lesions. Note the extension of the abnormal glandular mucosa into the gastric cardia above the rugal folds.

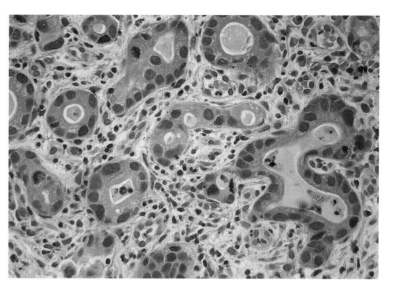

A

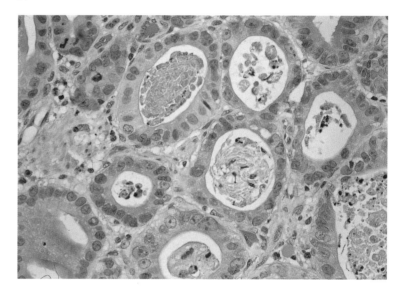

B

Figure 3–35. A: Adenocarcinoma of the esophagus, intestinal type, showing a tubular pattern with small irregular malignant tubules. B: Tubular adenocarcinoma, showing larger tubular structures lined by malignant epithelium.

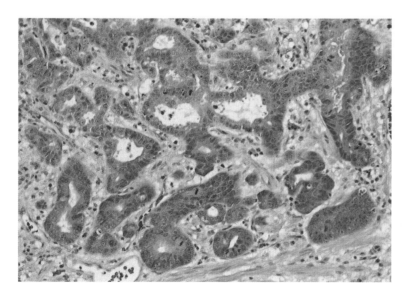

Figure 3–33. Early adenocarcinoma of the esophagus complicating Barrett's esophagus. The tumor shows a superficial ulceration. Note the grossly abnormal glandular epithelium in the gastric cardia between the tumor and the top of the gastric rugal folds.

adenocarcinoma of the esophagus are similar to those for gastric adenocarcinomas (see Chapter 5), with similar problems relating to biopsy interpretation. Intestinal-type carcinomas have to be distinguished from noninvasive high-grade dysplasia and regenerative glands associated with ulceration. The commonest pattern is a tubular pattern (Fig. 3–35); a variant of tubular adenocarcinoma is characterized by large irregularly infiltrating glands lined by cells that are cytologically bland (Fig. 3–36). This type of adenocarcinoma is associated with a significant false-negative

Figure 3–34. Esophageal biopsy specimen, showing adenocarcinoma, characterized by irregular malignant glands and cell nests surrounded by desmoplasia.

risk in small biopsy specimens. Papillary and clear cell features are common in Barrett's adenocarcinoma (Fig. 3–37). Poorly differentiated adenocarcinoma (Fig. 3–38) may require mucin stains to distinguish it from poorly differentiated squamous carcinoma. Signet ring cell carcinomas frequently occur in lower esophageal carcinoma complicating Barrett's esophagus (Fig. 3–38D). Other poorly differentiated carcinomas may have syncytial giant cells, resembling choriocarcinoma (Fig. 3–39) or have cells with eosinophilic cytoplasm resembling hepatocellular carcinoma ("hepatoid"), rhabdomyosarcoma, or rhabdoid tumors (Fig. 3–40). Immunoperoxidase staining is necessary to differentiate these adenocarcinoma variants from rare choriocarcinomas and rhabdoid tumors occurring in the esophagus.

Adenocarcinoma is frequently seen in the lamina propria underneath a squamous epithelial surface (Fig. 3–41). Note that in this regard the finding of glands under squamous epithelium

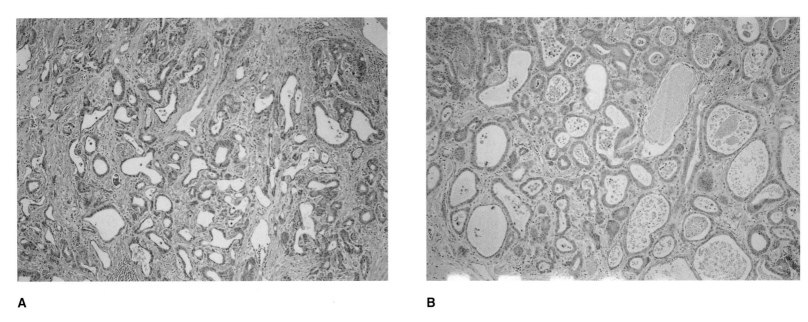

Figure 3–36. A: Adenocarcinoma of the esophagus, tubular type, characterized by malignant invasive tubule-shaped glandular structures and microcystic spaces lined by a cytologically bland cuboidal epithelium. B: Adenocarcinoma, microcystic type, showing bland cytologic features of the malignant cells.

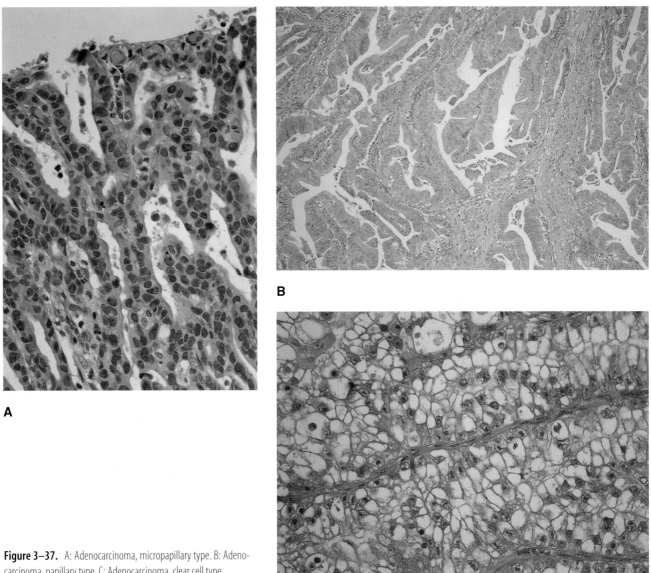

Figure 3–37. A: Adenocarcinoma, micropapillary type. B: Adenocarcinoma, papillary type. C: Adenocarcinoma, clear cell type.

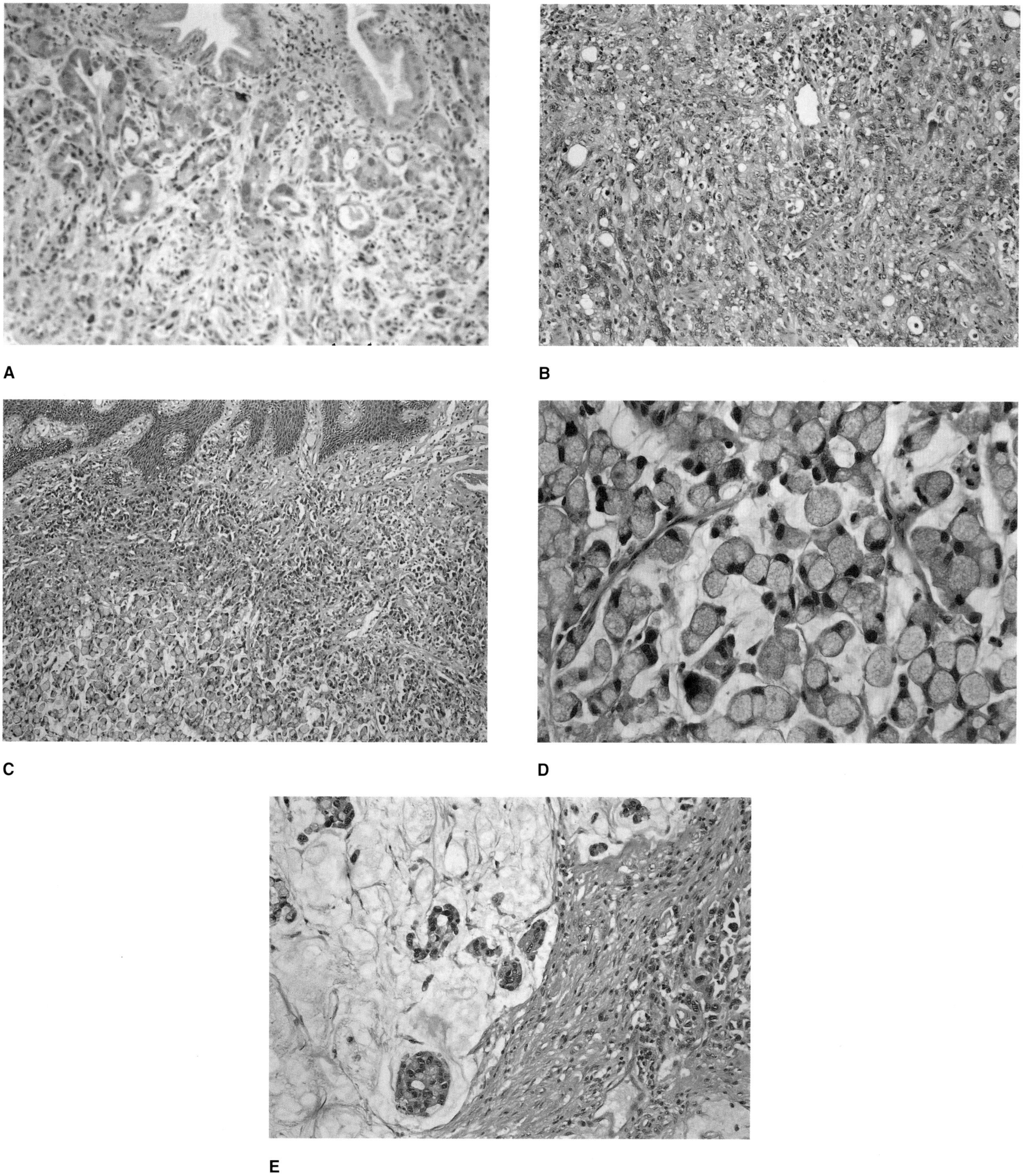

Figure 3–38. A: Adenocarcinoma, poorly differentiated, showing a tubular adenocarcinoma transforming into poorly differentiated carcinoma characterized by single infiltrating cells. B: Poorly differentiated adenocarcinoma, showing a diffuse proliferation of malignant cells without gland formation. Scattered signet ring cells are present. C: Adenocarcinoma of the esophagus, poorly differentiated, with desmoplasia. D: Signet ring cell adenocarcinoma occurring in Barrett's esophagus. E: Moderately differentiated adenocarcinoma with abundant extracellular mucin.

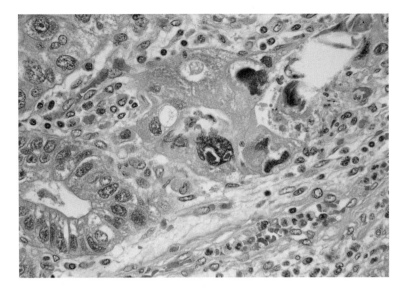

Figure 3–39. Adenocarcinoma with syncytiotrophoblast-like multinucleated giant cells. This was negative by immunoperoxidase for β-human chorionic gonadotropin.

is not a criterion of malignancy. Squamous epithelium overgrowth occurs over cardiac-type mucosa, nondysplastic Barrett's mucosa, and dysplastic Barrett's mucosa, as well as adenocarcinoma. The diagnosis of malignancy is based on histologic and architectural features of the glands concerned. Also, the fact that adenocarcinoma is present under the squamous epithelium does not mean that the tumor has invaded below the mucosa. The connective tissue immediately under the squamous epithelium of the esophagus is lamina propria and is separated from the submucosa by muscularis mucosae. The mucosa of the esophagus is a thicker structure than commonly realized (see Fig. 3–41).

Treatment

The treatment of advanced adenocarcinoma of the esophagus is identical to that for advanced squamous carcinoma.

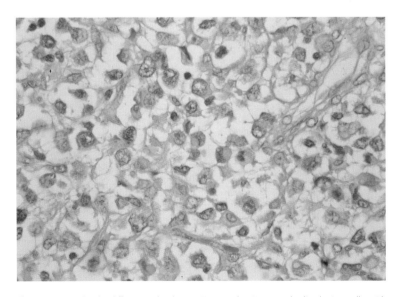

Figure 3–40. Poorly differentiated adenocarcinoma, showing round, discohesive cells with eosinophilic cytoplasm ("rhabdoid" features). This was positive for cytoplasmic mucin and, therefore, an adenocarcinoma.

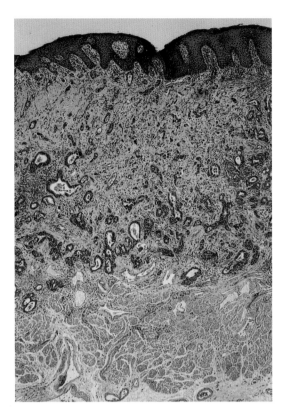

Figure 3–41. Adenocarcinoma in the lamina propria underneath a normal squamous epithelial surface lining. Note that the tumor is entirely within the mucosa, limited at its lower edge by a hyperplastic muscularis mucosae.

Localized forms of endoscopic mucosal resections and mucosal ablations are feasible for patients with high-grade dysplasia and intramucosal carcinoma. Local resections and ablation must be preceded by convincing endoscopic ultrasonography that shows the tumor confined to the mucosa. At present, the resolution associated with endoscopic ultrasound is inadequate to accurately exclude submucosal invasion,[38] and mucosal ablative procedures are rarely performed with curative intent. With improvement in the technology, these procedures are expected to proliferate.

Endoscopic ablation uses laser and photodynamically induced destruction of the abnormal epithelium. Both methods remove only the surface epithelium; healing may result in squamous overgrowth over residual Barrett's glands in the lamina propria, producing a suboptimal result. These therapies do not produce any specimens for pathologic examination.

Endoscopic treatment modalities are contraindicated when submucosal invasion is present because the incidence of nodal metastasis increases sharply.[24] These cases are treated with en bloc esophagectomy in centers where this procedure is accepted as being the treatment of choice for esophageal adenocarcinoma.

Pathologic Features and Prognosis

The pathologic examination of the resected specimen, staging, and prognosis are identical to that described for squamous carcinoma. Mucosal and submucosal lymphatic invasion is com-

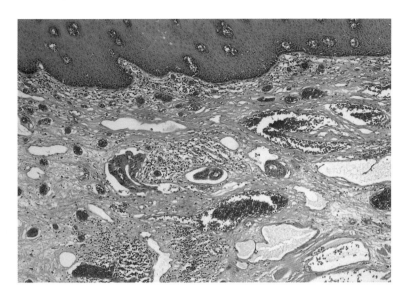

Figure 3–42. Mucosal lymphatic involvement by adenocarcinoma, showing well-differentiated adenocarcinoma in lymphatic vessel in the lamina propria away from the main tumor mass. Note the overlying normal squamous epithelium.

mon (Fig. 3–42) and mandates the same requirement for a 10-cm grossly clear mucosal margin at surgery.

Resections for high-grade dysplasia and early adenocarcinomas of the esophagus (see Figs. 3–31, 3–32, and 3–33) show the abnormal glandular mucosa extending up to a variable level of the esophagus. Frequently, there is minimal gross evidence of malignancy. The entire extent of glandular mucosa must be submitted for microscopic examination as serial transverse strips of the esophagus. Microscopic mapping of the extent of

intestinal metaplasia, low- and high-grade dysplasia, and invasive carcinoma is then possible. When invasive carcinoma is present, the depth of invasion must be assessed. Submucosal invasion is diagnosed when the tumor penetrates the muscularis mucosae completely (Fig. 3–43). We recommend that submucosal invasion be subdivided into superficial (involving the superficial 50% of the submucosa) and deep submucosal (involving the deeper half of the submucosa). Although this method is not yet recognized as a prognostic feature in early esophageal adenocarcinoma, it is becoming an important criterion in other sites, such as the rectum, with early cancers (see Chapter 13). In Barrett's esophagus, hypertrophy of smooth muscle in the lamina propria and muscularis mucosae is frequent, resulting in marked thickening of the muscularis mucosae, and care is needed to ensure complete penetration of this thickened muscle layer before a diagnosis of submucosal invasion is made. Intramucosal carcinoma has a low incidence of lymph node metastasis, but this increases when submucosal involvement is present.[24] In our cases, the presence of lamina propria lymphovascular invasion (Fig. 3–44) in intramucosal carcinoma is predictive for positive lymph nodes (Fig. 3–45).

In centers where endoscopic mucosal resections are performed, special pathologic methods are needed. These mucosal specimens are usually received as multiple small pieces of mucosa rather than as a large piece of intact mucosa. As such, complete pathologic evaluation is difficult, particularly as it relates to margins of excision. Every attempt must be made within the limitations of the specimen provided to assess the microscopic extent of intramucosal carcinoma and the presence or absence of submucosal extension and deep margin involvement. The

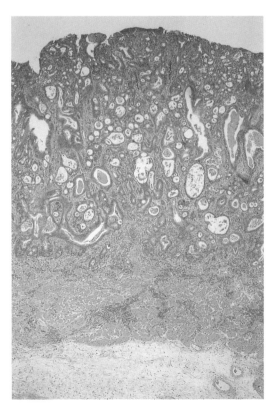

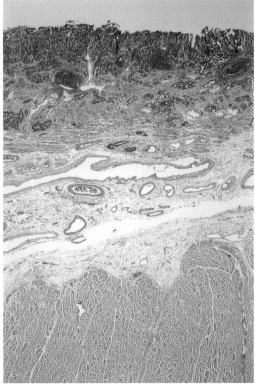

A **B**

Figure 3–43. A: Intramucosal adenocarcinoma in resection specimen. Note that the tumor extensively involves the mucosa but does not penetrate the muscularis mucosae. B: Minimal submucosal involvement by an esophageal adenocarcinoma, represented by two malignant glands below the level of the muscularis mucosae.

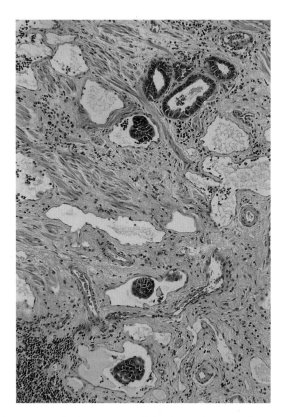

Figure 3–44. Intramucosal adenocarcinoma with lymphovascular invasion. This patient had two positive lymph nodes, despite the tumor being confined to the mucosa.

presence of an unexpectedly large volume of intramucosal carcinoma, submucosal extension, and positive resection margins are indications for considering more extensive surgery.

OTHER MALIGNANT NEOPLASMS

Unusual types of malignant esophageal neoplasms other than squamous carcinoma and adenocarcinoma complicating Barrett's esophagus account for less than 3% of esophageal can-

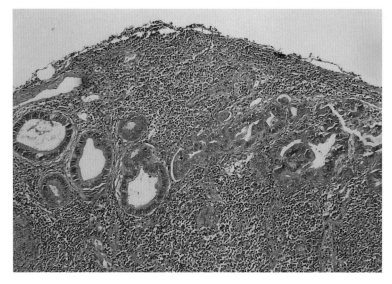

Figure 3–45. Positive lymph node in patient with intramucosal carcinoma.

cers.[39] The most common of these are malignant lymphoma (see Chapter 15), malignant GI stromal neoplasms (see Chapter 14), mucoepidermoid carcinoma, adenoid cystic carcinoma, malignant melanoma, and small-cell undifferentiated carcinoma. The other variants are extremely rare.

Variants of Squamous Carcinoma

Spindle Cell Squamous Carcinoma

These rare tumors, also called carcinosarcoma and polypoid squamous carcinoma, occur in elderly patients and typically present as a large polypoid mass in the lumen of the esophagus with a relatively narrow mucosal attachment (Fig. 3–46A). Not all carcinomas with a polypoid appearance are spindle cell squamous carcinomas; the majority are standard squamous carcinomas.[40] Spindle cell squamous carcinoma is characterized by squamous carcinoma associated with a prominent malignant spindle cell element, which is believed to represent metaplastic squamous carcinoma (Fig. 3–46B, C). The malignant spindle cell component usually resembles fibrosarcoma or malignant fibrous histiocytoma with pleomorphic giant cells; rarely, osteosarcomatous, chondrosarcomatous, and rhabdomyosarcomatous differentiation occurs. Immunoperoxidase staining shows the epithelial element to be cytokeratin+ and the spindle cell component to be vimentin+ with focal keratin positivity in some tumors.[41] When the tumor is composed entirely of spindle cells without a carcinomatous component, and cytokeratin immunoperoxidase fails to reveal a carcinomatous component, differentiation from a stromal neoplasm is virtually impossible.

Despite the large size of the intraluminal tumor at presentation, these neoplasms frequently show limited invasiveness. Infiltration is frequently intramural; transmural invasion and nodal metastases are seen in only about half the cases.[42] Stage for stage, they have the same prognosis as usual esophageal carcinomas. Size for size, however, the prognosis is better because of the frequency of cases of large tumors that have limited invasion.

Verrucous Carcinoma

Verrucous carcinoma is defined by its predominantly exophytic, warty gross appearance and the extremely well-differentiated histologic appearance. Microscopically, the tumor is difficult to distinguish from squamous papilloma, and establishing a diagnosis by endoscopic diagnosis can be difficult. Despite its low histologic grade, verrucous squamous carcinoma is a highly infiltrative tumor; most cases show transmural invasion, sometimes with involvement of adjacent structures. The prognosis is poor.[43]

Basaloid Squamous Cell Carcinoma

Basaloid squamous carcinoma is characterized by solid groups of cells in lobular configuration closely apposed to the surface mucosa that are composed of small basaloid cells with scanty

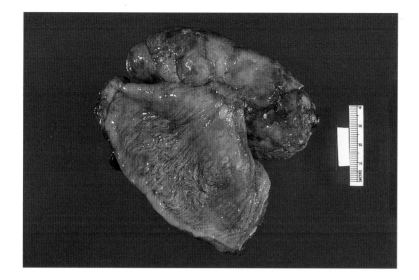

A

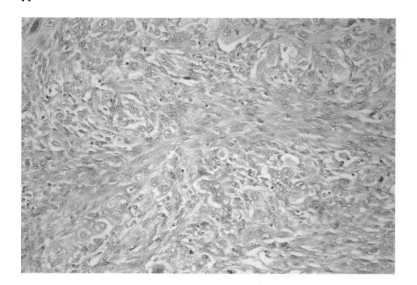

B

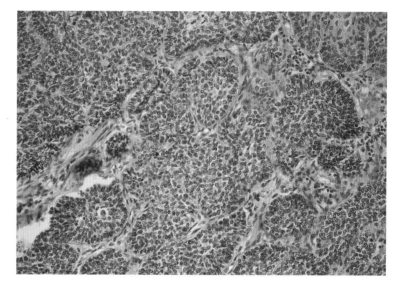

A

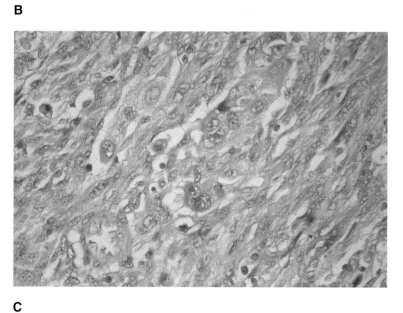

C

Figure 3–46. A: Spindle cell (polypoid) carcinoma of the esophagus, showing a large exophytic mass attached to the mucosa by a relatively narrow stalk. B: Spindle cell carcinoma of the esophagus, showing mixed spindle cell and recognizably squamous epithelial elements. C: Spindle cell carcinoma of the esophagus, showing malignant spindle cells admixed with more rounded epithelial cells showing focal keratinization.

cytoplasm and dark hyperchromatic nuclei without nucleoli (Fig. 3–47). The cell groupings may have small cyst-like spaces containing mucin-like material and comedo-like necrosis. Basaloid squamous carcinoma may coexist with more usual squamous carcinoma and squamous carcinoma in situ of the surface epithelium.[44] These neoplasms are aggressive and their prognosis is similar to that for usual squamous carcinomas.

EBV-Associated Undifferentiated Carcinoma with Lymphoid Stroma

Rare cases of Epstein-Barr virus (EBV) associated squamous carcinomas occur in the esophagus. These are histologically identical to nasopharyngeal lymphoepithelioma-like carcinoma, being composed of undifferentiated carcinoma with a rich lymphocytic admixture.[45]

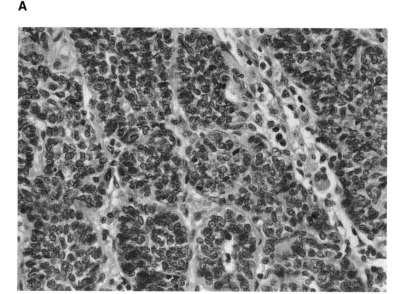

B

Figure 3–47. A: Basaloid carcinoma of the esophagus, showing irregular nests of small basaloid cells with high a nuclear-to-cytoplasmic (N:C) ratio and irregular hyperchromatic nuclei. B: Higher power micrograph of part A.

Variants of Adenocarcinoma

Mucoepidermoid Carcinoma

Mucoepidermoid carcinomas are believed to arise in the submucosal mucous glands of the esophagus. They resemble mucoepidermoid tumors that arise in salivary glands, being composed of nests of cells containing an admixture of mucous cells and more solid epidermoid cells. The tumor grows slowly; most patients have surgically resectable tumors at the time of presentation. Overall prognosis is poor, however, and not dissimilar to that for usual esophageal carcinoma.[46]

Rare cases of "mucoepidermoid" carcinomas have been reported to arise in Barrett's mucosa.[47] It is likely, however, that these differ from the majority of mucoepidermoid tumors of the esophagus. They represent squamous metaplasia in an adenocarcinoma arising in Barrett's esophagus, that is adenosquamous carcinoma (see later section). It is of interest that esophageal adenocarcinomas produced in experimental rats by surgical manipulations and carcinogens frequently show adenosquamous features.

Adenoid Cystic Carcinoma

Adenoid cystic carcinoma of the esophagus is also believed to arise in the esophageal mucous glands. These carcinomas have the histologic appearance of their salivary glands counterparts, being composed of nests of small basaloid cells with cribriform architecture. Unlike in the salivary gland, adenoid

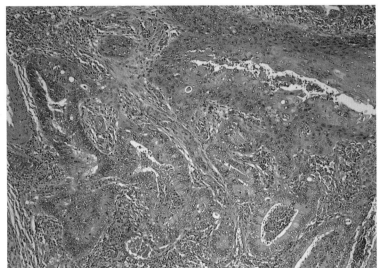

A

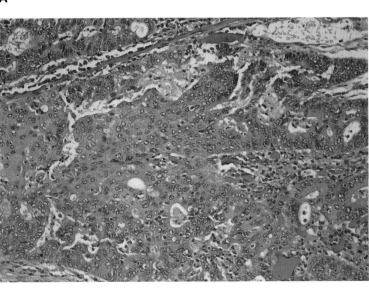

B

Figure 3–48. A: Poorly differentiated adenocarcinoma arising in Barrett's esophagus with squamous differentiation (adenosquamous carcinoma). B: Poorly differentiated adenosquamous carcinoma arising in Barrett's esophagus. The squamous component is less well differentiated than in part A.

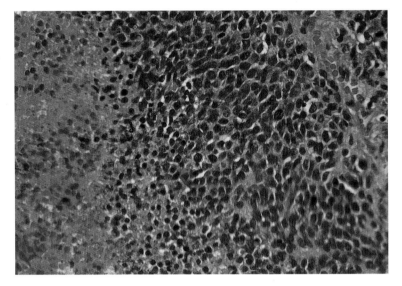

A

B

Figure 3–49. A: Small-cell undifferentiated carcinoma, showing typical cohesive small, ovoid cells with high ratio, and hyperchromatic nuclei without nucleoli. This appearance is indistinguishable from the same tumor that arises more commonly in the lung. B: Immunoperoxidase stain for keratin, showing the typical punctate, perinuclear cytoplasmic staining pattern typical of small-cell undifferentiated carcinoma.

cystic carcinomas of the esophagus have a high mitotic rate and necrosis. Squamous carcinoma is frequently present alongside the adenoid cystic carcinoma. These tumors have an aggressive behavior and the same prognosis as usual esophageal carcinomas.[48]

Adenocarcinoma of the Upper Esophagus Arising in Ectopic Gastric Mucosa ("Inlet Patch")

Grossly visible foci of ectopic gastric mucosa occur in approximately 3–5% of esophagi. These foci are usually oxyntic and contain parietal and chief cells; inflammation is usually absent. Intestinal metaplasia may occur, but is rare. These so-called "inlet patches" are etiologically different from Barrett's esophagus. The occurrence of adenocarcinoma in these foci of gastric mucosa in the upper esophagus is extremely rare.[49] When they occur, the adenocarcinomas are intestinal-type and usually well differentiated.

Adenocarcinoma with Germ Cell Elements

Adenocarcinomas of the esophagus rarely contain malignant germ cell elements such as choriocarcinoma and yolk sac carcinoma.[50] An association with Barrett's esophagus is usually present. The presence of a germ cell component is associated with elevation of serum beta-human chorionic gonadotropin (β-HCG) and α-fetoprotein. Adenocarcinomas with germ cell components respond to chemotherapeutic agents directed against the germ cell component, and their prognosis tends to be better

than that for the usual adenocarcinoma. Though rare, the fact that the presence of germ cell elements favorably affect survival has led to the recommendation that serum marker analysis be done on all patients with esophageal adenocarcinoma, particularly in patients younger than 50.

Adenocarcinoma with Squamous Differentiation

Rarely, adenocarcinoma arising in Barrett's esophagus shows squamous differentiation (Fig. 3–48). The squamous element may be poorly differentiated (adenosquamous carcinoma) or well differentiated (adenoacanthoma). The presence of squamous differentiation does not influence prognosis.

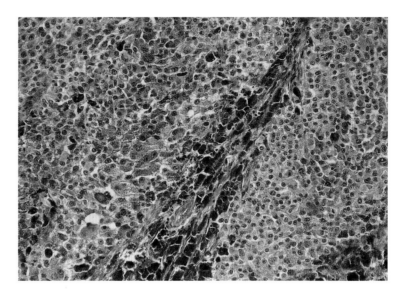

A

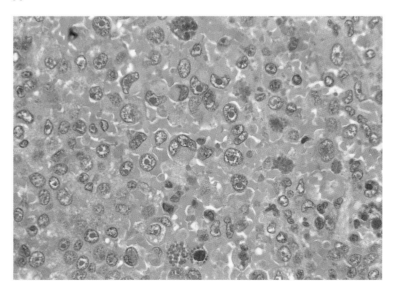

B

Figure 3–51. A: Malignant melanoma of the esophagus, showing pigmented malignant cells. Some of the more heavily pigmented cells are melanophages. B: Malignant melanoma, achromatic, showing undifferentiated malignant cells in sheets with round nuclei that have prominent nucleoli. The pigment-containing cells are siderophages containing hemosiderin. The diagnosis of melanoma must be confirmed by the immunophenotype of this neoplasm (vimentin+, keratin−, CD45−, S100 protein+, HMB45+).

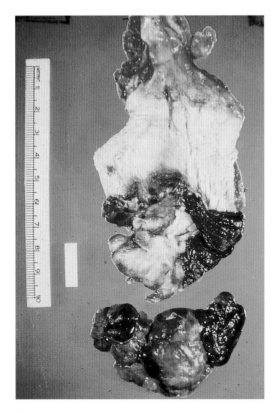

Figure 3–50. Primary malignant melanoma of the esophagus, showing a bulky pigmented malignant neoplasm.

Neuroendocrine Cell Tumors

Carcinoid Tumor

The occurrence of carcinoid tumors in the esophagus is extremely rare. Rare cases of atypical carcinoid tumor[51] and composite tumors composed of adenocarcinoma and carcinoid tumors have been reported.[52]

Small-Cell Neuroendocrine Carcinoma

Small-cell undifferentiated carcinoma constitutes 1% of all esophageal cancers. Located in the middle and lower third of the esophagus, it typically presents as a bulky tumor with evidence of systemic disease at the time of presentation.[53] Microscopically, the tumor is composed of small cells with scanty cy-

toplasm, nuclear molding, and round-to-oval hyperchromatic nuclei that show no nucleoli (Fig. 3–49A). The cells show immunohistochemical staining typical for neuroendocrine tumors with punctate perinuclear cytokeratin positivity (Fig. 3–49B), and stain positively with chromogranin A and neuron-specific enolase. These are highly aggressive neoplasms with a poor prognosis, but are important to recognize because meaningful improvement in survival occurs with chemotherapy. Small-cell carcinoma of the esophagus is believed to originate in neuroendocrine cells in the esophageal mucosa. Rarely, they are associated with squamous carcinoma and squamous dysplasia.[54]

Malignant Melanoma

The esophagus is a rare site for primary malignant melanoma, occurring mainly in patients older than 50. Melanocytes are normally found in the esophageal mucosa in 4–8% of patients. Melanosis esophagii, which is a rare benign condition of the esophagus, is believed by some to be a precursor to malignant melanoma.

Most tumors are at an advanced stage at presentation, with bulky tumors, located mainly in the lower esophagus (Fig. 3–50). Typically displaying a distinctive black gross appearance; microscopically, most tumors contain abundant melanin pigment in the cytoplasm, which makes diagnosis obvious (Fig. 3–51A). Achromatic tumors resemble carcinomas, from which they are distinguished by immunoperoxidase staining (Fig. 3–51B) (melanomas are cytokeratin±, vimentin+, S100 protein+, HMB45±) and demonstration of premelanosomes by electron microscopy. Esophageal malignant melanomas frequently show an in situ component at the edge of the invasive tumor, indicating their origin at this location. The prognosis is poor, though rare long-term survivals have been reported.[55]

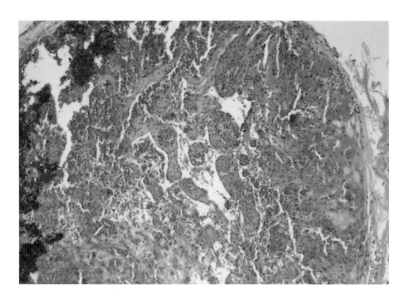

A

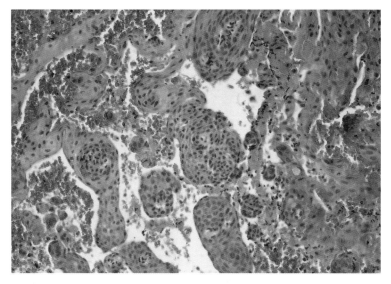

B

Figure 3–52. A: Unusual polypoid vascular lesion, characterized by cavernous spaces lined by flat endothelium separated by benign squamous epithelial elements. This was diagnosed as an angiokeratoma. B: Higher power micrograph of part A.

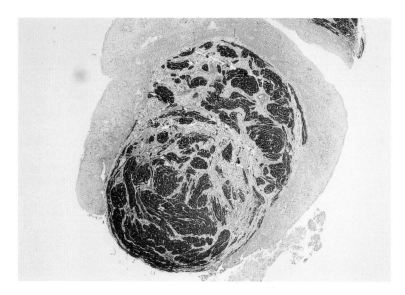

Figure 3–53. Esophageal neurofibroma, presenting as a polypoid lesion, and removed at endoscopy, stained by immunoperoxidase stain for S100 protein.

BENIGN NEOPLASMS

Benign neoplasms of the esophagus are usually small tumors detected incidentally during endoscopy. Rarely, they become large enough to present with dysphagia or ulcerate and cause upper GI bleeding.[56] A large variety of benign neoplasms have been reported; leiomyoma is the most common. They can be classified as follows:

1. Benign epithelial tumors, which include squamous papilloma and fibrovascular polyps lined by benign squamous epithelium.
2. Mesenchymal tumors, which include leiomyoma (see Chapter 14), hemangioma, angiokeratoma (Fig. 3–52), lymphangioma, lipoma, neurofibroma (Fig. 3–53), schwannoma, and granular cell tumor. Mesenchymal neoplasms are discussed more fully in Chapter 14. We have encountered two cases of granular cell tumor of the esophagus associated with squamous carcinoma,[57] and an unusual inflammatory pseudotumor that contained adipose tissue (Fig. 3–54).
3. Intramural cysts, which are most commonly foregut duplication cysts.
4. Thyroid or parathyroid epithelial rests rarely occur in the esophagus.

References

1. Kirby TJ, Rice TW. The epidemiology of esophageal cancer: The changing face of a disease. *Chest Surg Clin North Am.* 1994;4:217–225.
2. Parker SL, Tong T, Bolden S, et al. Cancer statistics, 1996. *CA Cancer J Clin.* 1996:65:5–27.
3. Boyce HW. Tumors of the esophagus. In Sleisenger MH, Fordtran J (eds): *Gastrointestinal Disease,* 5th ed. Philadelphia, WB Saunders, 1994. pp. 401–418.
4. Blot WJ, Devesa SS, Fraumen JF. Continuing climb in rates of esophageal adenocarcinomas: An update. *JAMA.* 1993;270:1320.
5. Blot WJ, Devesa SS, Kneller RW, et al. Rising incidence of adenocarcinoma of the esophagus and gastric cardia. *JAMA.* 265:1991;1287–1289.
6. Sugar PM. Aetiology of cancer of the oesophagus. Geographical studies in the footsteps of Marco Polo and beyond. *Gut.* 1989;30:561–564.
7. Chang F, Syrjanen S, Wang L, et al. Infectious agents in the etiology of esophageal cancer. *Gastroenterology.* 1992;103:1336–1348.
8. Brown LM, Blot WJ, Schuman SH, et al. Environmental factor and high risk of esophageal cancer among men in coastal South Carolina. *J Natl Cancer Inst.* 1988;80:1620–1625.
9. Isolauri J, Markkula H. Lye ingestion and carcinoma of the esophagus. *Acta Chir Scand.* 1989;155:269–271.
10. Harper PS, Harper RM, Howel-Evans AW. Carcinoma of the esophagus with tylosis. *QJ Med.* 1970;39:317–333.
11. Peracchia A, Segalin A, Bardini R, et al. Esophageal carcinoma and achalasia: Prevalence, incidence and results of treatment. *Hepatogastroenterology.* 1991;38:514–516.
12. Thomas CR. Biology of esophageal cancer and the role of combined modality therapy. *Surg Clin North Am.* 1997;77:1139–1167.
13. Stemmermann G, Heffelfinger SC, Noffsinger A, et al. The molecular biology of esophageal and gastric cancer and their precursors: Oncogenes, tumor suppressor genes, and growth factors. *Hum Pathol.* 1994;25:968.
14. Lazarus C, Jaskiewicz K, Sumeruk RA, et al. Brush cytology technique in the detection of oesophageal carcinoma in the asymptomatic, high risk subject: A pilot survey. *Cytopathology.* 1992;3:291–296.
15. Graham DY, Schwartz JT, Cain GD, et al. Prospective evaluation of biopsy number in the diagnosis of esophageal and gastric carcinoma. *Gastroenterology.* 1982;82:228–231.
16. Goldschmid S, Nord HJ. Endoscopic diagnosis and treatment or esophageal cancer. *Gastrointest Endosc Clin North Am.* 1994;4:827–850.
17. Sugimachi K, Ohno S, Matsui A, et al. Clinicopathologic study of early stage esophageal carcinoma. *Br J Surg.* 1989;76:759–763.

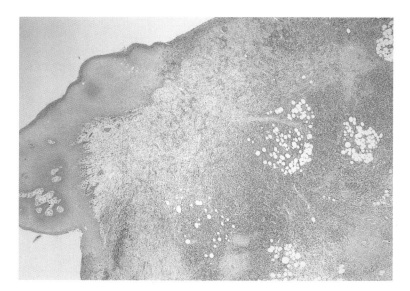

A

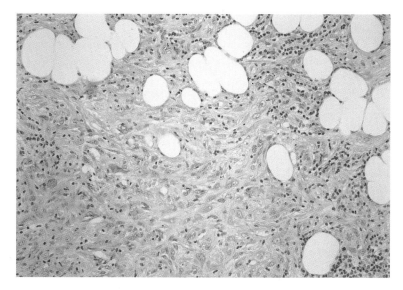

B

Figure 3–54. A: Inflammatory pseudotumor of the esophagus, showing a mixture of adipose tissue, vascular structures, and inflammatory cells under the squamous epithelium. B: Higher power micrograph of part A. The stromal cells show reactive atypia.

18. Sabik JF, Rice TW, Goldblum JR, et al. Superficial esophageal carcinoma. *Ann Thorac Surg.* 1995;60:896–902.

19. Sugimachi K, Ikebe M, Kitamura K, et al. Long-term results of esophagectomy for early esophageal carcinoma. *Hepatogastroenterology.* 1993;40:203–206.

20. Herskovic A, Martz K, Al-Sarraf M, et al. Combined chemotherapy and radiotherapy compared with radiotherapy alone in patients with cancer of the esophagus. *N Engl J Med.* 1993;326:1593–1598.

21. Beahrs OH, Henson DE, Hotter RVP, et al (eds). *Manual for Staging Cancer,* 4th ed. Philadelphia, JB Lippincott, 1992.

22. Skinner DB. En bloc resection for esophageal carcinoma. In Pearson FG, Deslauriers J, Ginsburg RJ, et al (eds): *Esophageal Surgery.* New York, Churchill Livingstone 1995. pp 709–718.

23. Clark GWB, Peters JH, Ireland AP, et al. Nodal metastases and sites of recurrence after en bloc esophagectomy for adenocarcinoma. *Ann Thorac Surg.* 1994;58:646–654.

24. Peters JH, Clark GWB, Ireland AP, et al. Outcome of adenocarcinoma arising in Barrett's esophagus in endoscopically surveyed and nonsurveyed patients. *J Thorac Cardiovasc Surg.* 1994;108:813–822.

25. Patti MG, Owen D. Prognostic factors in esophageal cancer. *Surg Clin North Am.* 1997;6:515–531.

26. Izbicki JB, Hosch SB, Pichlmeier, et al. Prognostic value of immunohistochemically identifiable tumor cells in lymph nodes of patients with completely resected esophageal cancer. *N Engl J Med.* 1997;337:1188–1194.

27. Bosher LH, Taylor FH. Heterotopic gastric mucosa in the esophagus with ulceration and stricture formation. *J Thorac Surg.* 1951;21:306–312.

28. Morson BC, Belcher JR. Adenocarcinoma of the esophagus and ectopic gastric mucosa. *Br J Cancer.* 1952;6:127–130.

29. Tytgat GNJ. Does endoscopic surveillance in esophageal columnar metaplasia (Barrett's esophagus) have any real value? *Endoscopy.* 1995;27:19.

30. Clark GWB, Smyrk TC, Burdiles P, et al. Is Barrett's metaplasia the source of adenocarcinomas of the cardia? *Arch Surg.* 1994;129:609.

31. Spechler SJ, Zeroogian JM, Antonioli DA, et al. Prevalence of metaplasia at the gastrooesophageal junction. *Lancet.* 1994;344:1533.

32. Oberg S, Peters JH, DeMeester TR, et al. Inflammation and specialized intestinal metaplasia of cardiac mucosa is a manifestation of gastroesophageal reflux disease. *Ann Surg.* 1997;226:522–532.

33. Stein HJ, Barlow AP, DeMeester TR, et al. Complications of gastroesophageal reflux disease: Role of the lower esophageal sphincter, esophageal acid and acid/alkaline exposure, and duodenogastric reflux. *Ann Surg.* 1992;216:35–43.

34. Reid BJ, Blount PL, Rubin CE, et al. Flow cytometric and histological progression to malignancy in Barrett's esophagus: Prospective endoscopic surveillance of a cohort. *Gastroenterology.* 1992;102:1212–1219.

35. Peters JH. The surgical management of Barrett's esophagus. *Gastroenterol Clin North Am.* 1997;26:647–668.

36. Souza RF, Meltzer SJ. The molecular basis for carcinogenesis in metaplastic columnar lined esophagus. *Gastroenterol Clin North Am.* 1997;26:583–597.

37. DeMeester TR. Surgical treatment of dysplasia and adenocarcinoma. *Gastroenterol Clin North Am.* 1997;26:669–684.

38. Peters JH, Hoeft SF, Heimbucher J, et al. Selection of patients for curative or palliative resection of esophageal cancer based on preoperative endoscopic ultrasonography. *Arch Surg.* 1994;129:534–539.

39. Lieberman MD, Franceschi D, Marsan B, et al. Esophageal carcinoma. The unusual variants. *J Thorac Cardiovasc Surg.* 1994;108:1138–1146.

40. Mori M, Mimori K, Sadanaga N, et al. Polypoid carcinoma of the esophagus. *Jpn J Cancer Res.* 1994;85:1131–1136.

41. Kuhajda FP, Sun T-T, Mendelsohn G. Polypoid squamous carcinoma of the esophagus. *Am J Surg Pathol.* 1983;7:495–499.

42. Gal AA, Martin SE, Kernen JA, et al. Esophageal carcinoma with prominent spindle cells. *Cancer.* 1987;60:2244–2250.

43. Biemond P, ten Kate FJW, van Blankenstein M. Esophageal verrucous carcinoma: Histologically a low grade malignancy but clinically a fatal disease. *J Clin Gastroenterol.* 1991;13:102–107.

44. Sarbia M, Verreet P, Bittinger F, et al. Basaloid squamous cell carcinoma of the esophagus: Diagnosis and prognosis. *Cancer.* 1997;79:1871–1878.

45. Mori M, Watanabe M, Tanaka S, et al. Epstein-Barr virus-associated carcinomas of the esophagus and stomach. *Arch Pathol Lab Med.* 1994;118:998–1001.

46. Bell-Thomson J, Haggitt RC, Ellis FH, Jr., et al. Mucoepidermoid and adenoid cystic carcinomas of the esophagus. *J Thorac Cardiovasc Surg.* 1980;79:438–446.

47. Pascal RR, Clearfield HR. Mucoepidermoid (adenosquamous) carcinoma arising in Barrett's esophagus. *Dig Dis Sci.* 1987;32:428–432.

48. Cerar A, Jutersek A, Vidmar S. Adenoid cystic carcinoma of the esophagus. A clinicopathologic study of three cases. *Cancer.* 1991;2159–2164.

49. Christensen WN, Sternberg SS. Adenocarcinoma of the upper esophagus arising in ectopic gastric mucosa. *Am J Surg Pathol.* 1987;11:397–402.

50. Wasan HS, Schofield JB, Krausz T, et al. Combined choriocarcinoma and yolk sac tumor arising in Barrett's esophagus. *Cancer.* 1994;73:514–517.

51. Lindberg GM, Molberg KH, Vuitch MF, et al. Atypical carcinoid of the esophagus: A case report and review of the literature. *Cancer.* 1997;79:1476–1481.

52. Chong FK, Graham JH, Madoff IM. Mucin-producing carcinoid ("composite tumor") of upper third of esophagus. *Cancer.* 1979;44:1853–1859.

53. Briggs JC, Ibrahim NBN. Oat cell carcinoma of the oesophagus: A clinicopathological study of 23 cases. *Histopathology.* 1983;7:261–277.

54. Sato T, Mukai M, Ando N, et al. Small cell carcinoma (nonoat cell type) of the esophagus concomitant with invasive squamous cell carcinoma and carcinoma in situ. *Cancer.* 1986;57:328–332.

55. De Mik JI, Kooijman CD, Hoekstra JBL, et al. Primary malignant melanoma of the oesophagus. *Histopathology.* 1992;20:77–79.

56. Fockens P, Bartelsman JFWM, Tytgat GNJ. Benign and malignant esophageal tumors other than squamous and adenocarcinoma. *Gastrointest Clin North Am.* 1994;4:791–801.

57. Joshi A, Chandrasoma P, Kiyabu M. Multiple granular cell tumors of the gastrointestinal tract with subsequent development of esophageal squamous carcinoma. *Dig Dis Sci.* 1992;37:1612–1618.

4

NONNEOPLASTIC DISEASES OF THE STOMACH

Helen Yen and Parakrama Chandrasoma

THE NORMAL STOMACH

The anatomically normal stomach extends from the gastroesophageal junction to the junction between the pylorus and duodenum. Physiologically, the proximal and distal limits of the stomach are defined by the lower end of the lower esophageal sphincter and the distal limit of the pyloric sphincter. The stomach is divided anatomically into the cardia, which is a small part of the stomach around the entry of the esophagus; the fundus, which is that part of the stomach situated above the level of the point of esophageal entry; the body; and the pyloric antrum, which ends in the pyloric sphincter. The body passes into the py-

loric antrum at a line drawn through a point of angulation on the lesser curvature known as the incisura angularis. The mucosal lining of the stomach is characterized by rugal folds (Fig. 4–1).

Microscopically, the surface is flat and characterized by shallow pits, or foveolae, into which the deep mucosal gastric glands drain (Fig. 4–2). The surface epithelium and foveolar region is lined by tall columnar cells with a basal nucleus and abundant neutral mucin in the apical region (see Fig. 4–2). The deepest cells of the foveolar region are the mucous neck cells, which represent the proliferative, or germinative, layer of the epithelium that is constantly dividing to replenish cells lost from the surface epithelium and gastric pit. The normal short length of the foveolar region reflects the steady state of cell turnover in the gastric mucosa. The surface epithelium and foveolar region is uniform throughout the stomach. In the thickest part of the mucosa (in the body), the foveolar region is about 25% of mucosal thickness; in the antral mucosa, it is about 40–50%.

The gastric mucosa is divisible into three parts, based on the nature of the glands present in the mucosa deep to the foveolar neck region. (1) Antral mucosa, which lines the distal stomach, is characterized by coiled glands that contain mucous cells with vacuolated cytoplasm (Fig. 4–3A), and specialized neuroendocrine cells. In the pyloric channel, the deep mucous glands are surrounded by fibers of the muscularis mucosae (Fig. 4–3B). (2) Oxyntic mucosa, which lines the gastric body and fundus (and is frequently termed body and fundic mucosae), is characterized by straight unbranched tubular glands that contain acid-secreting parietal cells, pepsinogen-secreting chief

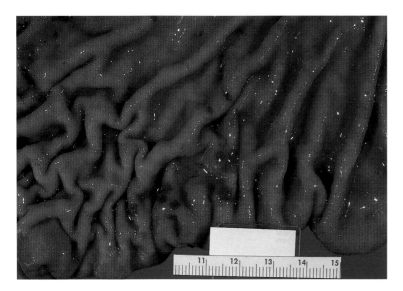

Figure 4–1. Nearly normal gastric mucosa, showing thin rugal folds. A few small hemorrhagic sports are evident, probably artifactual. This portion of the stomach was resected to treat a lower esophageal neoplasm. It was histologically normal.

cells, and neuroendocrine cells (Figs. 4–2 and 4–4). Mucous cells are not present in normal oxyntic glands. (3) Cardiac mucosa, which is the junctional mucosa immediately distal to the squamous epithelium of the esophagus. Cardiac mucosal glands are composed of mucous cells with a vacuolated cytoplasm.

The glands are separated by the connective tissue of the lamina propria. In oxyntic mucosa, lamina propria is very scanty, with the glands being packed tightly together, and lym-

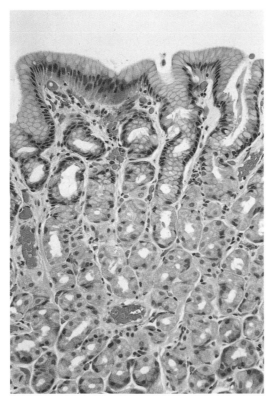

Figure 4–2. Normal oxyntic mucosa, showing the surface epithelium and foveolar region, which are lined by tall columnar cells with basal nuclei and apical mucin, and the straight tubular glands draining into the foveolar pit.

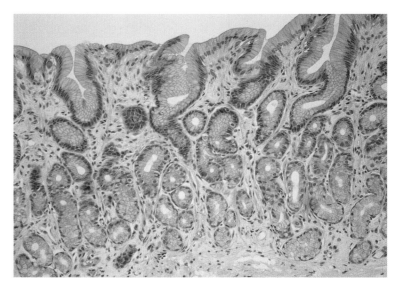

A

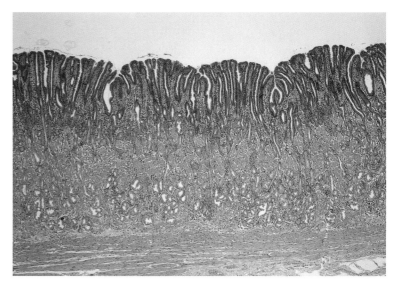

B

Figure 4–3. A: Normal antral mucosa, showing the foveolar region and mucous glands. B: Antral mucosa from the pyloric channel, showing mucous glands in the deep mucosa surrounded by smooth muscle of the muscularis muscosae. There is elongation of the foveolar region and inflammation in this antral mucosa.

phocytes are few in number, even in the superficial mucosa. In antral mucosa, the lamina propria normally contains up to five lymphocytes and plasma cells per 40× objective high-power field. Small nodular collections of lymphoid cells are normally present in the stomach, usually in the deep part of the mucosa. Normal lymphoid nodules in the stomach have no germinal centers.[1]

The mucosae described histologically do not correspond exactly to the anatomic divisions of the stomach. Antral mucosa lines a variable amount of the pyloric antrum. The junction between antral and oxyntic mucosa varies greatly among individuals; in the junctional region, the mucosal glands frequently contain a mixture of oxyntic and mucous cells (oxyntoantral mucosa) (Fig. 4–5).

Pathologic lesions of the stomach involve the antral and

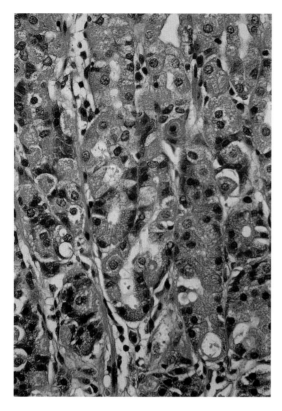

Figure 4–4. Oxyntic mucosa of the body and fundus of the stomach, showing parietal cells with eosinophilic cytoplasm and chief cells with basophilic cytoplasm.

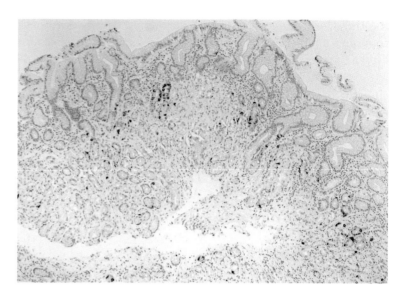

Figure 4–6. Gastric mucosa, immunoperoxidase stain for chromogranin A, showing distribution of neuroendocrine cells, which are seen scattered throughout the mucosa but, in this section, tend to be most numerous in the deep foveolar region.

oxyntic mucosae. Cardiac mucosal diseases are considered with the esophagus as gastroesophageal junctional disease. These are discussed in Chapter 2, where evidence is presented that cardiac mucosa represents an abnormal mucosa associated with gastroesophageal reflux rather than being part of the normal stomach mucosal lining.

Neuroendocrine cells are present throughout the gastric mucosa, being situated among the glandular epithelial cells, commonly toward the foveolar neck region and the gland base (Fig. 4–6). When numerous, they can be recognized as small round cells with clear cytoplasm, but are best identified in immunoperoxidase sections stained with specific markers (eg, chromogranin A, neuron-specific enolase). In the antrum, about half the neuroendocrine cells are gastrin-producing G cells, 30% are serotonin-producing enterochromaffin (EC) cells, and 15% are somatostatin-producing D cells. In the oxyntic mucosa of the body and fundus, the neuroendocrine cells are predominantly enterochromaffin-like (ECL) cells. Quantitation of neuroendocrine cells is difficult because their numbers are always determined in relation to the number of other cells present. When the number of oxyntic cells is reduced, for example, the number of neuroendocrine cells appear increased, giving the impression of neuroendocrine cell hyperplasia (pseudohyperplasia).

ANATOMIC ABNORMALITIES OF THE STOMACH

Congenital Pyloric Stenosis

This common disorder affects 1 in 150 newborns, predominantly firstborn male infants. Hypertrophy and hyperplasia of the smooth muscle of the pyloric sphincter occur associated with a functional failure of relaxation of the sphincter. Gastric outlet obstruction results, commonly presenting in the first month of life, with failure to thrive and projectile bile-free vomiting. The hypertrophic pylorus can usually be felt as a mass in the upper right abdomen. Treatment is with myotomy.

Gastroparesis

Gastroparesis results from hypomotility of the stomach, resulting in delayed gastric emptying. Acute transient gastroparesis occurs after abdominal surgery, abdominal trauma, and in peri-

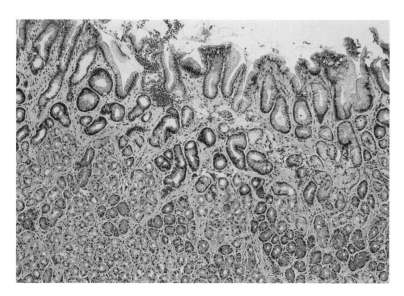

Figure 4–5. Oxyntoantral mucosa, showing a mixture of mucous and oxyntic cells in the glands beneath the foveolar region. There are rare lymphocytes in the lamina propria, within normal limits.

tonitis. Chronic gastroparesis occurs in autonomic neuropathies and is most commonly seen in diabetics. Progressive system sclerosis (see Chapter 2) and amyloidosis may also be associated with gastroparesis. Treatment of chronic gastroparesis with prokinetic drugs and direct electrical stimulation by gastric pacemakers is only partly successful; severe cases require some form of nutritional support.

Gastric Volvulus

Gastric volvulus is most commonly seen when the stomach is displaced into the thorax through the diaphragmatic hiatus as a paraesophageal hernia. In severe cases, ischemic necrosis of the gastric mucosa occurs, leading to pain, hematemesis, and shock. Gastric mucosal biopsies show acute ischemic necrosis of the entire mucosa. In less severe cases, ischemia may produce a histologic picture resulting from a combination of focal necrosis and regenerative change, resembling changes seen in reactive gastritis.

Gastric Bezoars

Gastric bezoars are associated with pica, a psychiatric disease in which patients swallow foreign material. Pica, including nail-biting, is very common, but the occurrence of bezoars is due to ingestion of material that has difficulty passing through the stomach. The most common of these are fruit and vegetable fibers and hair, producing phytobezoars and trichobezoars (Fig. 4–7), respectively.

The following case shows that the pathologist rarely encounters unusual cases in which diagnostic acumen apart from surgical pathology is needed. A schizophrenic man was admitted with a history of hematemesis associated with swallowing coins (Fig. 4–8). Endoscopy revealed the stomach to be filled with coins with associated mucosal ulcers. When expectant

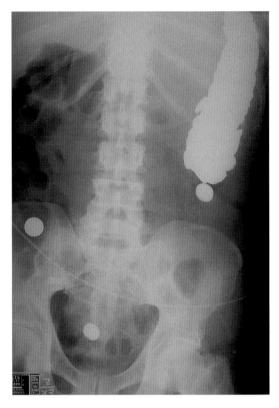

Figure 4–8. Plain roentgenogram of the abdomen showing a mass of coins in the stomach. A few coins have passed out of the stomach into the intestine.

treatment resulted in deterioration of the patient's general condition and the development of renal failure, gastrostomy was performed to remove the coins. Nearly 500 coins, mostly pennies, were recovered (Fig. 4–9). At the time of gastrostomy, a small piece of gastric wall was sent for pathologic examination. Histology showed reactive changes in the mucosa associated with an unusual degree of cytologic atypia of the lining epithelial cells (Fig. 4–10). The mucosal injury was initially thought to be caused by copper toxicity; however, upon investigation, it

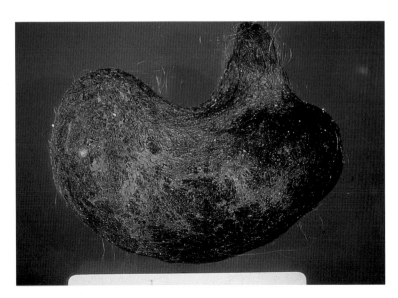

Figure 4–7. Trichobezoar of the stomach, composed of foreign material, including large amounts of hair.

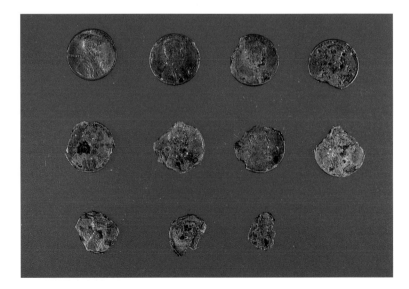

Figure 4–9. A selection of pennies from the nearly 500 coins removed from the stomach. Note that the pennies show varying degrees of corrosion due to gastric acid. The less eroded pennies predated 1981 when the U.S. Mint changed the composition of pennies from copper to predominantly zinc.

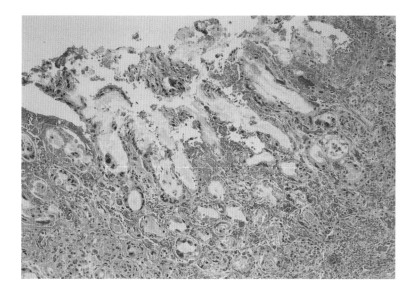

A

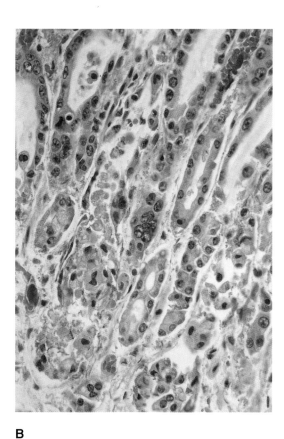

B

Figure 4–10. A: Gastric mucosa in patient with coin ingestion, showing reactive hyperplasia of the gastric mucosa. B: Higher power micrograph of part A, showing marked cytologic abnormality in the cells lining the foveolar region. The cells have enlarged, hyperchromatic nuclei with multinucleated forms.

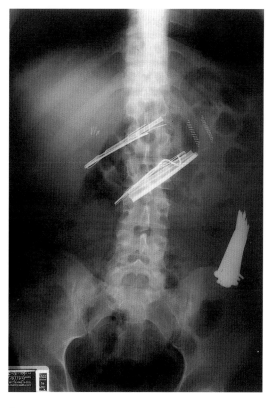

A

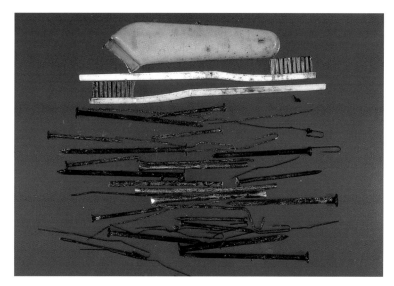

B

Figure 4–11. A: Plain roentgenogram of the abdomen showing a variety of ingested foreign material. The central opacities were in the stomach (see part B); the opacity on the left side of the abdomen is shown in Figure 4–12. B: Foreign material removed from the stomach at surgery, including nails, opened paperclips, two toothbrushes, and the handle of a urinal.

was learned that the U.S. Mint had changed the composition of the penny in the early 1980s from copper to predominantly zinc with a copper coating. Reexamination of the coins showed that all the pennies minted after 1981 showed evidence of erosion, whereas those before this date were intact, suggesting that those coins composed of zinc were more readily dissolved by gastric acid than the copper coins (Fig. 4–9). When the patient's serum zinc levels were examined, they were found to be greatly elevated, converting a case of coin bezoars to one of acute zinc poisoning.

A second case involved another psychotic male who swallowed a potpourri of objects (Fig. 4–11), among which were numerous 3-in. iron nails. The nails, unlike the coins in the previous case, were able to pass through the stomach into the small intestine, where they impacted and caused intestinal obstruction (Fig. 4–12).

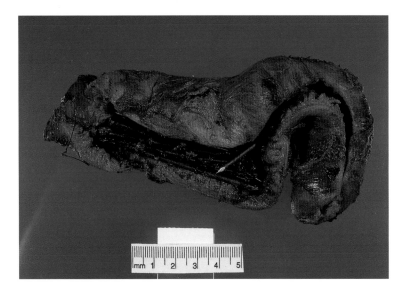

Figure 4–12. Small-bowel obstruction caused by impacted 3-in. nails.

Another unusual swallowed specimen that is not uncommon, particularly in areas of illicit drug trafficking, is heroin- and cocaine-filled condoms. These are swallowed by the carrier for transport across the U.S. border. These are encountered at autopsy, in cases where the condoms rupture in the intestine releasing lethal amounts of the drug, and in surgical pathology when the swallowed drugs are detected by the authorities.

Gastric Xanthelasma

Gastric xanthelasma is a common but clinically insignificant lesion, present in both normal stomachs and much more frequently, in patients who have had a partial gastrectomy. It is not associated with hyperlipidemia, and is believed to be related to bile reflux into the stomach, which is a source of cholesterol. They appear as small yellow spots on the mucosa on endoscopy and gross examination. Microscopically, the lesion shows a collection of foamy macrophages in the lamina propria beneath the surface epithelium (Fig. 4–13A). The cells are large, with small central nuclei. The only significance of this lesion is that it must be recognized as a benign lesion, differentiating it from signet ring cell carcinoma. Differentiation between the two is primarily by the morphologic features, but it can be confirmed by negative staining of the xanthelasma with digested periodic acid–Schiff (PAS) stain (Fig. 4–13B), mucicarmine, and keratin, as well as by positive staining with immunohistochemical markers for macrophages such as CD68.

Gastric Hemosiderosis

Patients ingesting large amounts of iron, usually as medication, may rarely show the presence of hemosiderin pigment in gastric epithelial cells (Fig. 4–14) and lamina propria macrophages. This is of little clinical significance and does not indicate that the patient suffers from hemochromatosis. The diagnosis of hemochromatosis must only be considered in a patient with clinical evidence of the disease.

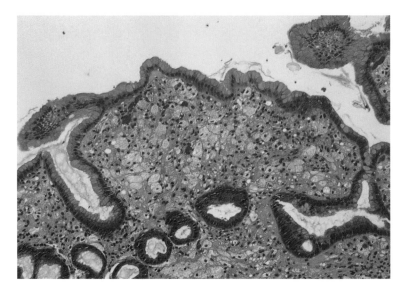

A

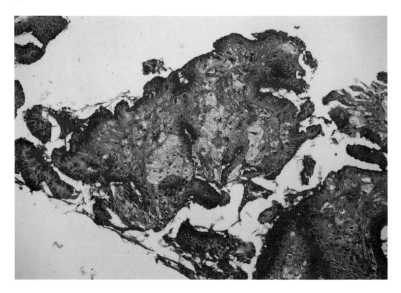

B

Figure 4–13. A: Gastric xanthelasma, showing a collection of foamy macrophages in the superficial gastric mucosal lamina propria. B: Gastric xanthelasma, periodic acid–Schiff (PAS) stain, showing negative staining of the lipid-containing foamy macrophages.

GASTRITIS

In the last decade, gastritis has evolved from a condition that was poorly understood to one with clear pathologic definitions and a rational method of diagnosis.[2] This progression resulted from the recognition of multiple etiologic factors, including *Helicobacter pylori* infection and nonsteroidal antiinflammatory drugs (NSAIDs) use, along with the cooperative effort of expert pathologists in the field.[2,3] The various terms used here have been defined precisely, and grading criteria for them have been established[2] (Table 4–1). Problems still exist in correlating the pathologic changes with the clinical and endoscopic findings and determining their clinical significance.[4] It has become clear, however, that certain morphologic types of gastritis are strongly associated with specific causal agents, resulting in an increas-

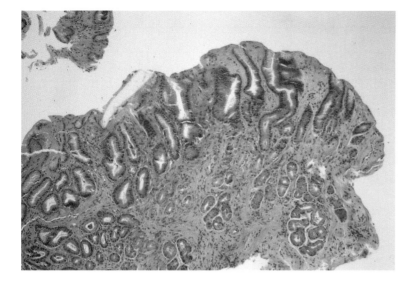

A

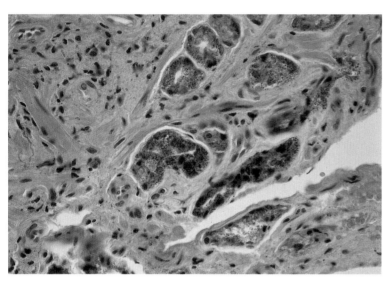

B

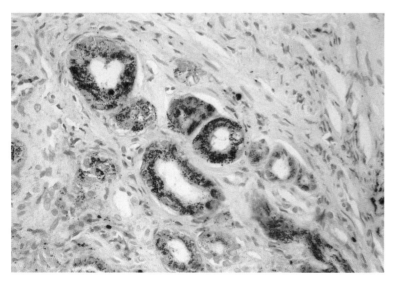

C

Figure 4–14. A: Gastric hemosiderosis, showing deposition of hemosiderin pigment in gastric mucosal epithelial cells. This patient gave a history of taking iron supplements and had no evidence of any disturbance in iron metabolism. B: Higher power micrograph of part A, showing hemosiderin in cells of gastric mucous glands. C: Gastric hemosiderosis, Prussian blue stain for iron.

ingly significant etiologic basis for the morphologic classification.

In gastritis the gastric mucosa is affected by two basic mechanisms:

1. Gastritis (see Table 4–1): Characterized by an inflammatory reaction, either acute or chronic, involving the gastric mucosa, most cases of gastritis are some form of chronic gastritis. Gastritis is caused by either an infection (eg, *Helicobacter pylori*) or an immunologic process (eg, autoimmune gastritis).
2. Reactive gastropathy (also called reactive gastritis): This condition results from an injury in which damage leads to an increased rate of loss of the surface epithelial cells. This induces a proliferation of the germinative foveolar neck cells in an attempt to compensate for the increased surface cell loss. If compensation fails, erosions occur (acute erosive gastritis). When compensation is successful, the surface remains intact. Evidence of increased foveolar proliferation can be recognized as elongation and serration of the foveolae and increased proliferative activity in the foveolar epithelial cells, which show reactive cytologic changes and increased mitotic activity. Erosions and reactive foveolar changes commonly coexist. Because inflammation is not the primary cause of this injury, "reactive gastropathy" is a more accurate term for this entity than reactive gastritis. Most cases of reactive gastropathy are caused by chemical injury from drugs, bile, and other toxic substances, leading to the alternative designation of chemical gastritis. A similar change occurs in mucosal ischemia, however, and for this reason, reactive gastropathy is the preferred term.[5]

The morphological classification of gastritis is based on topographic distribution of inflammation in the antrum and body. To properly classify gastritis, therefore, two labeled biopsy specimens should be taken. The first specimen should contain samples from the lesser and greater curvature from the antrum, 2–3 cm from the pylorus and from the incisura angularis. The incisura has the highest incidence of atrophy, intestinal metaplasia, and dysplasia.[6] The second specimen is taken from the gastric body 8 cm from the cardia at the lesser and greater curvature. In addition, any endoscopic lesions should be biopsied. The specimens should be submitted with pertinent clinical information, which must include endoscopic findings and a list of medications. Failure to provide clinical information frequently results in suboptimal pathologic interpretation of biopsies.

The routine use of special stains in gastric biopsies is not a universal practice. A routine stain for *Helicobacter pylori* is done in many laboratories, but it is adequate to carefully examine the hematoxylin and eosin (H&E)-stained slide and order special stains (Giemsa, Genta, or Steiner's silver stain) only when inflammation is present and *H. pylori* is not found. The vast majority of *H. pylori*-positive cases can be confidently diagnosed on the routine H&E section. Immunostains are available to demonstrate atypical coccoid forms of *H. pylori*,[7] but are rarely done. To demonstrate intestinal metaplasia, some laboratories perform a PAS–Alcian blue stain at pH 2.5. High-iron di-

TABLE 4–1. CLASSIFICATION OF GASTRITIS

Type of Gastritis	Defining Characteristics
Chronic Gastritis	Increased numbers of lymphocytes, plasma cells in lamina propria.
Autoimmune chronic atrophic gastritis	Corpus-predominant, with atrophy of parietal and chief cells; associated with autoimmunity and pernicious anemia.
Diffuse antral chronic gastritis	Antral-predominant nonatrophic chronic gastritis. Caused by *Helicobacter pylori* infection.
Multifocal chronic atrophic gastritis	Chronic gastritis characterized by multiple foci of atrophy and intestinal metaplasia throughout the stomach. *H. pylori* infection is very likely the major cause.
Reactive Gastropathy	Foveolar elongation and hyperplasia with smooth muscle proliferation.
NSAID gastropathy	
Bile reflux gastropathy	
Vascular gastropathies	
Special Morphologic Types of Gastritis	
Acute gastritis	True acute inflammation with neutrophils without significant chronic inflammation.
Acute erosive or hemorrhagic gastropathy	Acute mucosal injury characterized by erosion or lamina propria hemorrhage.
Lymphocytic gastritis	Infiltration of the surface epithelium and glands by >25 lymphocytes/100 epithelial cells.
Eosinophilic gastritis	Infiltration of mucosa by markedly increased numbers of eosinophils, with relative absence of other cells, also peripheral blood eosinophilia or allergic history.
Granulomatous gastritis	Presence of epithelioid granulomas.
Collagenous gastritis	Presence of a thick collagen band beneath the gastric surface epithelial basement membrane.
Hypertrophic gastritis (Ménétrier's disease)	
Special Etiologic Types of Gastritis	
Mycobacterial gastritis	
Gastric syphilis	
Cytomegalovirus gastritis	
Fungal gastritis	
Crohn's gastritis	

amine–PAS (HID–PAS) stain is useful for differentiating complete from incomplete intestinal metaplasia.

Chronic Gastritis

Chronic gastritis that does not fall within the special types of gastritis (see Table 4–1) is by far the most common pathologic process encountered in gastric biopsies. The mucosa commonly shows flattening of the rugal folds, sometimes with a fine nodularity (Fig. 4–15). It is defined by the presence of an increased number of lymphocytes and plasma cells in the lamina propria (Fig. 4–16A). Lymphoid follicles with reactive germinal centers are common (Fig. 4–16B). Sometimes, the plasma cells are very prominent with the cytoplasm distended by immunoglobulin (Russell bodies) (Fig. 4–16C, D). Eosinophils may also be present, but in much smaller numbers than is seen in eosinophilic gastritis. Chronic inflammation may be associated with the following changes:

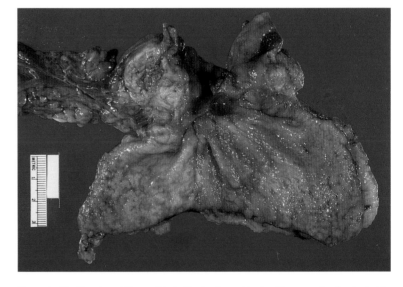

Figure 4–15. Chronic gastritis associated with a benign gastric ulcer. The mucosal surface has lost its rugal folds, appearing flat and granular.

1. Active inflammation (or, active chronic gastritis), which is characterized by the occurrence of congestion and edema of the mucosa (Fig. 4–17) and defined as the presence of neutrophils in the lamina propria or glands (Fig. 4–18).
2. Atrophy, which is a decrease in the normal glandular cells of the region. In antral mucosa, atrophy is defined by decreased numbers of mucous glands below the foveolae (Fig. 4–19); in oxyntic mucosa, atrophy is defined by decreased numbers of

parietal and chief cells in the glands (Fig. 4–20). The atrophic glands may disappear, causing thinning of the mucosa, or the parietal cells may be replaced by mucous cells (pseudopyloric metaplasia). Although the concept may be easy to understand, atrophy is difficult to establish, particularly in unoriented endoscopic biopsies.[8] Atrophy must be distinguished from simple displacement of glands by inflammation or lymphoid hyperplasia (Fig. 4–21). Visual analogues have been de-

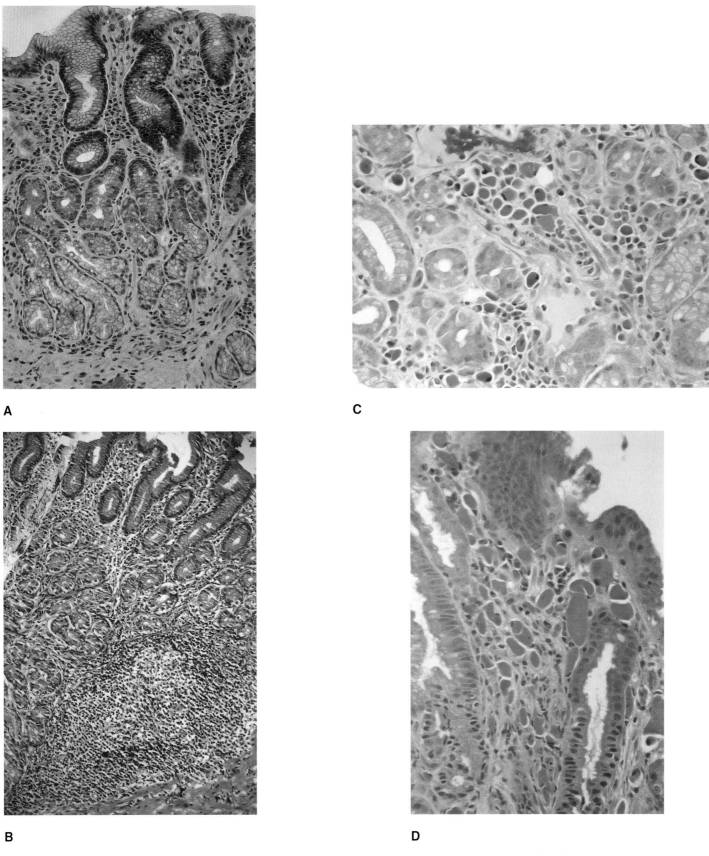

Figure 4–16. A. Chronic antral gastritis, showing an increase in the number of lymphocytes and plasma cells in the lamina propria. The inflammation is mild and involves the superficial mucosa around the foveolae more than the deep glandular region. The antral glands are normal without atrophy. B: Chronic gastritis, showing a reactive lymphoid follicle in the mucosa. C: Plasma cells distended with intracytoplasmic immunoglobulin (Russell bodies). This patient was evaluated for the possibility of a plasma cell disorder and was found to be negative. The immunoglobulins in the plasma cells had a polyclonal staining pattern for light chains. D: Large immunoglobulin deposits in the mucosa in chronic gastritis; same patient as in part C. It is difficult to determine whether the immunoglobulin occurs in markedly distended plasma cells or is extracellular.

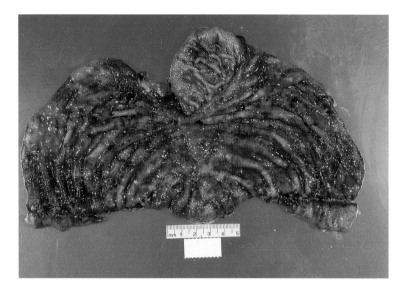

Figure 4–17. Active chronic gastritis, showing diffuse congestion and edema of the mucosa.

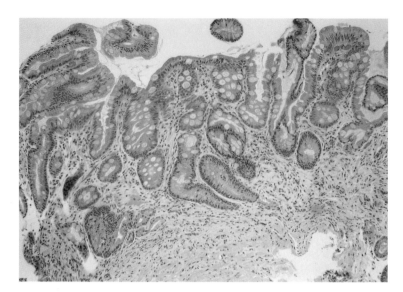

Figure 4–19. Atrophy of glands in the antral mucosa, showing a marked decrease in the number of mucous glands (a few mucous glands are present in the deep mucosa). Extensive intestinal metaplasia is evident as well as mild chronic inflammation.

veloped for evaluating atrophy that decrease the interobserver variation among experts, but these have not been evaluated in a general pathology setting. At present, atrophy is likely to be recognized only when the loss of glands is severe. The failure to recognize atrophy is not of great practical concern because it has no recognized association with any clinical feature and does not have an increased risk of malignancy, apart from its association with intestinal metaplasia.

3. Intestinal metaplasia, which is a replacement of the surface, foveolar, and glandular epithelial cells with intestinal goblet cells (Fig. 4–22). Intestinal metaplasia, when it is restricted to the surface and foveolar region, may occur without atrophy. Involvement of the glands, however, commonly indicates the presence of significant atrophy. Three types of intestinal

metaplasia are recognized, based on morphology and mucin type: type I, or complete intestinal metaplasia, consists of small intestinal type cells with brush borders and goblet cells with acidic mucin (positive with Alcian blue at pH 2.5), and has no increased risk of malignancy. Type II and type III, or incomplete-intestinal metaplasia, contain colonic-type goblet cells with either sialomucins (staining blue with HID–PAS stain) or sulfomucins (staining black with HID–PAS). Sulfomucin-positive type III intestinal metaplasia is associated with an increased risk of malignancy, but the degree and specificity of this risk is so small that it is of little practical value (see Chapter 5). In general pathology practice, special stains for intestinal metaplasia typing are rarely done because of the lack of clinical relevance.

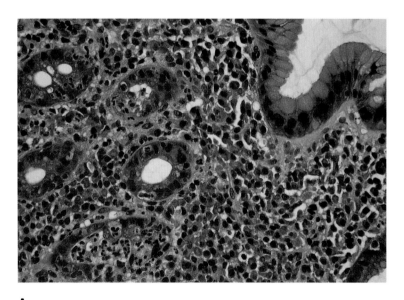

A

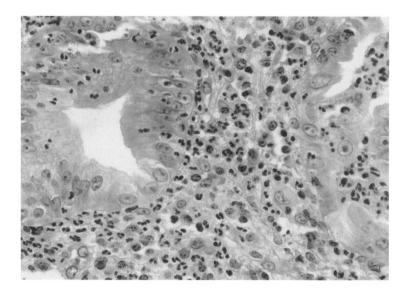

B

Figure 4–18. A: Active chronic antral gastritis, showing neutrophil infiltration of lamina propria and glands in addition to the background chronic inflammation. B: Active chronic gastritis, showing marked neutrophil infiltration of lamina propria and glands. The background chronic inflammation is minimal in this field.

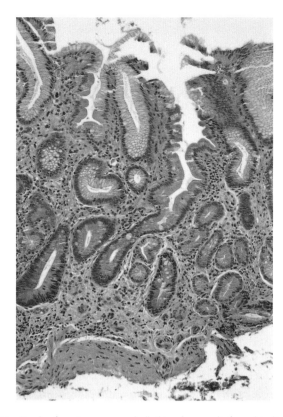

Figure 4–20. Atrophy of oxyntic mucosa, markedly thinned as a result of complete disappearance of parietal cells. The few residual glands are lined with mucous cells; the foveolar region is elongated and shows intestinal metaplasia. It is nearly impossible to identify this as oxyntic mucosa without knowing the location of the biopsy specimen.

Three topographically distinct types of chronic gastritis are recognized (Fig. 4–23)[9]: (1) Autoimmune chronic gastritis, involving oxyntic mucosa but sparing antral mucosa, is an autoimmune reaction directed at the parietal cells. This has also been called type A chronic gastritis. It is frequently associated with atrophy and rarely shows active inflammation. (2) Diffuse antral chronic gastritis (type B) is characterized by nonatrophic

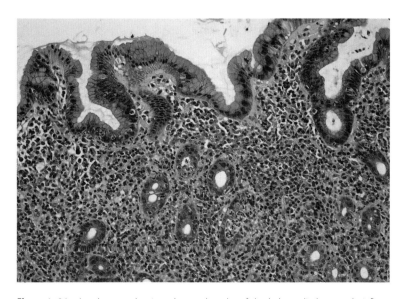

Figure 4–21. Antral mucosa showing a decreased number of glands due to displacement by inflammatory cells. This condition is difficult to distinguish from true atrophy, particularly in small endoscopic specimens.

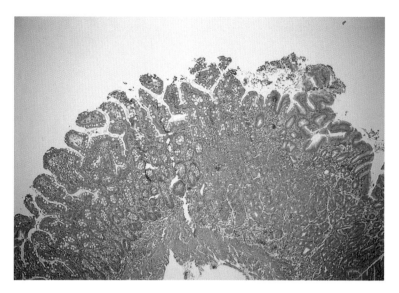

A

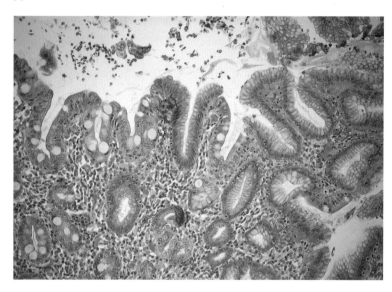

B

Figure 4–22. A: Intestinal metaplasia, showing the presence of goblet cells. Half of the mucosa shows almost complete intestinal metaplasia; the right half shows oxyntic mucosa. Chronic inflammation is evident, but the mucosal thickness is almost normal in the area of intestinal metaplasia. The presence of atrophy is difficult to evaluate. B: Intestinal metaplasia of the foveolar region and surface epithelium, contrasted with normal gastric foveolar and surface epithelium (on *right*). Chronic inflammation is evident.

active chronic inflammation involving predominantly the antral mucosa. The oxyntic mucosa may be involved but to a lesser extent than the antrum. (3) Multifocal chronic atrophic gastritis (type AB) begins at the incisura and involves the stomach diffusely, causing multifocal atrophy and intestinal metaplasia in the antral and oxyntic mucosae. Areas of atrophy and intestinal metaplasia commonly alternate with nonatrophic active chronic gastritis.

Diffuse antral gastritis and multifocal atrophic gastritis are both caused mainly by infection with *Helicobacter pylori* and are considered under the heading *H. pylori* gastritis.

In routine clinical practice, sampling at endoscopy rarely permits the detailed topographic analysis that is the basis of

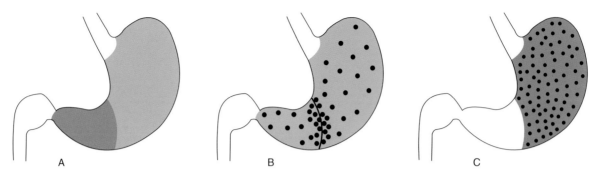

Figure 4–23. Topographic types of chronic gastritis. A: Diffuse antral chronic gastritis with predominant antral involvement and lesser degree of involvement of oxyntic mucosa. B: Multifocal chronic atrophic gastritis which begins at the incisura and involves the whole stomach with a patchy distribution of atrophy. C: Antral-sparing corporal chronic atrophic gastritis typical of autoimmune chronic gastritis.

classifying gastritis. When a single specimen is provided, the pathologist should provide information relating to the severity of chronic inflammation and the presence or absence of active inflammation, atrophy, intestinal metaplasia, and lymphoid hyperplasia. If significant inflammation occurs and *Helicobacter pylori* is not seen in routine sections, a special stain (eg, Giemsa, Genta) should be examined to exclude infection with this organism.

Autoimmune Chronic Gastritis

Autoimmune chronic gastritis (diffuse atrophic corporal gastritis; type A chronic gastritis) is a well-recognized clinicopatho-

logic entity that occurs worldwide, with a high frequency in northern Europe. It results from an autoimmune destruction of parietal cells in gastric oxyntic mucosa. Many different autoantibodies have been reported in serum and gastric juice, with activity directed against parietal cells or intrinsic factor. Destruction of the parietal cells results in hypochlorhydria. Clinical features relate to the failure of vitamin B_{12} absorption caused by the lack of intrinsic factor. Severe megaloblastic anemia and neurologic abnormalities, such as peripheral neuropathy and subacute combined degeneration of the spinal cord, can occur.

The oxyntic mucosa of the body and fundus of the stomach is selectively affected, with the pyloric antrum being spared. This "antral-sparing, body-predominant" pattern of chronic

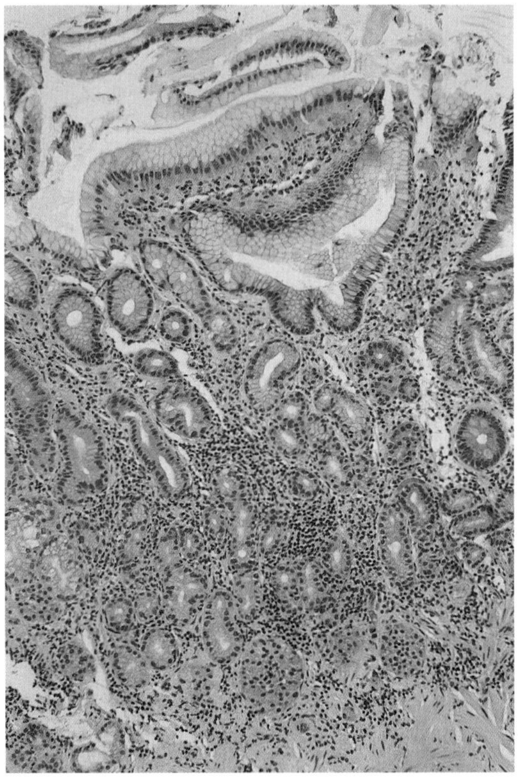

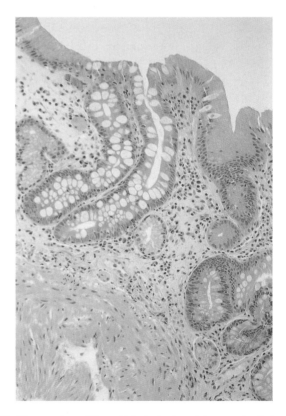

Figure 4–24. Biopsy sample from gastric body showing autoimmune chronic atrophic gastritis. Diffuse inflammation is evident predominantly in the deep mucosa, with lymphocytes and plasma cells present around glands. The glands are lined by mucous cells and show almost complete absence of parietal cells. Note the micronodules of neuroendocrine cells in the deep mucosa.

Figure 4–25. Biopsy specimen of the gastric body showing autoimmune chronic atrophic gastritis. Characterized by extreme thinning of the mucosa due to complete loss of parietal cell-containing glands, this condition is associated with intestinal metaplasia of the foveolar region. Note: The degree of chronic inflammation is minimal in this end-stage of the disease.

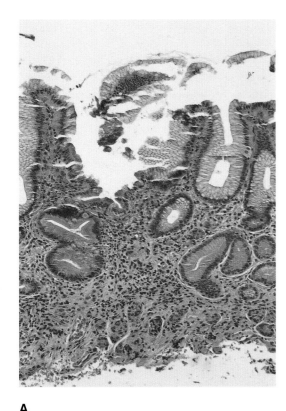

A

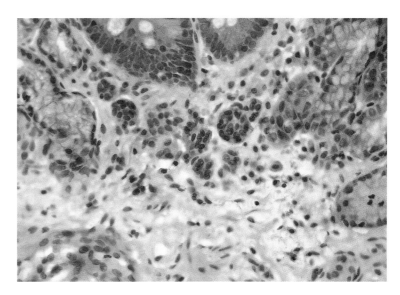

B

Figure 4–26. A: Gastric body biopsy specimen showing marked atrophy, chronic inflammation, absence of parietal cells, and presence of small rounded nests of cells in the deep mucosa, representing neuroendocrine cell hyperplasia. B: Neuroendocrine cell hyperplasia in autoimmune chronic atrophic gastritis, showing nests of small cells in the deep mucosa.

gastritis should always prompt clinical testing for autoimmune gastritis, particularly when active inflammation and *Helicobacter pylori* infection are absent. The pattern is not specific however; up to 14% of patients with *Helicobacter pylori* gastritis have a corpus-predominant pattern of gastritis.[10]

The involved oxyntic mucosa is diffusely affected and shows increased numbers of lymphocytes and plasma cells (Fig. 4–24). The inflammation involves the deep mucosa around the gastric glands more severely than in the superficial foveolar region.[11] The parietal cell numbers are markedly decreased in the well-established case and frequently completely absent (Figs.

4–24 and 4–25). The gastric glands become replaced by mucous cells, resembling antral mucosa ("pseudopyloric metaplasia") (see Fig. 4–24). Intestinal metaplasia is common, occurring in the surface, foveolar, and glandular epithelium (see Fig. 4–25). Epithelial dysplasia occurs in the atrophic mucosa, classified as low and high grade by criteria identical to those used for Barrett's esophagus and ulcerative colitis. The risk of adenocarcinoma complicating autoimmune atrophic gastritis is approximately 0.5% per year; at 20 years, 10% of patients are predicted to have developed adenocarcinoma.[4]

The mucosa of autoimmune chronic atrophic gastritis is

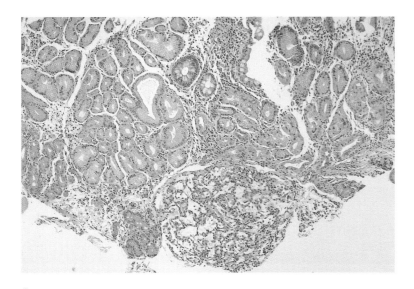

A

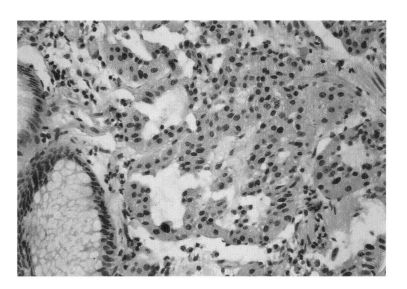

B

Figure 4–27. A: Microcarcinoid tumor in autoimmune chronic atrophic gastritis. The mucosa contains glands composed mainly of mucous cells with scattered residual parietal cells. B: Carcinoid tumor in autoimmune atrophic gastritis, showing small uniform cells with microacinar architecture.

characterized by a paucity of neutrophils. The lack of active inflammation is a feature at all stages of the disease, unlike in type B gastritis in which the early phase almost always shows neutrophil infiltration. *Helicobacter pylori* is rarely found, suggesting that an acid environment is necessary for optimal growth of this organism. Absence of *Helicobacter pylori,* however, is not very helpful in diagnosis because this organism is rarely seen when intestinal metaplasia is extensive, irrespective of etiology.

The achlorhydria stimulates antral G cells to produce increased amounts of gastrin, elevating serum gastrin levels. The gastrin excess, in turn, stimulates the enterochromaffin-like (ECL) cells of the oxyntic mucosa, which are normally situated at the basal region of the glands, resulting in ECL cell hyperplasia (Fig. 4–26). ECL hyperplasia, when severe, forms multiple small nodules that are visible on endoscopy. Biopsy shows multiple microcarcinoid tumors (Fig. 4–27A); more rarely, larger carcinoid tumors occur (Fig. 4–27B) (see Chapter 5). Cases in which the initial diagnosis of pernicious anemia is made by the finding of multiple microcarcinoids in a gastric biopsy are not unusual.

To summarize, the biopsy features that may suggest a diagnosis of autoimmune chronic atrophic gastritis in a patient not known to have this disease include: (1) predominant involvement of oxyntic mucosa of body and fundus, with sparing of the antrum; (2) marked atrophy, with severe and diffuse loss of parietal cells in the glands which show prepyloric and intestinal metaplasia; (3) absence of neutrophils and *Helicobacter pylori;* and (4) ECL cell hyperplasia, microcarcinoids, and larger carcinoid tumors.

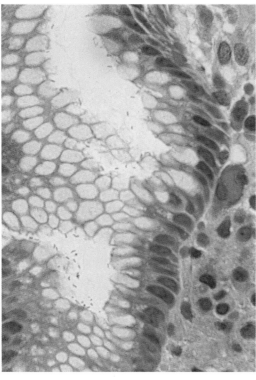

A

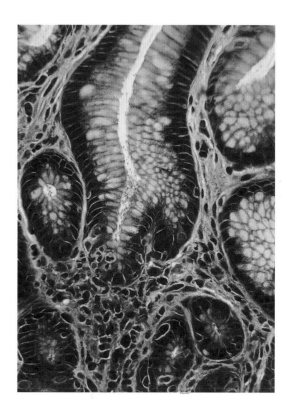

B

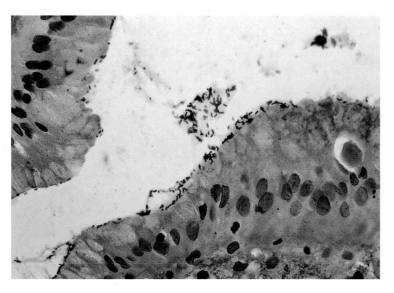

C

Figure 4–28. A: *Helicobacter pylori* in gastric mucosa, H&E stain, showing the curved rod-shaped organisms on the surface of the epithelial cells. B: *Helicobacter pylori,* Giemsa-stained section, showing the blue staining of the organisms. C: *Helicobacter pylori,* Genta's silver stain, showing the black staining of the organisms. The bacteria appear thicker in the Genta stain.

Helicobacter Pylori Gastritis

Helicobacter pylori is a common pathogen worldwide. The infection is most common in lower socioeconomic levels of the population and is more common in males. A large number of patients who harbor *H. pylori* and have evidence of chronic gastritis are asymptomatic.[12] *Helicobacter pylori* grows on the surface of the epithelial cells lining the surface and foveolar region and are seen in biopsies as short curved rods (Fig. 4–28A). The pyloric antral mucosa is the preferred site of infection, and it is unusual for *H. pylori* infection to spare the antrum.[13]

In most cases, the organisms can be seen in H&E sections, even when they are present in small numbers. Careful examination of the section for organisms is more important than special stains, which only slightly increase the yield of positive results.[4] The ease of finding the organism correlates with the number of neutrophils present. When significant chronic gastritis is present and *H. pylori* is not identified, it is advisable to perform any one of several special stains that facilitate identification of the organism. These include Giemsa (Fig. 4–28B), in which organisms appear blue, or any one of several silver stains, such as Steiner, Dieterle, Warthin-Starry, and Genta (Fig. 4–28C) in which organisms appear black.

Helicobacter pylori infection can also be diagnosed by the rapid urease test. The organism produces a potent urease, which hydrolyses urea to release ammonia; the consequent alkalinity can be detected by a pH indicator system. The CLO test is the most widely used urease test and has been shown to have a specificity of nearly 100% and a sensitivity of 80–85%. The test depends on the potency of *H. pylori* urease, which is greater than most other urease-producing bacteria. The test is performed in the endoscopy room immediately after the biopsy has been taken and can give a positive result in 30 min to 2 h.

Helicobacter pylori gastritis manifests as two distinctive topographic forms of chronic gastritis. Whether diffuse antral gastritis represents an earlier stage of multifocal atrophic gastritis is debatable, but the association of these two types of gastritis with different complications suggests that they represent two different forms of disease. It has been suggested that patients with a greater parietal cell mass and higher acid output levels are predisposed to developing diffuse antral gastritis, whereas those with a lower acid output are predisposed to developing multifocal atrophic gastritis.[13] Progressive atrophy in the latter group creates a vicious cycle by further decreasing acid output and facilitating infection of the body.

In addition to chronic gastritis, *Helicobacter pylori* infection of the stomach is associated with the following diseases: (1) gastric adenocarcinoma, particularly of the intestinal type, but also of the diffuse type (see Chapter 5); (2) malignant lymphoma arising in mucosal-associated lymphoid tissue (see Chapter 15); (3) duodenal ulcer and nonulcer dyspepsia (see Chapter 6); (4) gastric ulcer.

Diffuse Antral Chronic Gastritis.
Diffuse antral chronic gastritis (type B chronic gastritis) is most strongly associated with *Helicobacter pylori* infection.[9] Active inflammation is frequently ev-

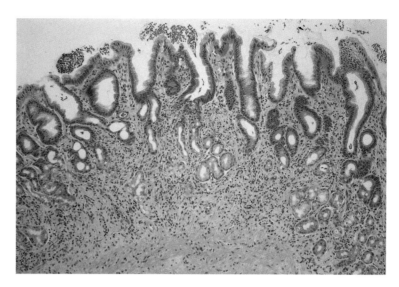

Figure 4–29. Active chronic antral gastritis. This was positive for *Helicobacter pylori.*

ident as well as hyperplastic lymphoid follicles (Fig. 4–29), but severe atrophy or extensive intestinal metaplasia are rare. The body may be involved but usually to a much lesser extent than the antrum; in most cases, the body shows a superficial inflammation restricted to the foveolar region, with sparing of the deep glandular zone (Fig. 4–30). Diffuse antral gastritis tends to be associated with peptic duodenitis and chronic peptic ulcers in the duodenum and prepyloric region. The risk of gastric adenocarcinoma is low.

Multifocal Chronic Atrophic Gastritis.
Multifocal chronic atrophic gastritis (type AB chronic gastritis or type B chronic atrophic gastritis) has an association with *H. pylori* infection that is not as strong as that for diffuse antral chronic gastritis, and there is evidence that dietary factors may also be involved.[14] It typically begins at the incisura and extends into both the antrum and the body in a radial manner (Fig. 4–23). Initially an active chronic gastritis, it tends to cause progressive atrophy of the antral mu-

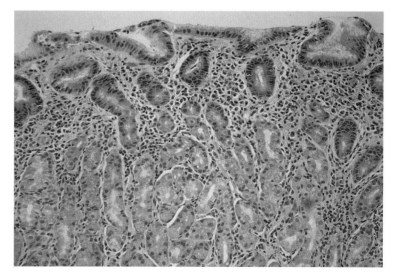

Figure 4–30. Involvement of oxyntic mucosa of the gastric body in diffuse antral gastritis, showing chronic inflammation restricted to the superficial foveolar region of the mucosa. This was positive for *Helicobacter pylori.*

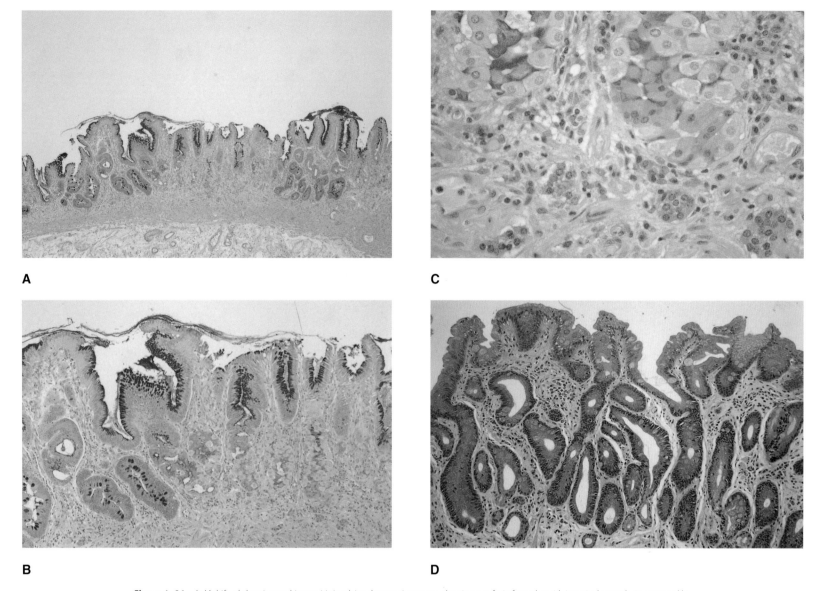

A

B

C

D

Figure 4–31. A: Multifocal chronic atrophic gastritis involving the oxyntic mucosa, showing two foci of atrophy with intestinal metaplasia separated by nonatrophic oxyntic mucosa (digested PAS stain). This was positive for *H. pylori*. B: Higher power micrograph of part A, showing atrophic mucosa adjacent to nonatrophic mucosa. C: Micronodular neuroendocrine cell hyperplasia in multifocal chronic atrophic gastritis of the oxyntic mucosa. D: Intestinal metaplasia and low-grade epithelial dysplasia in multifocal chronic atrophic gastritis.

cous glands and body oxyntic glands. Atrophy is commonly associated with extensive intestinal metaplasia (Fig. 4–31). In the early cases without atrophy and intestinal metaplasia, *H. pylori* is present; in cases with extensive intestinal metaplasia, this organism is often difficult to identify in biopsies. Multifocal chronic atrophic gastritis can be distinguished from autoimmune chronic atrophic gastritis by the fact that the antrum is commonly involved, the oxyntic gland atrophy is patchy, and active inflammation and *H. pylori* infection are frequent. When the antrum is spared and extensive intestinal metaplasia is present the distinction can be more difficult.

Multifocal chronic atrophic gastritis is also associated with gastric ulcers and is most at risk for developing gastric epithelial dysplasia (see Fig. 4–31D) and adenocarcinoma. With this condition patients also develop hypochlorhydria to an extent that depends on the degree of oxyntic gland atrophy. Hypochlorhydria stimulates gastrin production, which in turn causes ECL cell hyperplasia in the oxyntic mucosa. The ECL cells may form small aggregates in the glands and basal lamina propria, but have not been described to form microcarcinoid tumors (see Chapter 5).

Cases of multifocal chronic atrophic gastritis in which there is no evidence, either histologically or clinically, of *H. pylori* infection represent a problem. It is believed that many of these cases represent *H. pylori* infection in which the organisms can no longer be demonstrated because of atrophy and intestinal metaplasia. This viewpoint is favored by the finding that many of these patients have positive serologic tests for *H. pylori*.[15] Another cause of atrophic corporal gastritis that has recently become more common, diagnosed primarily by history, is that induced by long-term proton pump inhibitor (omeprazole) therapy. Omeprazole results in a decrease in the parietal cell mass associated with neuroendocrine hyperplasia and mild chronic inflammation, resembling multifocal chronic atrophic gastritis.

Benign Gastric Ulcer. Benign gastric ulcers usually complicate multifocal chronic atrophic gastritis and can occur in any part of the stomach, with the highest incidence in the region of the incisura angularis on the lesser curvature. The incidence of gastric ulcers is high, but modern acid suppressive agents, such as proton pump inhibitors, are highly effective treatment. Nowadays it is very uncommon to see a gastric resection for benign ulcer disease, unlike 20 years ago when peptic ulcer disease was the most common indication for gastrectomy. Benign gastric ulcers may be of varying size from small (Fig. 4–32) to very large (Fig. 4–33), solitary or multiple, and shallow or very deep (Figs. 4–32 and 33). They appear as punched-out ulcers with a necrotic floor and a base composed of granulation tissue and fibrosis. In deep ulcers, the base extends deep into the muscle wall; on occasion, they can extend through the gastric wall into adjacent organs such as the pancreas (penetrating gastric ulcer). The mucosal edge surrounding the ulcer is usually flat, but may show a slight elevation due to edema and inflammation. Fibrosis associated with the ulcer commonly causes the gastric folds to appear to radiate outward from the ulcer. Although the differences between benign and malignant gastric ulcers are well recognized, even gastric ulcers with endoscopic and radiologic features typical for benign ulcers can, in actuality, be malignant. Biopsy is therefore mandatory when a gastric ulcer is found at endoscopy. Specimens should be taken from the central part and edge of the ulcer. The ulcer base is composed of necrotic, inflamed debris or granulation tissue (Fig. 4–34A); the edge of the ulcer frequently shows regenerative glands distorted by fibrosis, sometimes superficially resembling adenocarcinoma (see Chapter 5). Gastric ulcers may present with complications such as hemorrhage and perforation (see Fig. 4–34B); most of these can be managed without surgical resection.

At present, because of the rarity of surgical resections for benign gastric ulcers, the possibility of unusual pathology must be considered when a gastrectomy specimen is received for a

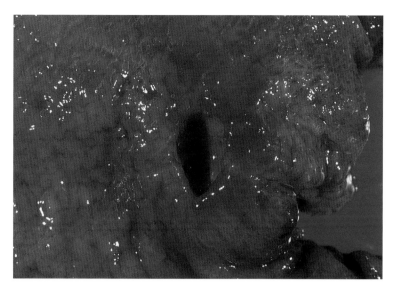

A

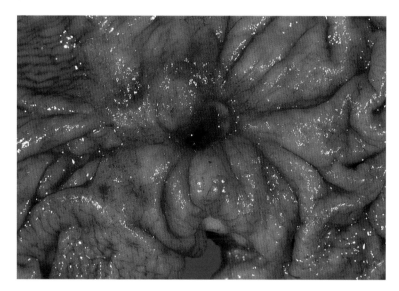

B

Figure 4–33. A: Chronic gastric ulcer complicating multifocal chronic atrophic gastritis. Note the punched-out appearance of the benign ulcer surrounded by atrophic, slightly granular gastric mucosa. B: Benign gastric ulcer. Note the gastric folds radiating out from the ulcer's edge; this is the result of fibrosis associated with the ulcer. The mucosa at the ulcer's edge is slightly raised due to edema. The ulcer has the typical punched-out appearance.

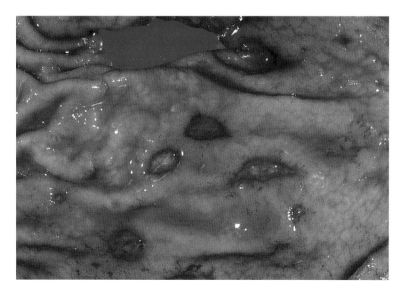

Figure 4–32. Chronic gastritis with multiple small benign gastric ulcers.

nonhealing gastric ulcer. A recent case of a 62-year-old patient who had a partial gastrectomy for a benign ulcer illustrates this point well. The specimen showed a benign gastric ulcer with evidence of hemorrhage in the wall. Microscopic examination showed a necrotizing vasculitis affecting small and medium-size arteries in the submucosa and muscle wall (Fig. 4–35). These vessels showed fibrinoid necrosis of the media, marked acute and chronic inflammation of the vessel wall, and focally ruptured microaneurysms. The histologic features suggested polyarteritis nodosa. The patient, while being evaluated for evidence of systemic vasculitis, had a sudden and fatal intracerebral hemorrhage, emphasizing the need for rapid diagnosis in such cases.

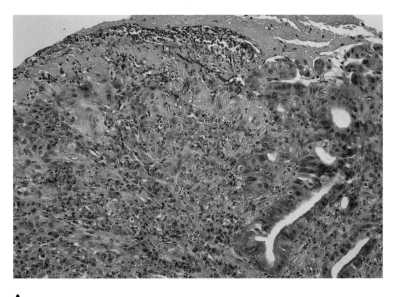

A

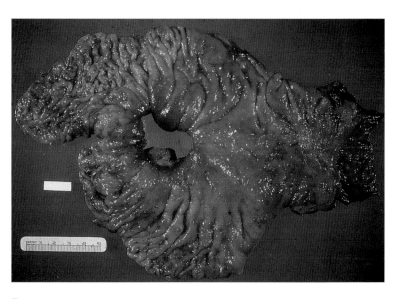

B

Figure 4–34. A: Biopsy specimen of chronic gastric ulcer, showing a necrotic base with underlying inflamed granulation tissue. The edge of the ulcer shows distorted glands with marked regenerative cytologic atypia. B: Perforated benign gastric ulcer.

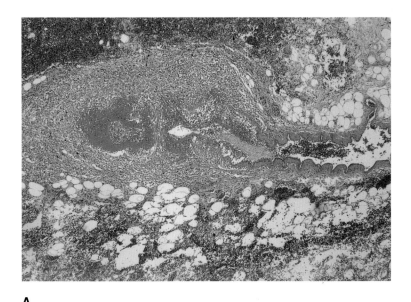

A

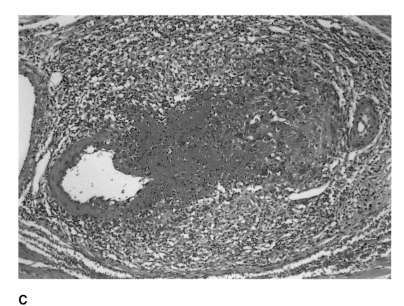

C

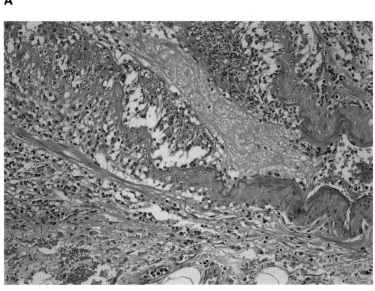

B

Figure 4–35. A: Vasculitis in the gastric submucosa in a benign gastric ulcer. The vessel shown is a medium-size artery, which is partially involved. The involved end of the artery shows marked inflammation in and around the vessel wall, microaneurysm formation, and rupture with evidence of perivascular hemorrhage. B: Higher power micrograph of part A, showing interphase between the normal and inflamed part of the artery. In the area of vasculitis, the internal elastic lamina and media are disrupted, and the full thickness of the vessel wall is infiltrated by acute and chronic inflammatory cells. C: Another affected artery in the muscle wall of the stomach, showing necrotizing vasculitis involving part of the vessel circumference, with microaneurysm formation and rupture associated with marked acute and chronic inflammation.

Reactive Gastropathy

Reactive gastropathy (also known as reactive gastritis or chemical gastritis) involves all parts of the stomach, may be either diffuse or focal, and may be associated with erosions. It is characterized by elongation and tortuosity of the foveolae, typically with serrated lumina (Fig. 4–36). The epithelial cells lining the foveolae and surface commonly show mucin depletion and reactive cytologic changes (Fig. 4–37). The foveolar abnormality is associated with lamina propria congestion and smooth muscle proliferation (Fig. 4–36B). Smooth muscle, which is derived from the muscularis mucosae, is seen as spindle cells with abundant eosinophilic cytoplasm in the mucosa. These are commonly seen perpendicular to the muscularis mucosae between the gastric glands, and can extend up to the mucosal surface. When cut in cross section, they may appear as rounded cells with eosinophilic cytoplasm.

Inflammation is not a feature of reactive gastropathy. Usually, a few lymphocytes and plasma cells are present. Reactive gastropathy superimposed on a preexisting chronic gastritis should be considered when significant active chronic inflammation coexists with reactive gastropathy (Fig. 4–38). In these cases, staining for *Helicobacter pylori* should be done. The simultaneous presence of chronic gastritis and reactive gastropathy is not surprising when one considers the frequency of *H. pylori* infection and use of nonsteroidal antiinflammatory agents (NSAIDs). *Helicobacter pylori* gastritis and NSAID gastropathy are independent injurious agents for the gastric mucosa; the presence of *H. pylori* gastritis does not represent a risk factor for NSAID gastropathy.[16]

Although intestinal metaplasia is sometimes present in the surface and foveolar region in reactive gastropathy, it is believed to be only a transient intestinal metaplasia that occurs during the healing phase of injury. There is no association between reactive gastropathy and gastric adenocarcinoma.

NSAID Gastropathy

Reactive gastropathy is most frequently caused by drugs, particularly NSAIDs. Commonly associated with acute erosive gastropathy (see later section), NSAID-associated gastropathy results from inhibition of prostaglandin synthesis in the gastric mucosa, which contributes to mucosal resistance to acid.[16] NSAID gastropathy is more common with the following risk factors:

1. Use of older NSAIDs such as, in order of decreasing gastric toxicity, piroxicam, naproxen, sulindac, indomethacin, diclofenac, and ibuprofen. Newer NSAIDs such as nabumetone, oxaprocin, and etodolic acid have a much lower gastric toxicity.
2. Increasing age, with individuals older than 60 years of age having the highest risk.
3. Female sex.
4. Concurrent use of other ulcerogenic substances such as corticosteroids and anticoagulants.[16]

NSAID gastropathy most commonly manifests as dyspepsia and epigastric pain, but serious consequences such as hemorrhage, chronic peptic ulcers, and perforation can also occur. NSAID gastropathy may occur within the first few weeks of initiating treatment, but may also be seen with long-term use.

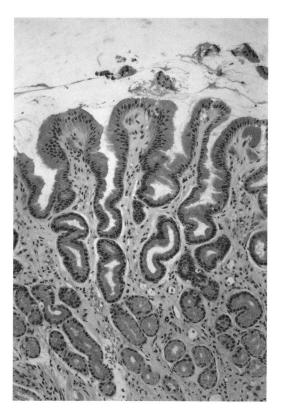

A

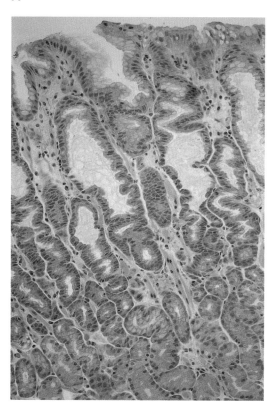

B

Figure 4–36. A: Mild reactive gastropathy, showing mild elongation and serration of foveolar region. Note the absence of significant inflammation. B: Hyperplastic, serrated foveolar region in a more severe degree of reactive gastropathy. Note the absence of inflammation and perpendicular smooth muscle fibers in the lamina propria.

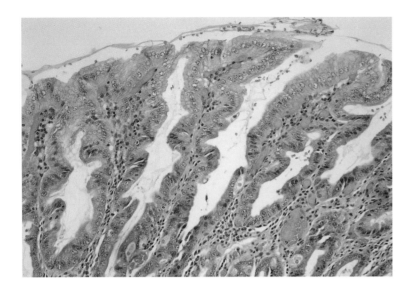

Figure 4–37. Reactive gastropathy showing reactive atypia in foveolar cells, characterized by mucin depletion, increased nuclear-to-cytoplasmic (N:C) ratio, and nuclear enlargement with prominent nucleoli.

Bile Reflux Gastropathy

Reactive gastropathy may also complicate excessive bile reflux ("bile reflux gastritis"). Bile reflux gastropathy occurs mainly after Billroth I partial gastrectomy with or without gastrojejunostomy. Although duodenogastric reflux occurs frequently in patients without prior surgery, the etiologic relationship of bile reflux to morphologic changes in gastric mucosa has not yet been clearly established. Bile reflux gastropathy is characterized by foveolar elongation and hyperplasia and smooth muscle proliferation.[17] Inflammation is usually mild, and erosions are not common.

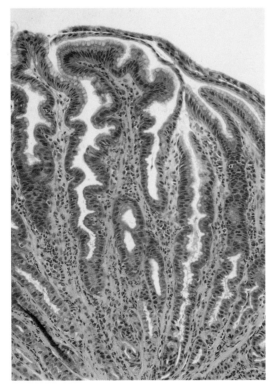

Figure 4–38. Reactive gastropathy associated with active chronic gastritis. This patient gave a history of NSAID use and was positive for *Helicobacter pylori*.

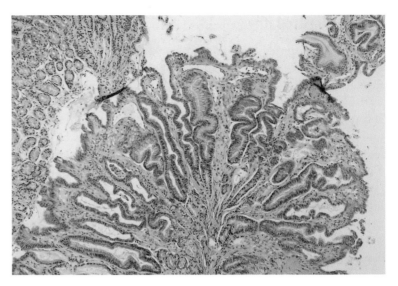

A

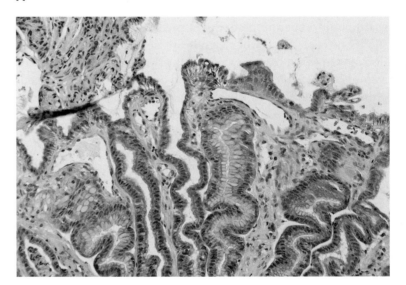

B

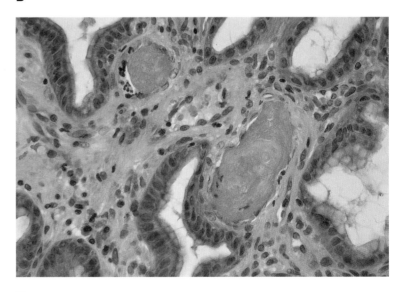

C

Figure 4–39. A: Gastric antral vascular ectasia, showing reactive foveolar changes associated with marked vascular ectasia in superficial lamina propria. B: Higher power micrograph of part A, showing marked ectasia of superficial lamina propria vessels. C: Fibrin thrombi in ectatic blood vessel in gastric antral vascular ectasia.

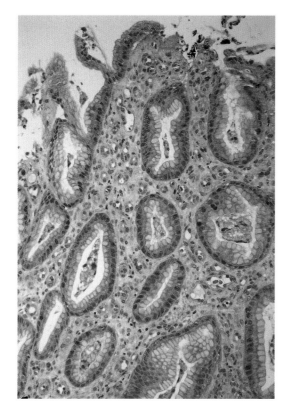

A

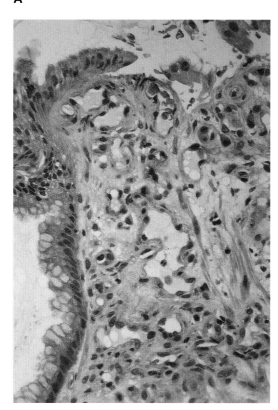

B

Figure 4–40. A: Portal hypertensive gastropathy in a patient with cirrhosis of the liver. The mucosa shows reactive changes and congestion, with many prominent vascular spaces in the lamina propria. B: Reactive gastropathy in portal hypertension, showing an increased number of vascular spaces in the superficial lamina propria.

Vascular Gastropathies

Reactive gastropathy also occurs in vascular lesions of the stomach, characterized by abnormalities in the mucosal blood vessels associated with reactive epithelial changes and minimal inflammation. All these conditions are associated with gastric bleeding, which may be severe enough to cause hematemesis and melena, or be occult, resulting in anemia.

Three entities are recognized within this category:

1. Gastric antral vascular ectasia (GAVE), which is characterized by fibromuscular hyperplasia of the lamina propria, reactive foveolar changes (Fig. 4–39A), and the presence of numerous markedly dilated mucosal capillaries in the antrum (Fig. 4–39B). Some of these capillaries show fibrin thrombi, a feature that is almost diagnostic for GAVE (Fig. 4–39C). GAVE is associated with a typical endoscopic appearance, which is known as "watermelon stomach" because of the linear streaks produced by the dilated blood vessels. GAVE is associated with autoimmune diseases. Cases associated with bleeding may need treatment, either endoscopic laser coagulation or, in more difficult cases, antrectomy.

2. Portal hypertensive gastropathy. This is a common cause of upper GI bleeding in patients with portal hypertension, which must be distinguished from the more severe esophageal variceal bleeding that also occurs in this population. The histologic features, which include reactive foveolar hyperplasia, smooth muscle proliferation, and marked vascular dilatation, particularly involving the proximal stomach, are nonspecific (Fig. 4–40).

3. Hepatic arterial chemotherapy may cause a reactive gastropathy associated with vascular ectasia. The chemotherapy may cause a reactive gastropathy associated with vascular ectasia. The chemotherapeutic agents act directly on gastric epithelial cells, resulting in focal necrosis, regenerative proliferation, and cytologic atypia. Very rarely, when collagen-based drug systems are used to deliver chemotherapeutic

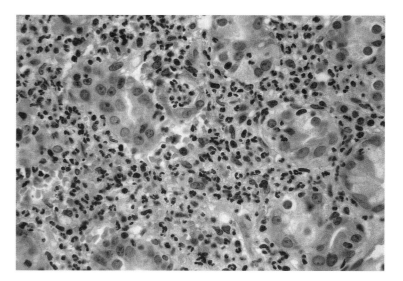

Figure 4–41. Acute gastritis, characterized by numerous neutrophils in the lamina propria and glands.

agents into the hepatic artery, these substances may be visible in the small blood vessels of the mucosa.

Specific Morphologic Types of Gastritis

Acute Gastritis

Acute gastritis is rare. It is characterized by the presence of neutrophils in the lamina propria and glands in the absence of significant chronic inflammation (Fig. 4–41). Acute gastritis is believed to occur in the acute phase of the initial infection with *H. pylori* characterized by a severe neutrophilic infiltration of the surface and foveolar epithelial cells with pit abscesses. Marked epithelial cell degeneration and reactive changes are present.[18] Acute *H. pylori* gastritis is rarely encountered at biopsy; in most patients, endoscopy is performed after the infection has been established, at which time features of chronic gastritis are evident.

Acute gastritis may also very rarely occur with acute pyogenic bacteria. The organisms cause a rapidly spreading acute suppurative and necrotizing inflammation centered in the submucosa, accompanied by intramural abscess formation (acute phlegmonous gastritis).[19] This form of gastritis is associated with severe bacteremia and is usually rapidly fatal. Most cases are diagnosed at autopsy. Biopsy specimens may not be diagnostic because the inflammation is centered in the submucosa and muscularis externa, with relative sparing of the mucosa.

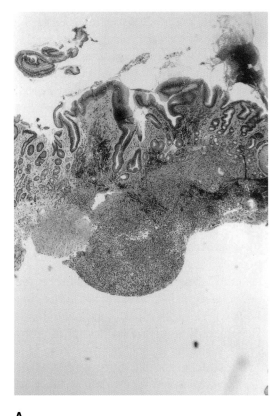

A

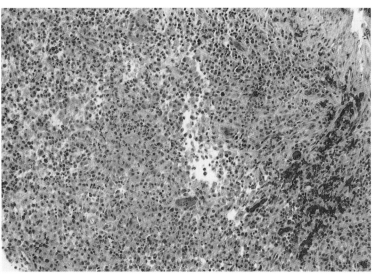

B

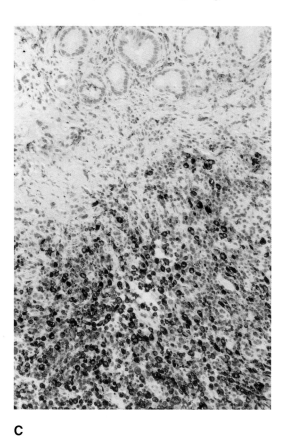

C

Figure 4–42. A: Unusual small rounded collection of cells in the deep mucosa of gastric biopsy specimen, with mild changes in the overlying intact mucosa. B: Higher power micrograph of part A, showing admixture of neutrophils and larger histiocyte-like cells, suggesting a mucosal microabscess. This specimen was *H. pylori*-negative, and the patient had no significant gastric pathology in a repeat biopsy 3 months later. C: Immunoperoxidase stain for CD68, a histiocyte marker, of the lesion shown in part A, confirming that the larger cells are histiocytes. Stain for cytokeratin was negative.

Rarely, small mucosal abscesses may be seen in the deep mucosa with an overlying intact mucosa (Fig. 4–42A), characterized by a focal accumulation of neutrophils and macrophages (Fig. 4–42B, C).

Acute Erosive, or Hemorrhagic, Gastropathy

Acute erosive gastropathy is a common form of acute gastric injury resulting from ingestion of a variety of chemicals, including NSAIDs, alcohol, corticosteroids, and corrosive substances (Figs. 4–43 and 4–44). Any cause of severe stress and shock associated with gastric hypoperfusion, most commonly that associated with major surgery, severe burns, sepsis, hypothermia, and myocardial infarction, can also cause acute erosive gastropathy. The mucosa shows multiple erosions throughout the stomach and duodenum with a tendency to involve the antrum maximally. The erosions are superficial, usually measure 2–10 mm, and are commonly associated with bleeding, which can be severe and life-threatening. Bleeding occurring from multiple erosions presents as an oozing of blood from the entire mucosa and can be difficult to control. Erosions differ from ulcers in that only part of the mucosal thickness is involved; ulcers involve the entire mucosa, including the muscularis mucosae.

Microscopically, erosions are characterized by denudation of the surface epithelium, which is replaced by a necrotic exudate (Fig. 4–45). Lamina propria hemorrhage is present. Inflammation is initially absent; however, neutrophils are attracted secondarily to areas of erosion and necrosis. In some cases, the mucosa shows marked lamina propria hemorrhage without erosion or significant inflammation (Fig. 4–46). These cases typically occur after excessive alcohol ingestion.[20] Hemorrhagic gastropathy is distinguishable from hemorrhage as an artefact of biopsy only by its severity.

Acute erosive gastropathy caused by chemical injury such as from a drug is associated with acute epigastric pain, nausea,

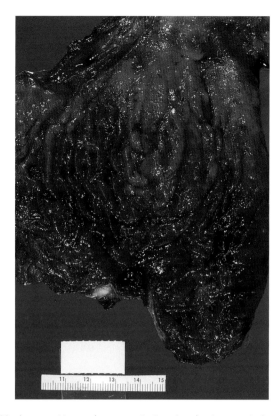

Figure 4–44. Acute gastritis secondary to corrosive ingestion, showing extensive hemorrhagic gastritis.

vomiting, and bleeding. These cases heal quickly by rapid regeneration of the epithelium (Fig. 4–47). When biopsies are performed in this regenerative phase, marked architectural and cytologic abnormalities may be present, with a significant risk of false-positive diagnosis of carcinoma (Figs. 4–48 and 4–49) (see Chapter 5). Cases of acute erosive gastropathy that occur in extremely ill patients as a result of shock and hypoperfusion are not as quickly reversible unless the precipitating cause is removed.

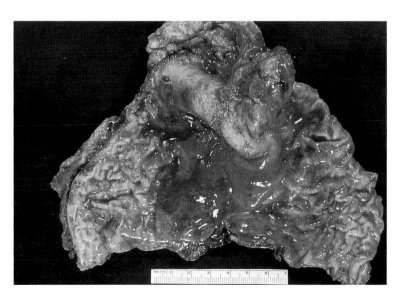

Figure 4–43. Acute erosive gastritis, showing congestion and denudation of a large part of the mucosal surface.

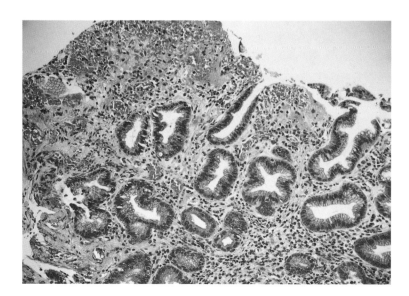

Figure 4–45. Acute erosive gastropathy, showing denudation of the surface, lamina propria hemorrhage, and reactive change in the foveolar region.

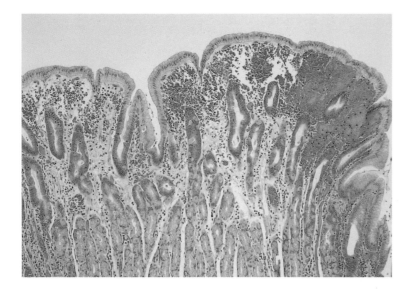

Figure 4–46. Acute hemorrhagic gastropathy, showing lamina propria hemorrhage. This biopsy specimen was taken from a patient with a clinical history of recent heavy alcohol intake.

Lymphocytic Gastritis

Lymphocytic gastritis is characterized by the presence of increased numbers of intraepithelial lymphocytes in the surface and foveolar epithelium (Fig. 4–50).[21] Normally, 4–7 lymphocytes are present per 100 epithelial cells; in lymphocytic gastritis, this number is greater than 25 lymphocytes per 100 epithelial cells. The intraepithelial lymphocytes are mainly CD8+ T suppressor cells. The lymphocytic infiltration of the epithelium is often associated with increased numbers of lymphocytes in the lamina propria, but this is not a consistently prominent feature.

Lymphocytic gastritis is associated with an endoscopic appearance known as varioliform gastritis. Varioliform gastritis is characterized by the presence of thickened rugal folds in the gastric body and small wart-like nodules with a central depres-

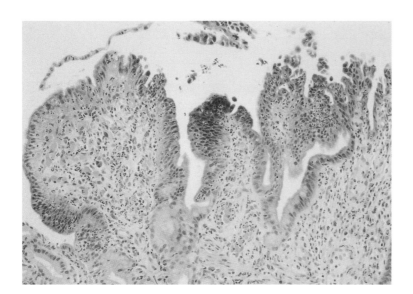

Figure 4–47. Early healing phase of a gastric erosion, showing a single layer of regenerated surface epithelium over the irregular surface. Marked acute inflammation is evident, probably representing the healing process.

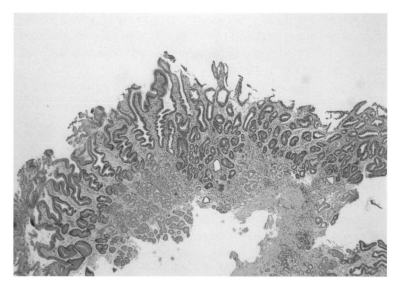

A

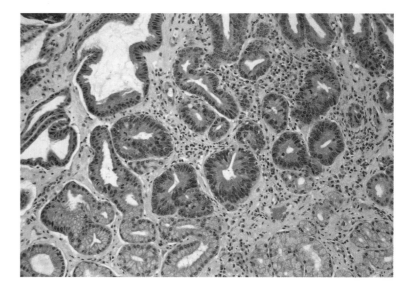

B

Figure 4–48. A: Healing phase of erosion with foveolar regeneration. B: Higher power micrograph of part A, showing regenerative atypia and increased mitotic activity in the deep foveolar region.

sion at the top of the mucosal folds. In some cases, the thickening of the rugal folds can be as prominent as those seen in Ménétrier's disease.[22] Lymphocytic gastritis is of unknown etiology and clinical significance, although evidence is emerging that many of these cases are caused by *Helicobacter pylori* infection.[23] There is also an association with celiac disease,[24] and the finding of lymphocytic gastritis in a biopsy should prompt the clinician to evaluate the patient for malabsorption and celiac disease.

Eosinophilic Gastritis

Eosinophilic gastritis is a rare condition for which morphologic diagnostic criteria are not well established. The presence of numerous eosinophils in an inflammatory cell infiltrate in the lamina propria is common in *H. pylori* gastritis (Fig. 4–51A). For a diagnosis of eosinophilic gastritis, the eosinophil must be the dominant cell with few other inflammatory cells present

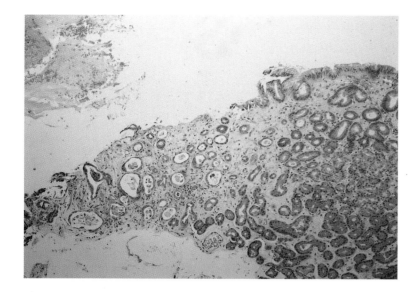

A

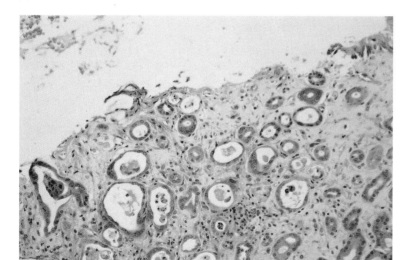

B

Figure 4–49. A: Healing erosion, showing a different healing pattern with a mucosa that is thinner and resembles ischemic change. B: Higher power micrograph of part A, showing dilated glands lined by flattened epithelial cells and containing necrotic debris in the lumen.

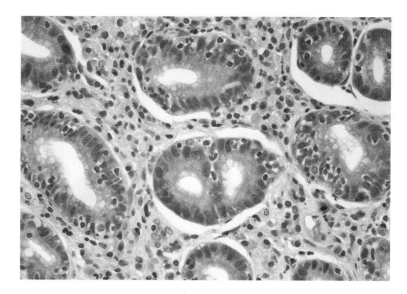

A

B

Figure 4–50. A: Lymphocytic gastritis, showing increased number of intraepithelial lymphocytes in the gastric glands. These are scattered in the glands without forming lymphoepithelial lesions. B: Lymphocytic gastritis, immunoperoxidase stain for CD45 (common leukocyte antigen), showing intraepithelial lymphocytes in the glands.

(Fig. 4–51B and C). A band of eosinophils immediately above the muscularis mucosae is present in some cases. The diagnosis is supported by clinical features, including an atopic history (asthma, atopic eczema, food intolerance), and by the presence of peripheral blood eosinophilia. In some cases eosinophilic gastritis is associated with eosinophilic infiltration of the esophageal and small-intestinal mucosa (eosinophilic gastroenteritis). The gastric antrum is usually the site of maximal involvement.

Granulomatous Gastritis

Nonnecrotizing epithelioid granulomas in gastric mucosa are rare (Fig. 4–52). Most cases are the result of Crohn's disease, sarcoidosis, or infections such as tuberculosis and fungal disease.[25] When these diseases have been excluded, a small number of patients remain in whom the granulomas have no cause. The term "idiopathic granulomatous gastritis" has been used for these cases, but there is no consistent clinical syndrome in these patients that justifies the use of this term. Most cases of isolated granulomatous gastritis coexist with *Helicobacter pylori* gastritis, leading to the suggestion that this may be a manifestation of *H. pylori* gastritis; this is not proven as yet. Both Crohn's disease and sarcoidosis may first manifest in the stomach,[25] and it seems preferable to use the descriptive designation "granulomatous gastritis" than to suggest that idiopathic granulomatous gastritis is a disease entity.

Collagenous Gastritis

This extremely rare condition is characterized by the presence of a thick band of collagen underneath the basement mem-

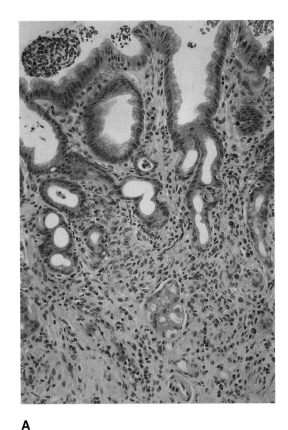

A

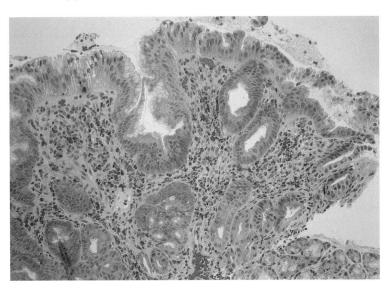

B

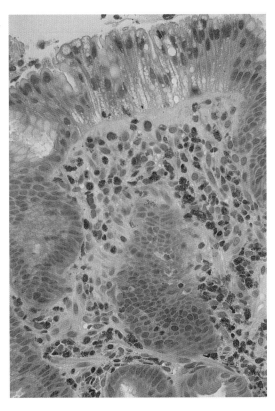

C

Figure 4–51. A: Eosinophils in the inflammatory infiltrate of active chronic *Helicobacter pylori* gastritis. B: Eosinophilic gastritis, showing predominantly eosinophil infiltration of the lamina propria. C: Eosinophilic gastritis, higher power micrograph of part B. Note the presence of rare intraepithelial eosinophils.

brane of the gastric and duodenal surface epithelium.[26] Some cases have been associated with collagenous colitis.[27]

Hypertrophic Gastritis

Ménétrier's disease (hypertrophic gastritis) is a poorly understood entity. It is characterized endoscopically and grossly by the presence of thickened rugal folds in the body of the stomach (Fig. 4–53). In most cases, the rugal hypertrophy involves much of the stomach, but more localized forms exist (Fig. 4–54). Rugae are diffusely involved, but polypoid forms have been described. Clinically the patients have evidence of hyposecretion of acid and protein-losing enteropathy. Microscopically,

marked foveolar hyperplasia is evident with cystic dilatation of the foveolae, associated with gland atrophy (Fig. 4–55A). Inflammation is mild, and smooth muscle proliferation is present in the lamina propria (Fig. 4–55B).

Grossly, Ménétrier's disease can be mimicked by pyloric hyperplasia that occurs in Zollinger-Ellison syndrome (Fig. 4–56); malignant neoplasms, particularly malignant lymphoma; cytomegalovirus gastritis in children; and lymphocytic gastritis. Microscopically the changes mimic a severe form of reactive gastropathy; when the change is more polypoid, Ménétrier's disease blends with multiple hyperplastic polyps.

In practice, the diagnosis of Ménétrier's disease is rarely made. It should probably be restricted to cases with the classic

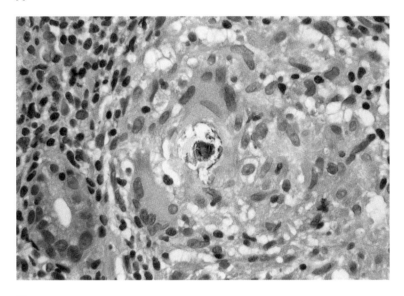

A

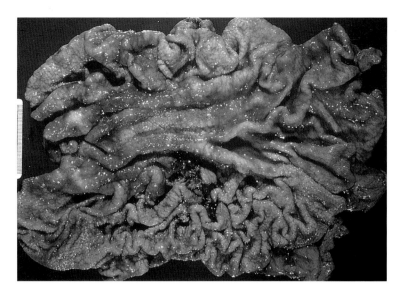

Figure 4–53. Ménétrier's disease, showing diffuse but irregular thickening of gastric folds.

B

Figure 4–52. A: Granulomatous gastritis, showing multiple nonnecrotizing epithelioid cell granulomas in the gastric mucosa. This patient had no history of Crohn's disease or sarcoidosis at the time of biopsy. Chest radiograph showed hilar lymph node enlargement suggestive of early sarcoidosis. B: Higher power micrograph showing nonnecrotizing epithelioid cell granuloma with a calcified Schaumann body.

combination of diffuse rugal hypertrophy, hypochlorhydria, protein-losing enteropathy, and marked foveolar hyperplasia with cystic dilatation of mucous glands.

Specific Etiologic Types of Gastritis

Mycobacterial Gastritis

Tuberculous gastritis is rare, even in patients with disseminated tuberculosis. It is characterized by the presence of caseating granulomas in the gastric mucosa. The gastric mucosa is also a rare site for infection with *Mycobacterium avium-intracellulare* (Fig. 4–57) (see also Chapters 6 and 8); this occurs in patients

with AIDS and is typified by the presence of macrophages containing numerous acid-fast bacilli.

Gastric Syphilis

In the past, gastric syphilis was a gummatous type of granulomatous inflammation that involved the stomach in the tertiary phase of the disease. With the decline in incidence of tertiary syphilis, gastric syphilis essentially became nonexistent. More recently, the occurrence of gastric lesions in early (secondary) syphilis has been recognized. This occurs mainly in otherwise healthy individuals with recent syphilis[28]; cases have also been reported in HIV-positive patients. Clinical features include epigastric pain, nausea, vomiting, and upper GI bleeding. The gastric mucosal injury is the result of a treponemal vasculitis, resulting in an erosive gastritis with thickened rugal folds involving mainly the antrum. Numerous spirochetes (*Treponema pallidum*) can be demonstrated by Warthin-Starry

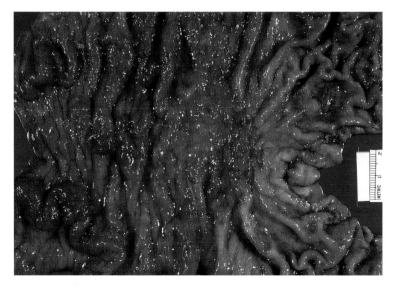

Figure 4–54. Ménétrier's disease, showing a more focal thickening of gastric folds, associated with some flattening of the mucosa.

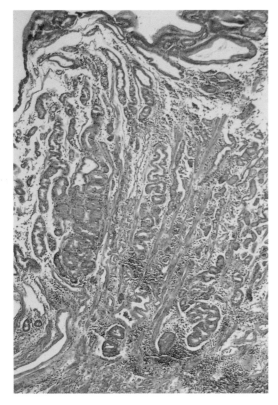

A

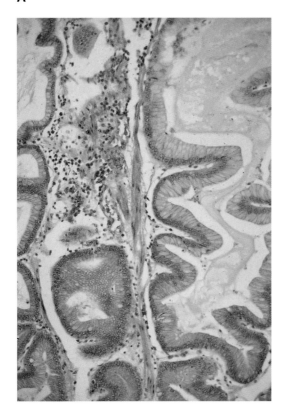

B

Figure 4–55. A: Ménétrier's disease, showing extreme foveolar hyperplasia with microcystic dilatation of glands. Smooth muscle hyperplasia is evident, and inflammation is minimal. B: Ménétrier's disease, showing the markedly elongated and serrated foveolar region. Note the smooth muscle fibers.

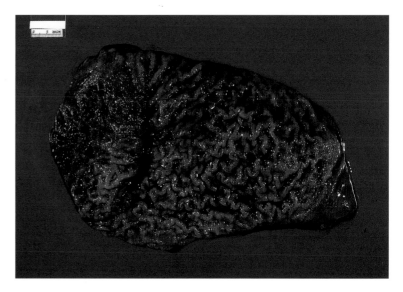

Figure 4–56. Gastric mucosa in a patient with Zollinger-Ellison syndrome. The diffuse and regular thickening of mucosal folds is due to parietal cell hyperplasia.

stain. Irregular large ulcers may be present, mimicking malignancy. Although most patients have evidence of secondary syphilis elsewhere in the body, gastric syphilis may represent the only manifestation of syphilis. Appropriate testing is indicated in any patient with an unremitting gastritis.

Cytomegalovirus Gastritis

Cytomegalovirus (CMV) gastritis occurs almost exclusively in infants and immunocompromised patients. In children, CMV gastritis is associated with thickening of rugal folds, resembling Ménétrier's disease. In immunocompromised patients, the gastric mucosa shows multiple shallow ulcers. Microscopically, the diagnosis is made on the basis of the typical cytomegalovirus cytopathic effect, consisting of enlargement of the cell, the

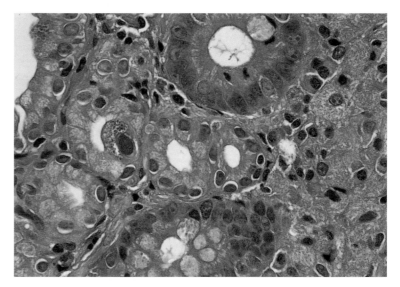

Figure 4–57. Mixed infection in a patient with AIDS. Cytomegalovirus-infected glandular cell is on the left; the right side shows macrophages with abundant fibrillary cytoplasm, indicative of *Mycobacterium avium-intracellulare* infection.

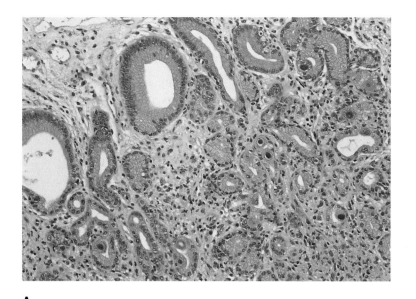

A

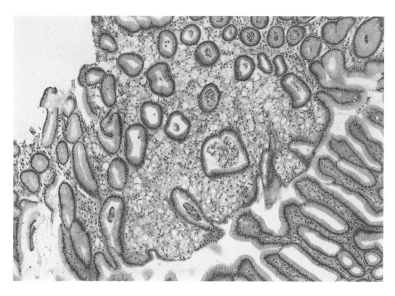

A

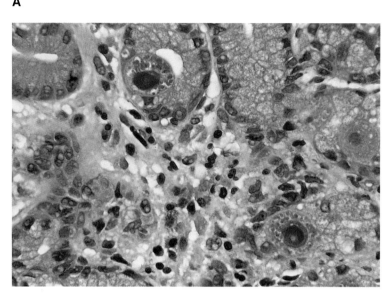

B

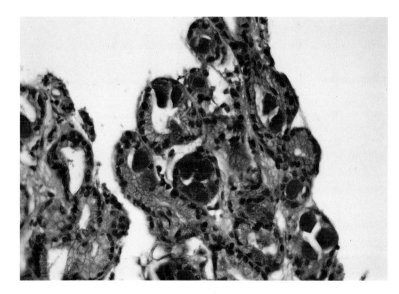

Figure 4–58. A: Cytomegalovirus gastritis, showing acute and chronic inflammation associated with numerous CMV-infected cells. B: Higher power micrograph of part A, showing typical CMV-infected cells, which are enlarged and show large Cowdry A intranuclear inclusions and small multiple cytoplasmic inclusions.

Figure 4–59. Cytomegalovirus infection of gastric mucosa in a neonate, showing numerous inclusions without significant inflammation.

B

C

Figure 4–60. A: Gastric mucosa infected with *Cryptococcus neoformans,* showing expansion of the lamina propria and separation of the glands by an infiltrate of cells with abundant pale cytoplasm. B: Higher power micrograph of part A, showing budding yeasts in the lamina propria. Note the clear space around the yeast due to the thick mucoid capsule. The yeasts are extracellular as well as within macrophages. C: Gastric cryptococcal infection; organisms stain positively with periodic acid–Schiff stain.

presence of a large intranuclear inclusion surrounded by a halo, and the presence of multiple granular basophilic cytoplasmic inclusions (Fig. 4–58). In children, epithelial cells are predominantly infected and inflammation is frequently minimal (Fig. 4–59). In immunocompromised patients, inclusions are seen in epithelial cells as well as vascular endothelial cells in the lamina propria; inflammation and erosion are common in these patients.

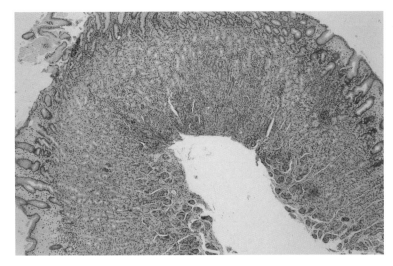

A

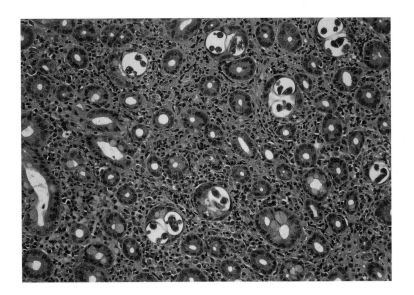

A

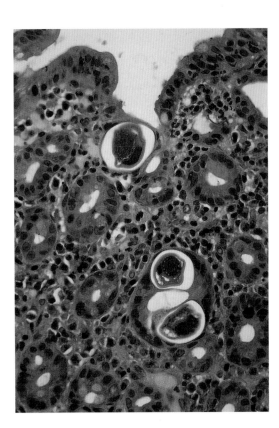

B

Figure 4–61. A: *Strongyloides stercoralis* in gastric mucosa, showing adult worms in the lumina of dilated glands. B: Higher power micrograph of part A, showing adult *Strongyloides stercoralis*.

B

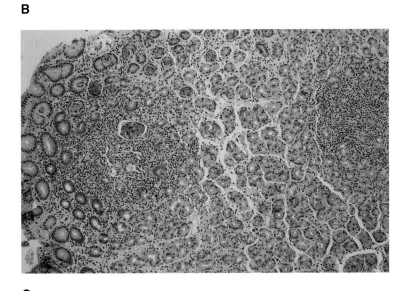

C

Figure 4–62. A: Crohn's disease of the stomach, showing focal acute gastritis with involvement of one area in the deep mucosa. The superficial mucosa and adjacent oxyntic mucosa are not inflamed. This patient had a prior history of ileocolic Crohn's disease. This pattern of gastric inflammation is typical of gastric involvement by Crohn's disease. B: Gastric involvement in Crohn's disease, higher power micrograph of part A, showing gland abscesses and lamina propria inflammation. C: Focal acute and chronic gastritis in Crohn's disease, showing a single focus of inflammation surrounded by normal oxyntic mucosa.

Fungal Gastritis

Several fungi may be found in the gastric mucosa, usually in patients with disseminated fungal infections, and predominantly in immunocompromised hosts. Among the fungi that may be seen are *Cryptococcus neoformans* (Fig. 4–60), *Histoplasma capsulatum, Candida* species, *Mucor,* and *Aspergillus* species. *Candida* species may also be present as a surface overgrowth in any large gastric ulcer.

Parasitic Gastritis

Parasitic infestation of the stomach is extremely uncommon. In immunocompromised hosts infected with *Cryptosporidium,* the gastric mucosa is sometimes affected. In patients with *Strongyloides stercoralis* infection adult worms can rarely be seen in the gastric mucosa (Fig. 4–61). Eating raw fish is rarely associated with ingestion of *Anisakis* larvae; these larvae enter the gastric wall and have been known to cause perforations.

Crohn's Disease of the Stomach

Crohn's disease rarely involves the stomach in a clinically relevant manner. Microscopic involvement may be more common than is realized. Gastric Crohn's disease manifests as focal gastritis in an otherwise normal mucosa. The foci of gastritis are characterized by focal erosion, acute and chronic inflammation involving the foveolar pits and glands, and lymphoid hyperplasia (Fig. 4–62). When nonnecrotizing epithelioid cell granulomas are present, the diagnosis of Crohn's disease can be made. When, however, granulomas are absent, the changes are considered to be nonspecific because focal gastritis is not an uncommon endoscopic and histologic abnormality. In a patient with Crohn's disease elsewhere in the bowel, the presence of focal gastritis represents suggestive evidence of gastric involvement.[29]

References

1. Owen DA. Stomach. In Sternberg SS (ed). Histology for Pathologists. Raven Press, New York, 1992. pp 533–545.
2. Dixon MF, Genta RM, Yardley JH, et al. Classification and grading of gastritis. The updated Sydney System. *Am J Surg Pathol.* 1996;20:1161–1181.
3. Price AB. The Sydney System: Histological Division. *J Gastroenterol Hepatol.* 1991;6:209–222.
4. Appleman HD. Gastritis: Terminology, etiology, and clinico-pathologic correlations: Another biased view. *Hum Pathol.* 1994;25:1006–1019.
5. Carpenter HA, Talley NJ. Gastroscopy is incomplete without biopsy: Clinical relevance of distinguishing gastropathy from gastritis. *Gastroenterol.* 1995;108:917–924.
6. Rugge M, Farinati F, Bafia R, et al. Gastric epithelial dysplasia in the natural history of gastric cancer: A multicenter prospective follow-up study. *Gastroenterol.* 1994;107: 1288–1296.
7. Chan WY, Hui PK, Leung KM, et al. Coccoid forms of *Helicobacter pylori* in the human stomach. *Am J Clin Pathol.* 1994;102:503–507.
8. Genta RM. Recognizing atrophy: Another step toward a classification of gastritis. *Am J Surg Pathol.* 1996;20: S23–S30.
9. Whitehead R. The classification of chronic gastritis: Current status. *J Clin Gastroenterol.* 1995;21:S131–S134.
10. Wyatt JI, Knight T, Wilson A, et al. *Helicobacter pylori* gastritis and serum pepsinogen A in a male non-patient population. *Gut.* 1995;37:A4.
11. Burman P, Kampe O, Kraaz W, et al. A study of autoimmune gastritis in the postpartum period and at a 5-year follow-up. *Gastroenterology.* 1992;103:934–942.
12. Dooley CP, Cohen H, Fitzgibbons PL, et al. Prevalence of *Helicobacter pylori* infection and histologic gastritis in asymptomatic persons. *N Engl J Med.* 1989;321:1562–1566.
13. Dixon MF. Histological responses to *Helicobacter pylori* infection: Gastritis, atrophy and preneoplasia. *Baillere's Clin Gastroenterol.* 1995;9:467–485.
14. Correa P. Chronic gastritis: A clinico-pathologic classification. *Am J Gastroenterol.* 1988;83:504–509.
15. Tucci A, Poli L, Donati M, et al. Value of serology (ELISA) for the diagnosis of *Helicobacter pylori* infection: Evaluation in patients attending endoscopy and in those with fundic atrophic gastritis. *Ital J Gastroenterol.* 1996;28:371–376.
16. Roth SH. NSAID gastropathy. A new understanding. *Arch Intern Med.* 1996;156:1623–1628.
17. Dixon MF, O'Connor HJ, Axon ATR, et al. Reflux gastritis: distinct histopathological entity. *J Clin Pathol.* 1986;39:524–530.
18. Rocha GA, Queiroz DM, Mendes EN, et al. *Helicobacter pylori* acute gastritis: Histological, endoscopical, clinical, and therapeutic features. *Am J Gastroenterol.* 1991;86:1592–1595.
19. Cruz FO, Soffia PS, Del Rio PM, et al. Acute phlegmonous gastritis with mural abscess: CT diagnosis. *AM J Roentgenol.* 1992;159: 767–768.
20. Laine L, Weinstein WM. Histology of alcoholic hemorrhagic "gastritis": A prospective evaluation. *Gastroenterology.* 1988;94: 1254–1262.
21. Haot J, Hamichi L, Wallez I, et al. Lymphocytic gastritis: A newly described entity: A retrospective endoscopic and histological study. *Gut.* 1988;29:1258–1264.
22. Wolfsen HC, Carpenter HA, Talley NJ. Ménétrier's disease: A form of hypertrophic gastropathy or gastritis? *Gastroenterology.* 1993; 104:1310–1319.
23. De Giacomo C, Gianatti A, Negrini R, et al. Lymphocytic gastritis: A positive relationship with celiac disease. *J Pediatr.* 1994;124: 57–62.
24. Niemela S, Karttunen T, Kerola T, et al. Ten year follow-up study of lymphocytic gastritis: Further evidence on *Helicobacter pylori* as a cause of lymphocytic gastritis and corpus gastritis. *J Clin Pathol.* 1995;48:1111–1116.
25. Shapiro JL, Goldblum JR, Petras RE. A clinicopathologic study of 42 patients with granulomatous gastritis. Is there really an "idiopathic" granulomatous gastritis? *Am J Surg Pathol.* 1996;20: 462–470.
26. Colletti RB, Trainer TD. Collagenous gastritis. *Gastroenterology.* 1989;97:1552–1555.
27. Stolte M, Ritter M, Borchard F, et al. Collagenous gastroduodenitis on collagenous colitis. *Endoscopy.* 1990; 22:186–187.
28. Kolb JC, Woodward LA. Gastric syphilis. *Am J Emerg Med.* 1997;15:164–166.
29. Danesh BJZ, Park RHR, Upadhyay R, et al. Diagnostic yield in upper gastrointestinal endoscopic biopsies in patients with Crohn's disease. *Gastroenterology.* 1989;96:A108.

5

GASTRIC NEOPLASMS

Roger Der and Parakrama Chandrasoma

POLYPS

Gastric polyps are commonly encountered during upper gastrointestinal endoscopy (Table 5–1). In most cases, the polyps are small and solitary and occur in patients with gastritis; many of these represent reactive processes. More rarely, multiple polyps are present (Fig. 5–1).

The most common reactive polyp is called focal foveolar hyperplasia, characterized by hyperplasia of the cells of the foveolar region. Focal foveolar hyperplasia represents a healing superficial erosion and is identical to reactive gastropathy (see Chapter 4), except that it is perceived as a polypoid lesion at endoscopy. Intestinal metaplasia, limited to the focal hyperplastic lesion, is sometimes present. In some cases, the reactive epithelial atypia in the foveolar cells can mimic adenomatous change. Focal foveolar hyperplasia is very likely a transient lesion that regresses to normal mucosa when healing is complete.

Lymphoid hyperplasia associated with chronic gastritis, particularly *Helicobacter pylori* gastritis, commonly presents a polypoid appearance of the gastric mucosa. The polyps present as nodular elevations, and the mucosa is commonly described as having a "cobblestone" appearance or looking like "goose-pimples." Microscopically, multiple lymphoid follicles with reactive centers are present. Histologically distinguishing gastric lymphoid hyperplasia in chronic gastritis from low-grade lymphomas arising in mucosal-associated lymphoid tissue (MALT) can be difficult (see Chapter 15). Endoscopically, MALT lymphomas rarely present as solitary polypoid lesions; they are characterized by rugal thickening over a larger area of mucosa, often with ulcers.

The polyps considered in the following sections represent the differential diagnosis of gastric polyps and include epithelial polyps (hyperplastic polyp, fundic gland polyp, and gastric adenoma), polyps derived from neuroendocrine cells (carcinoid tumor, composite adenocarcinoma-carcinoid tumor), choristoma (heterotopic pancreas, ectopic Brunner's glands), inflammatory fibroid polyps, and polyps of mesenchymal origin.

Epithelial Polyps

Hyperplastic Polyps

Hyperplastic polyps constitute about 75% of gastric polyps. Increasing in frequency with age, they are generally considered to be reactive lesions rather than true neoplasms. Hyperplastic polyps differ from focal foveolar hyperplasia (reactive gastropathy associated with healing erosion) by the fact that they are larger and, theoretically at least, do not regress. In a single small lesion, the distinction is academic; in patients with multiple

TABLE 5–1. GASTRIC POLYPS

Reactive Polyps
    Focal foveolar hyperplasia
    Reactive lymphoid hyperplasia
    Inflammatory fibroid polyp
Polyps Derived from Epithelial Cells
    Hyperplastic polyp
    Fundic gland polyp
    Adenoma
    Polypoid adenocarcinoma
Polyps Derived from Neuroendocrine Cells
    EC cell hyperplasia
    Carcinoid tumor
    Composite carcinoid–adenocarcinoma
Choristomas
    Heterotopic pancreas
    Ectopic Brunner's glands
Mesenchymal Polyps
    Leiomyoma
    Granular cell tumor
    Glomus tumor
    Lipoma
    GI stromal neoplasm

Abbreviations: EC = enterochromaffin; GI = gastrointestinal.

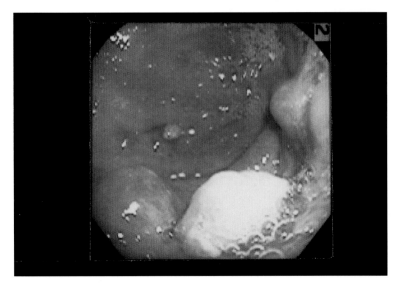

A

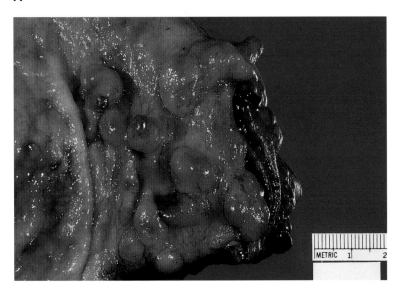

B

Figure 5–1. A: Multiple gastric polyps at endoscopy. B: Gastric mucosa showing multiple polyps. (Figure A courtesy of Aslam Godil, MD, Department of Gastroenterology, Loma Linda University, CA)

small polypoid lesions, the distinction between the two is sometimes impossible without a repeat endoscopy to evaluate regression. According to some authorities focal foveolar hyperplasia is the precursor lesion for hyperplastic polyps.

Hyperplastic polyps can occur anywhere in the stomach. Thirty percent are multiple[1]; they may occur in otherwise normal-appearing mucosa or in a background of chronic gastritis. Endoscopically, they are sessile or pedunculated and are usually less than 2 cm in size.

Histologically, hyperplastic polyps are characterized by a markedly elongated foveolar region; the underlying glands are not prominent and are usually mucous glands, irrespective of the location of the polyp (Fig. 5–2). The foveolar region shows tortuosity, luminal serration, and microcystic change. The lining cells are columnar, with a basally situated small nucleus and mucin distending the apical cytoplasm. Focal intestinal metaplasia is seen in 20%. There is marked lamina propria edema and inflammatory cell infiltration. Smooth muscle cells are present, often as thin bands, between the hyperplastic foveolae and are typically seen extending toward the surface perpendicular to the muscularis mucosae. Larger polyps may show focal surface ulceration.

Varying degrees of chronic gastritis are commonly present in the nonpolypoid gastric mucosa. In some cases, the flat gastric mucosa between hyperplastic polyps also shows similar hyperplastic features histologically ("polypoid hypertrophic gastritis" or "gastritis cystica polyposa"); these cases have similarities with Ménétrier's disease (see Chapter 4).

Hyperplastic polyps very rarely transform into carcinomas; the prevalence of malignancy is 0.3–1%.[2] Dysplasia and cancer are more commonly seen in hyperplastic polyps that are larger than 2 cm. The nonpolypoid mucosa of a stomach harboring multiple hyperplastic polyps has a greater premalignant potential, with a 4–13% prevalence of cancer. Endoscopic surveillance has been recommended for patients with multiple hyperplastic polyps and complete excision for any polyps exceeding 2 cm in size.[3]

Fundic Gland Polyps

Fundic gland polyps (also called fundic gland hamartomas and glandular cysts) are the second most common gastric polyps. They occur in oxyntic mucosa of the fundus and body and are found in about 2% of all endoscopies.[3] Their etiology is uncertain; the possibility that they may represent a reactive process associated with injury is suggested by the fact that they some-

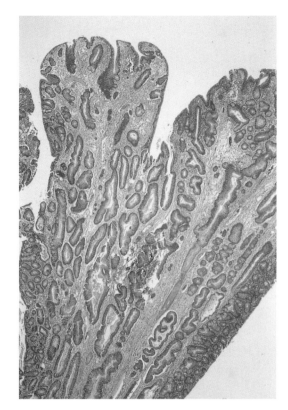

A

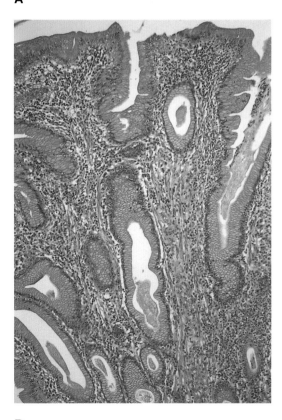

B

Figure 5–2. A: Hyperplastic polyp of the stomach, showing polypoid architecture, foveolar hyperplasia, mild inflammation, and edema. B: Hyperplastic polyp, showing dilated glands lined by hyperplastic epithelium. Inflammation and smooth muscle proliferation are evident in the lamina propria.

times regress spontaneously. More common in women, fundic gland polyps have no malignant potential, even when multiple. They are not associated with *Helicobacter pylori* infection.

Fundic gland polyps are not known to be associated with symptoms; they are found incidentally at endoscopy as small (<8 mm) smooth-surfaced mucosal polyps or nodules in an otherwise normal gastric mucosa. Usually numbering fewer than three, fundic gland polyps can be multiple and even very numerous polyps can occur. Fifty percent of patients who have multiple fundic polyps have familial adenomatous polyposis; in the others, the polyps represent the sole abnormality in the gastrointestinal tract.

Microscopically, fundic gland polyps show two abnormalities: (1) The part of the gland immediately below the normal or shortened foveolar region shows distortion and budding, resulting in a cloverleaf arrangement. (2) The deeper part of the gland shows cystic dilation; the most common diagnostic criterion is the presence of microcysts lined by chief and parietal cells (Figs. 5–3 and 5–4).

Gastric Adenoma

Although adenoma is the third most common type of gastric polyp, it is relatively rarely encountered in a gastric biopsy. Adenomas tend to occur in the pyloric antrum and are commonly solitary. They may be sessile or pedunculated and vary considerably in size and endoscopic appearance[4]; adenomatous polyps greater than 2 cm have a significant risk of harboring adenocarcinoma (Fig. 5–5). Flat or depressed adenomas have also been described; in Japan these constitute 10% of all gastric adenomas.[5] Flat adenomas are distinguished from gastric epithelial dysplasia by the fact that they are endoscopically visualized discrete lesions unlike dysplasia, which is a histologic finding in a gastric mucosa not perceived endoscopically as being abnormal.

Adenomas are defined, as in the colon, by the histologic presence of adenomatous change that is identical to low-grade epithelial dysplasia (Fig. 5–6A, B). Adenomatous change occurs in the foveolar mucous cells and is characterized by mucin depletion, increased nuclear size and chromaticity, and stratification of nuclei. The elongated, cigar-shaped nuclei retain a normal polarity, being perpendicular to the basement membrane of the gland. Mitotic figures are common. Most gastric adenomas have a tubular architecture (see Fig. 5–6); tubulovillous and villous adenomas are rare and they tend to be large (>2 cm) and have a high risk of malignancy. Adenomas have also been reported to arise in the deep pyloric glands and parietal cells of the oxyntic mucosa, but these are extremely rare.

Adenomas pass through increasing dysplasia to adenocarcinoma. High-grade dysplasia in an adenoma is defined by criteria identical to those for colonic adenomas, that is, severe cytologic abnormalities of high-grade dysplasia associated with loss of nuclear polarity of the lining cells or the presence of gland complexity characterized by cribriform change. High-grade dysplasia is followed by intramucosal adenocarcinoma, which is characterized by irregularity of the malignant glands and the

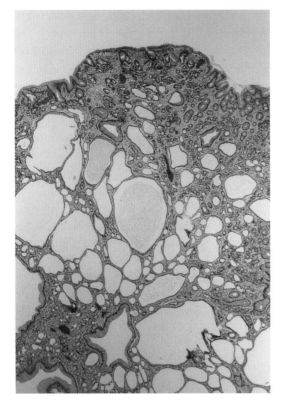

A

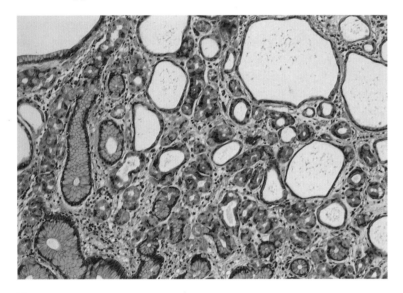

B

Figure 5–3. A: Fundic gland polyp, showing mixture of glands and cystic spaces of varying size. B: Fundic gland polyp, showing glands lined by foveolar mucous cells in addition to the oxyntic glands. The dilated cystic structures are lined by flattened parietal cells.

presence of small groups of invasive malignant cells in the lamina propria. Adenomas with intramucosal carcinoma are equivalent to early gastric cancer of the polypoid type. Dysplasia and carcinoma occurring in adenomas is discussed further in the section on gastric dysplasia and early gastric cancer.

The risk of malignancy in a gastric adenoma is closely related to size; 40% of malignant adenomas are larger than 2 cm.[3] The estimated overall risk of malignancy in gastric adenomas varies greatly from study to study; the most commonly quoted

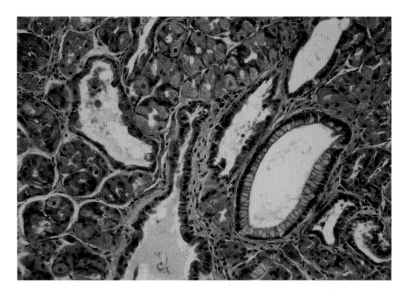

Figure 5–4. Small fundic gland polyp, showing dilated deep gastric glands lined by parietal cells. One microcyst is lined by mucous cells. The surrounding glands are normal oxyntic glands.

risk is 11%.[4] The risk of cancer in adenomas is the highest among all types of gastric polyps; complete endoscopic removal of an adenoma is indicated, even when this entails repeat endoscopy after the histologic nature of the polyp has been defined.

In addition to cancer developing in adenomas, the presence of gastric adenomas is associated with an increased cancer risk in the nonpolypoid gastric mucosa. This cancer risk is probably related to the fact that gastric adenomas commonly occur in patients with chronic atrophic gastritis, which is very likely the premalignant condition for most gastric carcinomas. The risk of gastric cancer associated with adenomas is variously estimated as 3–25%.[3] The presence of a gastric adenoma is therefore an indication for gastric cancer surveillance.

Gastric Polyps in Polyposis Syndromes

Familial Adenomatous Polyposis. Gastroduodenal adenomas occur in 35–100% of patients with familial adenomatous polyposis

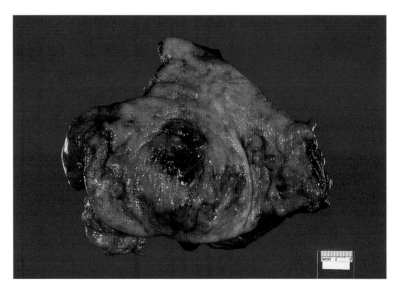

Figure 5–5. Multiple adenomas associated with a gastric adenocarcinoma.

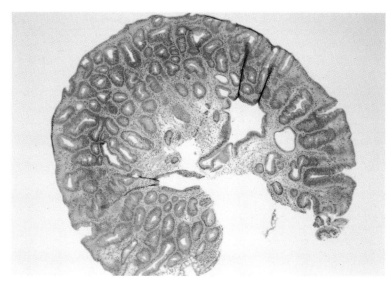

A

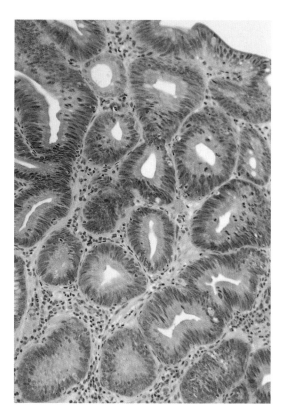

B

Figure 5–6. A: Gastric adenoma, showing a focal lesion (endoscopically recognized as a small polyp), showing adenomatous change. B: Gastric adenoma, showing adenomatous change (=low-grade dysplasia) of lining epithelium. The glands are tubular without serration and show enlarged cells with increased nuclear:cytoplasmic (N:C) ratio and enlarged nuclei. Mitotic figures are present.

(FAP) and Gardner's syndrome, with a higher prevalence in the duodenum than stomach. The prevalence increases with increasing duration of follow-up. Gastric adenomas in FAP occur at a younger age, are more frequently multiple, and have a higher risk of malignancy than sporadic gastric adenomas. The overall risk of gastric adenocarcinoma in patients with FAP, however, is reported to be similar to that in controls, except in Japan.[6]

Fundic gland polyps occur in up to 50% of patients with FAP and Gardner's syndrome. Compared with sporadic fundic gland polyps, patients with FAP tend to have multiple (over 50) polyps, but they do not have any risk of malignant transformation.

Patients with attenuated adenomatous polyposis coli (AAPC) also have an increased risk of developing gastric adenomas and fundic gland polyps. There is no increased risk of gastric cancer in these patients.[7]

Peutz-Jeghers Syndrome. Sessile hamartomatous polyps occur in the stomach of patients with Peutz-Jeghers syndrome. These polyps can be found anywhere in the stomach and may be multiple. The presence of an unusually large polyp or multiple polyps should raise the possibility of Peutz-Jeghers syndrome (Fig. 5–7A). Histologically, they resemble hyperplastic polyps with foveolar elongation, serration, and tortuosity with mucinous microcysts associated with inflammation and smooth muscle proliferation (Fig. 5–7B). Malignant transformation is very rare.

Juvenile Polyposis. Gastric polyps that are indistinguishable histologically from hyperplastic polyps occur in 10–15% of patients with familial juvenile polyposis and Cowden's disease. Multiple polyps are the rule. Polyps also occur in the Cronkhite-Canada syndrome, which is an acquired syndrome in adults with juvenile polyps throughout the gastrointestinal tract.

Carcinoid Tumors

Gastric carcinoid tumors occur by two pathogenetic mechanisms (Table 5–2): (1) as a response to hypergastrinemia (types 1 and 2 in Table 5–2) (75%) and (2) as sporadic tumors in normogastrinemic states (type 3 in Table 5–2) (25%). Carcinoid tumors occurring in conditions of hypergastrinemia are of enterochromaffin-like (ECL) cell origin, occur in a background of ECL cell hyperplasia, are multiple, and have a much lower rate of malignancy compared with sporadic carcinoid tumors that occur in normogastrinemic states, are of G-cell origin, and are larger solitary lesions without associated ECL cell hyperplasia.[8]

Gastric neuroendocrine cells are not reliably identified in routine histologic sections, unless they form nodules. They are best evaluated with immunoperoxidase stains (Fig. 5–8A). Chromogranin A is the best stain; neuron-specific enolase and synaptophysin are other choices. Identification of hormone products in gastric carcinoids is not usually necessary in practice; however, if necessary, immunoperoxidase stains are available for demonstrating gastrin (G cells), 5-hydroxytryptamine (antral enterochromaffin [EC] cells), histamine (oxyntic ECL cells), somatostatin (D cells), and α chain of human chorionic gonadotropin (ECL cell subset).

Carcinoid Tumors in Hypergastrinemic States

Gastrin is secreted physiologically by G cells in the gastric antrum; secretion rates are normally controlled by gastric acid

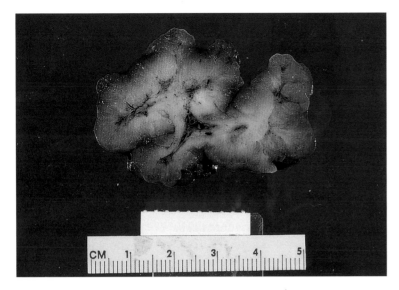

A

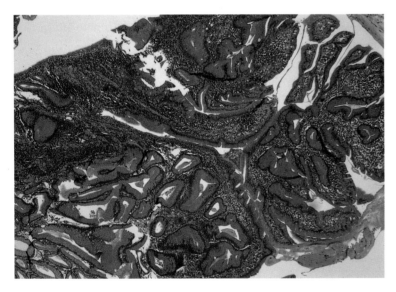

B

Figure 5–7. A: Gastric polyp in Peutz–Jeghers syndrome. This is a cut section of the polyp illustrated in Chapter 12. B: Peutz–Jeghers gastric polyp, showing hyperplastic foveolar mucous cells, inflammation, and smooth muscle in the lamina propria. The features are identical to those of hyperplastic polyp of the stomach. Hamartomatous and hyperplastic polyps of the stomach are not distinguishable histologically.

levels. Increased gastric secretion by G cells resulting in hypergastrinemia occurs when gastric acid secretion is decreased, such as in chronic autoimmune atrophic gastritis (type A chronic gastritis; pernicious anemia), multifocal chronic atrophic gastritis associated with *Helicobacter pylori* infection, and prolonged iatrogenic acid suppression with proton pump inhibitors such as omeprazole. Hypergastrinemia may also occur in patients with Zollinger-Ellison syndrome and multiple endocrine neoplasia (MEN), type I. In these cases, the source of gastrin is a gastrin-secreting neoplasm, commonly of the pancreas.

Gastrin is trophic to the ECL cells in the oxyntic mucosa, whether this is atrophic (as in the various types of chronic at-

TABLE 5–2. GASTRIC CARCINOID TUMORS AND NEUROENDOCRINE CARCINOMAS

TYPE 1: Carcinoid Tumors Associated with Chronic Atrophic Gastritis, type A.
    Well-differentiated (typical and atypical) and mixed, up to 2 cm in size: endoscopic surveillance; removal of polyps endoscopically.
    Well-differentiated (typical and atypical) and mixed, up to 2 cm in size, too numerous to remove or >2 cm in size: confirm ECL cell derivation by immunohistochemistry and consider antrectomy.
    Poorly differentiated neuroendocrine carcinoma (very rare): treat as malignant gastric neoplasm.

TYPE 2: Carcinoid Tumors Associated with Zollinger-Ellison Syndrome or MEN, type 1
    Treat gastrinoma; when treatment is successful, gastric tumors regress; when treatment is not successful, prognosis depends on the uncontrolled gastrinoma.
    Gastric carcinoids treated by regular polyp removal and surveillance.

TYPE 3. Sporadic Carcinoid Tumors in Normogastrinemic Patients
    Well-differentiated carcinoid (typical or atypical): treat with complete resection as soon as the biopsy diagnosis is made, on the assumption that it is a malignant neoplasm; assess prognosis on characteristics of the resected tumor: size, cytologic atypia, invasion, metastasis.
    Poorly differentiated neuroendocrine carcinoma: treat as for gastric carcinoma.

Abbreviations: ECL = enterochromaffin-like; MEN = multiple endocrine neoplasia.

rophic gastritis) or hyperplastic (as in Zollinger-Ellison syndrome) resulting in ECL cell hyperplasia progressing to carcinoid tumors.[9,10]

ECL cell hyperplasia passes through the following stages:

1. Simple or diffuse hyperplasia, which is defined as an increase in the number of ECL cells in oxyntic mucosa greater than two standard deviations as compared with age- and sex-matched controls (Fig. 5–8B). The cells are seen scattered in the mucosa, either singly or as aggregates of fewer than five cells.
2. Linear hyperplasia, characterized by linear sequences of more than four cells lying inside the basement membrane, either at the gland base or in the mucous neck region.
3. Micronodular hyperplasia is characterized by the presence of more than four ECL cells arranged in a nodular cluster not exceeding 150 μm in diameter, occurring within the glandular basement membrane or in the lamina propria (Fig. 5–9). Simple, linear and microglandular hyperplasia must be distinguished from pseudo-hyperplasia of ECL cells; this refers to an increased density of ECL cells without an absolute increase in their number that results from atrophy of other cells in the gland. Simple and linear ECL cell hyperplasia are rarely diagnosed in practice unless specifically looked for in a patient with known hypergastrinemia or a disease known to be associated with ECL cell hyperplasia. Micronodular ECL cell hyperplasia can be recognized with difficulty when the cell collections are within the basement membrane and more easily when they are separate from the glands in the lamina propria. Sometimes, the micronodules are buried in the muscularis mucosae and may even extend into the superficial submucosa (Fig. 5–10). Their recognition is important because it may provide the first clue that the patient has a condition associated with hypergastrinemia.

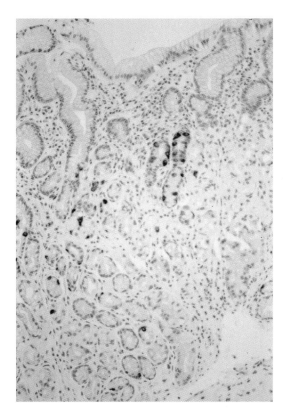

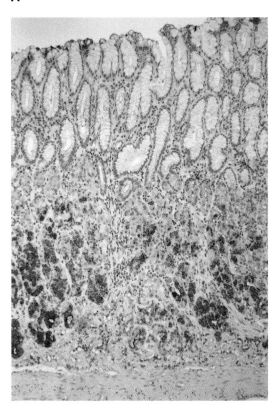

Figure 5–8. A: Gastric mucosa stained by immunoperoxidase technique for chromogranin A, showing scattered neuroendocrine cells in the gastric mucosa. B: Gastric mucosa in chronic atrophic gastritis stained with chromogranin A, showing diffuse hyperplasia of the neuroendocrine cells in the deep glands.

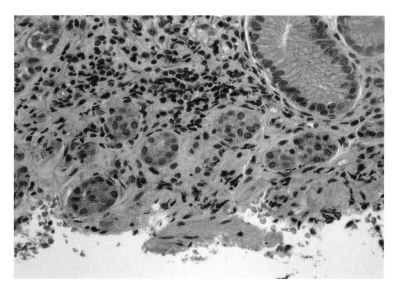

Figure 5–9. Micronodular ECL cell hyperplasia in a patient with autoimmune atrophic gastritis. The ECL cell nodules are seen as small nests of round cells in the deep lamina propria.

Lesions intermediate between ECL cell hyperplasia and carcinoid tumors are called ECL cell micronodules (or dysplastic lesions) (Fig. 5–11). ECL cell micronodules are nodular collections of ECL cells between 150 μm and 5 mm in size; they are usually in the lamina propria outside the gland basement membrane, but are restricted to the mucosa. They have no metastatic potential.

Hypergastrinemia-associated gastric carcinoid tumors are defined as ECL cell proliferations that exceed 5 mm in size (Fig. 5–12A). They are endoscopically visible as polyps and usually sessile. In practice, these occur in chronic autoimmune at-

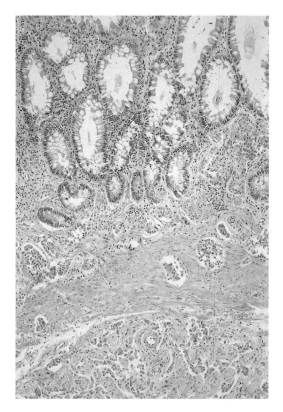

Figure 5–10. Micronodular ECL cell hyperplasia in autoimmune atrophic gastritis, showing small nests of neuroendocrine cells in deep mucosa, muscularis mucosae, and submucosa.

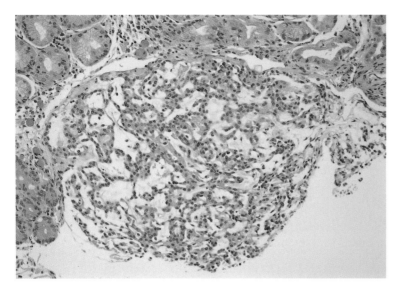

Figure 5–11. Microcarcinoid tumor in a patient with autoimmune atrophic gastritis. The tumor has a trabecular and microacinar pattern and consists of uniform small round cells. This patient had multiple microcarcinoid tumors, numbering in the hundreds.

rophic gastritis and Zollinger-Ellison syndrome, and although theoretically possible, carcinoid tumors have not yet been reported in patients with multifocal *H. pylori* atrophic gastritis or as a complication of proton pump inhibitor therapy.

Carcinoid tumors that occur in chronic atrophic gastritis are usually (over 90%) smaller than 1 cm and remain localized to the mucosa and submucosa. These tumors are predominantly well differentiated, cytologically benign carcinoid tumors; rarely, focal areas that are less differentiated and atypical are present. Multiple tumors are common. The rare larger tumors can infiltrate muscle, serosa, and lymphatics, but even then they almost never metastasize.[8] Treatment of patients with multiple carcinoid tumors associated with chronic atrophic gastritis consists of endoscopic removal of tumors and endoscopic surveillance (see Table 5–2). If tumors are too numerous to control endoscopically, antrectomy should be considered. Antrectomy removes the G cells, which are the source of gastrin, and results in regression of the carcinoid tumors. If a tumor larger than 2

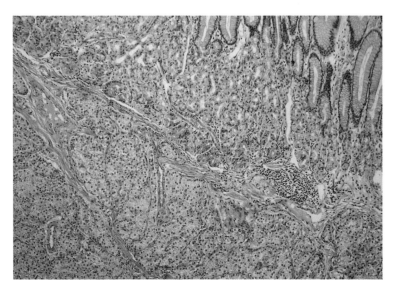

Figure 5–12. Carcinoid tumor of the stomach.

cm is found, there is enough uncertainty about this rare occurrence to recommend excision of the tumor plus antrectomy. Before antrectomy is performed, immunoperoxidase confirmation that the carcinoid tumors are of ECL cell derivation is essential.

Carcinoid tumors in patients with Zollinger-Ellison syndrome and MEN, type I, are also small and tend to remain localized to the mucosa and submucosa (see Table 5–2). Most are well-differentiated tumors, but some have atypical foci within them. Larger and more invasive tumors occur with about the same frequency as in chronic atrophic gastritis. In Rindi's series,[8] two cases showed regional lymph node metastases, but these patients were long-term survivors. The possibility exists in the two cases with nodal metastases that these were not true metastases but independent primary neoplasms; primary nodal gastrinomas are known to occur in patients with MEN (type I) and Zollinger-Ellison syndrome. The treatment of patients with Zollinger-Ellison syndrome is the surgical removal of the gastrinoma, which is a potentially malignant neoplasm. Survival of these patients depends on the gastrinoma; the gastric carcinoids are irrelevant because when the gastrinoma is successfully treated, the gastric carcinoids regress (see Table 5–2).

Sporadic Gastric Carcinoid Tumors. Gastric carcinoid tumors that occur in normogastrinemic patients are true neoplasms arising from ECL cells (the vast majority), G cells (unusual), or EC cells (very rare). Hormone production (serotonin or gastrin) may occur. They are almost always solitary, occur anywhere in the stomach, and are unassociated with hyperplasia of the gastric neuroendocrine cells. They occur in the 50–70-year age group and are more common in men. Sporadic gastric carcinoid tumors should be regarded as malignant neoplasms. When sporadic gastric carcinoid tumors are diagnosed at endoscopy, they should be completely resected either endoscopically or surgically (see Table 5–2).

Sporadic gastric carcinoids are classified as well-differentiated carcinoid tumors, poorly differentiated neuroendocrine carcinomas, and mixed tumors.[8]

WELL-DIFFERENTIATED CARCINOID TUMORS. Both the typical and atypical kinds of well-differentiated carcinoid tumors are composed of nests and anastomosing trabeculae of small cells with uniform round nuclei that have the typical granular ("salt-and-pepper") chromatin distribution (Fig. 5–12). A microacinar architecture is uncommon in gastric carcinoids and, when present, is usually focal. Typical carcinoid tumors have less than 1 mitotic figure per 10 hpf. Atypical carcinoid tumors have an architecture that is typical, but their cytology is atypical, characterized by nuclear irregularity and pleomorphism, and a mitotic rate of 2–9/10 hpf. Well-differentiated gastric carcinoid tumors are positive for chromogranin A and neuron-specific enolase and show argyrophilia (positive Grimelius stain); they tend to be well circumscribed but are not encapsulated. The presence of cords of cells with an invasive pattern at the periphery is common, particularly with atypical carcinoids.

Well-differentiated sporadic gastric carcinoid tumors tend to be large (median size of 2 cm); tumors with atypical cytologic features are more often larger than 2 cm than those with typical cytology. Lymphovascular invasion and infiltration of muscularis externa and serosa occurs. Sporadic gastric carcinoids metastasize to regional lymph nodes and the liver; the risk of metastasis is greatest in larger, more atypical tumors that show greater degrees of invasion. In an individual case, however, there is never a guarantee that metastasis will not occur. Complete excision is therefore mandatory.

POORLY DIFFERENTIATED NEUROENDOCRINE CARCINOMA. Poorly differentiated neuroendocrine carcinoma is characterized by poorly formed trabeculae, ill-defined nests, and diffuse sheets of cells. The neoplastic cells are small, round to oval, and show varying pleomorphism. The more malignant neoplasms of this type merge with poorly differentiated gastric adenocarcinomas and can be distinguished from them only with immunohistochemical staining for chromogranin A or the ultrastructural demonstration of dense core granules. The distinction is only of academic interest because poorly differentiated neuroendocrine carcinomas have a biologic behavior that is identical to gastric adenocarcinomas.

MIXED CARCINOID TUMORS. Composed of both well-differentiated and poorly differentiated areas, mixed carcinoid tumors are rare. When the poorly differentiated component is focal and the tumor is associated with hypergastrinemia, the risk of metastasis is low, and the prognosis is good.[8] In sporadic carcinoid tumors, however, the presence of even a small focus of poorly differentiated tumor indicates a significantly higher risk of metastasis.

Composite Glandular–Endocrine Cell Carcinoma

Gastric adenocarcinomas frequently have focal endocrine cells, and carcinoid tumors not uncommonly have an acinar pattern. The term "composite (or mixed) glandular-endocrine cell carcinoma" is applied to rare tumors that have both adenocarcinoma and carcinoid tumor, each comprising at least one third of the tumor mass.[11] The two elements may be well or poorly differentiated. Poorly differentiated tumors of this group behave in a manner similar to other gastric adenocarcinomas. Well-differentiated tumors present as a polypoid mass (Fig. 5–13) and has a biologic behavior that is similar to sporadic gastric carcinoid tumors, although the number of cases in the literature is too small to permit definite conclusions.

We have experienced a case of a well-differentiated composite glandular-endocrine cell carcinoma in which the superficial part was composed of adenocarcinoma with carcinoid elements restricted to the deep part of the tumor (Fig. 5–14). Endoscopic biopsies revealed only adenocarcinoma; the composite nature of the tumor was appreciated only in the resection specimen.[12]

Choristomas of the Stomach

Heterotopic Pancreas

Small submucosal nodular lesions composed of pancreatic elements are not uncommon in the stomach as incidental findings (Fig. 5–15A). Rarely they reach a size that renders them visible

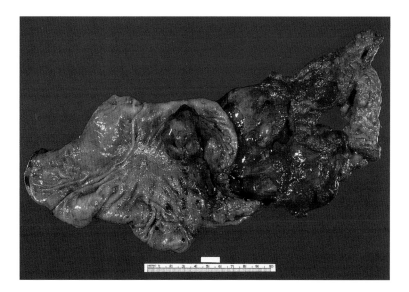

Figure 5–13. Composite adenocarcinoma–carcinoid tumor of the stomach, presenting as a polypoid mass.

at endoscopy or on radiologic studies. Microscopically, these lesions may resemble normal pancreatic parenchyma with well-organized acini and ducts, when they are referred to as heterotopic pancreas (Fig. 5–15B). At the other extreme, pancreatic acini are not present, and the lesion is composed of a disorganized mass of pancreatic ductal structures admixed with smooth muscle, in which case they are called adenomyomas (Fig. 5–15C). In most lesions, pancreatic acini, ducts, and smooth muscle are present in a disorganized mass. The term "pancreatic choristoma" appears to be an accurate designation for this entity.

Brunner's Gland Heterotopia

These insignificant lesions are commonly small and always located in the antrum. They are usually ignored because the heterotopic Brunner's glands can be differentiated from the nor-

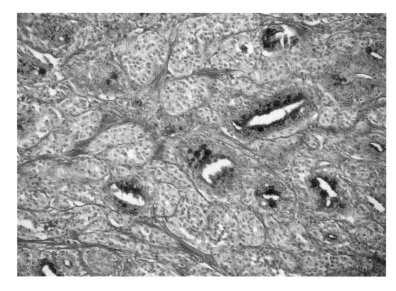

Figure 5–14. Composite adenocarcinoma–carcinoid tumor of the stomach, stained with Alcian blue, showing intimate admixture of mucin-positive, well-differentiated adenocarcinoma and nested carcinoid tumor.

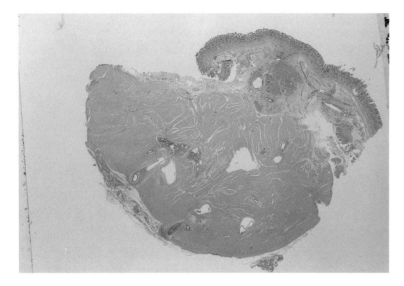

A

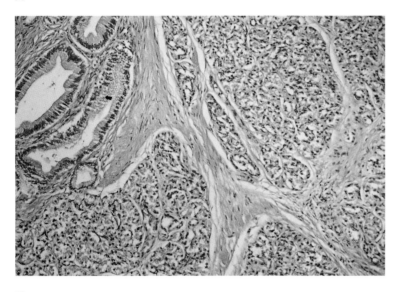

B

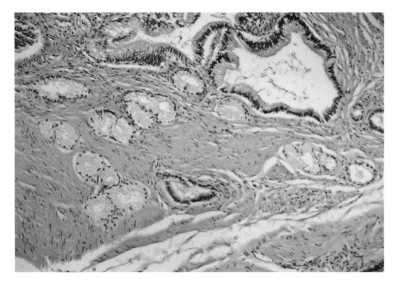

C

Figure 5–15. A: Heterotopic pancreatic tissue, showing a nodular mass in the submucosa of the stomach with an overlying normal mucosa. B: Heterotopic pancreatic tissue, showing serous acinar structures. C: Heterotopic pancreatic tissue, showing the lesion composed entirely of ducts and smooth muscle ("adenomyoma").

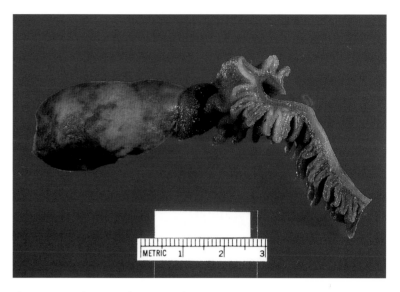

Figure 5–16. Inflammatory fibroid polyp of the stomach, showing a large, oval mass lesion. This prolapsed into the pyloric channel, causing gastric outlet obstruction. Note the congestion at the tip of the polyp.

mal mucous glands of the pyloric region only by their submucosal location. In normal antrum, the muscularis mucosae is normally split and encircles the mucous glands, making distinction of mucosal and submucosal location almost impossible on a biopsy. The diagnosis of Brunner's gland hyperplasia can only be made in a resection specimen, where it is usually an inconsequential incidental finding.

Other Polyps

Inflammatory fibroid polyps occur both in the stomach (Fig. 5–16) and small intestine (See Chapter 8). Mesenchymal polyps of various types, including lipoma (Fig. 5–17), leiomyoma, neurofibroma, granular cell tumor (Fig. 5–18A–D), and gastrointestinal stromal neoplasm also occur (See Chapter 14). Most mesenchymal neoplasms are submucosal and not seen in mucosal biopsies. The exception is granular cell tumor, which has

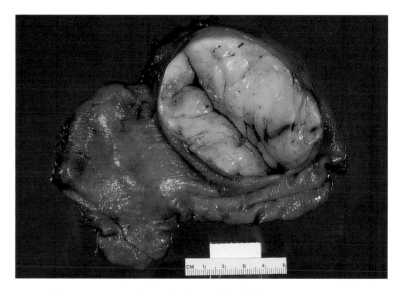

Figure 5–17. Gastric lipoma. The large size (8 cm) of this lesion is very unusual.

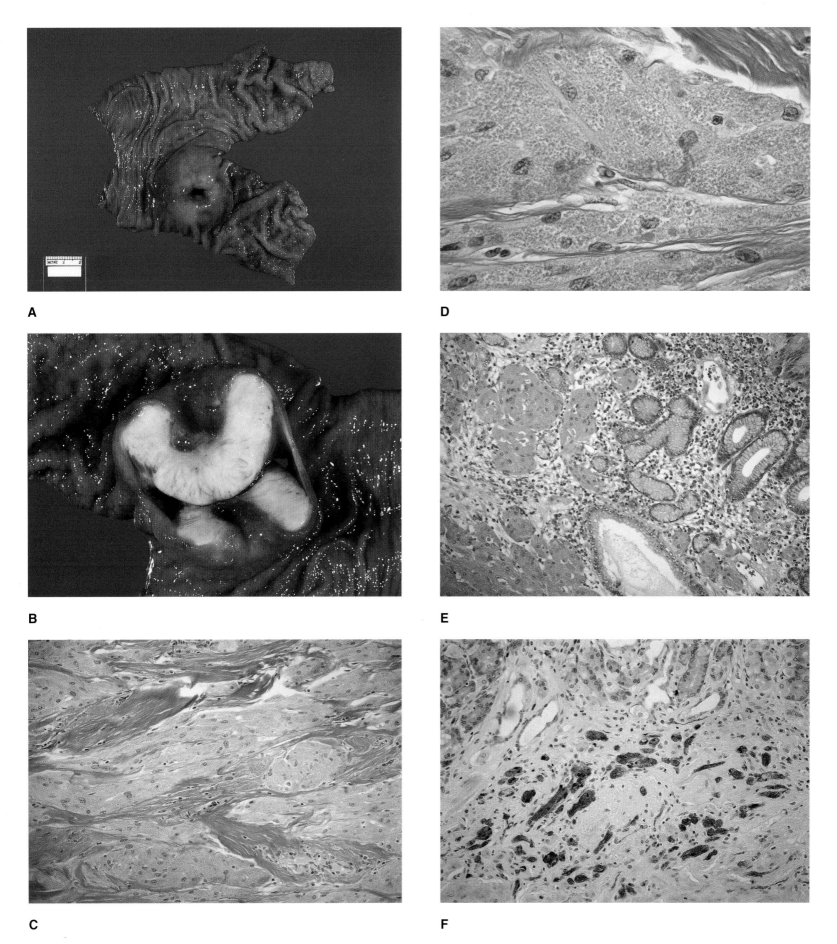

Figure 5–18. Granular cell tumor of the stomach. A: Submucosal mass projecting into the lumen, covered by mucosa with ulceration at dome. B: Tumor shown in part A bisected to show dense white appearance typical of granular cell tumor. C: Tissue characterized by nests of large spindle-shaped cells with abundant granular cytoplasm separated by collagen. D: Higher power micrograph of part C, showing neoplastic granular cells. E: Gastric biopsy specimen showing large cells with granular eosinophilic cytoplasm. These are easily missed in a biopsy specimen because they are commonly few in number. F: Neoplastic granular cells showing S100 protein positivity in immunoperoxidase-stained section.

an irregularly infiltrating edge, with neoplastic cells being frequently present in the overlying gastric mucosa (Fig. 5–18E). Their presence in mucosal biopsy can be confirmed with positive staining for S100 protein by immunoperoxidase (Fig. 5–18F). Very rarely, the stomach is the site for histiocytosis X, hemangioma, lymphangioma, eosinophilic granuloma, glomus tumor, osteoma, and osteochondroma.

Metastatic tumors very rarely involve the stomach, but those that do include malignant melanoma and carcinomas

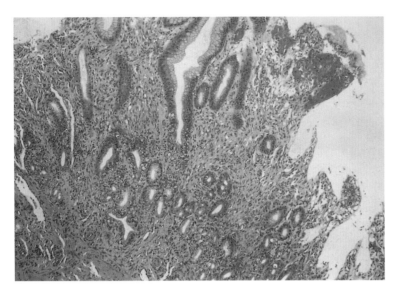

A

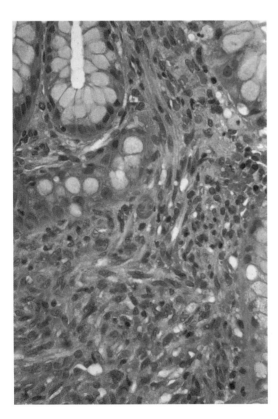

B

Figure 5–19. Kaposi's sarcoma of the stomach. A: Expansion of the lamina propria by a spindle cell proliferation. B: Higher power micrograph of part A, showing spindle cells with slit-like spaces in lamina propria between gastric glands.

from other sites. The latter are difficult to distinguish from primary gastric carcinomas unless there is a history of disseminated malignancy (particularly at autopsy) or the tumor clearly does not have a mucosal origin. Malignant lymphoma of the stomach is considered in Chapter 15. Immunocompromised patients, particularly those with AIDS, develop gastric lymphomas and Kaposi's sarcoma. Kaposi's sarcoma appears endoscopically as a red submucosal nodule. Biopsies show a spindle cell proliferation in the lamina propria with slit-like spaces, erythrocyte extravasation, and hemosiderin pigment. When the involvement is minimal, the diagnosis can be quite difficult (Fig. 5–19).

ADENOCARCINOMA

Classification

Many classifications of gastric carcinoma based on tumor location, invasiveness, histologic features, and growth patterns exist (Table 5–3). The recognition of true gastric carcinomas must exclude tumors that occur in the gastroesophageal junctional region because these behave epidemiologically like esophageal adenocarcinomas. Distinction into early and late gastric carcinoma is crucial, particularly in countries like Japan where screening protocols exist for gastric cancer.

TABLE 5–3. CLASSIFICATIONS OF GASTRIC CARCINOMA

By Location of Tumor	
Proximal vs. distal	*Proximal:* Occur in cardiac mucosa and gastroesophageal junction; not true gastric carcinomas.
	Distal: Occur in oxyntic and pylori mucosa; location within this area is irrelevant except in the choice of surgery.
By Invasiveness	
Early vs. late	*Early:* Invasion restricted to submucosa; further divided into intramucosal (EGC-m) and submucosal (EGC-sm) types.
	Late: Invasion of muscularis externa present.
By Differentiation	
Well, moderately, poorly	*Well:* Well-developed tubular glands, uniform cytologic features.
	Moderately: Complex glands with cribriform change; irregular small glands. Cytologic abnormalities severe.
	Poorly: Solid nests, single cells, signet ring cells; cytologic abnormalities variable.
By Histologic Features	
World Health Organization	Adenocarcinoma (papillary, tubular, mucinous, signet ring cell).
	Adenosquamous, and squamous cell carcinoma.
	Undifferentiated and unclassified carcinoma.
Lauren classification	Intestinal and diffuse (see text).
By Growth Pattern	
Ming	Expanding and infiltrative (see text).

Abbreviation: EGC = early gastric carcinoma.

In most centers, gastric adenocarcinoma is classified according to its degree of differentiation and histologic types according to the World Health Organization classification. The Lauren[13] and Ming[14] classifications have more value from an epidemiologic and prognostic standpoint. The Lauren classification is used in Europe but, although recommended for use, it has not yet gained universal acceptance in the United States.

Distal Versus Proximal Gastric Carcinoma

Gastric carcinoma consists of two separate entities: (1) that occurring in the body and pyloric antrum (distal carcinomas) and (2) that occurring in the cardia and gastroesophageal region (proximal carcinomas). Proximal cardiac carcinomas are epidemiologically similar to adenocarcinoma complicating Barrett's metaplasia in the lower esophagus and are considered in Chapter 3. When the term "gastric carcinoma" is used without qualification, it refers only to distal gastric carcinoma, excluding carcinoma of the gastroesophageal junctional region.

Considerable controversy surrounds whether a carcinoma in the gastroesophageal region represents gastric or esophageal carcinoma. The present recommendation is that if more than 50% of the tumor is located in the esophagus, it is esophageal, and if more than 50% is located in the stomach, the carcinoma is gastric. If the tumor equally occupies the esophagus and stomach, it is classified as esophageal if the histology is squamous, small-cell, or undifferentiated, and gastric if the histology is adenocarcinoma.[15] This method is very unsatisfactory for two reasons; first, it is difficult if not impossible to identify the lower end of the lower esophageal sphincter (which represents the true physiologic gastroesophageal junction) in a specimen; second, with the increasing incidence of adenocarcinoma complicating short-segment Barrett's esophagus, definition of any adenocarcinoma straddling the gastroesophageal region as gastric is very likely to be incorrect.

Early Versus Late Gastric Carcinoma

The most important classification of gastric carcinoma from a treatment and prognostic standpoint is into early and late gastric carcinoma. Early gastric carcinoma is defined as a carcinoma restricted to the mucosa and submucosa, irrespective of any other factor. Such tumors vary in size from 0.3 mm (minute gastric cancer) to a surface involvement exceeding 5 cm (superficial spreading cancer). Intramucosal carcinomas have a 0–5% risk of lymph node metastases and have a 5-year survival rate that exceeds 95%; submucosal invasion is associated with a rate of nodal metastasis of 10–20%. With resection, the overall 5-year survival rate for this group is 93%; patients with submucosal tumors and positive lymph nodes have a 5-year survival rate of 85%.

In contrast, late gastric carcinoma, which is defined as a carcinoma that infiltrates the muscularis externa has a less than 20% overall 5-year survival rate.

The Lauren Classification

The Lauren histologic classification of gastric adenocarcinoma into intestinal and diffuse has been emphasized in epidemiologic studies.[13] Intestinal-type gastric carcinoma is characterized by the following features:

1. A male:female ratio of 2:1 and a mean age of detection of 55 years.
2. Commonly presents as an exophytic intraluminal mass with an expansile growth pattern as it infiltrates the wall.
3. Characterized by tubular (Fig. 5–20), papillary (Fig. 5–21), and solid (Fig. 5–22) microscopic patterns, with mucin being restricted to the gland lumina. Squamous metaplasia may rarely occur (Fig. 5–23)
4. A 5-year survival rate of approximately 20%.
5. An almost 100% association with intestinal metaplasia and *Helicobacter pylori* infection.

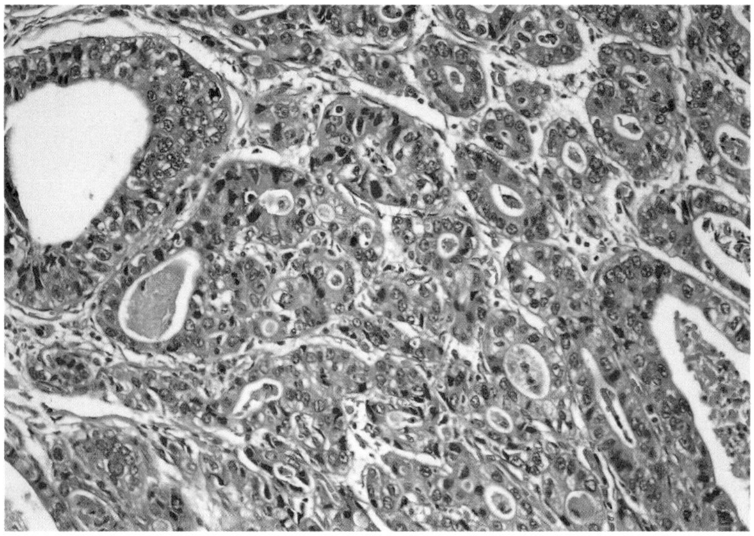

Figure 5–20. Adenocarcinoma of the stomach, intestinal type, showing moderately differentiated tubular structures.

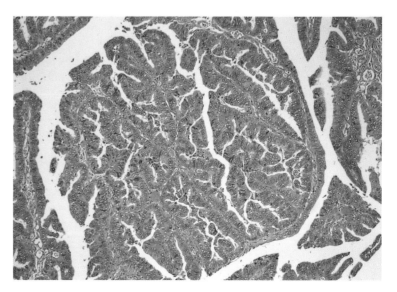

Figure 5–21. Adenocarcinoma of the stomach, intestinal type, showing papillary architecture.

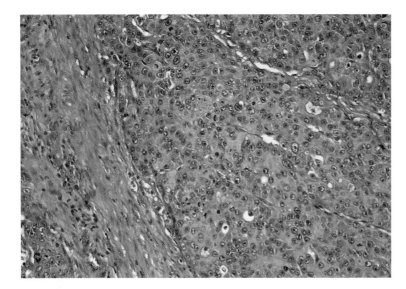

Figure 5–22. Adenocarcinoma of the stomach, intestinal type, showing solid architecture.

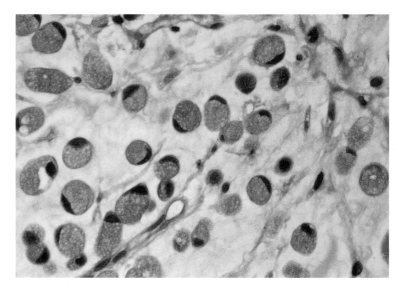

Figure 5–24. Adenocarcinoma of the stomach, diffuse type, showing signet ring cells.

Dietary and environmental factors are believed to be crucial to the development of intestinal-type gastric carcinoma.

In contrast, the diffuse type of gastric carcinoma has the following characteristics:

1. An equal sex distribution and tends to occur in younger patients (mean age at diagnosis is 48 years).
2. Commonly presents as an ulcerative, infiltrative tumor with a diffusely infiltrative pattern of growth in the gastric wall.
3. Characterized microscopically by poorly differentiated, discohesive cells, often signet ring cell type (Fig. 5–24), and often associated with intra- and extracellular mucin.
4. A poor prognosis, with the 5-year survival rate less than 10%.
5. Lower association with intestinal metaplasia and *Helicobacter pylori* infection than for intestinal type of gastric carcinoma.

Factors in the causation of the diffuse type of gastric carcinoma are less strongly related to diet and environment; genetic factors are thought to play a greater role.

The Ming Classification

The Ming classification[14] divides tumors by their growth pattern into (1) expansile tumors that grow as cohesive cell groups (Fig. 5–25) and (2) infiltrative tumors that have a diffusely infiltrative edge (Fig. 5–26). Most expansile carcinomas are of the intestinal type, but these also include poorly differentiated carcinomas growing as solid cell nests, which are difficult to classify in the Lauren classification. Infiltrative carcinomas are mostly of the diffuse type with signet ring cells but include infiltrative tumors composed of tubular structures (see Fig. 5–26). The Ming classification has prognostic value; patients with ex-

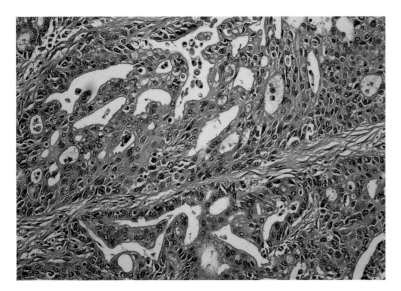

Figure 5–23. Adenocarcinoma of the stomach, intestinal type, showing solid area admixed with tubular element, suggesting focal squamous differentiation (adenosquamous carcinoma).

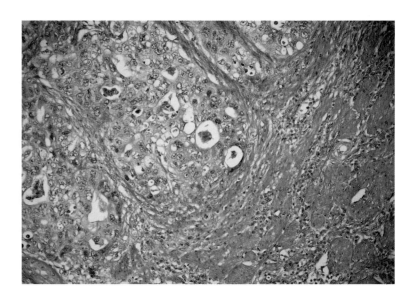

Figure 5–25. Expansile growth pattern in the Ming classification, showing a broad base of a solid tumor nest as it infiltrates the muscle wall. In the Lauren classification, this would be an intestinal-type, poorly differentiated carcinoma of solid pattern.

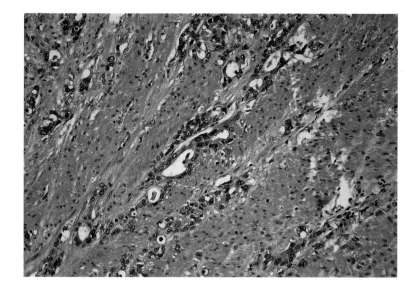

Figure 5–26. Infiltrative growth pattern in the Ming classification, showing a poorly differentiated carcinoma with tubule formation diffusely infiltrating the muscle wall.

pansile tumors have a higher survival rate than those with infiltrative tumors.

Epidemiology

In the United States, the incidence of gastric carcinoma declined dramatically from 1930 to 1985 and has remained stable since. Gastric carcinoma, with a death rate of 30/100,000 population, was a leading cause of cancer-related death in 1930. At present, the death rate is 6/100,000 population. Approximately 22,000 new cases are diagnosed annually in the United States; more than 90% of these are diagnosed at an advanced stage of disease, accounting for an overall 5-year survival rate of 17%. This overall survival statistic has not changed over the past two decades. The inability to identify high-risk groups has prevented the development of any relevant and cost-effective screening protocols for gastric carcinoma; until this is done, gastric carcinoma will continue to be detected at an advanced stage and the survival rates will remain low.

The decline in gastric carcinoma in the past few decades has been almost entirely due to the decrease in the incidence of intestinal-type carcinoma; the incidence of the diffuse type has not changed. Approximately 30% of gastric carcinomas diagnosed today are of the diffuse type, a considerable increase when compared to 20 years ago. This has resulted in gastric carcinoma being seen more frequently in younger patients and in women.

The reason for the decline in intestinal gastric carcinoma has been attributed to the more widespread availability of refrigeration and fresh produce, which have decreased the need for use of food preservatives. Use of nitrites as food preservatives and the lack of dietary antioxidants such as vitamin C resulting from a deficiency of fresh fruit and vegetables are believed to increase production of carcinogenic substances such as nitroso compounds in the stomach.

More recently, *Helicobacter pylori* infection has been implicated in the etiology of gastric carcinoma (see following section). *Helicobacter pylori* has an almost 100% association with intestinal-type gastric carcinoma, but is also significantly associated with the diffuse type.

Gastric carcinoma is uncommon in patients younger than 40 years; its incidence increases with age, peaking in the seventh decade. Men are affected about twice as frequently as women. In the United States, gastric carcinoma is more common among African-Americans, Native-Americans, and Hispanic-Americans than among Caucasians. There is a marked geographic variation in the incidence of gastric carcinoma. The incidence is highest in Japan (80/100,000 population) followed by Central and South America, China, and Eastern Europe. The high incidence of gastric carcinoma in these populations has been attributed to dietary and environmental factors that have not yet been clearly defined. The incidence in Japan has declined since 1960. In all populations the risk of gastric carcinoma increases with decreasing socioeconomic level.[16] This may be due to occupational factors[17] and the higher incidence of *H. pylori* infection in the lower socioeconomic sector of the population.

The frequency of gastric carcinoma is sufficiently high in Japan to recommend annual endoscopic or radiologic screening of persons older than 50 years. In Japanese endoscopy screening programs, more than 40% of cases are diagnosed before invasion of the muscle wall has taken place. This compares with less than 10% of early gastric cancers at time of diagnosis in the United States. These early gastric carcinomas have a 5-year survival rate exceeding 90% and account for the overall survival rates for gastric carcinoma being better in Japan. Diagnostic criteria for intestinal-type adenocarcinoma, however, appear to be different in Japan[18]; cases diagnosed as high-grade dysplasia and even low-grade dysplasia/adenoma by pathologists in the United States and Europe are frequently diagnosed as adenocarcinoma in Japan. In the United States and Europe, evidence of invasion is considered necessary to make a diagnosis of adenocarcinoma; in Japan, the diagnosis is made on cytologic criteria. These differences in diagnostic criteria between Japan and other countries may account for some of the variances in incidence, percentage of early cases, and survival rates from gastric carcinoma.

Although the role of genetic factors in gastric carcinoma is probably small, familial clustering does occur. The best known example of this is the Bonaparte family; Napoleon, several of his siblings, his father, and grandfather all died of gastric cancer.[19] Gastric carcinoma occurs in Lynch syndrome (hereditary nonpolyposis colorectal cancer), which results from a germline defect in DNA mismatch repair genes, and in patients with familial adenomatous polyposis (FAP). The first-degree relatives of patients with sporadic gastric carcinoma have a two- to threefold increase in developing gastric carcinoma.[20] A higher risk exists among persons of blood group A, suggesting genetic linkage. The genetic association with gastric carcinoma is higher in the diffuse type than the intestinal type of gastric carcinoma.

Premalignant Lesions

Many premalignant conditions put the stomach at increased relative risk for carcinoma. In the United States, however, the magnitude of risk associated with most of these conditions is so small that their recognition does not mandate either population screening or endoscopic surveillance. Endoscopic surveillance for gastric carcinoma is presently indicated for patients with gastric adenomas, FAP (where endoscopic surveillance is directed more at periampullary duodenal carcinoma), hyperplastic polyps, and high-grade gastric dysplasia when this has not led to gastric resection. Although *Helicobacter pylori* infection; chronic atrophic gastritis of all types, including pernicious anemia; intestinal metaplasia; the postgastrectomy gastric remnant, and low-grade gastric dysplasia, have known associations with gastric cancer, the low specificity of this association and the relatively low risk of cancer make surveillance not cost-effective in these populations. Benign gastric ulcer and Ménétrier's disease have been considered premalignant conditions in the past, but it is now generally accepted that patients with these conditions have no increased cancer risk.

Helicobacter Pylori Gastritis

Chronic atrophic gastritis caused by *Helicobacter pylori* is a common accompaniment of gastric carcinoma. Serologic evidence of *H. pylori* infection is more common in gastric cancer patients than in controls[21] and in populations of countries at high risk for gastric cancer.[22] *Helicobacter pylori* infection is associated with both the intestinal and the diffuse histologic type of gastric carcinoma, and with carcinomas involving the pyloric antrum and body but not the cardia and gastroesophageal junction. The association between *H. pylori* infection and gastric carcinoma is so strong that the World Health Organization has classified this organism as a major carcinogen.

Three mechanisms have been postulated to explain how *H. pylori* causes gastric carcinoma[23]:

1. *Helicobacter pylori* stimulates mucosal cell proliferation as shown by higher expression of nucleolar organizer regions and proliferating cell nuclear antigen in *H. pylori*-infected mucosa. Cell proliferation markers decline when *H. pylori* is eradicated.[24] This mitogenic effect of *H. pylori* is due to the organism's production of urease, which generates intraluminal ammonia, a compound known to stimulate cell proliferation. Increased cell proliferation results in an increase in the risk of mutations produced by carcinogenic agents.
2. Vitamin C is normally present in the stomach. *Helicobacter pylori* infection results in lowering of gastric luminal vitamin C concentration, an abnormality that is reversed when *H. pylori* is eradicated.[25] Vitamin C has well-known antioxidant properties, which may reduce the conversion of nitrites to carcinogenic nitroso compounds in the stomach. Antioxidants also prevent oxidative damage to DNA.
3. *Helicobacter pylori* infection is associated with increased neutrophils in the mucosa and gastric lumen. Neutrophils

are a known source of oxygen-based free radicals, which are capable of carcinogenesis. Infection with *H. pylori* is the most common cause of prolonged neutrophil infiltration of the gastric mucosa.

The sequence of change that leads to carcinoma in *H. pylori* infection is believed to be as follows: severe active gastritis → multifocal atrophic gastritis → intestinal metaplasia → increasing dysplasia → invasive carcinoma. This sequence is likely for the intestinal type of gastric carcinoma, which is associated with atrophic gastritis, intestinal metaplasia, and *H. pylori* infection. Although diffuse signet ring cell carcinoma and *H. pylori* are also associated statistically, the mechanism whereby infection causes this type of carcinoma is unclear.

From a practical standpoint, *Helicobacter* gastritis is not a useful marker for future gastric cancer despite the strong association. *Helicobacter pylori* gastritis is an extremely common infection in many populations, and the incidence of gastric carcinoma among this group is very small. The risk is small even in those patients with chronic atrophic gastritis and intestinal metaplasia. The presence of *H. pylori* gastritis in the absence of dysplasia is not an indication for surveillance in the United States and Western Europe.

Chronic Autoimmune Atrophic Gastritis

Chronic autoimmune atrophic gastritis (pernicious anemia) has long been considered a significant risk factor for gastric carcinoma; the prevalence of gastric carcinoma in this group is 1–3%. Recent evidence suggests that the risk of carcinoma results not from the presence of autoimmune gastritis, but from associated dietary factors. Atrophic gastritis causes achlorhydria, which permits overgrowth of anaerobic bacteria in the lumen; these metabolize nitrites in the food to produce carcinogenic nitroso compounds.

In Scandinavia, the incidence of gastric carcinoma in pernicious anemia is high enough to warrant surveillance. In the United States patients with pernicious anemia have an incidence of gastric carcinoma not significantly higher than that for the control population,[26] and endoscopic surveillance is therefore not considered necessary.

Intestinal Metaplasia

Intestinal metaplasia is characterized by the appearance of goblet cells in the mucosa. These may occur in the surface epithelium, foveolar region or the mucous glands of the pyloric antrum, or in the mucous glands that occur in atrophic oxyntic mucosa. Intestinal metaplasia is commonly a permanent change that occurs in atrophic gastritis, but it may also occur as a transient change in healing erosions, being associated with reactive gastropathy.

Intestinal metaplasia is associated with changes in mucin types and staining properties. Gastric surface and foveolar cells normally contain neutral mucin, which stains positively with periodic acid–Schiff (PAS) stain and negatively with Alcian blue

(AB) stain at pH 2.5. Goblet cells in intestinal metaplasia contain acid mucin, which stains a deep blue color with Alcian blue at pH 2.5. The acid mucin in intestinal metaplasia can be further classified by means of the combined high-iron diamine (HID)–PAS stain at pH 2.5 into sialomucins (blue cytoplasmic staining with HID–PAS) and sulfomucins (brown-black cytoplasm on HID–PAS).[27] The presence of sulfomucin indicates colonic-type intestinal metaplasia, which is believed to have the highest association with gastric carcinoma.

From a practical standpoint, the finding of sulfomucin-positive, intestinal metaplasia has a low predictive value for future malignancy. Sulfomucin-positive intestinal metaplasia is associated with benign conditions in 75% of cases,[28] and it is absent in 70% of patients with gastric carcinoma. The recognition of sulfomucin-positive intestinal metaplasia in the stomach is therefore not a useful marker to recommend screening for gastric carcinoma. As such, special staining to characterize mucin types is rarely undertaken in the routine evaluation of gastric biopsies. Complex classifications of different types of gastric intestinal metaplasia have been proposed; these are not presented here because they have little practical value.

Gastric Adenoma and Hyperplastic Polyps

These two premalignant lesions are discussed in the previous section on polyps.

Congenital Immunodeficiency Syndromes

The incidence of gastric carcinoma is higher in patients with immunodeficiency syndromes than in the general population. The incidence is highest in common variable immunodeficiency; 9% of these patients develop gastric carcinoma.[29] Gastric carcinoma also occurs in X-linked agammaglobulinemia. In both these diseases, chronic gastritis is common and may explain the predisposition to cancer. Gastrointestinal malignant lymphomas also occur with increased frequency in many congenital immunodeficiency syndromes.

Gastric Remnant After Partial Gastrectomy

The gastric remnant left after partial gastrectomy and enterogastric anastomosis for peptic ulcer disease is considered at increased risk for developing carcinoma. Although it is generally held that patients with a gastric remnant have a twofold increase in gastric carcinoma compared with the general population,[30] some authorities question the presence of any risk.[31] Theoretically, patients with partial gastrectomy are not at sufficiently proven increased risk to mandate routine endoscopic surveillance. Practically speaking, however, it is not uncommon for the pathologist to receive gastric biopsies from patients with prior gastrectomy.

The gastric mucosa in a gastric remnant commonly shows histologic abnormalities, both in and out of the region of the anastomotic site. Reactive gastropathy, inflammation, and lesions resembling hyperplastic polyps are common at the stoma; gastritis cystica polyposa is a specific change at the stoma associated with reactive change, fibrosis, and gland distortion with microcystic change.[32] Diffuse chronic gastritis, sometimes with atrophy, is common in the mucosa away from the stoma. Diffuse reactive changes induced by bile reflux gastritis also occur. Reactive epithelial abnormalities probably account for most cases in which significant cytologic atypia is seen. Cases in which low-grade dysplasia is diagnosed tend to remain stable, with a less than 10% rate of progression to high-grade dysplasia. High-grade dysplasia is rarely seen, but represents the only significant indicator of cancer risk. Resection should be considered when high-grade dysplasia is found in a gastric remnant.

Gastric Dysplasia

Gastric dysplasia is a rare diagnosis in gastric biopsies. It is distinguished from adenoma because it occurs in mucosa not perceived as being abnormal at endoscopy, whereas adenoma represents the identical histologic change occurring in an endoscopically visible lesion. This distinction is not made in many published studies of gastric dysplasia, making statistics difficult to interpret. Also, as endoscopic techniques improve, the frequency of recognizing small flat adenomas increases, converting lesions previously classified as dysplasia to adenomas.

The above-mentioned distinction between gastric dysplasia and adenoma has practical importance. In an adenoma, the pathologist can recommend repeat biopsy, endoscopic surveillance, or complete endoscopic excision of the visible lesion; in dysplasia, repeat biopsy does not guarantee sampling in the same area because no lesion is visible and biopsies are random. Also, dysplasia cannot be excised completely without resection because it is potentially a diffuse or multifocal abnormality.

Gastric dysplasia is divided into low-grade and high-grade dysplasia. Previously, three grades of dysplasia—mild, moderate, and severe—were used; the present division into two grades is independent of the three-tiered system, with some cases previously called moderate dysplasia now being designated low-grade and some high-grade dysplasia. Two histologic types of gastric dysplasia occur: the first resembles a tubular adenoma of the colon (Fig. 5–27); the second occurs in the setting of chronic atrophic gastritis with intestinal metaplasia.[33] The diagnosis of gastric dysplasia excludes all reactive and regenerative epithelial changes and is restricted to those cases in which the histologic abnormality is believed to be precancerous. The grading of gastric dysplasia into low and high grade is based on cytological and histological criteria.

Low-Grade Gastric Dysplasia. Low-grade dysplasia usually occurs in the foveolar region and surface (Fig. 5–27). The normal simple tubular foveolar structure is maintained, and the underlying deep foveolar region and glands are normal. Low-grade dysplasia is characterized by pseudostratification, cells with an increased nuclear:cytoplasmic (N:C) ratio, depletion of mucin, enlarged and hyperchromatic nuclei, and small numbers of typical mitotic figures. Nuclear polarity is maintained (see Fig. 5–27).

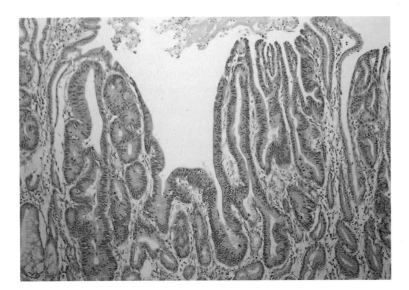

Figure 5–27. Gastric dysplasia, low grade, showing cells with cytoplasmic mucin depletion, nuclear enlargement, and disturbed nuclear chromatin in a mucosa showing no significant erosion or active inflammation. This was an area of a lesion that showed adenocarcinoma elsewhere, making it highly likely that this is true low-grade dysplasia.

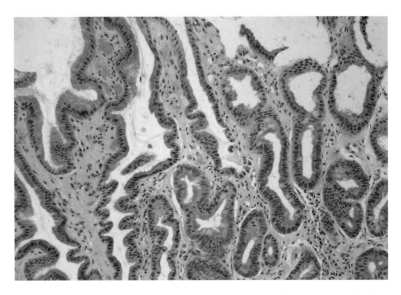

Figure 5–29. Reactive gastropathy, showing cytologic changes similar to low-grade dysplasia. These changes reversed on a repeat biopsy.

Low-grade dysplasia is difficult to differentiate from reactive epithelial changes associated with active inflammation and regeneration associated with reactive gastropathy and healing erosions (Figs. 5–28 and 5–29). Cytologically, the changes associated with reactive processes can almost exactly mimic low-grade dysplasia. The diagnosis of low-grade dysplasia is most confidently made when active inflammation and erosion are absent. In cases of doubt, a category of "indeterminate for dysplasia" can be used, but this has questionable practical value.

The significance of low-grade gastric dysplasia is questionable. Many studies suggest that it is a lesion that reverses in 60–70% of cases, persists in 20–30%, and has a low risk of progression to high-grade dysplasia and cancer.[3] The management of low-grade dysplasia is controversial. It has been suggested

that the finding of definite low-grade dysplasia warrants a rapid follow-up endoscopy with greater random sampling of the mucosa. If the low-grade dysplasia is widespread and persistent, surveillance may be indicated.

High-Grade Gastric Dysplasia. High-grade dysplasia is characterized by the presence of severe cytologic abnormalities in the epithelial cells with loss of nuclear polarity (Figs. 5–30 and 5–31). The affected foveolar region may remain simple, but frequently shows increasing complexity, with luminal bridging and cribriform change (Figs. 5–32 and 5–33). When gland crowding and complexity are present, the diagnosis of carcinoma in situ is sometimes made; this should be discouraged, however, because carcinoma in situ has the same significance as high-grade dys-

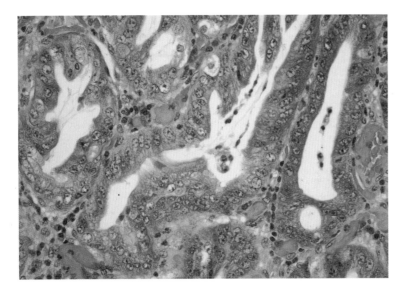

Figure 5–28. Reactive gastropathy, showing cytologic changes in the reactive foveolar epithelium that are similar to low-grade dysplasia. These changes reversed on a repeat biopsy.

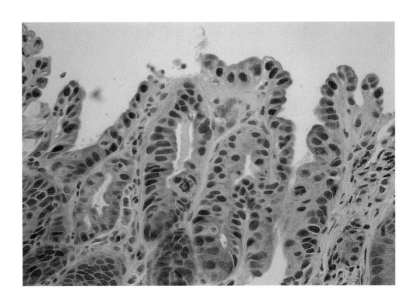

Figure 5–30. Gastric dysplasia, high grade, showing loss of polarity associated with moderate-to-severe cytologic abnormality. Significant observer variation can occur in this case, ranging from low-grade dysplasia to adenocarcinoma.

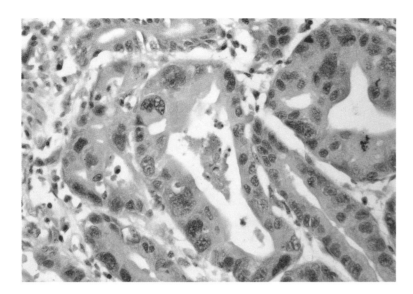

Figure 5–31. Gastric dysplasia, high grade, showing marked loss of polarity associated with severe cytologic abnormality. The diagnosis of high-grade dysplasia with this degree of abnormality is highly reliable.

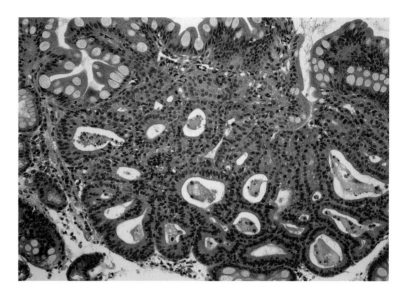

Figure 5–33. Gastric dysplasia, high grade, showing cribriform architecture of a complex glandular structure immediately below the surface epithelium, which shows intestinal metaplasia.

plasia and only adds to the confusion of the terminology. Intramucosal adenocarcinoma should be diagnosed when invasion of the lamina propria is evident (Fig. 5–34).

The finding of high-grade gastric dysplasia is always significant. It tends to persist, and progression to cancer occurs, although estimates of cancer risk are widely discrepant in different studies.[34,35] The management of high-grade dysplasia associated with a visible endoscopic lesion is generally considered to be excision, either by endoscopy or some form of gastrectomy.[33] When high-grade dysplasia is found in a random biopsy without a grossly visible lesion, however, the choice is between a large gastric resection and careful surveillance. Some authorities recommend careful surveillance because some studies suggest that the rate of progression to cancer is not high.[3,35] It should be recognized that diagnostic criteria for high-grade

dysplasia and adenocarcinoma are different in Japan; many cases called high-grade dysplasia by Western pathologists are called adenocarcinoma in Japan,[18] resulting in more aggressive surgical resection of these lesions in Japan. Whether this discrepancy is due to underdiagnosis of early gastric cancer by Western pathologists or overtreatment of high-grade dysplasia by Japanese physicians is not yet settled.

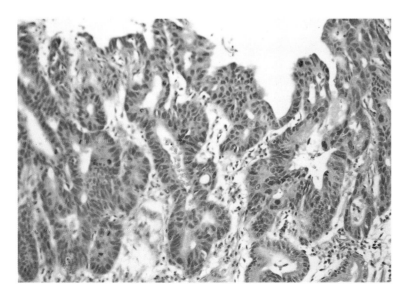

Figure 5–32. Gastric dysplasia, high grade, showing marked cytologic atypia associated with gland complexity characterized by luminal bridging and cribriform change. This degree of gland complexity is a highly reliable criterion for high-grade dysplasia.

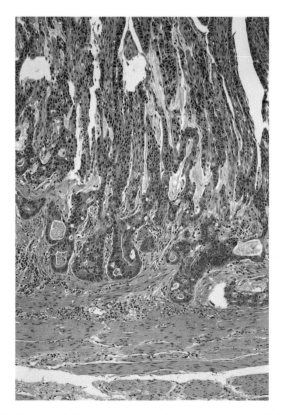

Figure 5–34. Intramucosal adenocarcinoma, intestinal type, showing irregular tubular malignant glands with complexity and irregularity. Rare single cells occur in the lamina propria. The carcinoma is limited at the lower edge by the muscularis mucosae.

Diagnosis

Endoscopic biopsy is the only method of diagnosing gastric carcinoma. The decision to perform endoscopy depends on the presence of suggestive symptoms and radiologic findings. Increasing the incidence of upper GI endoscopy for any reason increases the likelihood of early detection of gastric cancer. When symptoms typical for gastric carcinomas—anorexia, loss of weight, anemia, pyloric channel obstruction, hematemesis—occur, the tumor is invariably at an advanced stage. A significant number of early gastric carcinomas present with symptoms and endoscopic features of benign peptic ulcer; carcinoma is found at the ulcer edge on biopsy.

Rarely, adenocarcinoma of the stomach presents with evidence of metastasis, usually in the liver, a cervical lymph node (the left supraclavicular Virchow's node involvement is classical), or lung. When the metastasis includes signet ring cells, the stomach can be suggested as the most likely primary site (Fig. 5–35). Rare sites of metastasis from gastric carcinoma have been reported as a first presentation; these include uterine cervix (detected by a routine Pap smear),[36] the tonsil,[37] a congenital melanocytic nevus of the skin,[38] and microemboli to the lung causing cor pulmonale.[39] Peritoneal involvement manifests as ascites, ovarian masses (Krukenberg tumor) (Fig. 5–36), a mass in the rectovaginal pouch (Blumer's shelf on rectal examination), and a periumbilical nodule (Sister Mary Joseph's nodule).

Paraneoplastic syndromes are uncommon in patients with gastric cancer. Those reported are microangiopathic hemolytic anemia, membranous nephropathy, migratory thombophlebitis (Trousseau's sign), dermatomyositis, acanthosis nigricans, and sudden seborrheic keratosis (Leser-Trélat sign).

Endoscopic–Macroscopic Features

Gastric carcinomas are most commonly located in the pyloric antrum and the incisura angularis, which is the antrum–body

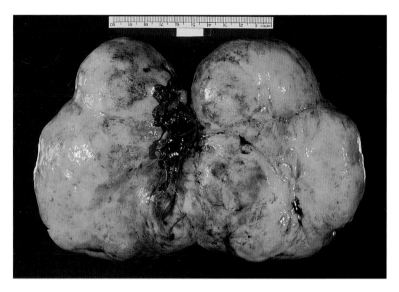

Figure 5–36. Krukenberg tumor of the ovary. Histologically, this had the typical appearance of a desmoplastic signet ring cell adenocarcinoma.

junction on the lesser curvature. The greater curvature and body are less common sites.

The gross appearance of advanced gastric carcinomas are classified into four types[40]: Type I is a nodular, broad-based, polypoid lesion without ulceration (Fig. 5–37); type II is a malignant ulcer or fungating tumor with an ulceration at the dome (Figs. 5–38 and 5–39); type III is an ulcerated tumor with an infiltrative base (Fig. 5–40); and type IV is a diffuse thickening of the gastric wall without a mucosal mass or ulcer, the classical linitis plastica type (Figs. 5–41 and 5–42).

Endoscopically 60–70% are large polypoid masses with or without ulceration (Types I and II). Biopsy specimens should be taken from the rim and the central ulcerated slough.[41] A prospective study[42] showed that a single biopsy sample yielded a positive diagnosis in 70% of cases; this increased to 95% when four specimens were taken and greater than 98% when seven

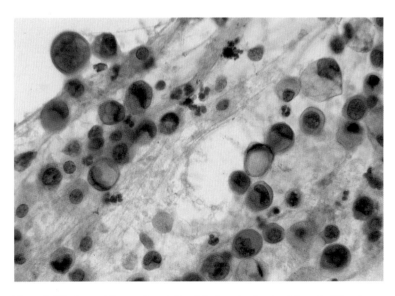

Figure 5–35. Smear of fine-needle aspiration of the liver, showing signet ring cells. Although nonspecific, this type of adenocarcinoma most commonly represents a metastasis from a gastric primary.

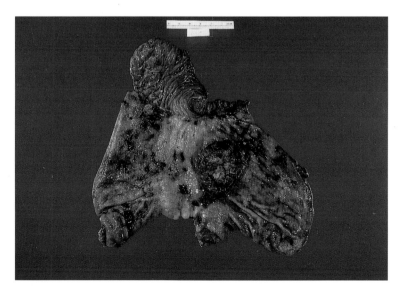

Figure 5–37. Gastric carcinoma, type I appearance, showing large, nodular, broad-based mass without significant ulceration.

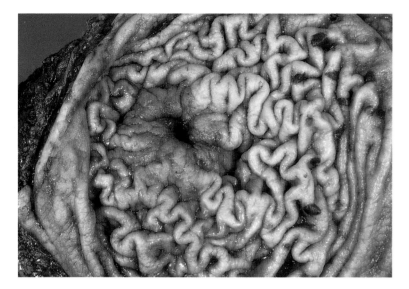

Figure 5–38. Gastric carcinoma, type II appearance, showing typical malignant ulcer with heaped edges.

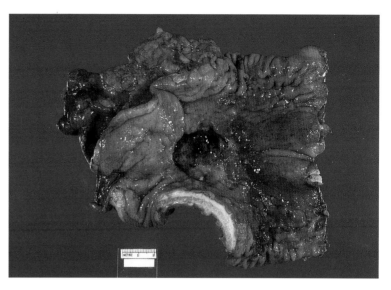

Figure 5–40. Gastric carcinoma, type III appearance, showing an ulcerated mass with an infiltrative base. This ulcer has a punched-out appearance, resembling a giant peptic ulcer. There was tumor, however, at the edges, base, and throughout the wall. The cut section of the wall of the pylorus shows thickening by the tumor.

were taken. Brush cytology samples increase the yield of positive diagnoses and is recommended.[43] It is not uncommon for a biopsy diagnosis of adenocarcinoma to be made when the endoscopic impression was of a benign lesion, particularly in ulcers.[42] The endoscopist should therefore obtain seven biopsy samples and a brush cytology specimen from any polypoid or ulcerative lesion of the stomach.

Thirty to 40% of advanced gastric carcinomas are diffusely infiltrative lesions. Many of these have obvious mucosal abnormalities that can be seen and biopsied (Types I–III). Some cases of linitis plastica-type cancer may have limited mucosal abnormalities (type IV); in these cases, false-negative diagnoses may occur even with multiple specimens. The use of jumbo biopsy

forceps with multiple specimens from any area of nodularity is recommended for lesions of this type. Endoscopic fine-needle aspiration may also be used in this situation.

Although brush cytology has been shown to improve diagnostic accuracy in gastric carcinoma, this technique has not received widespread acceptance. Cytologic interpretation is difficult, particularly in the presence of acute reactive processes (see Chapter 18). A positive cytologic test in the absence of a positive biopsy creates a problem. On the one hand, false-positive cytology occurs, albeit rarely[43]; on the other hand, it is difficult to ignore any positive diagnosis of malignancy. It is crucial, however, not to treat a patient for gastric carcinoma on the basis of a positive cytology without biopsy confirmation.

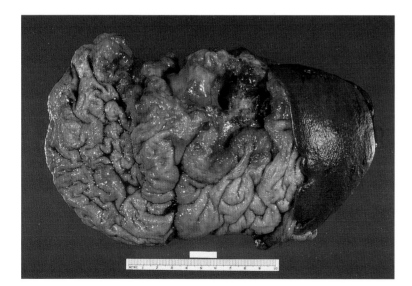

Figure 5–39. Gastric carcinoma, type II appearance, showing a large fungating mass with an extensive area of central ulceration.

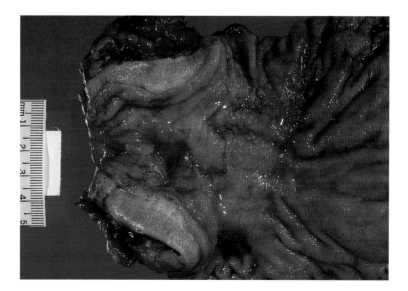

Figure 5–41. Gastric carcinoma, type IV appearance, with predominant infiltrative tumor causing thickening of the wall. In this case, the infiltrative tumor is restricted to the region of the pyloric antrum.

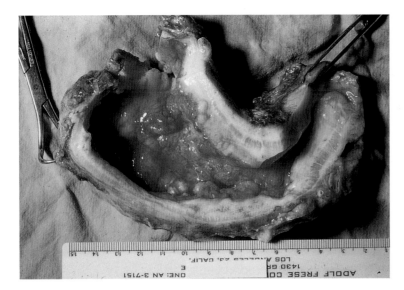

Figure 5–42. Gastric carcinoma, type IV appearance, showing the typical diffuse linitis plastica appearance. The entire gastric wall is thickened due to infiltrating cancer, resulting in a shrunken, nondistensible "leather-bottle" stomach.

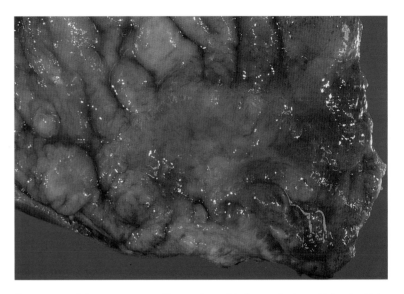

Figure 5–44. Early gastric carcinoma. The central part of the lesion is flat, but multiple polypoid elevations occur at the edge (mixed type I and IIb).

Early gastric carcinomas are much more subtle and require careful endoscopy. The gross classification of early gastric carcinoma recognizes the following types (Fig. 5–43)[44]:

1. Type I: protruding, or polypoid, type (Fig. 5–44).
2. Type II: superficial type characterized by unevenness of the mucosal surface. This is divided into an elevated type, which is essentially a plaque raised a few millimeters from the surface (type IIa) (Fig. 5–45); a flat type, which can be recognized only by a focal change in color of the mucosa (type IIb) (Fig. 5–46); and a depressed type, in which the surface is depressed a few millimeters from the surface and either has an intact or minimally eroded mucosal surface (Fig. 5–47) (type IIc).
3. Type III: excavated type, which is essentially a gastric ulcer (Fig. 5–48A). When these lesions are recognized endoscopically, biopsy can be done and has a high yield of positivity. Multifocal early gastric carcinomas occur in 5–15% of patients[45]; when one is found, it is imperative to carefully examine the rest of the gastric mucosa for subtle flat type IIb carcinomas.

The type III, excavated type of early gastric carcinoma is important to recognize (Fig. 5–48A). It differs from ulcerated advanced carcinoma in that, whatever the depth of the ulcer, the carcinomatous element is restricted to the mucosa and submucosa at the ulcer edge (Fig. 5–48B). The ulceration probably represents peptic ulceration caused by a loss of mucosal resis-

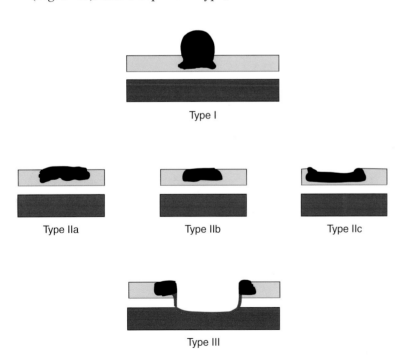

Figure 5–43. Classification of morphologic/endoscopic types of early gastric carcinoma. Type 1: polypoid; type IIa: elevated; type IIb: flat; type IIc: depressed; type III: excavated. The malignant element is shown in black. Note that in deeply excavated lesion in type III shown, the carcinoma is restricted to the mucosa.

Type I

Type IIa   Type IIb   Type IIc

Type III

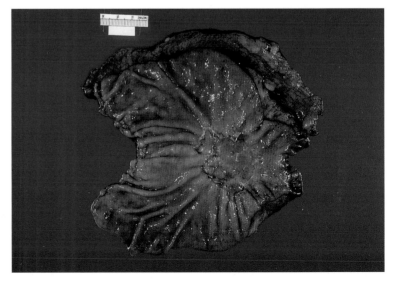

Figure 5–45. Early gastric carcinoma, type II (mixed), flat type with focal elevated and eroded areas.

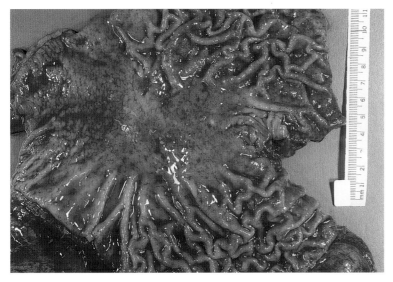

A

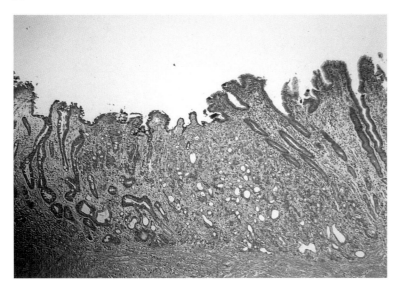

B

Figure 5–46. A: Early gastric carcinoma, type IIb, flat type. Grossly, the mucosa shows loss of rugal folds and fine granularity. Sections from this area showed a small area of intramucosal signet ring cell carcinoma. B: Intramucosal signet ring cell adenocarcinoma seen in sections taken from part A. Note that the area involved by adenocarcinoma is the same thickness as the surrounding mucosa.

tance resulting from the early gastric carcinoma. These ulcers resemble benign peptic ulcers of the stomach in their clinical symptoms, radiologic, and endoscopic features, and they frequently respond to medical therapy for peptic ulcer disease with healing of the ulcer. Understanding these factors is important because it emphasizes the need to take multiple specimens from all quadrants of benign gastric ulcers encountered at endoscopy. Four to 7% of benign-appearing ulcers are proven to be malignant histologically.

Biopsy Features

Approximately 70% of gastric carcinomas are of the intestinal type (Figs. 5–49 and 5–50); the other 30% are diffuse, often with signet ring cells (Figs. 5–51 and 5–52). There is some correlation between macroscopic appearance and histologic type. The polypoid lesions, both advanced and early, tend to be intestinal. The

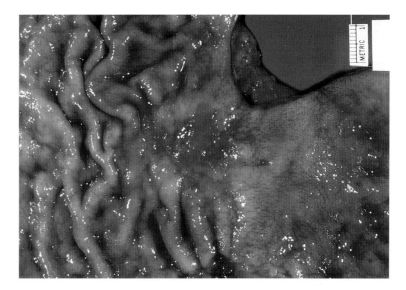

Figure 5–47. Early gastric carcinoma, type IIc, depressed type, showing a flat, depressed area with focal erosion of the surface.

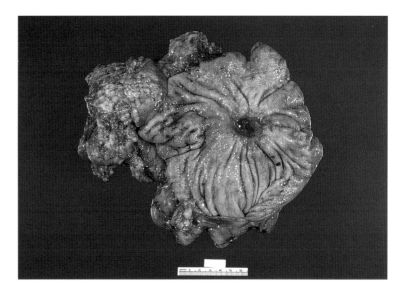

A

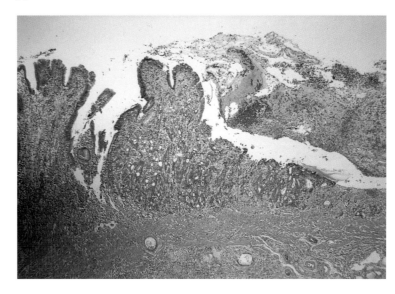

B

Figure 5–48. A: Early gastric carcinoma, type III, excavated type, showing gross features that are indistinguishable from a benign gastric ulcer. B: Biopsies from the edge of the ulcer shown in part A, showing intramucosal signet ring cell carcinoma at the ulcer's edge. No tumor is evident in the ulcer's base or in any submucosal location.

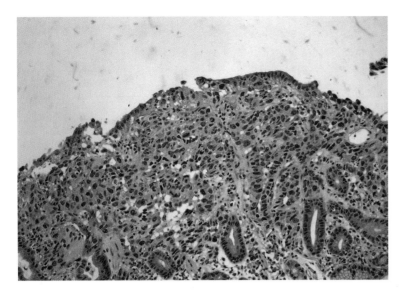

Figure 5–49. Gastric biopsy specimen showing a solid type of intestinal adenocarcinoma without signet ring cells in the superficial mucosa. Note that the surface epithelium is intact, although thin.

infiltrative late lesions and the depressed and excavated (types IIc and III) early lesions tend to be signet ring cell carcinomas.

Intestinal-type adenocarcinoma may present the pathologist with difficulty in the following situations:

1. Its differentiation from high-grade epithelial dysplasia depends on the presence of lamina propria invasion. Invasion is certain when irregular malignant glands are surrounded by desmoplasia, but can be difficult in early carcinomas in which invasion is restricted to the lamina propria (Fig. 5–53). This distinction is usually not important, particularly in centers where resection is considered to be the treatment of choice for high-grade dysplasia.
2. More troublesome, however, is the differentiation of intestinal type carcinoma from severe regenerative atypia associated with healing erosions. Healing erosions may show papilliform (Fig. 5–54) and complex glandular architecture (Fig.

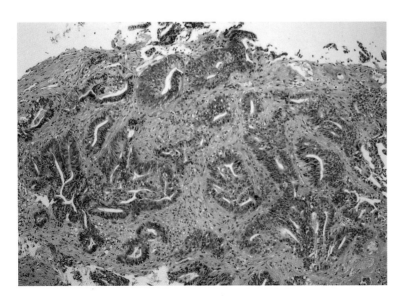

Figure 5–50. Gastric biopsy specimen showing invasive, moderately differentiated adenocarcinoma, intestinal type, with irregular infiltrative malignant glands surrounded by desmoplastic reaction.

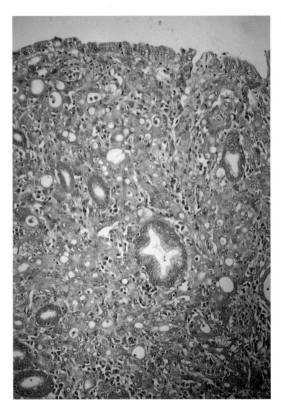

Figure 5–51. Gastric biopsy specimen, showing signet ring cell adenocarcinoma. The lamina propria is distended with malignant cells that show signet ring change focally. Normal glands are scattered throughout the slide.

5–55) and a pseudo-infiltrative appearance with fibrosis (Fig. 5–56). When these are associated with the cytologic changes of reactive atypia, the risk of a false-positive diagnosis of adenocarcinoma is significant. The presence of necrotic cells in the lumina of the atypical glands, glands lined with flattened epithelium (Fig. 5–56C), and the presence of parietal cells in the atypical glands are helpful indications of reactive change.

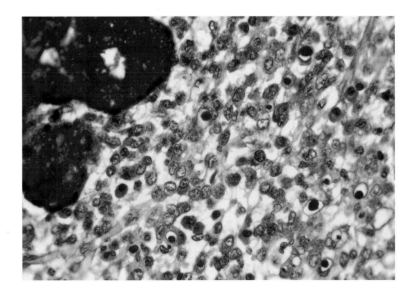

Figure 5–52. Gastric biopsy specimen, showing signet ring cell adenocarcinoma, periodic acid–Schiff stain after diastase digestion. The malignant cells show globules of mucin, often surrounded by a halo ("target" appearance). Note the positive staining of neutral mucin in the benign epithelial cells.

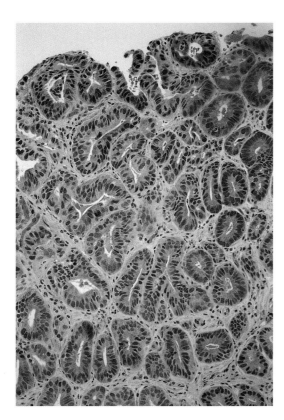

Figure 5–53. Complex dysplastic glandular proliferation in a gastric biopsy from a endoscopically suspicious lesion. This is difficult to interpret with a differential diagnosis of adenoma with high grade dysplasia and intramucosal adenocarcinoma. The diagnosis made was intramucosal tubular adenocarcinoma. leading to a gastrectomy which contained a residual early gastric adenocarcinoma with focal submucosal invasion.

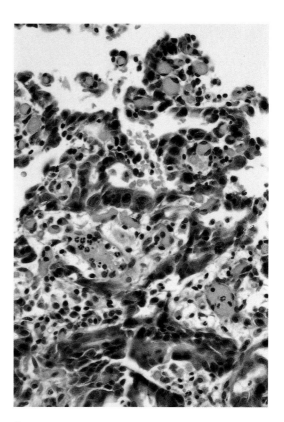

A

B

Figure 5–54. A: Healing erosion, showing a papillary surface with marked cytologic atypia. This patient was reexamined 3, 6, and 12 months later and had no gastric abnormality. B: Healing erosion, deeper area with regenerative glands, showing marked cytologic atypia contrasting with the adjacent normal glands.

Although early carcinoma can show erosions (Fig. 5–57), a diagnosis of adenocarcinoma must be made with caution in the presence of surface erosion because the majority of these lesions will be reactive. The recognition of parietal cells in an atypical gland argues strongly against adenocarcinoma, which involves the foveolar region and has little tendency to spread in Pagetoid fashion into the oxyntic glands.

3. Regenerative changes in gastric glands at the edge of a benign peptic ulcer may be difficult to differentiate from ulceration associated with an excavated (type III) intestinal-type early gastric carcinoma (Fig. 5–58). This distinction depends entirely on cytologic criteria.

Diffuse signet ring cell carcinoma rarely causes diagnostic problems, except that sometimes the number of cells present can be very small (Fig. 5–59) or obscured by inflammation in an ulcer base (Fig. 5–60), and the lesion can be completely missed. In most cases, the signet ring cells are easily recognizable at an ulcer base or between glands in the lamina propria. Although cytologic features of malignancy are usually obvious, signet ring cell carcinoma can sometimes have a bland cytologic appearance, with the cells resembling muciphages (Fig. 5–61). Muciphages almost never occur in gastric mucosa. Presence of cells resembling muciphages almost always indicates signet ring cell adenocarcinoma. Other macrophage lesions of the mucosa, such as gastric xanthelasma, and infectious diseases, such as

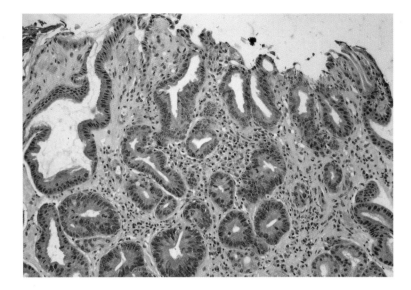

A

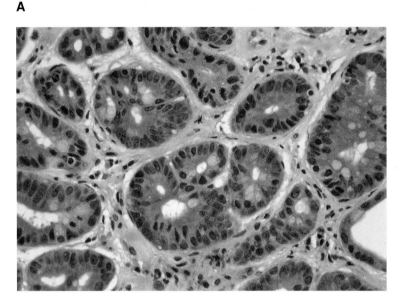

B

Figure 5–55. A: Healing erosion with reactive change. The glands show severe regenerative cytologic atypia. This lesion was also shown to have reversed on follow-up examination. B: Higher power micrograph of part A, showing early gland complexity associated with regenerative atypia. This has features that are easily mistaken for high-grade dysplasia or malignancy.

atypical mycobacterial infection and cryptococcal infection of the mucosa, may have a superficial resemblance to signet ring cell adenocarcinoma. In any case of doubt, staining for mucin (mucicarmine or hyaluronidase-digested PAS stain) (Fig. 5–62) or, better, immunoperoxidase stain for cytokeratin (Fig. 5–63), are diagnostic. Cytokeratin stain is preferable because it shows positivity in poorly differentiated malignant cells that do not contain mucin as well as in signet ring cell carcinomas.

Infiltrative gastric carcinomas of the linitis plastica type without much mucosal change at endoscopy require deep biopsies to demonstrate malignant cells. In these cases, the superficial part of the specimen can be normal, and the diagnosis depends on identifying small numbers of malignant signet ring cells in the deepest part of the mucosa (Fig. 5–64).

Difficulty is sometimes encountered when detached signet

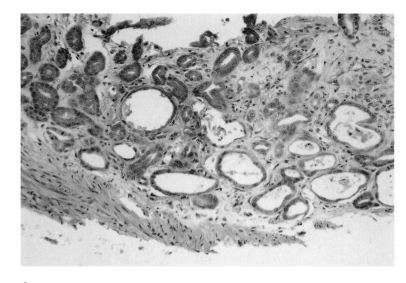

A

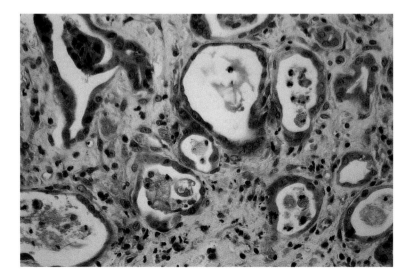

B

C

Figure 5–56. A: Healing erosion, with irregular glands showing an infiltrative pattern. Note that the thickness of the mucosa is much less than normal. B: Higher power micrograph of part A, showing severe reactive cytologic changes associated with regeneration. This patient has remained without gastric lesions in follow-up examinations. C: Higher power micrograph of part A, showing irregular glands lined by flattened epithelial cells and containing necrotic debris in the gland lumen.

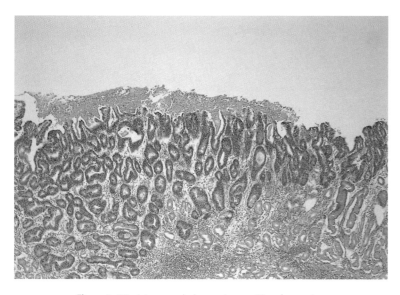

Figure 5–57. Intramucosal adenocarcinoma with surface erosion.

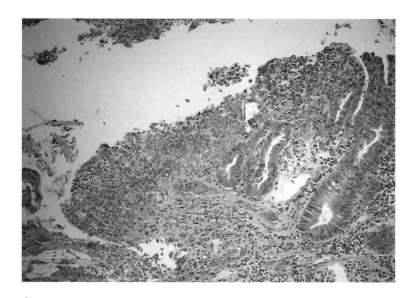

A

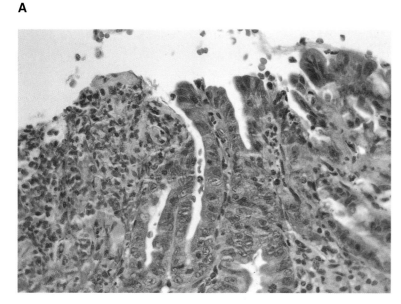

B

Figure 5–58. A: Edge of benign peptic ulcer, showing irregular glands with distortion. B: Higher power micrograph of part A, showing severe regenerative atypia at the edge of a benign peptic ulcer.

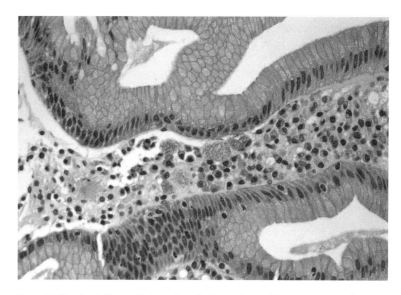

Figure 5–59. Gastric biopsy with signet ring cell adenocarcinoma. Only rare signet ring cells are evident in the mucosa. This specimen was from a patient who had advanced linitis plastica-type carcinoma.

ring cells are present in a biopsy specimen of the superficial necrotic debris of an ulcerated lesion (Fig. 5–65A and B). Detached, degenerated mucous cells from normal mucosa can resemble signet ring cells, so care is needed before a diagnosis of adenocarcinoma is made on the basis of such detached cells (Fig. 5–65C). When the detached cells are well preserved and show cytologic features of malignancy, however, a confident diagnosis is possible (Fig. 5–65D).

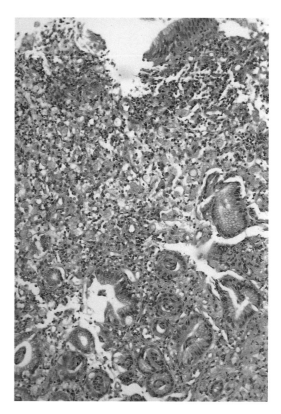

Figure 5–60. Gastric biopsy with signet ring cell carcinoma, showing an abnormal cell proliferation in the lamina propria. Careful examination is necessary to recognize the signet ring cells in this cellular infiltrate, which is associated with inflammation and granulation tissue.

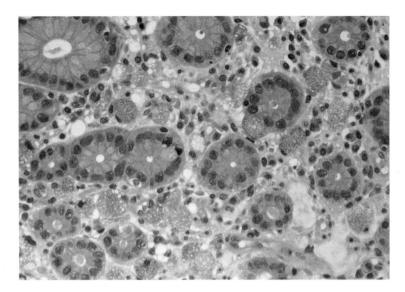

Figure 5–61. Signet ring cell carcinoma. The malignant cells have a deceptively bland cytologic appearance. They should never be mistaken for muciphages, which almost never occur in gastric mucosa.

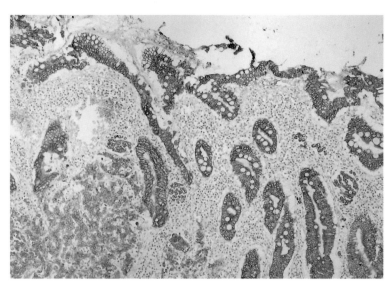

Figure 5–63. Gastric adenocarcinoma, stained by immunoperoxidase for cytokeratin, showing positive staining in both normal and malignant cells. The malignant cells appear as several small irregular cell groups, which can be recognized by their lack of organization.

Degeneration of cells lining glands can sometimes result in the cells becoming detached and falling into the gland (Fig. 5–66A). Cytoplasmic degeneration can result in an appearance that closely mimics signet ring cells (Fig. 5–66B). Staining for cytokeratin also shows a superficial resemblance to carcinoma (Fig. 5–66C). The crucial feature to recognize in these cases to avoid a false-positive diagnosis is the preservation of the gland outline (Fig. 5–66D). Signet ring cell carcinoma must not be diagnosed without the presence of signet ring cells in the lamina propria outside the glands.

Another situation associated with the potential for false-positive diagnosis of signet ring cell carcinoma is in a gastric malignant lymphoma. At the end stage of destruction of gastric glands by infiltrating lymphoma cells, the epithelial cells in lymphoepithelial lesions can simulate signet ring cells. The recognition of the malignant lymphoma prevents misdiagnosis.

Cases in which the biopsy features are worrisome but not diagnostic for carcinoma should be rare. In these cases, repeat biopsy can be recommended if an endoscopically defined focal lesion is present. This may be particularly indicated if the number of specimens taken in the original endoscopy is fewer than seven because some data show an increase in the yield of carcinoma diagnoses for up to seven biopsies.[42] When the atypical histologic changes are seen in a random biopsy, repeat biopsy is frequently not a satisfactory option because it is difficult to identify the original biopsy site accurately for a repeat biopsy. Attempts to identify the most subtle endoscopic changes asso-

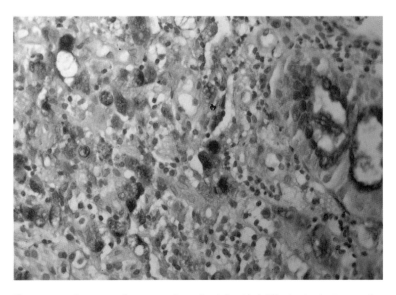

Figure 5–62. Signet ring cell carcinoma, digested periodic acid–Schiff stain, showing intracytoplasmic mucin. The mucin is diffusely distributed in the cytoplasm of these signet ring cells.

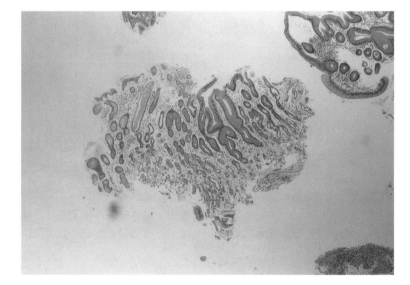

Figure 5–64. Signet ring cell carcinoma in the deep mucosa with overlying normal mucosa in a patient with advanced linitis plastica-type carcinoma.

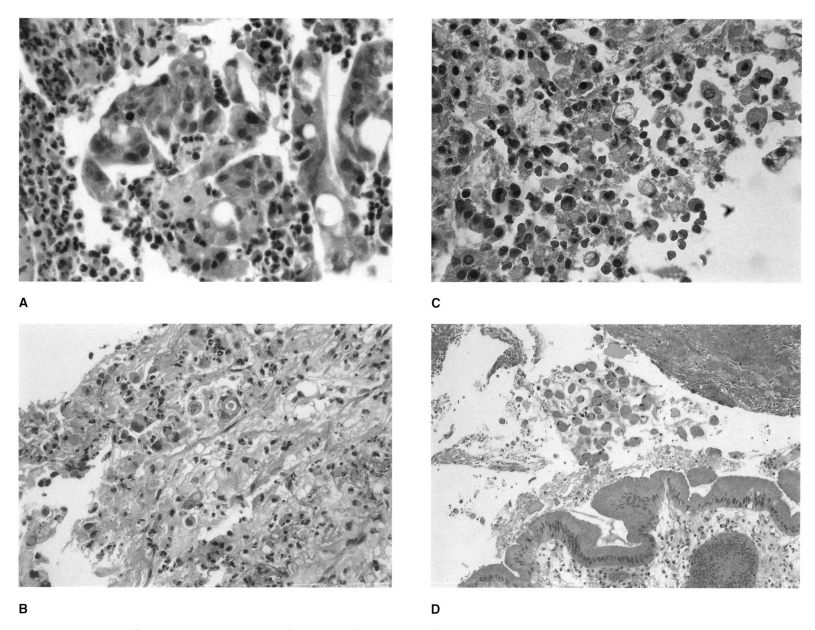

Figure 5–65. A: Detached signet ring cells in ulcer debris. This specimen was called "suspicious and atypical" but showed adenocarcinoma in a subsequent specimen. B: Degenerating cells in a gastric erosion. Some of the degenerated cells have a resemblance to signet ring cells. This patient did not have carcinoma. C: Degenerating cells in the necrotic debris of an erosion resembling signet ring cells. This patient did not have carcinoma. D: Detached cluster of signet ring cells overlying normal mucosa in a gastric biopsy specimen. This shows features that permit definitive diagnosis.

ciated with early gastric carcinoma may provide definition of a previously unseen lesion.

Tumor Markers

A large number of tumor markers, including tumor-associated antigens (carcinoembryonic antigen, CA 19-9, CA 125, tumor-associated glycoprotein) and oncogenes (K-*ras,* C-*erb* B-2, c-*myc*); as well as evaluation of DNA content of cells, aneuploidy, and expression of proliferation markers, such as nucleolar organizer regions and proliferative cell nuclear antigen, have been studied in gastric carcinoma. To date, no tumor marker has proven to be of value in diagnosis, screening, staging, or prognosis assessment in gastric carcinoma.[46]

A large number of genetic abnormalities have been identified in gastric carcinoma cells.[47] These include microsatellite instability; K-*ras* mutations; c-*erb* B-2, c-*met,* and K-*sam* amplification; *bcl*-2 loss of heterozygosity; *p53* mutation and loss of heterozygosity; *APC* (5p) gene mutation and loss of heterozygosity; and *DCC* (18q) loss of heterozygosity. Molecular changes appear to differ between well-differentiated (intestinal) and poorly differentiated (diffuse) gastric carcinomas, suggesting different carcinogenetic pathways (Table 5–4). Some of these genetic abnormalities are also present in premalignant lesions, such as adenoma and hyperplastic polyps. Unlike colon cancer, no constant sequence of genetic change has been detected in gastric carcinoma. These genetic abnormalities are not constant enough to provide diagnostic or prognostic information.

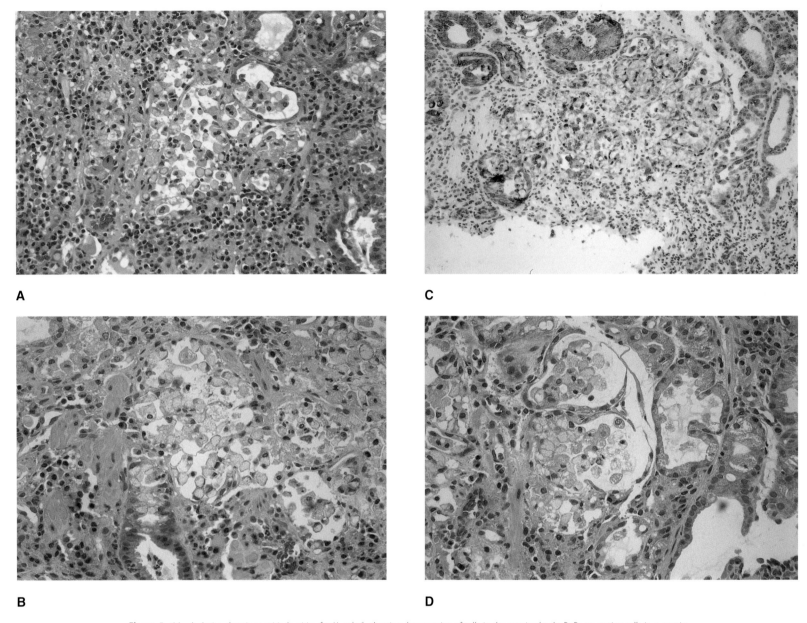

Figure 5–66. A: Active chronic gastritis (positive for *H. pylori*), showing degeneration of cells in the gastric glands. B: Degenerating cells in a gastric gland in gastritis, showing the cells to have rounded up with eccentric nuclei and cytoplasmic mucin, bearing a close resemblance to signet ring cells. C: Immunoperoxidase stain for cytokeratin in area of biopsy shown in part B, showing disorganized appearance that mimics signet ring cell carcinoma. Careful examination is necessary to recognize that the degenerated cells are confined within the gland basement membrane. D: Higher power micrograph of part B, showing the degenerated cells within the lumen of the gland.

Preoperative Staging

Preoperative staging is important in determining appropriate treatment. Endoscopic ultrasound (EUS) permits recognition of five layers, which correlate with mucosa, submucosa, muscularis externa, subserosa, and serosa. Evaluation of adjacent organs and perigastric lymph nodes is also possible. EUS permits accurate assessment of the depth of invasion of gastric carcinomas and detection of gross lymph node involvement. Fine needle aspiration biopsy of endoscopically defined lesions is feasible at endoscopy.

In early gastric carcinomas, treatment depends on whether the tumor is restricted to the mucosa or has infiltrated the submucosa, the latter being evidenced by disruption of the echo-

rich submucosal layer on EUS. Endoscopic resection is feasible in types I, IIa, and IIb intramucosal gastric carcinomas that are less than 2 cm in size. It is contraindicated in excavated or ulcerated lesions (types IIc and III) and when submucosal involvement occurs because of the difficulty in establishing a plane of mucosectomy and the increased incidence of lymph node involvement. Endoscopic treatment methods include strip biopsy, photodynamic therapy, and endoscopic aspiration mucosectomy.[44,48] Endoscopic resection specimens are difficult to evaluate for surgical margins because they are rarely in one piece; if a mucosal resection is ever received as a complete mucosal piece, it should be inked appropriately, carefully pinned out, and fixed before sections are cut.

Preoperative staging of advanced gastric cancer may use a

TABLE 5–4. MOLECULAR ABNORMALITIES IN GASTRIC CARCINOMAS

	Well Differentiated* (Intestinal)	Poorly Differentiated (Diffuse)
Microsatellite instability	+	++
K-*ras* (mutation)	+/−	−
c-*met* (amplification)	+	++
K-*sam* (amplification)	−	++
c-*erb* B-2 (amplification)	+	−
bcl-2 (LOH)	++	−
p53 (mutation, LOH)	+++	+++
APC gene (mutation, LOH)	+++	−
DCC gene (LOH)	+++	−
Epidermal growth factor	++	−
Cadherin (deletion)	−	++

Abbreviations: LOH = loss of heterozygosity; APC = adenomatous polyposis coli; DCC = deleted in colon cancer.

* − = 0; +/− = 1–9%; + = 10–24%; ++ = 25–49%; +++ = >50%.

combination of computed tomography (CT) scan to detect liver metastases and lymph node involvement, EUS to establish the depth of wall invasion, and laparoscopy. Laparoscopy increases detection of extragastric spread, including peritoneal seeding, which may prevent futile attempts at curative surgery in these patients.[49] Laparoscopy also permits peritoneal lavage for cytologic examination, which is a sensitive method of detecting occult peritoneal involvement.

Treatment

Surgery

Radical surgical resection of gastric carcinoma represents the only chance for cure. This should be undertaken in all patients after a biopsy diagnosis of carcinoma has been made, unless there is evidence of disseminated disease or a contraindication to surgery. For pyloric antral tumors, partial gastrectomy with resection of adjacent nodes is the surgery of choice. Total gastrectomy is often needed for more proximal tumors. Splenectomy increases complications and gives no survival benefit and should not be done routinely.

Surgical management of gastric carcinoma in Japan uses an extended lymph node resection, which includes all lymph nodes within 3 cm of the tumor and nodes adjacent to the left gastric, splenic, common hepatic, and celiac arteries.[50] The value of this extended lymph node resection is presently being evaluated in prospective clinical trials.

In patients with disseminated disease, several nonsurgical endoscopic treatment modalities, including laser ablation of tumor tissue and the use of plastic and metal stents to overcome obstructive symptoms, are available for palliation. The ability to palliate without surgery has increased the need for accurate preoperative detection of disseminated disease.

Intraoperative staging can change the course of planned surgery in patients with gastric carcinoma. Frozen section of enlarged lymph nodes and lesions in the liver and peritoneum can provide evidence of disseminated disease that was not detected preoperatively. Frozen section of margins in the resected specimen is important in verifying the adequacy of resection, especially when partial gastrectomy has been performed.

Other Treatment Modalities

Gastric carcinomas are resistant to radiation. Radiation is only of value in end-stage disease for temporary tumor control.

Chemotherapy regimens that include multiple drugs (fluorouracil, doxorubicin, mitomycin, etoposide, cisplatin, etc) have been reported as having response rates of up to 40%. Rare cases have shown complete histologic response and tumor downstaging when chemotherapy has been used preoperatively. In these cases, areas of tumor necrosis are represented by histiocyte collections and fibrosis (Fig. 5–67).[51] No definite survival benefit has yet been shown.

Pathologic Features

Histologic Types

Over 99% of gastric carcinomas are adenocarcinomas,[52] and 70% of these are of the intestinal type by the Lauren classification (see Figs. 5–20 through 5–23). These have cytologic features resembling colorectal carcinoma, being composed of tubular glands that are lined by columnar cells. Papillary architecture and gland complexity are common. Solid areas also occur. Mucinous carcinomas have well-differentiated glands in extracellular mucin lakes. These intestinal carcinomas are commonly well and moderately differentiated, but many have areas within them that are poorly differentiated and solid, making their designation as intestinal difficult. The frequency with which poorly differentiated areas are admixed with the more classical intestinal type is one reason why Lauren's classification is difficult to apply uniformly. Most intestinal carcinomas, even those with solid areas, commonly have an expansile growth pattern without single-cell infiltration.

Thirty percent of gastric adenocarcinomas are of the diffuse type, being composed of poorly differentiated singly infiltrative signet ring cells (see Fig. 5–24 and Figs. 5–59 through 5–64). Signet ring cell carcinomas are commonly associated with marked desmoplasia, producing highly scirrhous tumors. In these, the malignant epithelial cells can be so obscured by the desmoplasia that they are difficult to recognize without mucin stains (Fig. 5–68). This fact is relevant, particularly at frozen sections for margins, nodal involvement, and peritoneal cavity involvement, where it causes frequent false-negative diagnosis. The use of smears and toluidine blue-stained, air-dried, frozen sections are helpful in these cases. Toluidine blue accentuates mucin in the epithelial cells. Some tumors have large amounts of extracellular mucin (Fig. 5–69); these tumors differ from mucinous carcinomas by having signet ring cells suspended in the

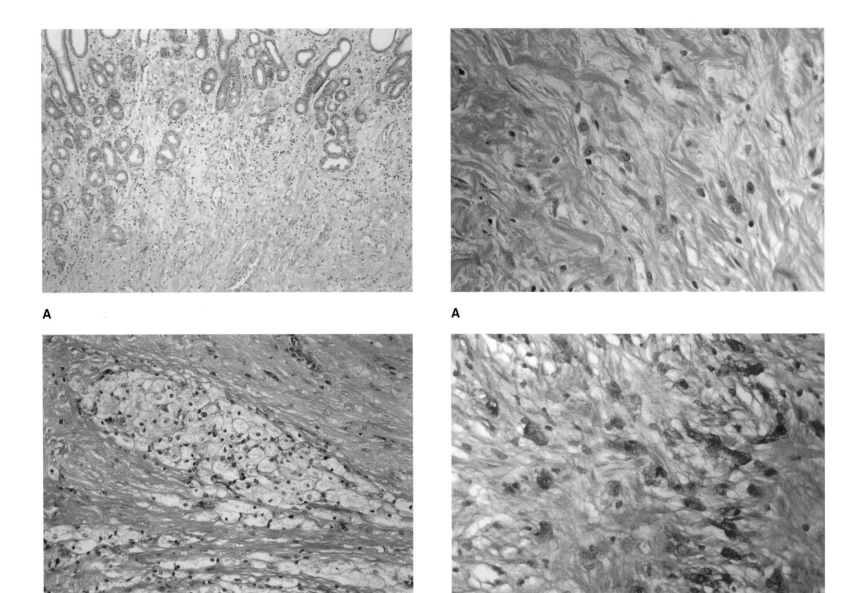

Figure 5–67. A: Area of regressed carcinoma in a gastrectomy specimen in a patient treated with preoperative chemotherapy, showing fibrosis in the mucosal lamina propria, most likely representing reaction to necrotic tumor. B: Chemotherapy-induced changes in the gastric wall, most likely representing histiocyte accumulation and fibrosis as a reaction to tumor necrosis. Staging is difficult in those cases where residual viable carcinoma is either minimal or not found.

Figure 5–68. A: Metastatic gastric adenocarcinoma in the omentum, showing tumor cells obscured by marked desmoplastic stromal reaction. B: Digested PAS stain showing mucin positivity in epithelial cells in the desmoplastic reaction.

mucin lakes. Mixtures of signet ring cell and better differentiated carcinomas also occur.

Most gastric carcinomas are histologically heterogeneous in terms of histologic type and degree of differentiation, producing a large variety of patterns that confound most attempts at classification. Approximately 25% of gastric carcinomas have both intestinal and diffuse types by the Lauren classification. It is recommended that these be classified as diffuse-type carcinomas.[13] This is not likely to be uniformly applied, however, particularly when the diffuse component is relatively small. Despite these difficulties, the Lauren classification is the best available histologic classification for gastric carcinoma.

A few (1%) gastric carcinomas are unusual histologically. Among the unusual histologic types described in the stomach are adenosquamous carcinoma (Fig. 5–70),[53] pure squamous cell carcinoma,[54] clear cell adenocarcinoma (Fig. 5–71), lymphoepithelioma-like carcinomas associated with Epstein-Barr virus,[55] primary gastric choriocarcinoma that produces β-human chorionic gonadotropin (Figs. 5–72 and 5–73),[56] adenocarcinomas with yolk sac carcinoma (endodermal sinus tumor) features that secrete α-fetoprotein,[57] hepatoid carcinoma with α-fetoprotein either in the tumor cells or in the serum (Fig. 5–74),[58] small-cell undifferentiated carcinoma of neuroendocrine derivation,[59] non-small-cell poorly differentiated carcinoma with neuroendocrine features,[8] sarcomatoid carcinoma,[60] and vimentin-positive gastric carcinoma with rhabdoid features.[61] Rare instances of mature and immature teratoma of the stomach have also been reported. These commonly occur in

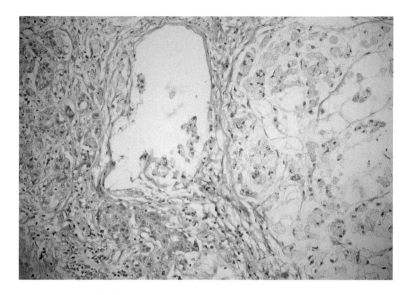

Figure 5–69. Signet ring cell adenocarcinoma with abundant extracellular mucin.

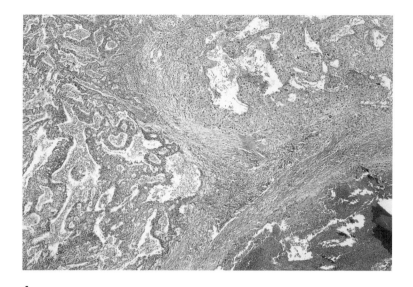

A

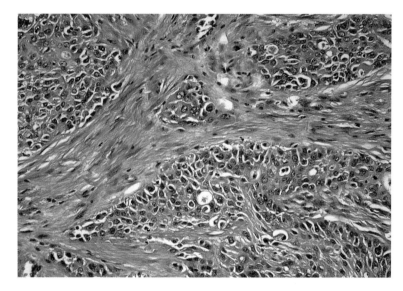

Figure 5–70. Adenosquamous carcinoma of the stomach. This was an area in a tumor that had better differentiated intestinal type adenocarcinoma.

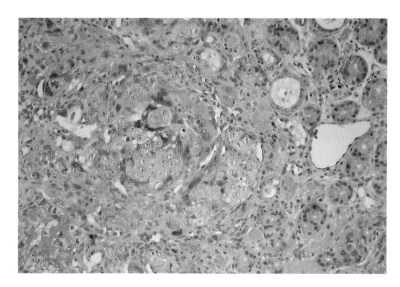

B

Figure 5–72. A: Gastric adenocarcinoma with choriocarcinomatous area. B: Higher power micrograph of the choriocarcinomatous area of part A, showing cytotrophoblastic cells with focal syncytiotrophoblastic cells. This was positive by immunoperoxidase for β-human chorionic gonadotropin.

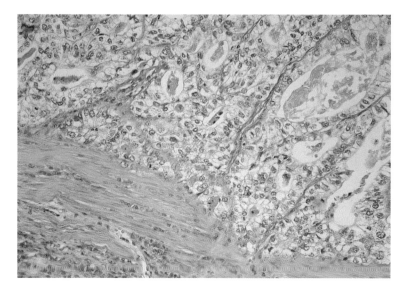

Figure 5–71. Clear cell adenocarcinoma of stomach.

Figure 5–73. Gastric mucosa with choriocarcinoma, showing cytotrophoblastic and syncytiotrophoblastic cells.

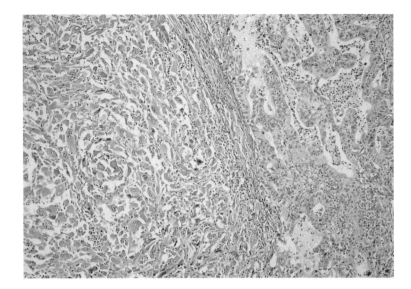

Figure 5–74. Gastric adenocarcinoma, hepatoid type, showing the poorly differentiated area with cells resembling hepatocytes adjacent to the better differentiated carcinoma.

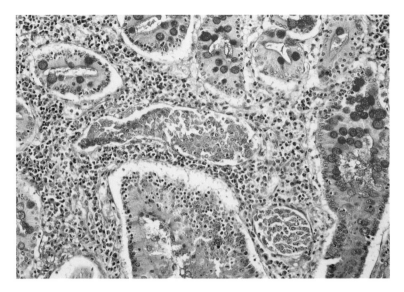

Figure 5–75. Invasion of the lymphatic in the mucosa by gastric adenocarcinoma, digested PAS stain. This shows dilated lymphatics in the lamina propria distended by tumor. The mucosal glands are normal.

children. One case of an adenocarcinoma arising in a gastric teratoma has been reported in an elderly man.[62]

Rare adenocarcinomas also occur in heterotopic pancreas[63] and in parietal cells of the oxyntic mucosa. Parietal cell carcinomas of the stomach are very rare; they present as deep mucosal or intramural nodules and resemble epithelioid stromal neoplasms microscopically. They are cytokeratin-negative and vimentin-positive, but on electron microscopy have cell junctions and dilated intracellular canaliculi with villi that are distinctive components of parietal cells.[64] Electron microscopy is essential for this diagnosis. Parietal cell carcinomas may metastasize to regional nodes, but in general have a better prognosis than usual gastric adenocarcinoma.

Rarely, gastric adenocarcinomas coexist with malignant lymphomas arising in mucosal-associated lymphoid tissue.[65] This is not totally unexpected because of the common etiologic association these two neoplasms have with *Helicobacter pylori* infection.

Mechanisms of Spread

Gastric carcinoma spreads by four different means:

1. Local infiltration through the wall in both a horizontal and vertical direction. Direct horizontal spread may occur at all levels, but is relatively limited in that its microscopic extent is not far from the gross edges of the tumor. Gastric carcinomas rarely spread directly into the duodenum.
2. Lymphovascular extension, which is common and represents the major reason for many treatment failures (Fig. 5–75). Submucosal lymphatic extension (Fig. 5–76) can extend horizontally for long distances outside the gross tumor edges (Fig. 5–77), and is the reason why a mucosal margin of 5 cm is deemed necessary for a curative resection in gastric carcinoma. Vertical lymphatic invasion through and outside the gastric wall also represents a common source of noncontigu-

ous ("satellite") tumors. Lymphatic invasion results in lymph node involvement, which may be regional or distant (Fig. 5–78). Involvement of the left supraclavicular lymph node at the point of entry of the thoracic duct into the jugular vein (Virchow's node) is a classical presenting manifestation of gastric cancer. Perineural invasion also occurs (Fig. 5–79).
3. Transcelomic spread is a risk in all tumors that infiltrate the full thickness of the gastric wall with serosal involvement. Peritoneal involvement results in ascites (with positive cytol-

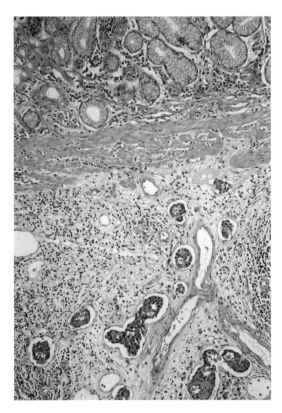

Figure 5–76. Submucosal lymphatic permeation in gastric adenocarcinoma, showing tumor extensively involving dilated lymphatic spaces. The overlying mucosa is normal.

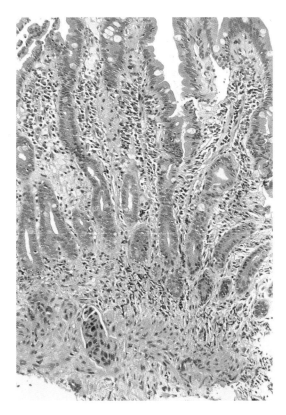

Figure 5–77. Extension of submucosal lymphatic carcinomatosis into the duodenum. Several tumor emboli are present in the submucosal lymphatics.

ogy), multiple peritoneal nodules (visible at laparoscopy), bilateral ovarian involvement as Krukenberg tumors (see Fig. 5–36), and deposits in the rectovesical or rectovaginal pouch as Blumer's shelf palpable on rectal examination.
4. Hematogenous spread to the liver, lungs, and other organs usually occurs late in the course of the disease.

Pathologic Staging

The pathologic stage is the most important determinant of prognosis in gastric carcinoma. The confusion regarding clini-

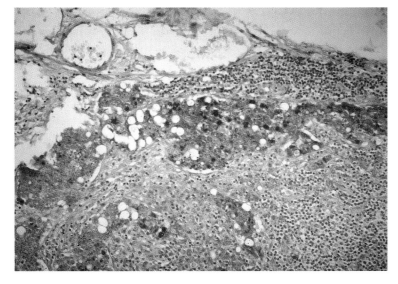

Figure 5–79. Gastric adenocarcinoma in perigastric connective tissue showing perineural invasion.

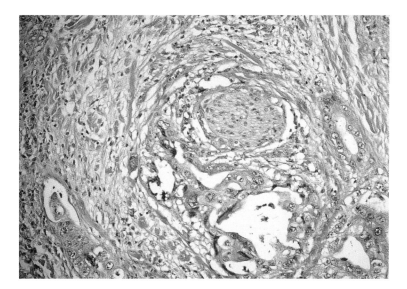

Figure 5–78. Perigastric lymph node, stained with digested PAS stain, showing gastric adenocarcinoma distending the peripheral sinus of the node.

copathologic staging systems has been somewhat resolved by the general acceptance, at least in the United States, of the 1992 revision of the tumor, node, metastases (TNM) classification of gastric cancer (Table 5–5).[66] Although this system is accepted, it continues to provide difficulties because of its complexity. It is a rare pathologist that can accurately assign a stage to a gastric carcinoma without consulting the staging manual.

One problem frequently encountered by pathologists in staging is the appropriate designation of tumor satellites in the perigastric tissues. Tumor satellites are tumor nodules that are discontinuous with the primary tumor but not within lymph nodes. The rules developed for satellite nodules are as follows: (1) if recognized macroscopically, satellite nodules are classified as lymph node metastases, irrespective of whether residual nodal tissue is present; (2) when the satellite is microscopic, with a size less than 3 mm, it is classified as subserosal invasion.

This staging system complements the basic classification of gastric carcinoma into early (all T1 lesions including N0 and N1) and late (all lesions that are T2 and higher).

Examination of the Gastrectomy Specimen

Two types of gastrectomy are performed to treat gastric carcinoma. Most pyloric antral tumors are treated by partial gastrectomy, in which the distal margin is the duodenum and the proximal margin is the gastric body. Tumors that involve the gastric body are commonly treated with total gastrectomy, in which the distal margin is the duodenum and the proximal margin is the esophagus. The nature of the specimen should be identified by the pathologist and the dimensions of the stomach, duodenum, and esophagus present should be recorded. When the spleen and greater omentum are present in the specimen, this should be recorded.

The Primary Tumor. The gross examination of the specimen is ideally done in the fresh state and should document the following:

TABLE 5–5. TNM SYSTEM FOR STAGING OF GASTRIC CANCER

Primary Tumor (T Stage)

Tis	Carcinoma in situ (=high-grade dysplasia).
T1*	Invasion of lamina propria or submucosa.
T2	Invasion of muscularis externa or subserosa.
T3	Invasion of the serosa.
T4[†]	Invasion of contiguous structures.

Regional Lymph Nodes (N Stage)

Nx	Lymph nodes cannot be assessed.
N0	No evidence of nodal metastases.
N1	Metastases in perigastric lymph nodes within 3 cm of the edge of the primary tumor.
N2	Metastases in perigastric lymph nodes >3 cm of the edge of the primary tumor *or* nodes along the left gastric, common hepatic, splenic, or celiac arteries.

Distant Metastases (M Stage)

M0	No evidence of distant metastases.
M1	Distant metastases present (includes extraregional lymph nodes).

Clinical Stage Groupings

Stage 0	Tis N0 M0
Stage IA	T1 N0 M0
Stage IB	T1 N1 M0 or T2 N0 M0
Stage II	T1 N2 M0 or T2 N1 M0 or T3 N0 M0
Stage IIIA	T2 N2 M0 or T3 N1 M0 or T4 N0 M0
Stage IIIB	T3 N2 M0 or T4 N1 M0
Stage IV	T4 N2 M0 or AnyM1

Abbreviation: TNM = tumor, node, metastases.
*In the Japanese literature T1 lesions are further subdivided into T1-m (= intramucosal) and T1-sm (submucosal) lesions.
[†]Extension of tumor intramurally into the esophagus or duodenum with clear surgical margins does not represent invasion of contiguous structures.

1. The exact mucosal location and extent of the tumor
2. The distance of tumor edges from proximal and distal margins
3. The gross appearance of the tumor, including size and, in the case of early lesions, the morphologic type
4. Gross examination of a vertical cut section through the wall, with a description of the changes observed

Sections must be submitted to permit adequate microscopic evaluation of the tumor, recognizing that gastric carcinomas are frequently heterogeneous. The exact number of sections submitted depends on the size of the tumor.

The pathologist should type the tumor microscopically according to whether it is intestinal or diffuse (Lauren classification), its degree of differentiation, and the WHO microscopic patterns (ie, tubular, papillary, mucinous, signet ring cell adenocarcinoma). The presence or absence of lymphovascular invasion should be noted.

Pathologic staging requires microscopic documentation of the maximum level of invasion by the tumor (see Table 5–5).

Microscopic examination of the nontumor gastric mucosa should document any associated lesions, such as from gastritis, intestinal metaplasia, *Helicobacter pylori* infection, polyps, and dysplasia.

Evaluation of Surgical Margins. The gastrectomy specimen has only proximal and distal mucosal margins. Being completely covered by peritoneum, the outer surface of the resected stomach represents a surface, not a resection margin. The surgical margin status of the gastrectomy specimen is indicated by an R designation as follows: R0 = surgical margins clear; R1 = surgical margins microscopically involved; R2 = surgical margins grossly involved. A positive microscopic surgical margin reduces the expected survival of stage II disease by 50%.[67]

In attempted curative gastric resections, microscopically positive margins are found in 13–22% of cases.[67] The positive margin is almost always the proximal one. To avoid a positive microscopic surgical margin, it is recommended that the surgeon includes a length of 5 cm from the proximal edge of gross tumor in planning the proximal limit of the gastrectomy. Intraoperative frozen sections of margins should be done routinely.

Lymph Node Evaluation. The Japanese Research Society for Gastric Cancer (JRSGC) has recommended a precise and detailed method of evaluation of lymph nodes in a gastrectomy specimen. This details exact nodal locations in terms of four nodal stations (N1–N4) based on the location of the primary tumor (Table 5–6).[68] Complete nodal evaluation requires evaluation of nodes in the gastrectomy specimen as well as nodes submitted separately from the various sites used in the classification. Based on this system of nodal classification, the extent of lymph node dissection association with gastrectomy is classified as follows: D0 lymphadenectomy = not all the N1 lymph nodes have been removed; D1 lymphadenectomy = all N1 nodes have been removed, but not all N2 nodes; D2 lymphadenectomy = all N2 nodes have been removed but not all N3 nodes.

Less than 5% of patients with gastric carcinoma in the United States undergo a D2 lymphadenectomy, which is considered the routine surgery in Japan. Most patients in the United States undergo a D1 or D0 lymphadenectomy; the frequent N1 lymph nodes that are not sampled in those patients having a D0 lymphadenectomy are nodes in the proximal part of the left gastric artery (station 7) and infrapyloric nodes near the head of the pancreas (station 6).

The degree of precision advocated by the JRSGC is rarely followed in the United States. Labeled sampling of different nodal stations is rarely done. The pathologist commonly receives the gastrectomy specimen with the nodes in situ. The TNM staging requirement for the pathologist is to divide the lymph nodes in the specimen into those within 3 cm from the edge of the primary tumor and those beyond this distance. The only reason to document the location of individual nodes is to evaluate the extent of lymphadenectomy; at this time, this procedure is not considered essential in the pathologic examination of the gastrectomy specimen in the United States.

There is a positive correlation between the number of

TABLE 5–6. LYMPH NODE LOCATIONS AND NODAL STATIONS IN GASTRIC CARCINOMA

Number	Description	Location of Primary Tumor			
		Pangastric	Antral	Middle	Cardiac
Nodes Present in the Usual Gastrectomy Specimen					
1	Right cardial	N1	N2	N1	N1
2	Left cardial	N1	N3	N2	N1
3	Lesser curvature	N1	N1	N1	N1
4sa	Short gastric	N1	N1	N1	N1
4sb	Left gastroepiploic	N1	N1	N1	N1
4d	Right gastroepiploic	N1	N1	N1	N2
5	Suprapyloric	N1	N1	N1	N2
6	Infrapyloric	N1	N1	N1	N2
Nodes Present with an Extended Lymphadenectomy					
7	Left gastric arterial	N2	N2	N2	N2
8a	Ant common hepatic arterial	N2	N2	N2	N2
8b	Post common hepatic arterial	N3	N3	N3	N3
9	Celiac arterial	N2	N2	N2	N2
10	Splenic hilar	N2	N3	N2	N2
11	Splenic arterial	N2	N3	N2	N2
Extraregional Nodal Groups					
12	Hepatoduodenal ligament	N3	N3	N3	N3
13	Retropancreatic	N3	N3	N3	N3
14A	Superior mesenteric arterial	N4	N4	N4	N4
14V	Superior mesenteric venous	N3	N3	N3	N3
15	Middle colic arterial	N4	N4	N4	N4
16	Para-aortic	N4	N4	N4	N4
17	Anterior pancreatic	N3	N3	N3	N3
18	Inferior pancreatic	N3	N3	N3	N3
19	Infradiaphragmatic	N4	N4	N4	N3
20	Esophageal hiatus	N3	N4	N4	N2

lymph nodes examined and the incidence of node positivity.[15] Because the extent of nodal dissection differs so greatly in different gastrectomy specimens, it is important to record the total number of nodes identified in the specimen.

The Pathology Report for Gastric Carcinoma

The elements that must be present in the pathology report of a gastric carcinoma resection specimen are shown in Table 5–7.[69]

Prognostic Indicators

The prognosis of gastric carcinoma correlates best with pathologic stage. Patients with early gastric cancer have a 5-year survival of 90% compared with the overall 17% 5-year survival rate for patients with all gastric carcinomas in the United States. These rates indicate considerable room for improvement of survival in gastric cancer with early detection.

TABLE 5–7. SURGICAL PATHOLOGY REPORT IN GASTRIC CANCER

Pathology Laboratory Information
[Patient Demographic Information]   [Dates]
[Pathology Number]
[Clinical Data (including physicians involved)]
[Specimens Submitted]

Intraoperative Consultation Results (including frozen sections)
Gross Description
 Tumor
  Obligatory: Location: Upper third/ middle third/ lower third/ upper and middle third/ middle and lower third/ pangastric.
  Desirable: Tumor size; gross type.
 Extent of Surgery
  Obligatory: Total/ partial proximal/ partial distal gastrectomy.
   Removal of greater omentum/ spleen/ pancreas/ other organs.
   Length of removed duodenum and esophagus.
  Desirable: Extent of lymphadenectomy
Microscopic Description/Diagnosis
 Histomorphology
  Obligatory: Lauren type, WHO type and degree of differentiation.
   Lymphovascular invasion.
 Staging/primary tumor.
  Obligatory: Depth of infiltration (Tis–T4).
 Staging/lymph nodes.
  Obligatory: TNM lymph node status (N0, N1, or N2).
  Desirable: Number of nodes examined and number involved; topography of involved nodes in accordance with the JRSGC system.
 Surgical margin involvement (residual tumor).
  Obligatory: Surgical margin status (R0–R2); when margins are clear, the extent of margin clearance.
  Other lesions in the specimen, if any: Gastritis, *Helicobacter pylori,* intestinal metaplasia, polyps, dysplasia, etc.

Histologic type also influences prognosis. Well-differentiated adenocarcinomas of intestinal type have the best prognosis, and poorly differentiated diffuse carcinomas with signet ring cells have the worst.

Stage for stage, the prognosis is better in Japan than it is in the United States (Table 5–8). The better prognosis in stage 1

TABLE 5–8. SURVIVAL RATES AFTER RESECTION OF GASTRIC CARCINOMA AMONG U.S. AND JAPANESE CENTERS

	United States (1982–1987)*		Japan (1971–1985)†	
Stage	Number of Cases (%)	5-yr Survival	Number of Cases (%)	5-yr Survival
I	2004 (18.1%)	50.0%	1453 (45.7%)	90.7%
II	1796 (16.2%)	29.0%	377 (11.9%)	71.7%
III	3945 (35.6%)	13.0%	693 (21.8%)	44.3%
IV	3342 (30.1%)	3.0%	653 (20.6%)	9.0%

*Based on data from 11,087 patients treated at 700 U.S. hospitals.
†Based on data from 3176 patients treated at the National Cancer Center Hospital, Tokyo, Japan.

TABLE 5–9. PROGNOSTIC INDICATORS IN GASTRIC CARCINOMA

Pathologic stage	Correlates best with survival.
Histologic type	Intestinal type has better prognosis than diffuse type.
Degree of differentiation	Well differentiated has a better prognosis than poorly differentiated.
Extent of lymphadenectomy[68]	D2 better than D1; under debate.
Angiogenesis in tumor[70]	Number of vessels in tumor correlate with hematogenous and peritoneal metastases.
Perineural invasion[71]	Presence correlates with increased recurrence and lower survival rate.
Serum β-HCG[72]	Serum β-HCG >4 IU/L correlate with poor prognosis.
Serum CA-125[73]	Serum CA-125 >350 U/mL correlate with poor prognosis.
Aneuploidy[74]	Aneuploid tumors have a worse prognosis.
Lymph node micrometastasis[75]	Correlate with poor prognosis in early gastric carcinomas.
Bone marrow micrometastases[76]	Detected in patients with gastric carcinoma; not correlated with prognosis.
EGF receptor[76]	Expression correlates with poor prognosis.
p53 protein, c-erb B-2, K-ras	Expressed in gastric cancer; conflicting evidence as to prognostic value.
PCNA[76]	Conflicting results.

Abbreviations: HCG = human chorionic gonadotropin; EGF = epidermal growth factor; PCNA = proliferative cell nuclear antigen.

disease may relate to the larger number of intramucosal tumors detected in Japan and the more aggressive diagnosis of intramucosal cancer in Japan.[18] The better prognosis in the more advanced stages of gastric cancer may relate to the more extended lymph node resections performed in Japan.

Pathologic staging exerts such a dominant influence in the prognosis of gastric cancer that other prognostic criteria are of little practical value, particularly in the United States, where the majority of cancers are found in an advanced stage, in which the prognosis is very poor. In early gastric carcinomas, these prognostic indicators may be useful in identifying a subset of patients at risk for recurrence. The prognostic criteria that have been shown to have any value in gastric carcinoma are listed in Table 5–9.[68,70–76]

References

1. Graeme-Cook F. Pathology neoplastic and non-neoplastic. *Surg Clin North Am.* 1996;5:487–512.
2. Schmitz JM, Stolte M. Gastric polyps as precancerous lesions. *Gastrointest Clin North Am.* 1997;7:29–46.
3. Antonioli DA. Precursors of gastric carcinoma: A critical review with a brief description of early (curable) gastric cancer. *Hum Pathol.* 1994;25:994–1005.
4. Kamiya T, Morishita T, Asakura H, et al. Long term follow-up study on gastric adenoma and its relation to gastric protruded carcinoma. *Cancer.* 1982;50:2496–2503.
5. Xuan ZX, Ambe K, Enjoji M. Depressed adenoma of the stomach revisited: Histologic, histochemical and immunohistochemical profiles. *Cancer.* 1991;67:2382–2389.
6. Offerhaus GJA, Giardiello FM, Krush AJ, et al. The risk of upper gastrointestinal cancer in familial adenomatous polyposis. *Gastroenterology.* 1992;102:1980–1982.
7. Lynch HT, Smyrk TC, Lanspa SJ, et al. Upper gastrointestinal manifestations in families with hereditary flat adenoma syndrome. *Cancer.* 1993;71:2709–2714.
8. Rindi G. Clinicopathologic aspects of gastric neuroendocrine tumors. *Am J Surg Pathol.* 1995;19:S20–S29.
9. Solcia E, Fiocca R, Villani L, et al. Hyperplastic, dysplastic, and neoplastic enterochromaffin-like-cell proliferations of the gastric mucosa: Classification and histogenesis. *Am J Surg Pathol.* 1995;19:S1–S7.
10. Bordi C, D'Adda T, Azzoni C, et al. Hypergastrinemia and gastric enterochromaffin-like cells. *Am J Surg Pathol.* 1995;19:S8–S19.
11. Yang GCH, Rotterdam H. Mixed (composite) glandular–endocrine cell carcinoma of the stomach. *Am J Surg Pathol.* 1991;15:592–598.
12. Wheeler D, Chandrasoma PT, Carriere CA, et al. Cytologic diagnosis of composite gastric adenocarcinoma-carcinoid. *Acta Cytol.* 1984;28:706–708.
13. Lauren P. The histological main types of gastric carcinoma: Diffuse and so-called intestinal-type carcinoma. *Acta Pathol Microbiol Scand.* 1965;64:31–49.
14. Ming S-C. Gastric carcinoma. A pathobiological classification. *Cancer.* 1977;39:2475–2485.
15. Hermanek P, Wittekind C. News of TNM and its use for classification of gastric cancer. *World J Surg.* 1995;19:491–495.
16. Fuchs CS, Mayer RJ. Gastric carcinoma. *N Engl J Med.* 1995;333:32–41.
17. Cocco P, Ward MH, Buiatti E. Occupational risk factors for gastric cancer: An overview. *Epidemiol Rev.* 1996;18:218–234.
18. Schlemper RJ, Itabashi M, Kato Y, et al. Differences in diagnostic criteria for gastric carcinoma between Japanese and Western pathologists. *Lancet.* 1997;349:1725–1729.
19. Sokoloff B. Predisposition to gastric cancer in the Bonaparte family. *Am J Surg.* 1938;40:673–678.
20. Zanghieri G, Di Gregorio C, Sacchetti C, et al. Familial occurrence of gastric cancer in the 2 year experience of a population-based registry. *Cancer.* 1990;66:2047–2051.
21. Parsonnet J, Friedman GD, Vandersteen DP, et al. *Helicobacter* infection and the risk of gastric carcinoma. *N Engl J Med.* 1991;325:1127–1131.
22. Correa P, Fox J, Fontham E, et al. *Helicobacter pylori* and gastric carcinoma: Serum antibody prevalence in populations with contrasting cancer risks. *Cancer.* 1990;66:2569–2574.
23. Correa P. *Helicobacter pylori* and gastric carcinogenesis. *Am J Surg Pathol.* 1995;19:S37–S43.
24. Correa P, Ruiz B, Shi T, et al. *Helicobacter pylori* and nucleolar organizer regions in the gastric antral mucosa. *Am J Clin Pathol.* 1994;101:656–660.
25. Ruiz B, Rood JC, Fontham ETH, et al. Vitamin C concentration in gastric juice before and after anti-*Helicobacter pylori* treatment. *Am J Gastroenterol.* 1994;89:533–539.
26. Schafer LW, Larson DE, Melton LJ, et al. Risk of development of gastric carcinoma in patients with pernicious anemia. A population-based study in Rochester, Minnesota. *Mayo Clin Proc.* 1985;60:444–448.

27. Antonioli DA. Esophagus. *In* Henson DE, Albers-Saavedra J (eds): *Pathology of Incipient Neoplasia,* 2nd ed. Philadelphia, WB Saunders, 1994, pp. 64–84.

28. Filipe MI, Potet F, Bogomoletz WV, et al. Incomplete sulfomucin-secreting intestinal metaplasia for gastric cancer. Preliminary data from a prospective study from three centres. *Gut.* 1985;26:1319–1326.

29. Paller AS. Immunodeficiency syndromes. *Dermatol Clin.* 1995;13:65–71.

30. Offerhaus GJA, Tersmette AC, Tersmette KWF, et al. Gastric, pancreatic, and colorectal carcinogenesis following remote peptic ulcer surgery: Review of the literature with the emphasis on risk assessment and underlying mechanism. *Mod Pathol.* 1988;1:352–356.

31. Hermanek P, Reimann JF. The operated stomach—still a precancerous condition? *Endoscopy.* 1982;14:113–114.

32. Bogolometz WV, Molas G, Potet F, et al. Pathologic features and mucin histochemistry of primary gastric stump carcinoma associated with gastritis cystica polyposa. *Am J Surg Pathol.* 1985;9:401–410.

33. Goldstein NS, Lewin KJ. Gastric epithelial dysplasia and adenoma: Historical review and histological criteria for grading. *Hum Pathol.* 1997;28:127–133.

34. Saraga EP, Gardiol D, Costa J. Gastric dysplasia. A histological follow-up study. *Am J Surg Pathol.* 1987;11:788–796.

35. Serck-Hanssen A, Osnes M, Myren J. Epithelial dysplasia in the stomach: The size of the problem and some preliminary results of a follow-up study. *In* Ming SC (ed): *Precursors of Gastric Cancer.* New York, Praeger, 1984, pp. 53–71.

36. McGill F, Adachi A, Karimi N, et al. Abnormal cervical cytology leading to the diagnosis of gastric cancer. *Gynecol Oncol.* 1990;36:101–105.

37. Benito I, Alvarez-Gago T, Morais D. Tonsillar metastasis from adenocarcinoma of the stomach. *J Laryngol Otol.* 1996;110:291–293.

38. Betke M, Suss R, Hohenleutner U, et al. Gastric carcinoma metastatic to the site of a congenital melanocytic nevus. *J Am Acad Dermatol.* 1993;28:866–869.

39. Cheung TC, Ng FH, Chow KC, et al. Occult gastric cancer presenting as cor pulmonale resulting from tumor cell microembolism. *Am J Gastroenterol.* 1997;92:1057–1059.

40. Brenes F, Correa P. Pathology of gastric cancer. *Surg Oncol Clin North Am.* 1993;2:347–370.

41. Hatfield ARW, Slavin G, Segal AW, et al. Importance of the site of endoscopic gastric biopsy in ulcerating lesions of the stomach. *Gut.* 1975;16:884–886.

42. Graham DY, Schwartz JT, Cain GD, et al. Prospective evaluation of biopsy number in the diagnosis of esophageal and gastric carcinoma. *Gastroenterology.* 1982;82:228–231.

43. Qizilbash AH, Castelli M, Kowalski MA, et al. Endoscopic brush cytology and biopsy in the diagnosis of cancer of the upper gastrointestinal tract. *Acta Cytol.* 1980;24:313–318.

44. Ellis KK, Fennerty MB. Gastric malignancy. *Gastrointest Endosc Clin North Am.* 1996;6:545–563.

45. Isozaki H, Okajima K, Hu X, et al. Multiple early gastric carcinomas, Clinicopathologic features and histogenesis. *Cancer.* 1996;78:2078–2086.

46. Nava HR, Arredondo MA. Diagnosis of gastric cancer. Endoscopy, imaging, and tumor markers. *Surg Oncol Clin North Am.* 1993;2:371–392.

47. Tahara E. Molecular biology of gastric cancer. *World J Surg.* 1995;19:484–490.

48. Fujino MA, Morozumi A, Kojima Y, et al. Gastric carcinoma, An endoscopically curable disease. *Bildgebung.* 1994;61:38–40.

49. Lowy AM, Mansfield PF, Leach SD, et al. Laparoscopic staging of gastric cancer. *Surgery.* 1996;119:611–614.

50. Noguchi Y, Imada T, Matsumoto A, et al. Radical surgery for gastric cancer: A review of the Japanese experience. *Cancer.* 1989;64:2053–2062.

51. Kiyabu M, Leichman L, Chandrasoma P. Effects of preoperative chemotherapy on gastric adenocarcinomas: A morphologic study of 25 cases. *Cancer.* 1992;70:2239–2245.

52. Wanebo HJ, Kennedy BJ, Chmiel J, et al. Cancer of the stomach. A patient care study by the American College of Surgeons. *Ann Surg.* 1993;218:583–592.

53. Mori M, Iwashita A, Enjoli M. Adenosquamous carcinoma of the stomach. A clinicopathologic analysis of 28 cases. *Cancer.* 1986;57:333–339.

54. Lissens P, Peprstraete L, Mulier K, et al. Primary pure squamous cell carcinoma of the antrum of the stomach: A case report. *Acta Chir Belg.* 1995;95:184–186.

55. Adachi Y, Yoh R, Konishi J, et al. Epstein-Barr virus-associated gastric carcinoma. *J Clin Gastroenterol.* 1996;23:207–210.

56. Saigo PE, Brigati DJ, Sternberg SS, et al. Primary gastric choriocarcinoma. An immunohistologic study. *Am J Surg Pathol.* 1981;5:333–342.

57. Motoyama T, Saito K, Iwafuchi M. Endodermal sinus tumor of the stomach. *Acta Pathol Jpn.* 1985;39:497–505.

58. deLorimier A, Park F, Aranha GV, et al. Hepatoid carcinoma of the stomach. *Cancer.* 1993;71:293–296.

59. Hussein AM, Otrakji CL, Hussein BT. Small cell carcinoma of the stomach. Case report and review of the literature. *Dig Dis Sci.* 1990;35:513–518.

60. Iezzoni JC, Mills SE. Sarcomatoid carcinomas (carcinosarcomas) of the gastrointestinal tract: A review. *Semin Diag Pathol.* 1993;10:176–187.

61. Ueyama T, Nagai E, Yao T, et al. Vimentin positive gastric carcinomas with rhabdoid features. A clinicopathologic and immunohistochemical study. *Am J Surg Pathol.* 1993;17:813–819.

62. Matsukuma S, Wada R, Daibou M, et al. Adenocarcinoma arising from gastric immature teratoma. *Cancer.* 1995;75:2663–2668.

63. Jeng KS, Yang KC, Kuo SHF. Malignant degeneration of heterotopic pancreas. *Gastrointest Endosc.* 1991;37:196–198.

64. Capella C, Figerio B, Cornaggia M, et al. Gastric parietal cell carcinoma—A newly recognized entity. Light microscopic and ultrastructural features. *Histopathology.* 1984;8:813–824.

65. Wotherspoon AC, Isaacson PG. Synchronous adenocarcinoma and low grade B cell lymphoma of mucosa associated lymphoid tissue (MALT) of the stomach. *Histopathology.* 1995;27:325–331.

66. American Joint Committee on Cancer. *Manual for Staging of Cancer,* 4th ed. Philadelphia, JB Lippincott, 1993.

67. Kirkwood KS, Khitin LM, Barwick KW. Gastric cancer. *Surg Oncol Clin North Am.* 1997;6:495–514.

68. Hundahl SA. Gastric cancer nodal metastasis. Biologic significance and therapeutic implications. *Surg Oncol Clin North Am.* 1996;5:129–144.

69. Hermanek P. A pathologist's checklist for evaluation of patients with gastric carcinoma. *Scand J Gastroenterol.* 1987;22:40–42.

70. Tanigawa N, Amaya H, Matsumura M, et al. Extent of tumor vas-

cularization correlates with prognosis and hematogenous metastsis in gastric carcinomas. *Cancer Res.* 1996;56:2671–2676.

71. Tanaka A, Watanabe T, Okuno K, et al. Perineural invasion as a predictor of recurrence of gastric cancer. *Cancer.* 1994;73: 550–555.

72. Webb A, Scott-Mackie P, Cunningham D, et al. The prognostic value of serum and immunohistochemical tumour markers in advanced gastric cancer. *Eur J Cancer.* 1996;32A:63–68.

73. Korenaga D, Okamura T, Saito A, et al. DNA aneuploidy is closely linked to tumor invasion, lymph node metastasis, and prognosis in clinical gastric cancer. *Cancer.* 1988;62:309.

74. Maehara Y, Oshiro T, Endo K, et al. Clinical significance of occult micrometastasis in lymph nodes from patients with early gastric cancer who died of recurrence. *Surgery.* 1996;119:397–402.

75. Maehara Y, Yamamoto M, Oda S, et al. Cytokeratin-positive cells in bone marrow for identifying distant micrometastasis of gastric cancer. *Br J Cancer.* 1996;73:83–87.

76. D'Agnanao I, D'Angelo C, Savarese A, et al. DNA ploidy, proliferative index, and epidermal growth factor receptor: Expression and prognosis in patients with gastric cancers. *Lab Invest.* 1995;72:432–438.

6

THE DUODENUM

Gail Wehrli and Parakrama Chandrasoma

▶ CHAPTER OUTLINE

NORMAL STRUCTURE

The duodenum begins at the distal end of the pyloric sphincter and ends at the ligament of Treitz. The duodenum is divided into four parts. The first part, the duodenal bulb and horizontal portion, is suspended from the inferior surface of the liver by the gastroduodenal ligament, which contains the portal vein, hepatic artery, and common bile duct. The second, or descending, part of the duodenum curves around the head of the pancreas in the retroperitoneum. This portion of the duodenum contains the papilla of Vater into which opens the ampullary part of the duct created by the joining of the common bile duct and pancreatic duct. The third and fourth parts of the duodenum are related to the inferior aspect of the body of the pancreas. At the ligament of Treitz, the duodenum ends and becomes the jejunum, which is entirely in the peritoneal cavity.

The duodenal mucosa begins abruptly at the distal end of the pyloric sphincter. It has villi, which are lined by absorptive and goblet cells, and crypts, which contain goblet cells and Paneth cells. Submucosal Brunner's glands are typical of the duodenum and are most prominent in the proximal part (Fig. 6–1). The mucosa over Brunner's glands commonly have short, blunt villi (Fig. 6–2). Neuroendocrine cells are present in the crypts, but can be identified only in sections that are stained for

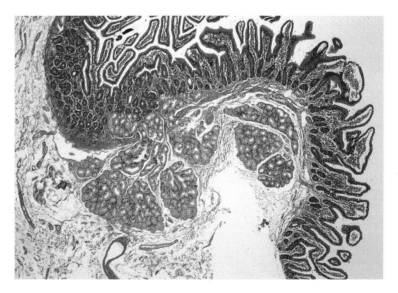

Figure 6–1. Normal duodenal mucosa with Brunner's gland.

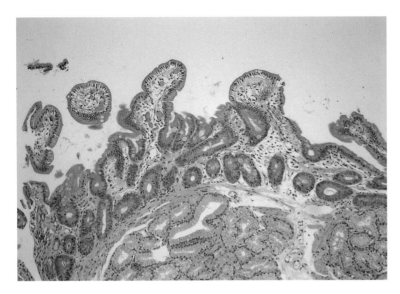

Figure 6–2. Normal duodenal mucosa with blunted villi over a Brunner's gland.

chromogranin A by immunoperoxidase. Duodenal endocrine cells secrete cholecystokinin and secretin, hormones that are major regulators of the digestive process. Rarely, macrophages are distended with black pigment in the duodenal mucosa; these are usually present at the tips of the villi, producing a brown speckling of the mucosa seen during endoscopy. This condition is called melanosis duodeni. The pigment is probably lipofuscin and not melanin. This condition is of unknown cause and has no clinical significance.

DUODENITIS

Nonspecific Duodenitis

Nonspecific duodenitis is a common condition that affects the duodenal bulb. It is frequently associated with erosions and probably represents a pre-ulcerative stage in the pathogenesis of peptic duodenal ulceration. Most patients with histologic features of nonspecific duodenitis have active duodenal ulcers, recently healed ulcers, or a history of duodenal ulcer.[1]

The clinical associations of nonspecific duodenitis are not clear. Duodenitis occurs in many asymptomatic patients, and nonulcer dyspepsia is an extremely common symptom without endoscopic or histologic evidence of duodenitis. It is therefore difficult to ascribe a causal relationship when duodenitis coexists with dyspeptic symptoms in a patient. The etiology of nonspecific duodenitis is identical to that of peptic duodenal ulcer; many patients have diffuse antral gastritis associated with *Helicobacter pylori* infection.

Endoscopic features of duodenitis correlate well with the presence of histologic changes. Focal erythema and edema are present in the duodenal bulb, features which are associated with superficial erosions in more severe cases.

Histologic examination of biopsies shows infiltration of the lamina propria and epithelium by neutrophils (Fig. 6–3);

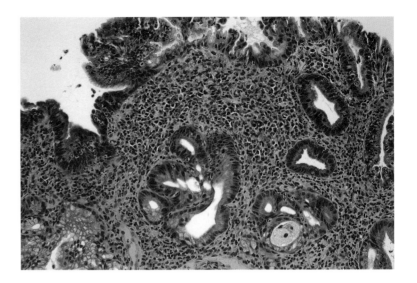

A

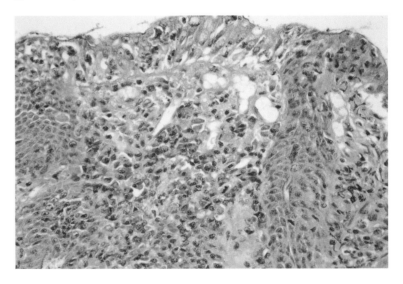

B

C

Figure 6–3. A: Acute nonspecific duodenitis, showing blunting of villi and acute and chronic inflammation in the lamina propria. B: Acute nonspecific duodenitis, showing neutrophil infiltration in lamina propria, crypts, and surface epithelium. C: Acute nonspecific duodenitis, periodic acid–Schiff (PAS) stain, showing neutrophils infiltrating the surface epithelium. The blunted villi and surface epithelial infiltrate bear a superficial resemblance to celiac disease; the infiltrating cells are, however, neutrophils.

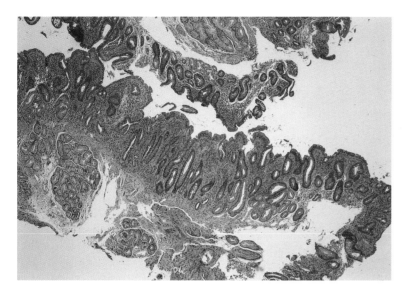

Figure 6–4. Acute and chronic nonspecific duodenitis with blunted villi and marked inflammation in the lamina propria.

lymphocytes and plasma cells are also increased in number. The villi are blunted to a variable extent (Fig. 6–4). Surface erosions are common and consist of denudation of the superficial part of the mucosa (Fig. 6–5), the eroded superficial mucosa is covered by inflammatory exudate, and the underlying deep mucosa shows acute inflammation. Gastric surface metaplasia is almost invariably evident in nonspecific duodenitis (Fig. 6–6).[2] The gastric metaplasia is easily recognized by the presence of cells with the typical eosinophilic appearance of apical mucin of gastric surface epithelium, which contrasts with the denser amphophilic cytoplasm of the absorptive cells and the vacuolated cytoplasm of goblet cells. In some patients with duodenitis, gastric surface metaplasia is accompanied by the appearance of parietal cells in the deep mucosal glands (Fig. 6–6). The presence of active inflammation in cases of gastric metaplasia help distinguish this condition from heterotopic gastric mucosa in the duodenum.

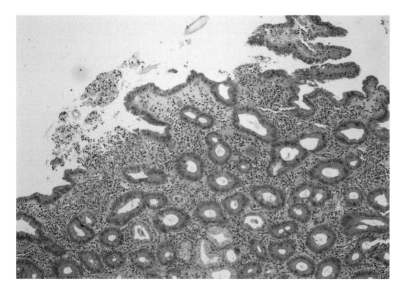

Figure 6–5. Acute duodenitis with early surface erosion.

It has been suggested that the inflammation is the result of infection of metaplastic gastric surface epithelium by *H. pylori*. The reported incidence of *H. pylori* in metaplastic gastric mucosa in the duodenum varies from 8% to 92% in different series, however.[3] Our experience is that *H. pylori* can only be demonstrated rarely in duodenal biopsies with gastric metaplasia.

Reactive changes may be present in the duodenal epithelial cells in the regenerative phase of erosions (Fig. 6–7). These can be associated with significant cytologic atypia; however, this is not likely to be mistaken for malignancy because adenocarcinoma is so rare in the duodenal bulb that it is rarely a diagnostic consideration.

Duodenal Involvement in Diseases of the Small Intestine

The duodenum is commonly affected in diseases of the small intestine, such as celiac disease, tropical sprue, and Whipple's disease (see Chapter 7). In these cases, the changes affect the second part of the duodenum as well as the duodenal bulb. These changes permit differentiation from nonspecific duodenitis, which is a process restricted to the duodenal bulb.

Less than 5% of patients with Crohn's disease of the ileum and colon show involvement of the duodenum.[4] Duodenal Crohn's disease manifests as ulceration resembling peptic ulcers except for their location distal to the first part of the duodenum, diffuse inflammation and thickening of the duodenum, and fistulas. Most patients give a prior history of Crohn's disease elsewhere in the intestine. In most patients, duodenal biopsies show nonspecific acute and chronic inflammation of varying severity; granulomas are rarely seen. The presence of significant nonspecific inflammation in the second or third part of the duodenum in a patient with a history of Crohn's disease elsewhere is suggestive of duodenal involvement when there is no other obvious cause for the inflammation. In a patient without a history of Crohn's disease, the possibility of Crohn's disease of the duodenum can be suggested when severe inflammation is associated with nonnecrotizing epithelioid cell granulomas. In these cases, the presence of clinical evidence of duodenal thickening is helpful. Also, tuberculosis must be excluded by appropriate studies before a diagnosis of Crohn's disease is made.

Chronic segmental duodenitis with formation of strictures has also been reported to occur very rarely in patients with ulcerative colitis.[5]

Infections

In the Immunocompetent Host

Giardia lamblia is an intestinal flagellate that lives in the duodenum, usually as a commensal. The prevalence of *Giardia* in the general population is high; serologic testing suggests that as much as 15% of the population in the United States may have harbored the organism. The prevalence is much higher in Cen-

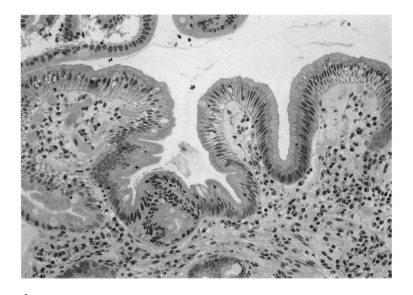

Figure 6–6. A: Gastric metaplasia of duodenal surface epithelium in nonspecific duodenitis. The gastric epithelium shows apical mucin without goblet cells. B: Gastric metaplasia, showing gastric-type surface cells with apical mucin. The gastric metaplastic epithelium contrasts with the goblet cell containing intestinal epithelium. C: Gastric metaplasia in nonspecific duodenitis, showing metaplasia of the surface and the presence of a focus of oxyntic glands between the surface and the Brunner's glands.

tral America where rates reach 50%. Most patients with *Giardia,* particularly in endemic areas, are asymptomatic. Host factors are important in pathogenesis. Hypogammaglobulinemia and IgA deficiency produce severe disease. Giardiasis is manifested clinically by watery diarrhea, often profuse and associated with cramping abdominal pain. Chronic infections result in malabsorption. Duodenal biopsies show the trophozoites on the surface of the epithelium (Fig. 6–8A, B); these are 10–20 μm in size and appear pear-shaped with two nuclei or sickle-shaped when seen in profile. Organisms are numerous in patients with hypogammaglobulinemia, but can be difficult to find in immunocompetent hosts. The sensitivity of finding organisms is greatest with a duodenal aspirate; stool examination is less sensitive (Fig. 6–8C, D). The mucosa may be normal, but commonly shows mild villous blunting and an increase in the number of lymphocytes in the lamina propria.

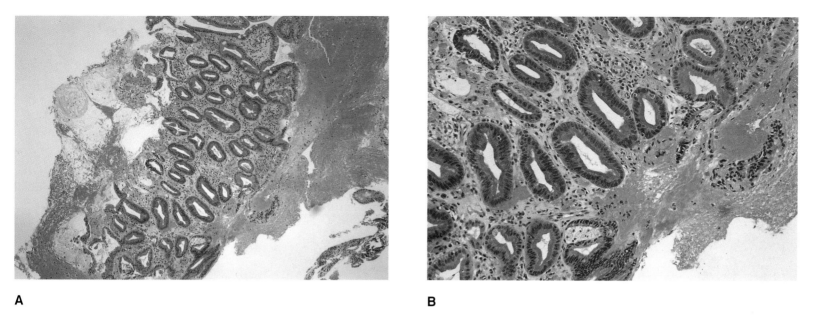

Figure 6–7. A: Reactive change in duodenal epithelium associated with erosion. B: Higher power of part A showing cytologic atypia in reactive crypts.

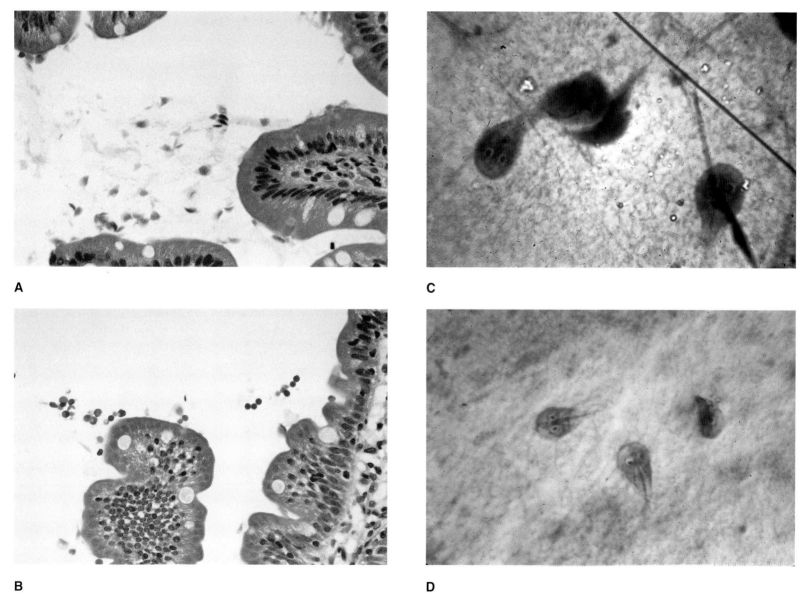

Figure 6–8. A: *Giardi lamblia* infection of the duodenum, showing numerous trophozoites in and around the surface of the cells. *Giardia* has a pear shape with two nuclei when seen en face, but has a flattened appearance when seen on end. This was a biopsy specimen from a patient with hypogammagobulinemia. B: Giardiasis, showing smaller number of trophozoites. When scarce, the organisms can be difficult to identify. C: *Giardia lamblia* in stool preparation. D: *Giardia lamblia* in stool preparation, showing typical pear-shaped organism with two nuclei and prominent flagella.

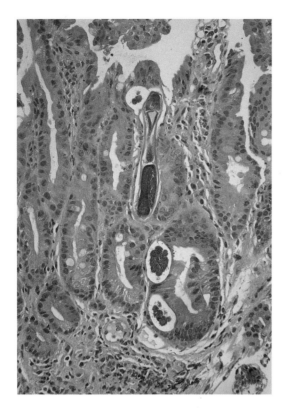

Figure 6–9. *Strongyloides stercoralis*, adult worm in duodenal mucosa, associated with acute duodenitis.

Other infectious diseases such as tuberculosis and helminth diseases such as strongyloidiasis (Fig. 6–9) can affect the duodenum and are encountered in duodenal biopsies; these are more common in the ileum and are described in Chapter 8.

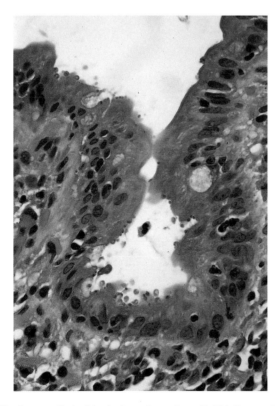

Figure 6–10. Cryptosporidiosis of the duodenum in a patient with AIDS. The organisms are small, rounded structures on the surface of the cells.

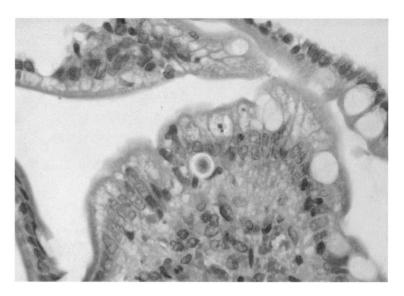

Figure 6–11. *Isospora belli* infection of the duodenum in patient with AIDS. The organism is the large rounded body in the epithelium, seen between the base of the cell and the basement membrane.

In the Immunocompromised Host

Duodenal biopsies frequently show infectious agents in patients with watery diarrhea who are immunodeficient; acquired immunodeficiency syndrome (AIDS) is the most common immunodeficiency. These agents include:

1. *Cryptosporidium*, which appears as 2–5 μm round oocysts on the surface of the epithelial cell (Fig. 6–10). Large numbers of oocysts are commonly present.
2. *Isospora belli*, which is rarely seen in the mucosal cell as a rounded oocyst and is larger than *Cryptosporidium*, measuring 10–12 μm (Fig. 6–11).
3. *Microsporidium*, which is a minute intracellular organism that is difficult to identify by routine light microscopy. Silver stains such as Warthin-Starry stain and modified trichrome stain facilitate light microscopic diagnosis; electron microscopy is more effective in identifying the organisms (see Chapter 17).
4. *Mycobacterium avium-intracellulare*, which is characterized by the presence in the lamina propria of macrophages that contain large numbers of acid-fast bacilli (Fig. 6–12).

The diagnosis of all of these agents is more commonly made by examination of stool specimens than by histologic examination of biopsy samples.

PEPTIC DUODENAL ULCER

Peptic ulcer disease of the duodenum affects 10% of the population of developed countries at sometime during their lifetime. In the past decade, however, medical management of peptic ulcer disease has improved dramatically because of the avail-

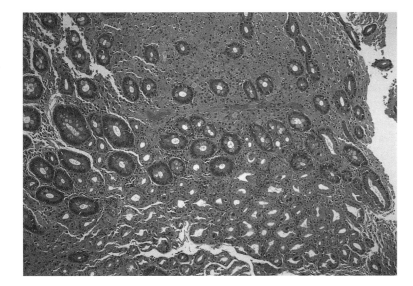

A

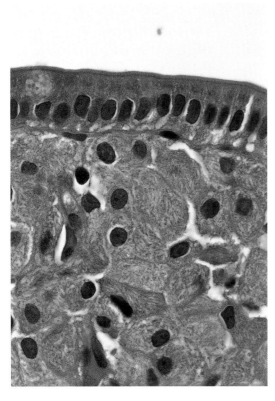

B

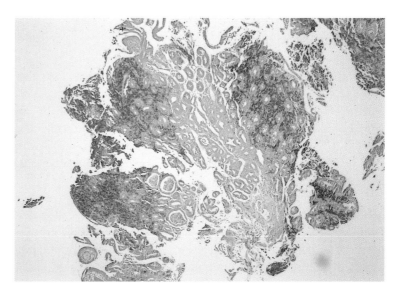

C

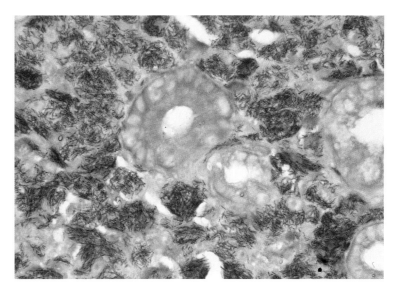

D

Figure 6–12. A: *Mycobacterium avium-intracellulare* infection of the duodenum, showing distension of the lamina propria, which is filled with macrophages with abundant fibrillary cytoplasm. B: Higher power micrograph of part A, showing macrophages with the typical fibrillary cytoplasm. C: Acid-fast stain of mucosa showing patchy involvement of the mucosa, with macrophages containing massive numbers of mycobacteria. D: Higher power micrograph of part C, showing lamina propria macrophages distended with mycobacteria.

ability of more effective acid-suppressing agents, such as proton pump inhibitors,[6] and the recognition that duodenal peptic ulcers are etiologically related to *Helicobacter pylori* infection. Eradication of *H. pylori* infection increases the likelihood of healing and decreases recurrence of duodenal ulceration after healing.[7] Peptic ulcers occurring in the prepyloric region have the same pathogenesis as duodenal ulcers.

Although acid and *H. pylori* are central to the pathogenesis of duodenal ulcers, the exact mechanism by which these two factors cause duodenal ulcers is uncertain. Virtually all patients with duodenal ulcers have evidence of diffuse antral gastritis associated with *H. pylori*.[8] Not all patients with *H. pylori* gastritis develop duodenal ulcers, however, suggesting that other factors

play a role. The link between *H. pylori* gastritis and duodenal ulcer has been explained as follows:

1. *Helicobacter pylori* gastritis affects normal inhibition of gastrin secretion, resulting in hypersecretion of acid and increased acid load in the duodenal bulb.[9]
2. Increased acid exposure in the duodenum is believed to be the stimulus for gastric metaplasia of the surface epithelium of the duodenum.[10]
3. These metaplastic foci provide sites for colonization by *H. pylori*, which evokes an active chronic duodenitis (nonspecific duodenitis).
4. Nonspecific duodenitis results in a lowering of the duodenal

mucosal resistance against acid and pepsin, resulting in erosion and ulceration.[10]

Patients with Zollinger-Ellison syndrome (caused by a gastrin-secreting neoplasm, usually of the pancreas, and associated with marked acid hypersecretion by the stomach) develop severe duodenal peptic ulcers. Ulcers are commonly multiple and tend to involve the second part of the duodenum. Disease in these patients is also well controlled with proton pump inhibitor therapy.

The success of medical treatment for duodenal ulcers has greatly decreased the pathologist's function in this disorder. Duodenal ulcers are diagnosed by endoscopy; biopsies are not considered necessary because endoscopically typical duodenal ulcers are almost never malignant. In the past, a significant number of patients failed medical treatment, leading to surgical procedures; this has become extremely uncommon, and today's pathologists hardly ever receive surgical specimens relating to duodenal ulcers.

Grossly, duodenal ulcers are typically solitary, punched-out ulcers in the duodenal bulb, measuring between 0.5 and 2 cm, but rare giant ulcers larger than 3 cm do occur. Two ulcers involving anterior and posterior walls of the duodenal bulb ("kissing ulcers") are not uncommon. Histologically, the ulcer floor consists of necrotic tissue (Fig. 6–13); its base consists of granulation tissue with fibrosis, and its edge shows reactive epithelium. Complications of duodenal ulcers include hemorrhage and perforation. Complications are usually controlled without surgery; when surgery is performed, vagotomy rather than resections are performed and the specimens received by the pathologist, if any, are vagus nerves.

Surgical treatment of duodenal peptic ulcer consists of one of several acid-reducing procedures. When the surgery is an antrectomy (which is done to remove the gastrin-producing re-gion of the stomach), the pathologist has an important intraoperative role in determining the adequacy of the procedure. It is advisable in this procedure to perform a frozen section of the entire distal surgical margin to ensure that it consists of duodenum. An incomplete antrectomy may result in "retained antrum syndrome" if a Billroth II operation is performed. The gastrin-producing cells in the retained antrum in the afferent duodenal loop, removed from the inhibitory effect of acid by the fact that it is disconnected from the stomach, secrete excess gastrin, causing acid hypersecretion and peptic ulceration in relation to the gastrojejunostomy stroma.

DUODENAL POLYPS

Adenoma

The duodenum is the most common location for adenomas in the small intestine, but duodenal adenomas are much less common than colonic and gastric adenomas, evident as incidental findings only in 0.4% of upper endoscopies.[11] Adenomas occur throughout the duodenum but have the highest incidence in the periampullary region (Fig. 6–14). Periampullary adenomas are a rare cause of obstructive jaundice. Adenomas in other areas of the duodenum are usually asymptomatic and found incidentally at endoscopy. Rarely, they cause bleeding.

Duodenal adenomas are usually solitary, sessile, and small (<1 cm). Rarely, they are large and pedunculated; multiple adenomas are uncommon. Large sessile villous adenomas are difficult to distinguish from adenocarcinomas. Duodenal adenomas are associated with an increased risk of malignancy; the exact magnitude of the risk is unknown. Cancer risk increases with periampullary location, size, and villous architecture.

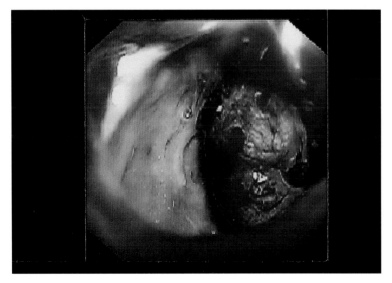

A

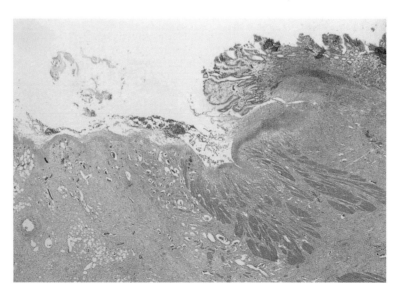

B

Figure 6–13. A: Duodenal ulcer seen at endoscopy. B: Chronic duodenal ulcer, showing edge and base of the ulcer. The muscle wall is drawn up to the ulcer base, and adipose tissue is present in the ulcer base, indicating that the ulcer has penetrated through the duodenal wall. (Figure A courtesy of Aslam Godil, Department of Gastroenterology, Loma Linda University, CA)

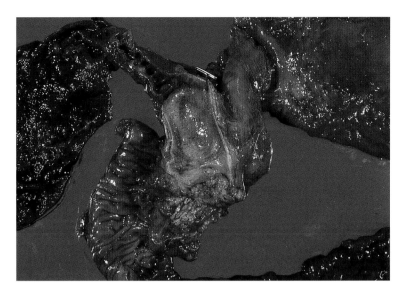

Figure 6–14. Small polypoid mass at the papilla of Vater. This was a tubulovillous adenoma.

In Familial Polyposis Syndromes

Patients with familial adenomatous polyposis (FAP), including Gardner's syndrome, frequently develop duodenal adenomas.[12] In these patients, adenomas develop at an earlier age, are commonly multiple, and increase in number with time. In addition to adenomas, dysplasia has been found incidentally in biopsy specimens taken of endoscopically normal mucosa in these patients.[13,14] The risk of developing duodenal adenocarcinomas, particularly in the periampullary region, is greatly increased in

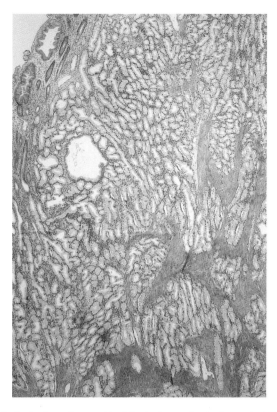

Figure 6–16. Section from a 2-cm nodule of the duodenum, showing Brunner's gland hyperplasia. The overlying mucosa is greatly thinned. The hyperplastic Brunner's glands are admixed with smooth muscle.

patients with FAP compared with the general population. Periampullary carcinoma represents the most common cause of death from cancer in patients with FAP who have had a prophylactic colectomy.[15] Upper gastrointestinal surveillance is indicated for all patients with FAP.

Duodenal hamartomas occur in patients with Peutz-Jeghers syndrome. These patients are also at risk for developing duodenal adenomas and have a slightly increased risk of duodenal adenocarcinoma.[16]

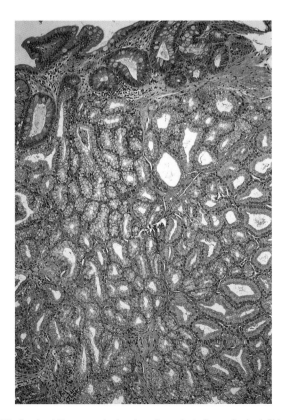

Figure 6–15. Duodenal biopsy sample showing a hyperplastic Brunner's gland. This sample was from a small sessile nodule in the first part of the duodenum.

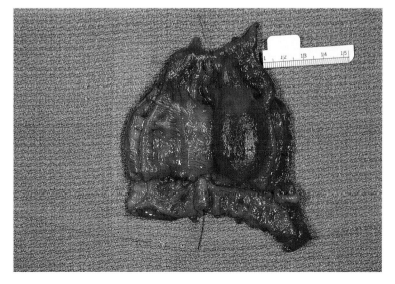

Figure 6–17. Polypoid mass in the duodenum.

Brunner's Gland Hyperplasia and Hamartoma

Brunner's glands occur in the submucosa of the duodenum, being most prominent in its proximal part. The size of Brunner's glands varies considerably; it is not unusual for hyperplastic Brunner's glands to be found incidentally as small nodules, often multiple, at endoscopy. These hyperplastic Brunner's glands extend upward to the mucosal surface; their superficial part is represented in mucosal biopsies (Fig. 6–15). More rarely, the hyperplastic glands form a larger mass that consists of histologically normal Brunner's glands with interspersed muscle (Fig. 6–16). The cause of Brunner's gland hyperplasia is unknown, but increased duodenal acid exposure is the most likely cause. Brunner's gland hyperplasia has no clinical significance.

Rarely, large polypoid mass lesions may occur in the second part of the duodenum, consisting predominantly of Brunner's glands (Fig. 6–17).[17] These may erode the surface and cause hemorrhage.[18] Grossly, these circumscribed mass lesions involve the submucosa and muscle of the duodenum. They can be distinguished from Brunner's gland hyperplasia by the fact that they are demarcated from the overlying mucosa by a fibrous capsule (Fig. 6–18A). Microscopically, it consists of a disorganized mass of hyperplastic Brunner's glands associated with irregular smooth muscle bands (Fig. 6–18B). Cystic change may be present (Fig. 6–18C). There is no atypia, mitotic activity, or necrosis. In many cases, other components are present, including heterotopic pancreatic tissue[18] and adipose tissue (see Fig. 6–18B).[17] The lack of cytologic atypia and the admixture of multiple tissue types suggest that these are hamartomatous lesions, and the term "Brunner's gland hamartoma" appears most appropriate. The diagnosis of Brunner's gland hamartoma can be made by mucosal biopsy only with the knowledge that a large mass lesion is present; otherwise, the mucosal biopsy features are indistinguishable from Brunner's gland hyperplasia. These benign tumors present no risk of malignancy.

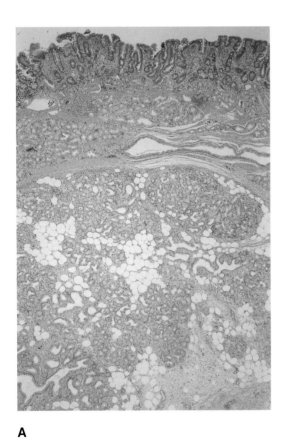

A

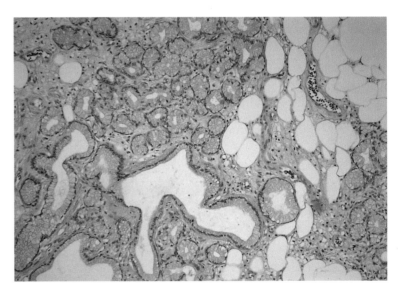

B

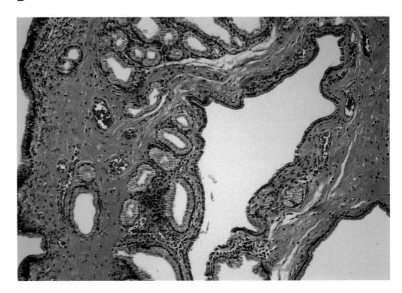

C

Figure 6–18. A: Brunner's gland hamartoma of the duodenum. The mass is circumscribed by a fibrous capsule and lies below the mucosa. B: Brunner's gland hamartoma, showing disorganized Brunner's glands, ducts, and adipose tissue. C: Brunner's gland hamartoma, showing cystic change.

Choristomas

Heterotopic Gastric Mucosa

Heterotopic gastric mucosa occurs commonly in the duodenal bulb. It presents endoscopically as a small mucosal nodule in an otherwise normal duodenum. Microscopically, it is characterized by the presence of gastric-type glands containing parietal cells (Fig. 6–19); the surface epithelium is predominantly flat and of gastric type, but there may be an admixture of normal duodenal mucosa. No active duodenitis is evident, unlike in gastric metaplasia. The finding of heterotopic gastric mucosa in the duodenum is of no clinical significance.

Heterotopic Pancreas

Pancreatic acinar and ductal tissue is frequently found in the duodenal wall (Fig. 6–20), particularly around the common bile duct as it exits the head of the pancreas and penetrates the duodenal wall en route to the papilla of Vater. Rarely, the heterotopic pancreatic tissue forms a clinically detectable nodular mass in the duodenal wall.

Mesenchymal Neoplasms

Benign mesenchymal neoplasms including lymphangioma, hemangioma, lipoma, and neurfibroma, occur very rarely in the duodenum. Malignant GI stromal tumors occur in the duodenum; these are considered in Chapter 15. In immunocompromised patients, particularly those with AIDS, Kaposi's sarcoma may occur in the duodenum. Endoscopically, Kaposi's sarcoma presents as a submucosal red nodule covered by mucosa that projects into the lumen (Fig. 6–21A). Microscopically, the lamina propria is infiltrated by a diffusely infiltrative spindle cell proliferation that separates the crypts (Fig. 6–21B, C). The spindle cells contain slit-like spaces, erythrocyte extravasation, and hemosiderin pigment.

NEUROENDOCRINE TUMORS

Five types of neuroendocrine tumors can be recognized in the duodenum[19] (Table 6–1).

Gastrin-Producing Tumor

Gastrin-producing tumors account for about two thirds of all duodenal neuroendocrine tumors. Mainly occurring in the proximal duodenum, these tumors are usually smaller than 1 cm when detected. Microscopically, they have an insular or trabecular pattern (Fig. 6–22). Although small, many show lymph node metastases at the time of diagnosis.[20] Metastasis to the

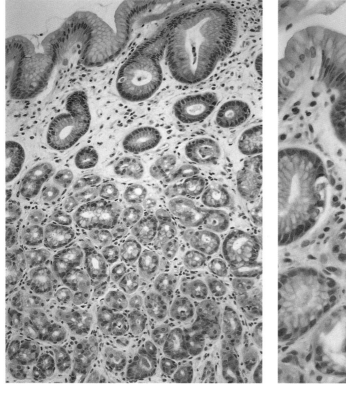
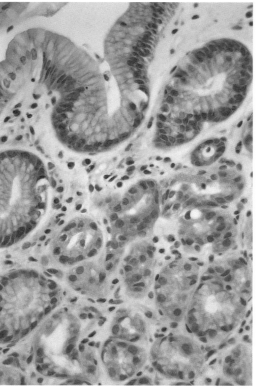

A   B

Figure 6–19. Gastric heterotopia of duodenum. A: The appearance is indistinguishable from normal gastric oxyntic mucosa when the surface is lined by gastric epithelium. This biopsy was from a small nodule in the duodenum, a history that is necessary for diagnosis. B: Higher power of 19A, showing gastric surface epithelium and oxyntic glands.

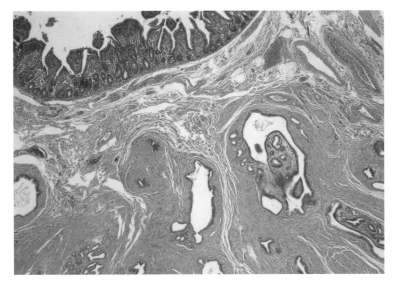

A

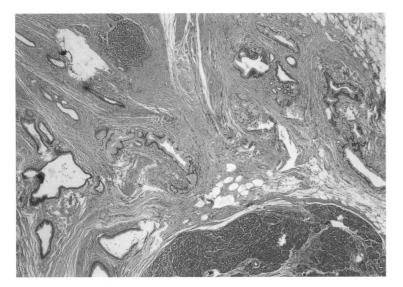

B

Figure 6–20. A: Pancreatic heterotopia of the duodenum, showing a nodular mass composed of distorted smooth muscle and pancreatic ductal tissue. B: Pancreatic heterotopia in the duodenal wall, showing pancreatic acinar tissue admixed with smooth muscle and irregular ducts.

TABLE 6–1. NEUROENDOCRINE TUMORS OF THE DUODENUM

Benign Behavior
Nonfunctioning, well-differentiated, carcinoid tumor; less than 1 cm in size; restricted to mucosa and submucosa; and without angioinvasion.
Serotonin-producing carcinoid tumor, less than 1 cm, outside the papilla of Vater.
Gangliocytic paragangliomas, any size.

Low-Grade Malignant Behavior
Nonfunctioning, well-differentiated, carcinoid tumor; greater than 1 cm in size; extending beyond submucosa; or with angioinvasion.
Gastrinoma, sporadic or MEN, type 1-associated.
Somatostatinoma, with or without neurofibromatosis, type 1.
Serotonin-producing carcinoid tumor, larger than 1 cm in the papilla of Vater.

High-Grade Malignant Behavior
Neuroendocrine carcinoma, functioning or nonfunctioning.

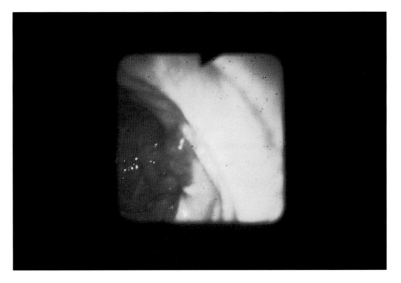

A

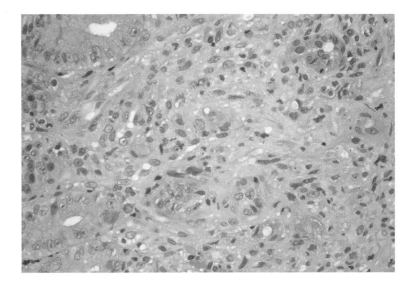

B

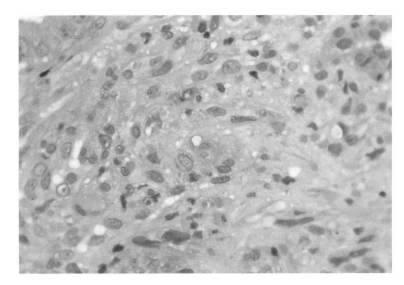

C

Figure 6–21. A: Kaposi's sarcoma of the duodenum at endoscopy, showing a submucosal red nodule covered by mucosa and protruding into the lumen. B: Kaposi's sarcoma of the duodenum, showing spindle cell proliferation in the lamina propria between crypts. C: Kaposi's sarcoma, higher micrograph power of part B.

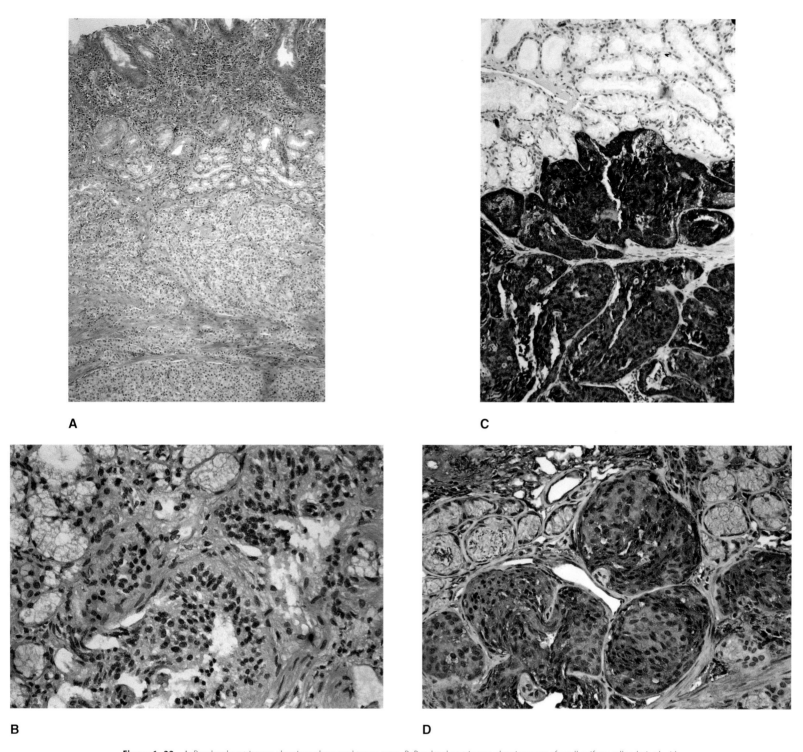

Figure 6–22. A: Duodenal gastrinoma, showing submucosal tumor mass. B: Duodenal gastrinoma, showing nests of small uniform cells admixed with normal mucous glands. C: Immunoperoxidase stain for synaptophysia showing strong positivity in the gastrinoma cells. D: Immunoperoxidase stain for gastrin, showing strong positivity in the gastrinoma cells.

liver, however, is rare and occurs late. Duodenal gastrinoma is often part of the multiple endocrine neoplasia, type 1, syndrome (MEN, type 1); in these patients, multiple duodenal and pancreatic tumors are frequently present. One third of duodenal gastrinomas produce Zollinger-Ellison syndrome.[21] Duodenal gastrinomas should be regarded as slowly growing, low-grade, malignant neoplasms because of their propensity to produce lymph node metastasis.

Somatostatin-Producing Tumor

These tumors constitute 15–20% of duodenal neuroendocrine tumors.[19] They almost always occur at the papilla of Vater and are frequently large mass lesions.[22] They have a low-grade malignant biologic behavior. Histologically, they commonly have a microacinar pattern and may show psammomatous calcification (Figs. 6–23 and 6–24). Somatostatin can be demonstrated

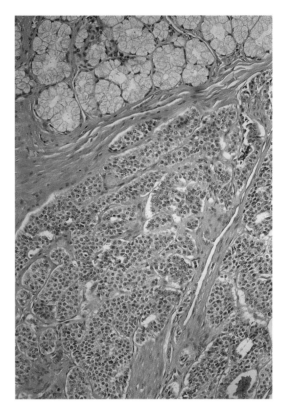

B

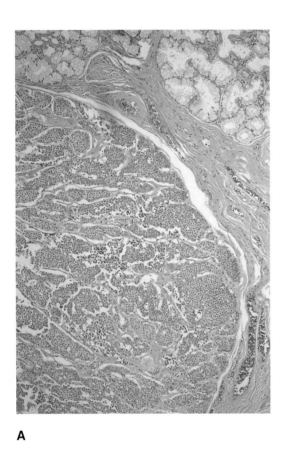

A

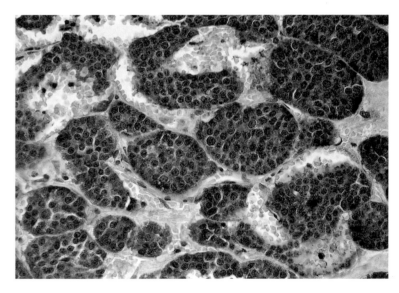

C

Figure 6–23. A: Duodenal somatostatinoma, showing submucosal tumor with trabecular and insular pattern. B: Duodenal somatostatinoma, higher power micrograph of part A, showing uniform cells. C: Duodenal somatostatinoma, stained by immunoperoxidase for somatostatin, showing strong cytoplasmic positivity in the neoplastic cells.

in the neoplastic cells by immunoperoxidase technique. One third of duodenal somatostatinomas are associated with neurofibromatosis, type 1 (von Recklinghausen's disease).

Carcinoid Tumor

Carcinoid tumors are either serotonin-producing or nonfunctioning. Tumors smaller than 1 cm in this category have a benign behavior, particularly if they are located proximal to the papilla of Vater. Larger tumors, and tumors involving the papilla of Vater, should be considered potentially malignant (see Table 6–1). Microscopically, carcinoid tumors have an insular or trabecular growth pattern composed of small cells with uniform round nuclei (Fig. 6–25).

Gangliocytic Paraganglioma

These tumors occur only in the second part of the duodenum. Histologically, they show a mixture of organoid paraganglioma, trabecular carcinoid tumor, and ganglioneuromatous elements,

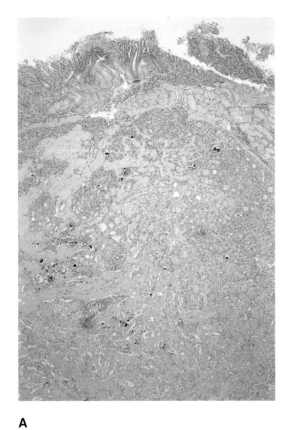

A

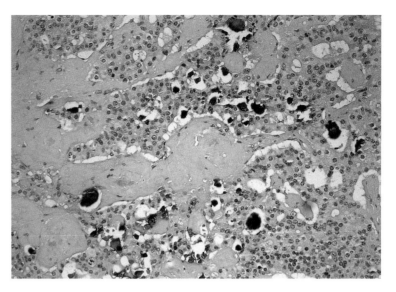

B

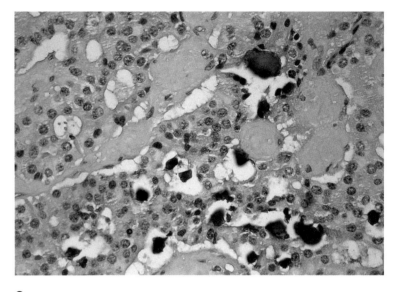

C

Figure 6–24. A: Duodenal somatostatinoma, sowing circumscribed nodular mass under the mucosa and Brunner's glands. B: Higher power micrograph of part A, showing irregular nests of small uniform neuroendocrine cells associated with psammomatous calcification. C: Higher power micrograph of part B, showing uniform appearance of the neuroendocrine cells and psammomatous calcification.

admixed in different proportions (Fig. 6–26) (see also Chapter 14). Although they often reach a large size (over 2 cm) and involve the muscularis externa, these tumors are invariably benign.

Neuroendocrine Carcinoma

These tumors are extremely rare in the duodenum; most reported cases have occurred in the region of the papilla of Vater. These undifferentiated, cytologically high-grade malignant neoplasms can be distinguished from poorly differentiated adenocarcinoma only because of their positivity with neuroendocrine markers by immunohistochemistry or electron microscopy.

DUODENAL ADENOCARCINOMA

Primary adenocarcinoma of the duodenum is rare, accounting for less than 0.5% of gastrointestinal carcinomas. The majority of duodenal carcinomas arise in the periampullary region, involving the papilla of Vater. Nonampullary duodenal carcinomas are distributed fairly evenly in the nonampullary second, third, and fourth parts of the duodenum. Primary carcinomas almost never occur in the duodenal bulb. When biopsies show adenocarcinoma in the duodenal bulb, the possibility of direct invasion of the duodenum by a gastric, pancreatic, or colon carcinoma must be considered (Fig. 6–27). We have encountered a case in which a colon adenocarcinoma directly invaded the

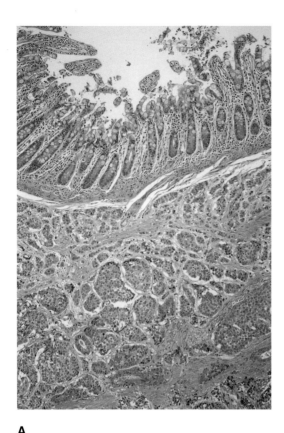

A

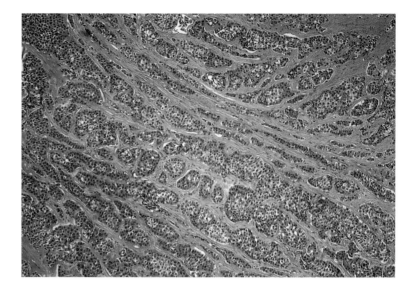

B

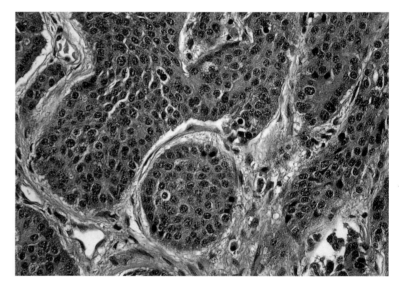

C

Figure 6–25. A: Duodenal carcinoid tumor, submucosal tumor with an insular pattern. B: Duodenal carcinoid tumor, showing mixed architecture with trabecular, insular, and microacinar patterns. C: Duodenal carcinoid tumor, showing nests of uniform cells typical for carcinoid tumor.

duodenum, causing mucosal ulceration in the duodenum. Biopsy specimens from the duodenal tumor gave a false impression of origin from the duodenal mucosa, including what appeared to be an in situ papillary component. Rarely, carcinomas from other sites metastasize to the duodenum (Fig. 6–28).

Periampullary Carcinoma

Periampullary carcinomas most likely arise in preexisting adenomas, passing through an adenoma–carcinoma sequence similar to that seen in the colon. A significant number of patients with villous adenomas and periampullary adenocarcinoma have familial adenomatous polyposis (usually Gardner's syndrome). Most patients present with obstructive jaundice.

Tumors are frequently papillary and endoscopically indistinguishable from villous adenomas (Fig. 6–29). Preoperative biopsies from such ampullary lesions confirm the diagnosis of a villous adenoma, but have a relatively low sensitivity in detect-

ing malignancy (Fig. 6–30); in tumors that ultimately prove to be malignant, preoperative biopsies are positive in approximately half the cases.[23] Malignancy should be strongly suspected in patients who have obstructive jaundice, even when biopsies are negative.

Treatment options for villous adenomas of the periampullary region in which biopsies have been negative for malignancy include local resections of the tumor (ampullectomy, submucosal resections) or pancreaticoduodenectomy (Whipple's procedure). When preoperative biopsies have demonstrated invasive carcinoma, pancreaticoduodenectomy is indicated, if the tumor is resectable.

Periampullary adenocarcinomas that arise from the duodenal mucosa can be difficult to distinguish from tumors arising in the terminal ampullary part of the common biliary and pancreatic duct (ampullary carcinoma) and from carcinoma of the head of the pancreas, particularly if these tumors are large and have grown into the duodenal mucosa at the papilla (Figs. 6–31 and 6–32). In early lesions of the ampullary part of the bile

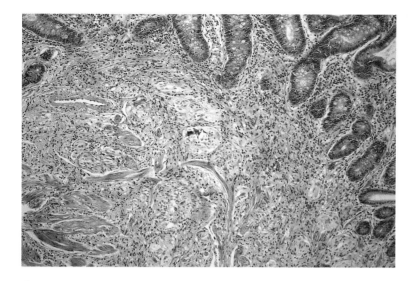

A

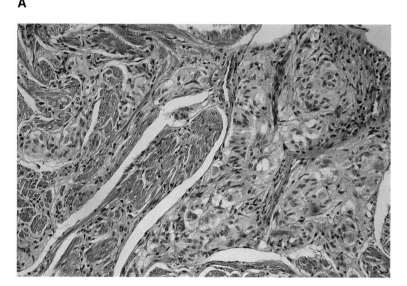

B

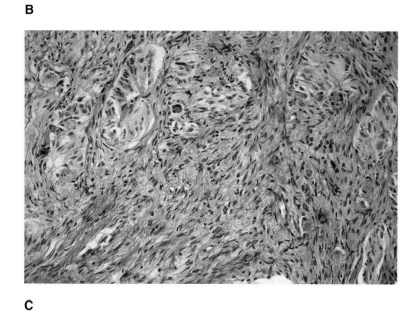

C

Figure 6–26. A: Gangliocytic paraganglioma of the duodenum, showing the organoid tumor nests under the mucosa. The tumor is not demarcated from the mucosa. B: Gangliocytic paraganglioma of the duodenum, showing organoid pattern with nests of large cells infiltrating between muscle fibers. C: Gangliocytic paraganglioma, mixed organoid and ganglioneuromatous pattern with scattered ganglion cells.

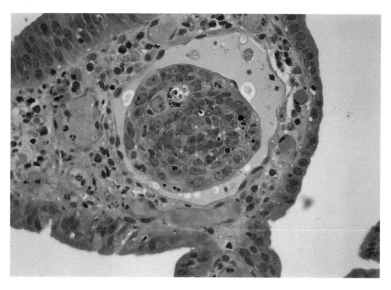

Figure 6–27. Intralymphatic carcinoma in the duodenal mucosa. This was a poorly differentiated gastric adenocarcinoma involving the duodenum.

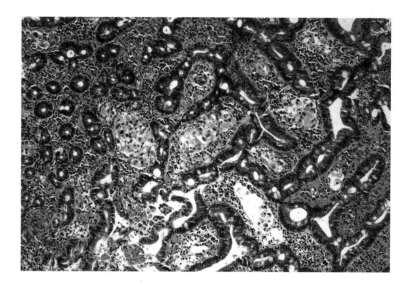

A

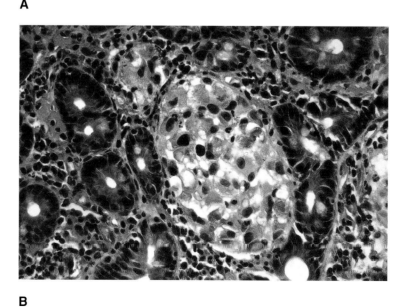

B

Figure 6–28. A: Intralymphatic clear cell adenocarcinoma in the mucosa of the duodenum. This was positive for cytokeratin and vimentin, and the patient had a history of renal adenocarcinoma, raising the possibility of metastatic renal adenocarcinoma. B: Higher power micrograph of part A.

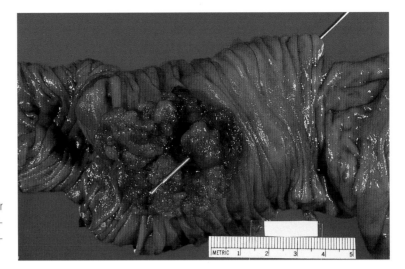

Figure 6–29. Papillary adenocarcinoma of the papilla of Vater (probe through the bile duct opening). This tumor is indistinguishable from a villous adenoma grossly. Biopsy showed invasive carcinoma.

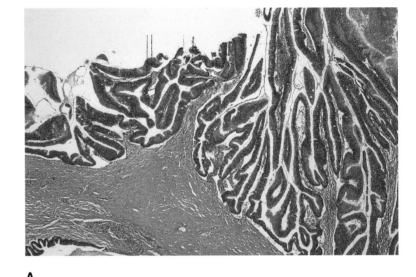

Figure 6–30. A: Villous adenoma of the papilla of Vater. B: Villous adenoma of the papilla of Vater with high-grade dysplasia. C: Villous adenoma of the papilla of Vater with early invasive carcinoma. D: Terminal bile duct adenocarcinoma involving the papilla of Vater and mimicking a carcinoma arising in the papilla of Vater. This patient had extensive involvement of the biliary system with multifocal adenocarcinoma.

A

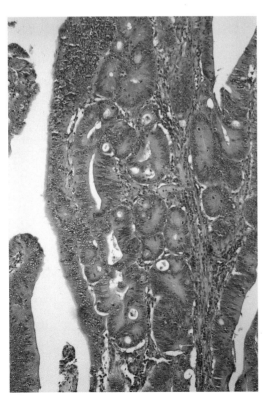

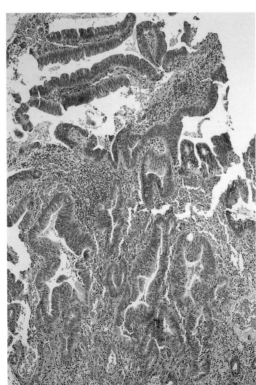

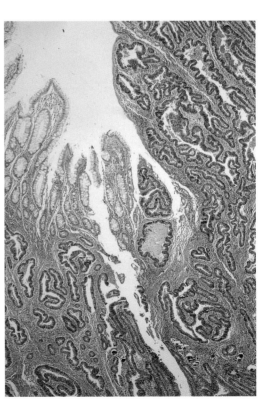

B

C

D

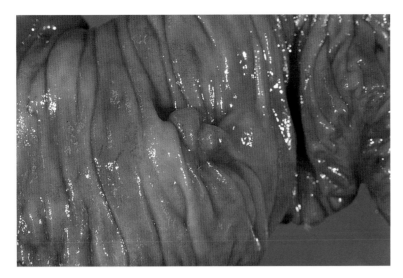

Figure 6–31. Nodularity and distortion of papilla of Vater by an underlying terminal bile duct carcinoma.

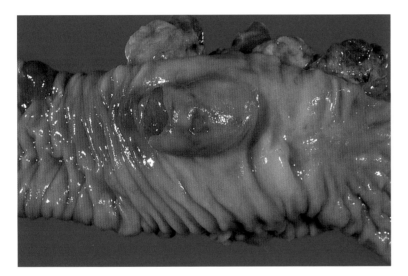

A

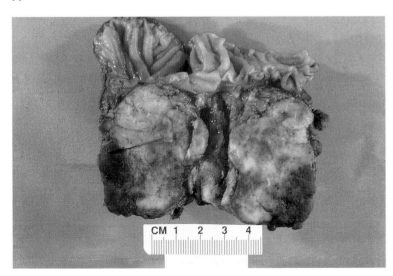

B

Figure 6–32. A: Large polypoid enlargement of the papilla of Vater due to an underlying terminal bile duct adenocarcinoma. B: Cross section across the papillary region of the duodenum, showing a large carcinoma of the head of the pancreas involving the duodenal wall and terminal common pancreaticobiliary duct.

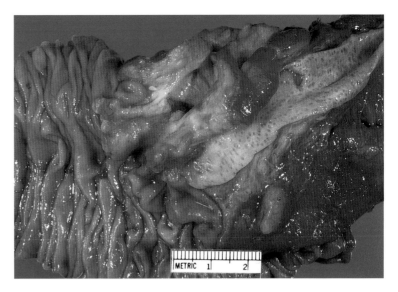

Figure 6–33. Carcinoma of the ampullary portion of the terminal bile duct. The bile duct is opened and shows a nodular mass in the terminal part of the bile duct extending to the papilla.

duct, the tumor is clearly seen to be in the terminal bile duct prior to its opening at the tip of the ampulla (Figs. 6–33 and 6–34). Histologically, periampullary adenocarcinomas tend to be well-differentiated papillary carcinomas (Fig. 6–30), compared with the ampullary and pancreatic adenocarcinomas, which are usually well-differentiated tubular carcinomas with a marked desmoplastic response (Fig. 6–35A, B). Although helpful, this feature is not totally reliable (Fig. 6–35C). Bile duct carcinoma also frequently shows evidence of in situ carcinoma of the bile duct epithelium proximal to the ampullary tumor (Fig. 6–36).

Assessment of invasion of the duodenal wall by a periampullary carcinoma can be difficult because of the complex anatomy of this region (Fig. 6–37). The common bile duct penetrates the muscle wall of the duodenum at this site, and it is frequently difficult to separate bile duct smooth muscle from duodenal wall, as well as to identify the outer limit of the duodenal

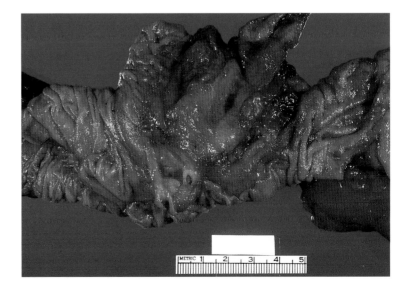

Figure 6–34. Carcinoma of the ampullary part of the terminal bile duct, showing diffuse thickening of the bile duct.

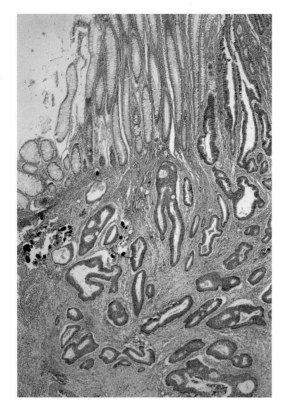

A

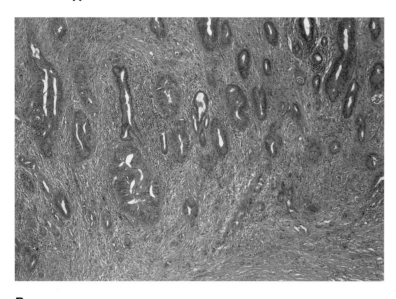

B

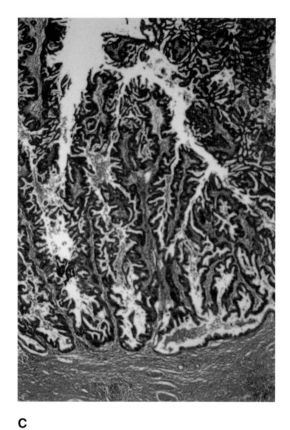

C

Figure 6–35. A: Bile duct adenocarcinoma, showing well-differentiated tubular structures associated with desmoplasia. B: Bile duct adenocarcinoma, showing well-differentiated malignant tubular structures. C: Papillary adenocarcinoma of the terminal part of the common pancreaticobiliary duct.

wall. Careful, well-oriented sections are crucial for accurate assessment and staging.

The prognosis of periampullary carcinoma depends on the type of surgery performed (patients who have a surgical resection with curative intent, usually a pancreaticoduodenectomy, are the only patients who have a chance of prolonged survival), the pathologic stage, and the histologic grade (poorly differentiated carcinoma has a poorer prognosis than that for well-differentiated tumor). Staging is done by tumor, node, metastasis (TNM) criteria, similar to that for colorectal carcinoma; the presence of invasion through the duodenal wall and nodal involvement are indicators of poor prognosis. Periampullary adenocarcinomas express p53, c-*neu,* and tumor growth factor-alpha (TGF-α). C-*neu* expression is predictive of a short survival.[24] The data relating to these prognostic criteria are open to debate because the numbers of cases in most studies has been small.

Nonampullary Duodenal Carcinoma

Duodenal adenocarcinomas not related to the papilla of Vater are extremely rare. Although similar pathologically to peri-

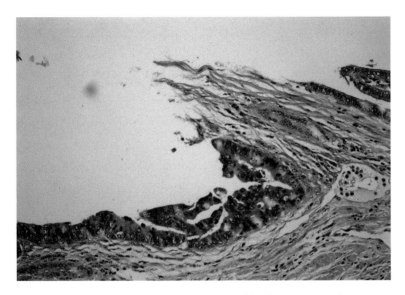

Figure 6–36. High-grade epithelial dysplasia in the proximal bile duct in a patient with a carcinoma of the ampullary region of the bile duct.

ampullary carcinoma, they have two differences: (1) they do not cause obstructive jaundice, and therefore tend to present at a later stage of disease, and (2) resection of the duodenal segment containing the tumor does not usually entail a pancreaticoduodenectomy. The mortality rate from segmental duodenectomy is much lower than for pancreaticoduodenectomy.[25]

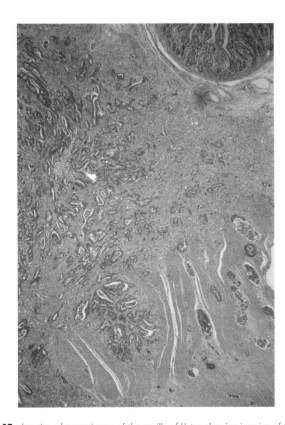

Figure 6–37. Invasive adenocarcinoma of the papilla of Vater, showing invasion of the duodenal wall.

References

1. Sircus W. Duodenitis: A clinical, endoscopic and histopathologic study. *Q J Med.* 1985;56:593–600.
2. Caselli M, Trevisani L, Aleotti A, et al. Gastric metaplasia in duodenal bulb and *Campylobacter*-like organisms in development of duodenal ulcer. *Dig Dis Sci.* 1989;34:1374–1378.
3. Lam SK. Etiology and pathogenesis of peptic ulcer. *J Gastroenterol.* 1994;29:39–54.
4. Poggioli G, Stocchi L, Laureti S, et al. Duodenal involvement of Crohn's disease: Three different clinicopathologic patterns. *Dis Colon Rectum.* 1997;40:179–183.
5. Mitomi H, Atari E, Uesugi H, et al. Distinctive diffuse duodenitis associated with ulcerative colitis. *Dig Dis Sci.* 1997;42:684–693.
6. Jones DB, Howden CW, Burget DW, et al. Acid suppression in duodenal ulcer: A meta-analysis to define optimal dosing with antisecretory drugs. *Gut.* 1987;28:1120–1127.
7. Hosking SW, Ling TKW, Chung SCS, et al. Duodenal ulcer healing by eradication of *Helicobacter pylori* without antacid treatment: Randomized, controlled trial. *Lancet.* 1994;343:508–510.
8. Sipponen P, Seppala K, Aarynen M, et al. Chronic gastritis and gastroduodenal ulcer: A case control study on risk of coexisting duodenal or gastric ulcer in patients with gastritis. *Gut.* 1989;30:922–929.
9. Hamlet A, Olbe L. The influence of *Helicobacter pylori* infection on postprandial duodenal acid load and duodenal bulb pH in humans. *Gastroenterology.* 1996;111:391–400.
10. Walker MM, Dixon MF. Gastric metaplasia: Its role in duodenal ulceration. *Aliment Pharmacol Ther.* 1996;10:119–128.
11. Perzin K, Bridge M. Adenomas of the small intestine: A clinicopathologic review of 51 cases and a study of their relationship to carcinoma. *Cancer.* 1981;48:799.
12. Bertoni G, Sassatelli R, Nigrisoli E, et al. High prevalence of adenomas and microadenomas of the duodenal papilla and periampullary region in patients with familial adenomatous polyposis. *Eur J Gastroenterol Hepatol.* 1996;8:1201–1206.
13. Sarre RG, Frost AG, Jagelman DG, et al. Gastric and duodenal polyps in familial adenomatous polyposis. A prospective study of the nature and prevalence of upper gastrointestinal polyps. *Gut.* 1987;28:306–314.
14. Iida M, Aoyagi K, Fujimura Y, et al. Nonpolypoid adenomas of the duodenum in patients with familial adenomatous polyposis (Gardner's syndrome). *Gastrointest Endosc.* 1996;44:305–308.
15. Offerhaus GJA, Giardiello FM, Krush AJ, et al. The risk of upper gastrointestinal cancer in familial adenomatous polyposis. *Gastroenterology.* 1992;102:1980–1982.
16. Ichiyoshi Y, Yao T, Nagasaki S, et al. Solitary Peutz-Jeghers type polyp of the duodenum containing a focus of adenocarcinoma. *Ital J Gastroenterol.* 1996;28:95–97.
17. de Silva S, Chandrasoma P. Giant duodenal hamartoma consisting mainly of Brunner's glands. *Am J Surg.* 1977;133:240–243.
18. Kouraklis G, Kostakis A, Delladetsima J. Hamartoma of Brunner's glands causing massive haematemesis. *Scand J Gastroenterol.* 1994;29:841–843.
19. Capella C, Heitz PU, Hofler H, et al. Revised classification of neuroendocrine tumors of the lung, pancreas and gut. *Digestion.* 1994;55:11–23.
20. Pipeleers-Marichal M, Donow C, Heitz PU, et al. Pathologic aspects of gastrinomas in patients with Zollinger-Ellison syndrome with and without multiple endocrine neoplasia type 1. *World J Surg.* 1993;17:481–488.

21. Norton JA. Neuroendocrine tumors of the pancreas and duodenum. *Curr Probl Surg.* 1994;31:77–156.
22. Dayal Y, Tallberg KA, Nunnemacher G, et al. Duodenal carcinoids in patients with and without neurofibromatosis. A comparative study. *Am J Surg Pathol.* 1986;10:348–357.
23. Pezet D, Rotman N, Slim K, et al. Villous tumors of the duodenum: A retrospective study of 47 cases by the French Association for Surgical Research. *J Am Coll Surg.* 1995; 180:541–544.
24. Ahu L, Kim K, Domenico DR, et al. Adenocarcinoma of duodenum and ampulla of Vater: Clinicopathologic study and expression of p53, c-*neu*, TGF-alpha, CEA, and EMA. *J Surg Oncol.* 1996;61:100–105.
25. Fronticelli CM, Borghi F, Gattolin A, et al. Primary adenocarcinoma of the angle of Treitz. Case report and review of the literature. *Arch Surg.* 1996;131:1109–1111.

7

MALABSORPTION SYNDROME

Evelyn Choo and Parakrama Chandrasoma

► CHAPTER OUTLINE

NORMAL ABSORPTION

Normal digestion of food begins in the stomach and is completed in the upper small intestine. Digestion involves the breakdown of complex molecules into simpler molecules that are capable of passage through the mucosal cells. Carbohydrates are broken down into monosaccharides and disaccharides, proteins into amino acids, and fats to monoglycerides and fatty acids. These molecules are transported across the intestinal cell by four basic mechanisms:

1. Active transport, which usually occurs against an electric or chemical gradient and requires an energy-dependent carrier mechanism.

2. Passive diffusion, which occurs along an electric or chemical gradient and is energy-independent.
3. Facilitated diffusion, which occurs along a gradient but is facilitated by a carrier mechanism.
4. Endocytosis, in which the molecule is taken up by the cell by a mechanism similar to phagocytosis, that is, the particle is surrounded by the cell membrane, which transports it across the cell to the opposite surface. Endocytosis is not a substantial mechanism of food absorption.

Most food products can be absorbed throughout the small intestine, but some selectivity is present in normal people. The proximal small intestine is a major area of absorption of iron, calcium, vitamins, and fat. Carbohydrates and amino acids are absorbed in the midintestine. Bile acids and vitamin B_{12} absorption is specifically restricted to the distal ileum. The intestine is highly efficient in the absorption of carbohydrates and proteins, and most malabsorptive states manifest as fat malabsorption.

The normal adult ingests 50–100 g of fat daily, mainly as long-chain triglycerides. In the small-intestinal lumen, triglycerides are hydrolyzed into fatty acids and monoglycerides by a complex of pancreatic and biliary secretions, which include pancreatic lipase, pancreatic colipase, and bile salts. The fatty acids and monoglycerides are then complexed with bile salts to form a globular structure called a mixed micelle. Fat-soluble vitamins are also associated with micelles. The micelles attach to the surface of the intestinal cell and dissociate: the fatty acids, vitamins, and monoglycerides enter the cell by a process of diffusion, and the bile salts remain in the lumen. The bile salts are finally reabsorbed in the terminal ileum for transport to the liver and resecretion (the enterohepatic circulation of bile salts).

In the endoplasmic reticulum of the mucosal cell, fatty acids and monoglycerides derived from long-chain (C16–18) triglycerides are immediately reesterified into triglycerides and complexed with apoproteins, cholestrol, and phospholipid to form chylomicrons and very low density lipoproteins (VLDL). Chylomicrons and VLDL are secreted by the cell into the lacteals in the lamina propria for transport via the thoracic duct to the bloodstream. Fatty acids derived from medium-chain (C8–12) triglycerides are not reesterified in the intestinal cell. Instead, they rapidly enter the portal venous system for direct transport to the liver as fatty acids complexed to albumin.

MECHANISMS AND CLINICAL FEATURES OF MALABSORPTION

Malabsorption may be a general failure of absorption of food in the small intestine or a specific failure to digest and absorb one specific food component. General failure of malabsorption is commonly manifested by a failure of fat absorption and defined as the excretion of more than 6 g/day of fat in a person with a normal fat intake. This is assessed in a 72-h stool sample. Fat malabsorption usually manifests clinically as steatorrhea, which is the passage of soft, yellowish, greasy stools that float in water. Many patients with steatorrhea also have diarrhea, but diarrhea is not a constant symptom in fat malabsorption.

In patients without diarrhea or stools recognized as being characteristic of steatorrhea, symptoms of malabsorption may be subtle and relate to malabsorption of vitamin A (night blindness, Bitot's spots in the conjunctiva), vitamin D (bone pain due to osteomalacia and tetany due to hypocalcemia), folic acid (anemia), thiamine (peripheral neuropathy), or vitamin K (bleeding tendency). Unexplained iron deficiency anemia, weight loss, short stature, and abdominal bloating are also common manifestations of malabsorption. In these cases, the diagnosis of malabsorption can be made by stool fat analysis. Other tests of malabsorption include xylose absorption (the most commonly used test for carbohydrate absorption), secretin test (for pancreatic function), bile acid breath tests (for bacterial overgrowth), and small-bowel radiography.

Malabsorption results from a large number of diseases, and it is useful to develop a classification of these diseases by recognizing the basic mechanisms that lead to malabsorption (Table 7–1).

NORMAL SMALL-INTESTINAL MUCOSA

The normal small intestine is perfectly designed for absorption. Its 5–6-m length is converted into an enormous mucosal surface area by the plicae circulares, or the intestinal folds, and the villi. The mucosa consists of a surface epithelium, which represents the barrier that controls entry of luminal contents into

TABLE 7–1. MECHANISMS OF MALABSORPTION

General Malabsorption with Steatorrhea

Pancreatic Enzyme (Lipase) Deficiency
  Failure of pancreatic secretion
    Cystic fibrosis
    Chronic pancreatitis
    Pancreatic resection
    Pancreatic carcinoma
  Failure of lipase activation
    Zollinger-Ellison syndrome (gastrinoma of pancreas)
Bile Salt Deficiency
  Failure of bile salt secretion
    Liver failure
    Biliary obstruction
  Bacterial overgrowth in small intestine
    Stasis from any cause: diverticula, blind loops, strictures, hypomotility (progressive systemic sclerosis, diabetes, intestinal pseudo-obstruction)
    Fistulas
  Failure of enterohepatic bile salt circulation
    Distal ileal resection
    Distal ileal disease (Crohn's enteritis)
  Drugs inhibiting bile salts (neomycin, cholestyramine)
Inadequate Small Intestine (Short-bowel syndrome)
  Intestinal resection (neonatal necrotizing enterocolitis, mesenteric ischemia with infarction, regional enteritis, trauma)
  Jejunoileal bypass (for treatment of obesity)
Hypermotility
  Carcinoid syndrome
  Hyperthyroidism
Primary Mucosal Diseases
  Celiac disease (gluten-induced enteropathy)
  Tropical sprue
  Collagenous sprue
  Whipple's disease
  Radiation enteritis
  Others (see Table 7–2)
Lymphatic Obstruction
  Intestinal lymphangiectasia, primary and secondary
  Malignant lymphoma

Specific Biochemical Disorders

  Disaccharidase (lactase) deficiency (lactose intolerance)
  Autoimmune gastritis (pernicious anemia—vitamin B_{12})

the cells, the lamina propria, and the thin muscularis mucosae. The mucosa is configured into villi that project up from the surface and crypts that extend down. The villi are normally 0.3–1 mm in height.

The surface epithelium lines the villi and the crypts. The villi tend to be broad and leaf-shaped in the duodenum (Fig. 7–1). They are taller, thinner, finger-like, and more numerous in the jejunum (Fig. 7–2) than in the ileum, where they are shorter, more club-shaped, and sparser (Fig. 7–3). At the base of the villi,

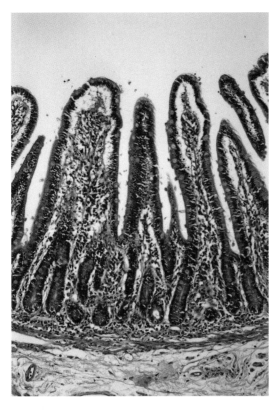

Figure 7–1. Normal mucosa from the proximal duodenum, showing relatively short, leaf-like villi typical for this region.

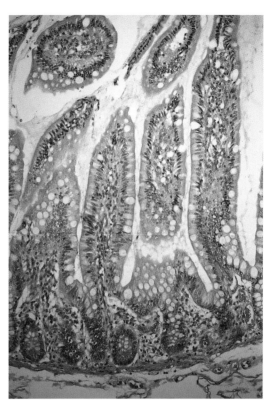

Figure 7–3. Normal ileal mucosa, showing shorter villi than in the jejunum with greater number of goblet cells.

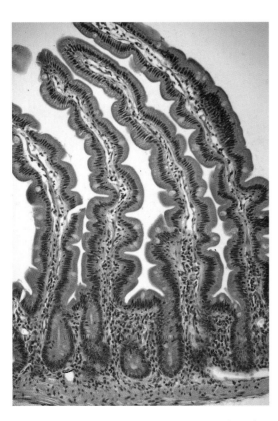

Figure 7–2. Normal jejunal mucosa, showing long, slender villi that are four to five times the length of the crypts.

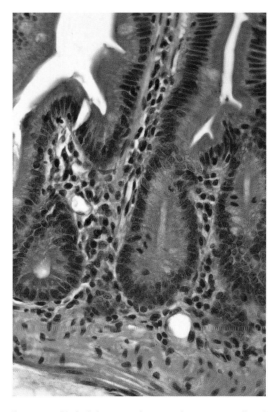

Figure 7–4. Short crypts of Lieberkühn in jejunal mucosa, showing active cells with mitotic figures in the germinative region of the mucosa.

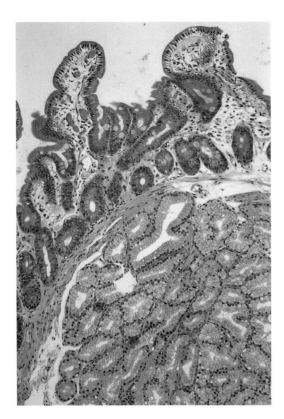

Figure 7–5. Proximal duodenal mucosa over a Brunner's gland, showing short, blunt villi.

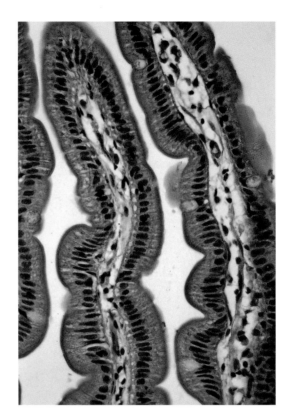

A

the epithelium dips down into the crypts of Lieberkühn, which extend vertically downward to the level of the muscularis mucosae (Fig. 7–4). In Western countries, the villi are normally at least three times the height of the crypts throughout the small intestine (ie, the villous:crypt ratio is greater than 3:1). The only exceptions to this are: (1) In the proximal duodenum, where villi in the mucosa overlying Brunner's glands may be shorter (Fig. 7–5). (2) Overlying lymphoid aggregates (Fig. 7–6), where the mucosa is flattened and the villi frequently attenuated. (3) In 30% of normal children in whom the villi are shorter and the crypts longer than in adults.[1]

The epithelial cells lining the villi form a continuous layer,

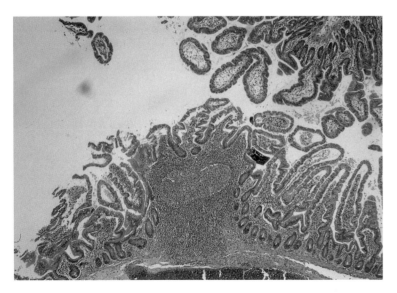

Figure 7–6. Lymphoid follicle in the ileal mucosa, showing shortened villi overlying it.

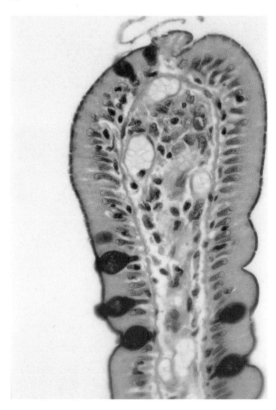

B

Figure 7–7. A: Jejunal villus, lined mainly by absorptive cells, which are tall columnar cells with a distinct brush border. Rare interspersed goblet cells are also evident. Note the rare intraepithelial lymphocytes between epithelial cells. B: Jejunal villi, PAS stain, showing the brush border of the absorptive cells and the positive staining of the mucus in the goblet cells. Again, note the scattered intraepithelial lymphocytes.

with tight cell junctions that prevent entry of molecules between cells. All absorption occurs through the mucosal cells. Several cell types are present in the epithelium. The villi are lined by differentiated absorptive cells (enterocytes) and goblet cells (Fig. 7–7A). The differentiated enterocytes lining the villi are columnar cells characterized by long microvilli, which are visible on light microscopy as a brush border on the surface. The brush border is accentuated by staining with periodic acid–Schiff (PAS) stain (Fig. 7–7B). Goblet cells are more numerous in the ileum than in the jejunum. The crypts are lined by undifferentiated germinative cells that continually replenish epithelial cells lost from the surface. The crypts show frequent mitotic figures, indicative of the very rapid cell turnover rate in the small-intestinal mucosa. Paneth cells, which are serous cells with eosinophilic granular cytoplasm, are present mainly along the crypt base (Fig. 7–8). M cells are specialized epithelial cells that are found interspersed between the absorptive cells, particularly over the lymphoid patches.[2] They are distinguished from absorptive cells by their short, fat microvilli, visible only on electron microscopy. M cells function to absorb and transport antigen, including intact large protein molecules and microorganisms from the lumen to the lamina propria by endocytosis. Staining with chromogranin shows the presence of scattered neuroendocrine cells in the mucosa, particularly in the crypts; these are of several different types and have the ability to secrete several hormones, including serotonin, somatostatin, and bombesin.

The lamina propria contains connective tissue; capillaries; absorptive lymphatics (lacteals); and many cells, predominantly lymphocytes and plasma cells, but also eosinophils, macrophages, mast cells, fibroblasts, and rare smooth muscle cells. Lymphocytes are also present above the basement membrane of the surface epithelium, between enterocytes (see Fig. 7). In normal mucosa, approximately 1 intraepithelial lymphocyte occurs for every 10 epithelial cells. The intraepithelial and lamina propria lymphocytes are predominantly T lymphocytes that recirculate continuously. The plasma cells produce all classes of immunoglobulin, but predominantly secretory IgA. IgA produced by the plasma cell combines with a glycoprotein receptor on the basal aspect of the epithelial cell membrane and is transported through the cell for release into the lumen; part of the glycoprotein receptor represents the "secretory piece" of the secretory IgA molecule.

Lymphoid aggregates are normally present in the intestinal mucosa and submucosa (Fig. 7–9). They are sparse in the je-

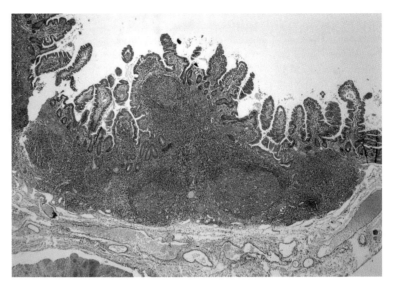

A

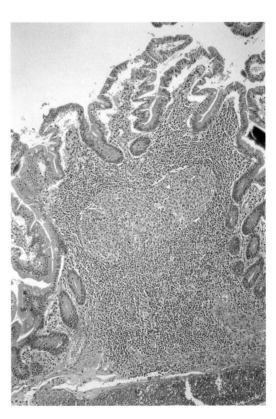

B

Figure 7–9. A: Lymphoid patch in the ileum, showing reactive follicles. Normal lymphoid patches are well circumscribed. Biopsy specimens from mucosa over these lymphoid patches should not be confused with chronic inflammation or lymphoma. B: Lymphoid patch in the ileal mucosa, showing a reactive germinal center.

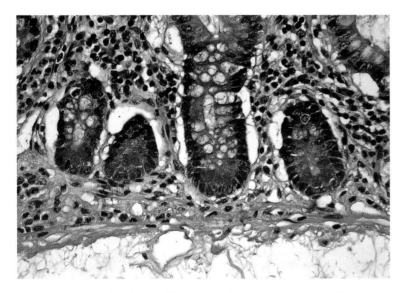

Figure 7–8. Paneth cells at the base of the crypts with their typical granular eosinophilic cytoplasm.

junum, and progressively increase in size and number toward the terminal ileum. The larger lymphoid aggregates (Peyer's patches) occur in the terminal ileum in children and may reach a size of 2 cm and appear as nodules covered by mucosa. They usually atrophy with increasing age. Microscopically, the lymphoid aggregates are well-circumscribed nodules in the deep mucosa and submucosa composed of reactive follicles with prominent germinal centers.

SMALL-INTESTINAL BIOPSY

Small-intestinal biopsy is most commonly performed via upper gastrointestinal (GI) endoscopy. The biopsy specimen should be taken as distal as possible in the duodenum, where the density of Brunner's glands decreases and the mucosal features become representative of the small intestine. In the second part of the duodenum where Brunner's glands are present, biopsy samples may be difficult to interpret because the mucosa overlying Brunner's glands is frequently thinner and the villi shorter than normal.

Biopsies are best done with a jumbo 3–4-mm diameter biopsy forceps; these produce specimens twice the size of a standard sample, have less crush artefact, and are easier to orient, and provide greater sampling area.[3] These specimens should ideally be oriented before being placed in formalin, but this requires an endoscopy unit with individuals trained in biopsy sample orientation. In units with untrained personnel, which represents the majority of community hospitals and many academic institutions, the sample should be placed in formalin without orientation. Clumsy attempts at orienting the specimen by individuals who do not routinely do so can lead to marked distortion and artefact. Unoriented biopsy samples can be interpreted because multiple-level sectioning always provides a well-oriented area in the biopsy adequate for histologic evaluation.

Another method of obtaining a biopsy of the small intestine is at colonoscopy. The endoscope can usually be passed into the terminal ileum and a mucosal biopsy sample obtained. Terminal ileal biopsies are most suited to evaluating for Crohn's disease. They are less suited as a method of evaluating diseases associated with malabsorption such as celiac disease. Many terminal ileal biopsies show reactive lymphoid hyperplasia because of the prominence of lymphoid aggregates in this region; this should not be mistaken for chronic inflammation or malignant lymphoma.

In occasional patients in whom upper GI endoscopy is not indicated, a sample can be obtained through one of many suction devices that can be passed orally into the jejunum. The most commonly used device in adults is Rubin's tube, which is a four-holed suction tube that is passed into the jejunum and yields four mucosal specimens of approximately 5 mm in diameter. Other biopsy instruments include the Crosby-Kugler and Carey capsules, which are used more commonly in children because of their safety and ease of oral passage.[4]

Small-bowel biopsy is indicated in a patient with steatorrhea, unexplained diarrhea, or anemia, and when clinical evaluation suggests the possibility of any disease that may be associated with an abnormal small-bowel biopsy (Table 7–2). By far the most common indication for small-bowel biopsy in practice is the evaluation of a patient for the possibility of celiac disease.

Evaluation of the small-intestinal biopsy requires the presence of a minimum of four consecutive vertically oriented villi and crypts. The examination should routinely evaluate the following characteristics:

1. Length, breadth, and shape of villi. Usually, these features are compared with the pathologist's impression of normal structure from past experience. Actual measurement is rarely undertaken, and no established criteria of normalcy are based on measurement. Decrease in villous height is classified subjectively by degree into partial, subtotal, and total villous atrophy.

TABLE 7–2. DISEASES ASSOCIATED WITH ABNORMALITIES IN A SMALL-BOWEL BIOPSY

Disease	Abnormality
Celiac disease	Villous atrophy, crypt hyperplasia, surface epithelial damage, intraepithelial lymphocytic infiltration; changes reverse with gluten withdrawal.
Collagenous sprue	Same as celiac disease plus collagen deposition in lamina propria.
Tropical sprue	Similar to celiac disease.
Kwashiorkor	Similar to celiac disease.
Familial enteropathy	Flat mucosa with moderate lamina propria inflammation; EM shows microvillus inclusions.
Whipple's disease	Distension of lamina propria with foamy macrophages containing PAS-positive bacilli.
Abetalipoproteinemia	Vacuolation of epithelial cell cytoplasm due to increased intracytoplasmic lipid.
Agammaglobulinemia	Villous atrophy; increased lymphocytes in lamina propria; absent plasma cells.
Systemic mastocytosis	Mast cell infiltration of lamina propria.
Amyloidosis	Amyloid deposition in vessels, lamina propria.
Macroglobulinemia	PAS-positive material in dilated lymphatics.
Malignant lymphoma	Infiltration of lamina propria and epithelium with malignant lymphoid cells.
Intestinal lymphangiectasia	Dilated lymphatics in lamina propria.
Giardiasis	Villous atrophy, lymphocytic infiltration; trophozoites present.
Folate deficiency	Villous atrophy, crypt atrophy, megalocytosis.
Vitamin B_{12} deficiency	Similar to folate deficiency.
Radiation enteritis	Similar to folate deficiency; hyalinized mucosal vessels.
Crohn's disease	Acute and chronic inflammation; villous damage and crypt distortion; granulomas.

Abbreviations: PAS = periodic acid–Schiff (stain); EM = electron microscopy.

2. Length of crypts, which are similarly compared with the pathologist's concept of normalcy.
3. The villous:crypt ratio, which is averaged over several villi and crypts in the biopsy sample, ensuring that only completely vertically sectioned villi and crypts are used for this assessment.
4. The morphologic features of the epithelial cells lining the villi for decrease in height, presence of visible intracytoplasmic lipid, and loss of brush border.
5. The number of intraepithelial lymphocytes.
6. Presence of abnormal cells in the lamina propria, including macrophages, lymphocytes, mast cells, eosinophils, plasma cells (absence of plasma cells is a feature of agammaglobulinemia), and neoplastic cells.
7. Presence in the lamina propria of abnormal connective tissue elements, such as collagen, amyloid, and lymphangiectasia.
8. Infectious agents, such as *Giardia lamblia, Cryptosporidium, Isospora*, and cytomegalovirus.

The relative and absolute height of villi and crypts provide useful information on the pathogenesis of small-intestinal diseases. The normal structure of the intestinal mucosa, with villi 0.3–1 mm in height and a villous:crypt ratio of 3:1, represents the normal steady state of intestinal surface cell loss and replacement (Fig. 7–10). Two basic mechanisms result in villous atrophy, which is a decrease in the height of villi:

1. Crypt hyperplastic villous atrophy (see Fig. 7–10). This condition is the result of an increased rate of surface epithelial cell loss due to diseases causing epithelial damage, such as celiac disease and tropical sprue. The crypts undergo hyperplasia in an attempt to replenish the increased cell loss at the surface, resulting in an elongation of the crypt and increased mitotic activity in the crypt cells. When crypt proliferation cannot compensate for the cell loss, the villi become shortened. These biopsy samples are characterized by absolute shortening of villi, crypt elongation, and a marked decrease in the villous:crypt ratio. In extreme cases, the surface is flat without villi, and the villous:crypt ratio is 0:1.

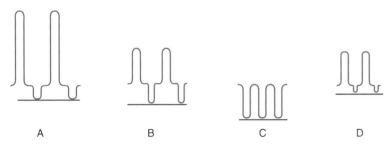

Figure 7–10. Diagram of villous atrophy. A: Normal small intestine. The villi are 3 to 5 times the length of the crypts (ie, villous:crypt ratio of 3–5:1). B: Partial villous atrophy (crypt hyperplastic type). The villi are shorter than normal and the crypts are slightly elongated, resulting in a villous:crypt ratio of 2:1. C: Total villous atrophy (crypt hyperplastic type), producing a flat surface without villi and elongated hyperplastic crypts. The villous:crypt ratio is 0:1. D: Partial villous atrophy (crypt atrophic type). Both villi and crypts are shorter than normal due to atrophy. The villous:crypt ratio is normal. Note that the interphase of the villi and crypts remains the same in the different sections of mucosa shown.

2. Crypt atrophic villous atrophy (see Fig. 7–10). This condition is the result of a failure of the crypt germinative epithelium to replenish normal surface epithelial cell loss. The crypts are shorter than normal and do not show normal mitotic activity. The villi show a decrease in the absolute height, but the villous:crypt ratio is usually maintained within normal limits. This pattern is seen in patients who have impairment of cell replication in the small intestine, as after radiation treatment or in folate and vitamin B_{12} deficiency.

DISEASES ASSOCIATED WITH MALABSORPTION

Celiac Disease

Celiac disease is the most common cause of malabsorption syndrome. It has been known by many other names: celiac sprue, nontropical sprue, gluten-sensitive enteropathy, gluten-induced enteropathy. Celiac disease is caused by small-intestinal epithelial cell damage by gluten. Although gluten is a wheat protein, it is also present in a variety of other cereal grains, including rye, barley, and oats.

Epidemiology

Celiac disease has a worldwide distribution, but is rare among African-Americans and in Japan.[5] Exact incidence and prevalence rates are difficult to establish because of a significant number of asymptomatic cases. The disease has a high (1 in 400 to 1 in 2000 population) prevalence in Northern Europe and the British Isles. In the United States, celiac disease affects 1 in 3000 to 1 in 10,000 people. Females are affected twice as commonly as males.

Celiac disease has its highest incidence in the first 3 years of life when cereals are introduced into the diet. A second incidence peak is seen in adults 20–40 years old; it is not unusual, however, for the disease to be first diagnosed in patients older than 60 years old.

Etiology

Celiac disease is caused by the gliadin fraction of gluten in genetically susceptible individuals. Genetic susceptibility is strongly related to the presence of human leukocyte antigens (HLA)-B8 and HLA-Dw 3, which are present in 80–90% of North European patients with celiac disease compared with 25% in the general population. The HLA associations with celiac disease may be different in other populations.[6] These HLA phenotypes have no value as diagnostic tests because of low sensitivity and specificity.

Celiac disease has a familial tendency, but there is no defined inheritance pattern. The incidence of celiac disease in first-degree family members of patients is probably less than 5%.[7] The presence of the specific celiac disease-associated HLA phenotypes in relatives does not increase the likelihood that they will have celiac disease.[6]

The HLA complex is linked to immune response genes that

govern the production of antigliadin antibodies. Antigliadin antibodies of IgA or IgG classes are present in the serum in most patients with active celiac disease. Serum antigliadin antibody levels decrease when patients are placed on a gluten-free diet.

IgA antigliadin antibody secreted by intestinal plasma cells is believed to be involved in the pathogenesis of celiac disease. One suggested mechanism is the binding of secretory Iga to gliadin at the surface of the mucosal epithelial cell, resulting in an antibody-dependent cell-mediated cytotoxic reaction against the mucosal epithelial cell.[8] Evidence for such a mechanism is provided by the increased numbers of IgA-producing plasma cells in the lamina propria in active disease,[9] the presence of increased local production of antigliadin antibody in active disease,[10] and the increased numbers of CD8+ suppressor T cells in the lamina propria and epithelium.[11]

Infection with adenovirus serotype 12 has been suggested as an etiologic factor in celiac disease.[5] Untreated celiac disease patients have a much higher incidence of prior infection with this virus than normal controls. Adenovirus type 12 contains an amino acid sequence in its protein that is identical to a part of the gliadin molecule; this provides a basis whereby the virus plays a role in the pathogenesis of celiac disease.

Pathologic Features

Although the entire small-intestinal mucosa is equally susceptible to damage by gliadin, the distal intestine is usually less affected because the toxic protein molecules are largely digested in the proximal intestine. In most patients, pathologic changes are restricted to the duodenum and proximal jejunum, with the distal small intestine being affected only in patients with severe disease.

At endoscopy, severe celiac disease can be suspected because of a loss in the normal mucosal folds of the duodenum. The absence of villi can also be confirmed with a hand lens or dissecting microscope, but these are rarely used. Histologic examination of the biopsy specimen shows a crypt hyperplastic-type of villous atrophy. During the active disease, the villi show total atrophy, resulting in a flat surface associated with greatly elongated crypts (Fig. 7–11). The surface-lining epithelial cells show evidence of damage characterized by decreased height from columnar to cuboidal cells, loss of normal basal nuclear polarity, cytoplasmic basophilia, and disappearance of the brush border (Fig. 7–12A, B). The surface epithelium and crypts are also infiltrated with increased numbers of lymphocytes relative to the number of epithelial cells (Fig. 7–12) (normally the intraepithelial lymphocyte:epithelial cell ratio is 1:10; in celiac disease, intraepithelial lymphocytes may equal or exceed the number of epithelial cells). The lamina propria shows an increase in lymphocytes, plasma cells, eosinophils, and mast cells (see Fig. 7–12A). Neutrophils are either absent or very scarce. The presence of numerous neutrophils in a flat mucosa should make the pathologist consider infectious diseases and bacterial overgrowth. Increased numbers of enterochromaffin cells have also been reported.[12]

The histologic changes of celiac disease are not specific;

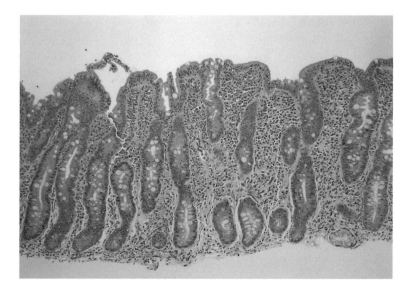

Figure 7–11. Distal duodenal biopsy specimen in celiac disease, showing flat mucosa with elongated crypts (crypt hyperplastic villous atrophy) typical of celiac disease.

they can also be seen in tropical sprue and collagenous sprue. Increased serum levels of antigliadin antibodies in conjunction with the typical histologic features, however, permit a confident diagnosis to be made. Final confirmation of the diagnosis is a therapeutic test of strict gluten withdrawal from the diet. Within a few days, the surface epithelial changes reverse, with columnar cells with basal nuclei and brush borders returning to normal, and the number of intraepithelial lymphocytes decreasing. Regeneration of normal villous height and regression of crypt hyperplasia and the lamina propria cellular infiltrate occurs over the next few months. In many patients, the mucosa does not return to complete normalcy even years after a gluten-free diet and reversal of symptoms.

Two other categories of patient present specific diagnostic problems:

1. Patients with a prior diagnosis of celiac disease who have been asymptomatic for many years, have a negative serum antigliadin antibody test, and now doubt the original diagnosis and question the need for a strict gluten-free diet. These individuals frequently have no abnormality on a baseline small-intestinal biopsy. The problem is most easily solved by examining the original small-bowel biopsy specimen. If this is not available, the diagnosis of celiac disease is best confirmed by a gluten challenge with repeat biopsy. The occurrence of symptoms of malabsorption or histologic features of surface epithelial damage and increase in intraepithelial lymphocytes confirms the diagnosis of celiac disease in these patients (Fig. 7–13). An increase in serum antigliadin antibody also occurs with gluten challenge.

2. Patients with a prior diagnosis of celiac disease who develop mild symptoms and the question of treatment failure arises. Many of these patients have been lax with their diet. Serology is frequently positive and small-intestinal biopsies show lesser degrees of villous atrophy, epithelial injury, and in-

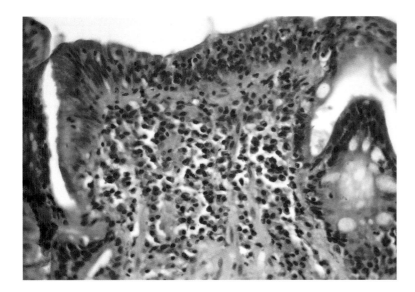

A

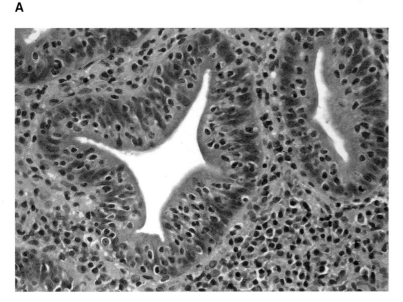

C

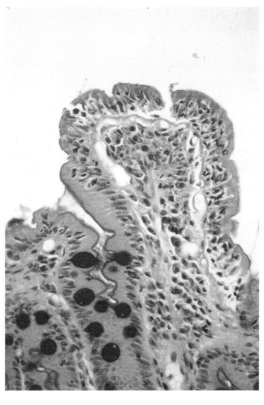

B

Figure 7–12. A: Surface epithelium in celiac disease, showing marked increase in intraepithelial lymphocytes associated with cell damage. The lamina propria also contains increased numbers of lymphocytes and plasma cells. B: Celiac disease, lesser degree of involvement in small-intestinal biopsy, stained with PAS. The short villus shows a normal brush border on the left, but the right side shows epithelial damage, loss of the brush border, and increased intraepithelial lymphocytes. C: Mucosa in celiac disease, showing infiltration of crypts by greatly increased numbers of lymphocytes, associated with lamina propria chronic inflammation.

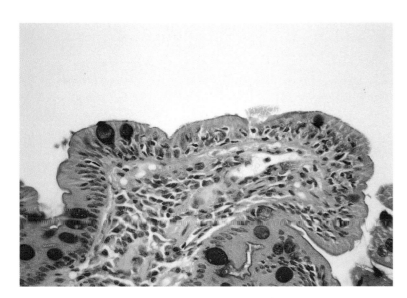

Figure 7–13. Small-intestinal biopsy in patient in remission after gluten challenge, showing early changes of damage characterized by focal loss of brush border, epithelial cell damage, and intraepithelial lymphocytic infiltration.

traepithelial lymphocytes than occur in untreated celiac disease. If strict gluten withdrawal does not lead to remission, the possibility of a complication such as a malignant neoplasm or ulcerative jejunoileitis (see below) should be considered. Rarely, refractory celiac disease needs treatment with corticosteroids or immunosuppressive agents. Patients who are refractory to all treatments need lifetime total parenteral nutrition.

Other Diagnostic Tests

Radiologic studies (barium follow through) are not specific. Changes are seen only in severe cases and consist of dilatation of the small intestine, loss of normal mucosal fold pattern, segmentation of the barium column, and prolonged transit time. A normal barium study does not exclude celiac disease.

Serologic tests are useful in diagnosis and monitoring response to and compliance with a gluten-free diet. Serum antigliadin antibodies of IgA and IgG types can be assayed by enzyme-linked immunosorbent assay (ELISA) and radioimmunoassay. Elevated levels are present in more than 90% of patients with active disease; levels decrease with treatment. Elevation of serum antigliadin antibody is not specific for celiac disease; it can occur in patients with other small-intestinal diseases such as Crohn's disease.[13] Other antibodies are also present in celiac disease; these include anti-reticulin antibody, which has a high specificity but low sensitivity, and IgA antiendomysial antibody, which has 100% specificity and 74% sensitivity and has been suggested as a definitive diagnostic test that obviates the need for small-bowel biopsy.[14] IgA antiendomysial antibody has also been recommended for screening populations at high risk for celiac disease such as those with Down syndrome, first-degree relatives of patients, and insulin-dependent diabetics.[15]

Diseases Associated with Celiac Disease

Dermatitis Herpetiformis. The majority of patients with dermatitis herpetiformis, which is a bullous dermatitis associated with IgA deposition at the dermoepidermal junction, have an enteropathy with features similar to celiac disease.[16] The mucosal changes are often patchy and not as severe as in untreated celiac disease, and most patients do not have overt malabsorption. Like celiac disease dermatitis herpetiformis has a high association with HLA-B8 and HLA-Dw3. Both the skin lesions and jejunal mucosal abnormalities respond to a gluten-free diet, but the skin lesion improvement is slow and is not seen in all patients. Only a minority of patients with celiac disease have dermatitis herpetiformis.

Other Diseases. Celiac disease is associated with insulin-dependent diabetes mellitus, Down syndrome, autoimmune thyroid diseases, selective IgA deficiency, an arthritis resembling ankylosing spondylitis, splenic atrophy, and several autoimmune diseases.[5] Many of these diseases are associated with HLA-B8 or HLA-D3 phenotypes, but the basis of their association with celiac disease is unknown. Patients with celiac disease sometimes show lymphocytic gastritis and microscopic colitis.

Complications

Ten to 15% of patients with celiac disease develop neoplasms. Approximately half of these are enteropathy-associated malignant lymphomas of the intestine that are of T-cell derivation (see Chapter 15). Other neoplasms include adenocarcinoma of the small intestine and carcinomas of the esophagus and oropharynx.[17]

Ulcerative jejunoileitis is a serious complication of celiac disease with a high mortality rate.[18] It is characterized by multiple chronic ulcers in the small intestine. The ulcers may perforate, result in severe hemorrhage, or be associated with fibrous strictures resulting in intestinal obstruction. The etiology of ulcerative jejunoileitis is unknown, but it has been suggested that the condition is an unusual manifestation of a malignant lymphoma which is difficult to diagnose in a manner analogous to polymorphous nasal lymphomas associated with lethal midline granuloma of the nose. Patients respond poorly to a gluten-free diet; if the response to corticosteroids is also poor, surgical resection may be necessary.

Neurologic complications are a recognized but unusual complication of celiac disease. They include neuromyopathy and cerebellar, posterior column, and lateral column degenerations.[19] Their cause and relationship to celiac disease are unknown.

Collagenous Sprue

Collagenous sprue is diagnosed by the presence of abundant collagen in the lamina propria, appearing either as a thick subepithelial band or diffuse collagenosis of the lamina propria (Fig. 7–14).[20] The amount of collagen necessary for diagnosis has not been quantitated. Collagenous sprue is characterized by clinical features and mucosal histologic changes that are similar to celiac disease. Collagenous sprue is associated with a failure to respond to a gluten-free diet and a progressive course with high morbidity that is difficult to control even with corticosteroids and immunosuppressive agents.

Collagenous sprue is particularly difficult to separate from celiac disease, and it is not certain whether it is a variant of celiac disease or a completely separate entity. Small amounts of subepithelial collagen may be present in both celiac disease and tropical sprue,[21] and these patients respond normally to a gluten-free diet. It is uncertain whether collagen itself determines failure of response to gluten withdrawal. Also uncertain is the exact amount of lamina propria collagen that distinguishes collagenous sprue from celiac disease. Practically speaking, all patients with changes characteristic of celiac disease who have collagen in the lamina propria are given a trial of gluten withdrawal, and treatment is determined by their response. Accordingly, the diagnosis of collagenous sprue at this time has little practical value, except to indicate a greater than usual likelihood of treatment failure at the time of initial biopsy.

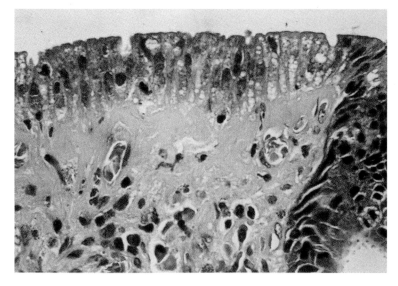

Figure 7–14. Collagenous sprue, trichrome stain, showing marked increase of the amount of collagen in the lamina propria.

Tropical Sprue

Tropical sprue is an uncommon disease of adults, which is restricted to certain tropical countries, mainly in South Asia, Philippines, West Indies, parts of Africa, the Middle East, and Central America. A history of travel to these countries is necessary for tropical sprue to be a viable diagnosis.

Tropical sprue is believed to be a chronic infectious disease caused by persistent colonization of the normally sterile proximal small intestine by toxigenic aerobic coliform bacteria, such as *Klebsiella, Escherichia,* and *Enterobacter* species.[22] No single infectious agent has been implicated, and the reason for bacterial colonization of the proximal small intestine in tropical sprue is unknown.

Patients with tropical sprue present with malabsorption syndrome and have a tendency to develop megaloblastic anemia due to combined deficiency of folic acid and vitamin B_{12}.

The pathologic changes involve the entire small intestine, but occur maximally in the jejunum. The changes are those of a crypt hyperplastic villous atrophy. The villi are shortened (Fig. 7–15A); total villous atrophy with a flat mucosa as is seen in untreated celiac disease is evident in only 10% of patients with tropical sprue. The surface epithelium shows cuboidal transformation and intraepithelial lymphocytes, but in lesser degree than in untreated celiac disease (Fig. 7–15B). The number of chronic inflammatory cells in the lamina propria is increased. The histologic features are indistinguishable from those for celiac disease, although, in general, the severity of the changes are less in tropical sprue.

Staining of frozen sections of biopsy samples for lipid with oil red O has been reported to show specific changes in tropical sprue that permit its distinction from celiac disease.[23] In tropical sprue, lipid droplets accumulate in the lamina propria immediately beneath the surface epithelium. In celiac disease, lipid droplets accumulate in the cytoplasm of the enterocyte. Because this test requires that biopsy tissue be submitted in the fresh state to permit frozen sections, oil red O staining is precluded in most small centers.

The nonspecific nature of the histologic findings and the absence of a specific diagnostic test makes tropical sprue a diagnosis of exclusion. Celiac disease should be excluded by serologic testing for antigliadin and IgA anti-endomysial antibodies. Specific infectious agents such as *Giardia lamblia,* which can also cause partial villous atrophy, should be excluded. The final test is the response to long-term antibiotic therapy, usually combined with folic acid and vitamin B_{12}. Reversal of gastrointestinal symptoms occurs in 1–2 weeks; mucosal abnormalities take several months to resolve.

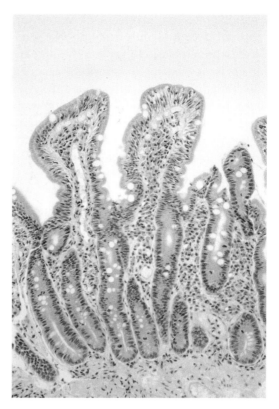

A

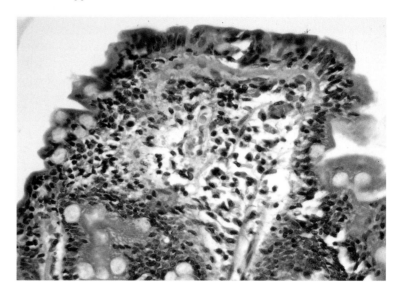

B

Figure 7–15. A: Partial villous atrophy with marked crypt hyperplasia (villous:crypt ratio is approximately 1:1). There is no obvious surface epithelial damage and only a minimal increase in intraepithelial lymphocytes. This patient was from the West Indies and was treated for tropical sprue with good clinical response. B: Tropical sprue, showing a shortened villus with patchy surface epithelial damage and increased intraepithelial lymphocytes.

Whipple's Disease

Whipple's disease is a chronic multisystem disease resulting from infection with *Tropheryma whippelii,* a rod-shaped bacterium that has not yet been cultured. The diagnosis can be established by detecting the presence of *T. whippelii* DNA in affected tissues using the polymerase chain reaction (PCR).[24]

Whipple's disease is uncommon, with only a few cases being reported each year in the world. There is a striking racial predominance in white people, and males are affected three times as frequently as females. The disease occurs in adults, being very rare below age 20 years; the median age at diagnosis is 50 years.[25]

Whipple's disease manifests primarily in the intestine and

mesenteric lymph nodes, but involvement of many other organs can occur without detectable intestinal disease. Clinical manifestations are extremely varied (Table 7–3), and considerable clinical acumen is needed for diagnosis in cases that do not have intestinal manifestations. Intestinal involvement manifests as weight loss, diarrhea, and fever. Steatorrhea is present in over 90% of cases with intestinal involvement, and gastrointestinal bleeding, both occult and gross, may occur. Mesenteric lymphadenopathy is detectable radiologically and may sometimes produce a palpable mass. Common extraintestinal clinical manifestations are arthralgia affecting large joints; pleural and pericardial effusion; lymphadenopathy; and central nervous system abnormalities, including dementia, hypothalamic dysfunction, ophthalmoplegia, and a rare but specific disorder called oculomasticatory myorhythmia.

When the diagnosis of Whipple's disease is suspected, the test of choice is a distal duodenal biopsy, which is the site of most frequent involvement. The entire small intestine can be involved, but the stomach and colon are usually spared. At endoscopy, the duodenal mucosa shows thickened mucosal folds that demonstrates a diffuse, white, granular covering or 1–2 mm yellow-white plaques. Biopsy specimens should be taken from areas of discoloration. If the endoscopy shows no gross abnormality, which is the rule in mild disease, five or six jumbo biopsy samples should be taken because the mucosal lesion is patchy in the early stages.

Histologic examination shows villi that are either normal or club-shaped owing to distension of the lamina propria, with the typical foamy macrophages (Fig. 7–16). PAS stain shows numerous PAS-positive granular inclusions distending the cytoplasm of the macrophages as well as lying free in the lamina propria (Fig. 7–17). The macrophages and PAS-positive bacilli

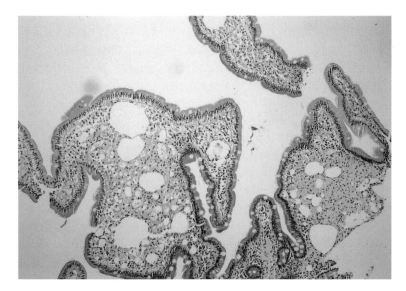

A

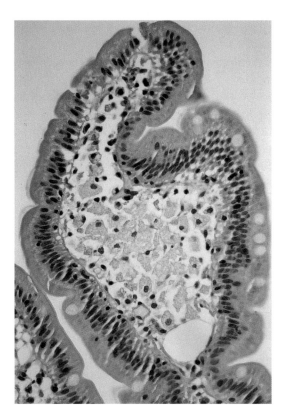

B

Figure 7–16. A: Whipple's disease, small-intestine biopsy. The villi are distended with macrophages. B: Villus in Whipple's disease showing distention of the lamina propria with macrophages characterized by abundant eosinophilic cytoplasm.

are most prominent at the apices of the villi, but not uncommonly involve the entire mucosa and rarely extend into the submucosa (Fig. 7–18). Involved mesenteric lymph nodes are enlarged and contain numerous macrophages. Electron microscopy, which shows rod-like bacilli within the macrophages, is not essential for diagnosis (Fig. 7–19).

Rarely, Whipple's disease is encountered in biopsies of extraintestinal organs in patients not suspected of having Whipple's disease. We recently encountered a case presenting as a

TABLE 7–3. ORGAN INVOLVEMENT AND CLINICAL MANIFESTATIONS OF WHIPPLE'S DISEASE

Site of Involvement	Clinical Manifestations
General symptoms	Weight loss, anemia; fever of unknown origin.
Intestine	Involves duodenum, jejunum and ileum; abdominal pain, diarrhea, steatorrhea.
Lymph nodes	Enlarged; mesenteric involvement maximal; generalized adenopathy.
Heart	Adhesive pericarditis; vegetative endocarditis and cardiac valve deformity; myocarditis; cardiac failure is rare.
Central nervous system	Cortical lesions with dementia, personality disorders, seizures; hypothalamic involvement with sleep and eating disorders; cerebellar ataxia; ophthalmoplegia; oculomasticatory myorhythmia; myoclonus; meningitis.
Eye	Uveitis, vitritis, retinitis, retrobulbar neuritis.
Skeletal system	Arthritis affecting large joints; sacroiliitis.
Lungs	Chest pain, chronic cough; focal and diffuse pulmonary infiltrates; pleural effusion.
Skin	Increased pigmentation.

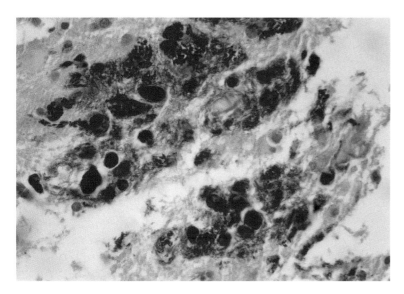

Figure 7–17. Whipple's disease, PAS stain, showing strong cytoplasmic positivity of macrophages.

brain mass lesion, which underwent stereotactic brain biopsy (Fig. 7–20).

The best method of confirming the diagnosis of Whipple's disease is by demonstrating *T. whippelii* DNA in mucosal biopsy samples using PCR.[24] PCR is positive even in mucosal areas that are negative histologically and represents a highly sensitive diagnostic technique for Whipple's disease. PCR testing of cerebrospinal fluid and brain biopsy material is extremely sensitive in detecting Whipple's disease of the central nervous system, even in patients without neurologic symptoms.[26] PCR testing of cerebrospinal fluid has been recommended in all patients with intestinal Whipple's disease as a staging method, because neurologic relapse is a common cause of treatment failure in Whipple's disease.[26]

Occasionally, involved tissues contain sarcoid-like, noncaseating, epithelioid cell granulomas. Their prominence in the mesenteric lymph nodes can cause confusion because they are PAS-negative.[27] The cause of these granulomas is unknown.

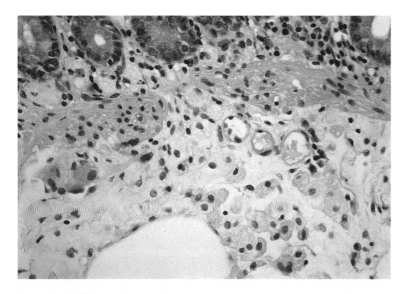

Figure 7–18. Whipple's disease, small intestine, showing submucosal macrophages with pale cytoplasm and small nuclei. Note the nest of ganglion cells.

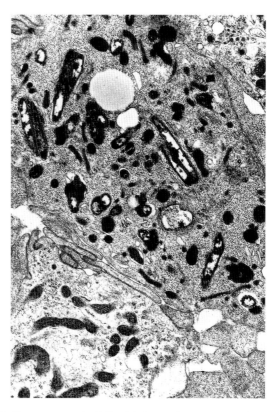

Figure 7–19. Electron micrograph of Whipple's disease, showing numerous bacteria in the cytoplasm.

Their presence may cause considerable diagnostic confusion, however, unless Whipple's disease is recognized as a cause of sarcoid-like granulomas.

Whipple's disease is treated with long-term antibiotic therapy; a 1-year course of trimethoprim-sulfamethoxazole is commonly used. The clinical response to treatment is usually dramatic. The intestinal pathology reverses slowly with progressively decreasing numbers of PAS-positive macrophages. A few macrophages remain after completion of treatment.[28] A significant number of patients who initially respond to antibiotic therapy have late relapses, most commonly in the central nervous system (see Fig. 7–20). The probability of treatment failure can be predicted by testing posttreatment biopsy samples using PCR; patients whose tissues become PCR-negative have a low risk of relapse, but those whose PCR remains positive after completion of antibiotic treatment are at risk to develop relapses.[24] PCR testing is therefore a powerful tool for the diagnosis and monitoring of treatment of patients with Whipple's disease.

Intestinal Lymphangiectasia

Intestinal lymphangiectasia is a condition characterized by obstruction of the lymphatic drainage of the small intestine. Two forms of disease are recognized:

1. Primary intestinal lymphangiectasia, which is an inherited disorder of lymphatics, occurs in children.[29] Most patients have disease limited to intestinal lymphatics; rarely, lym-

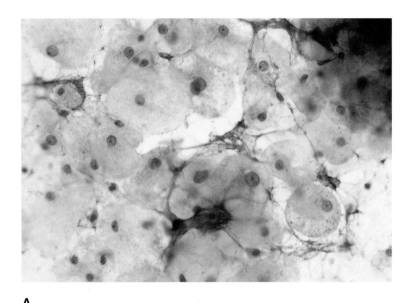

A

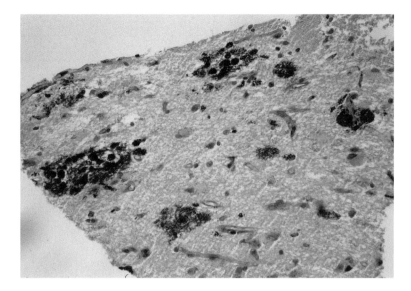

B

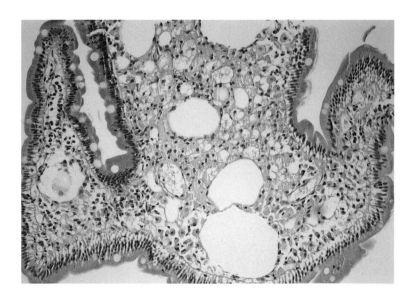

C

Figure 7–20. Whipple's disease of the brain. A: Smear from a stereotactic brain biopsy specimen showing numerous foamy macrophages. This appearance is not diagnostic of Whipple's disease; foamy macrophages also occur in infarcts, necrotizing inflammation, and demyelinating lesions. B: Stereotactic brain biopsy showing multiple small collections of PAS-positive macrophages in cerebral white matter. Strong PAS positivity such as this is highly suggestive of Whipple's disease. C: Electron micrograph of brain biopsy (shown in part B) showing numerous bacteria in the cytoplasm of macrophages, diagnostic of Whipple's disease.

phatic drainage of the extremities may also be defective (Milroy's disease).[30] Primary intestinal lymphangiectasia may also be associated with yellow nails[31] and with Hennekam's syndrome, in which associated peripheral lymphedema, facial anomalies, and mental retardation occur.[32]

2. Secondary intestinal lymphanciectasia is an acquired condition usually seen in adults in which an underlying disease causes obstruction of the intestinal lymphatics. Diseases reported to cause secondary intestinal lymphangiectasia are Crohn's disease, malignant neoplasms extensively involving the mesentery and retroperitoneum, mesenteric and retroperitoneal fibrosis, tuberculosis, sarcoidosis, abdominal radiation, Behçet's disease, constrictive pericarditis, and Whipple's disease (Fig. 7–21).

Histologic examination of biopsy samples shows dilated lacteals in the villi, lamina propria, and submucosa in both forms of intestinal lymphangiectasia (Fig. 7–22). When exten-

Figure 7–21. Whipple's disease, showing dilated lymphatics in the lamina propria (secondary lymphangiectasia).

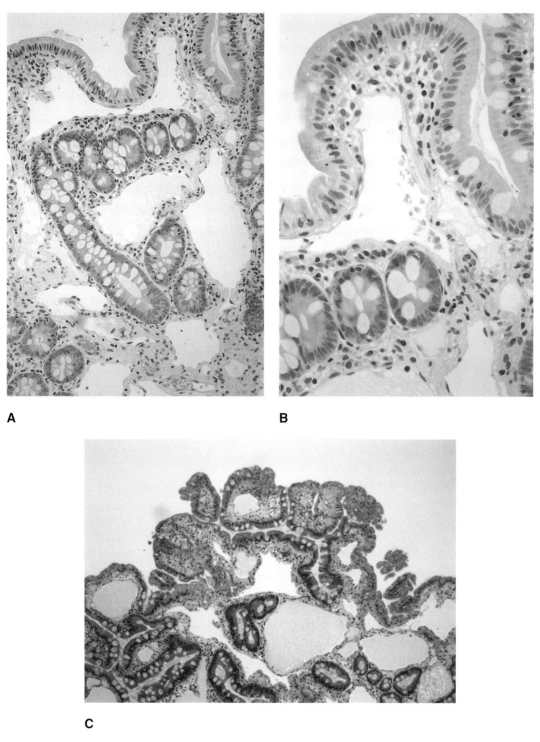

Figure 7–22. A: Intestinal lymphangiectasia, small-bowel biopsy specimen, showing marked dilatation of lymphatics in the mucosa. B: Higher micrograph power of part A, showing dilated lymphatic in villus. C: Duodenal biopsy with dilated lacteals in the villi. This was an incidental finding in a patient without evidence of malabsorption. This patient had gastric carcinoma. Altered lymphatic flow with secondary lymphangiectasia is a possibility.

sive, these dilated lacteals result in a white discoloration of the villi or the presence of multiple white spots on the mucosa. Radiologic studies may also reveal lymphatic dilatation in the serosa and mesentery; rarely these extraintestinal lymphatics rupture into the peritoneal cavity and cause chylous ascites. The lymphangiectasia is often patchy, and multiple specimens are often necessary for diagnosis. In some cases, the histologic features are subtle, with very few dilated lacteals being present. The histologic features of primary and secondary lymphangiec-

tasia are indistinguishable by biopsy. Use of clinical data (age, family history, peripheral lymphedema) and radiologic features (identification of a cause of lymphatic obstruction on computed tomography [CT] scan) are necessary for the differential diagnosis. When the cause of lymphatic obstruction is localized, secondary lymphangiectasia may affect only a segment of the bowel. Primary lymphantgiectasia, although its changes can be patchy, involves the entire small intestine without a segmental distribution.

Intestinal lymphangiectasia of all causes, if severe enough, produces the following clinical effects:

1. Obstruction of the lymphatics causes impairment of chylomicron transport, resulting in malabsorption of fat and fat-soluble vitamins. Chylomicrons accumulate in the dilated lymphatics and lamina propria. Despite malabsorption, gastrointestinal symptoms are not common.
2. Recirculation of intestinal lymphocytes into the peripheral circulation is impaired, resulting in lymphopenia, particularly of the T lymphocytes. Despite lymphopenia, opportunistic infections are not common.
3. The dilated lymphatics in the villi, which are under increased pressure, leak lymph containing chylomicrons, protein, and lymphocytes into the intestinal lumen, probably through small lymph-enteric fistulas. This results in protein-losing enteropathy with peripheral edema and hypoalbuminemia, which are the common clinical manifestations in most patients with intestinal lymphangiectasia.

The biopsy diagnosis of intestinal lymphangiectasia must be made with caution. Ideally, the diagnosis must be made in a patient who has some of the background clinical features of intestinal lymphangiectasia. In this situation, even a rare dilated lacteal is of significance. In the absence of suggestive clinical features, the finding of a few dilated lymphatics in a duodenal biopsy should be reported, but not interpreted as being diagnostic of intestinal lymphangiectasia (Fig. 7–22). The diagnosis should be made if dilated lymphatics occur in several adjacent villi or if the lymphatic dilatation involves the subvillous lamina propria and submucosa (Fig. 7–23).

In a single biopsy specimen that shows massively dilated lymphatics involving the mucosa and submucosa, the possibility of a lymphangioma should also be considered. Lymphangiomas are focal lesions recognized at endoscopy as distinctly circumscribed, small, white plaques or nodules. More rarely, they form large-mass lesions recognized during radiology.[33] When the history of a focal lesion is available, diagnosis is easy. In cases when severe lymphangiectasia is present and there is no history of a focal lesion, the best way to differentiate intestinal lymphangiectasia from a lymphangioma is by examining a second biopsy specimen some distance from the first. The specimen will be normal in a lymphangioma and usually show at least some lymphatic dilatation in lymphangiectasia. In cases of persisting doubt, it is necessary to test for protein-losing enteropathy by gastrointestinal clearance of α_1-antitrypsin.[34]

Treatment of intestinal lymphangiectasia is directed at the cause of lymphatic obstruction in secondary cases. Primary lymphangiectasia and secondary lymphangiectasia in which the cause cannot be treated benefit from restricting long-chain triglycerides from the diet and substituting short-and medium-chain triglycerides, which are absorbed directly into the portal system without incorporation into chylomicrons in the intestinal cell. This reduces intestinal protein loss and causes a rise in the serum albumin level.[35]

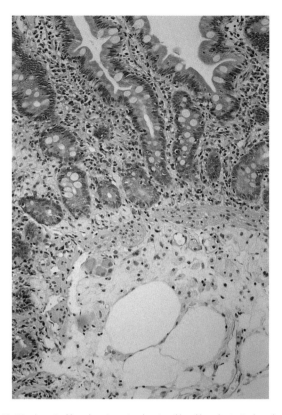

Figure 7–23. Intestinal lymphangiectasia, showing dilated lymphatics in the submucosa.

Abetalipoproteinemia

Abetalipoproteinemia is an autosomal-recessive inherited disease caused by an inability of the intestinal cell to secrete apolipoprotein B (Apo B). The failure to secrete apo B is believed to be due to a mutation involving the microsomal triglyceride transfer protein (MTP) gene.[36] Absence of MTP results in a failure of synthesis of Apo B-containing triglycerides in the intestinal cell. This causes the retention of triglycerides in the intestinal mucosal cell, leading to fat malabsorption and steatorrhea. Onset of disease is in infancy. Small-intestinal biopsy done in the fasting state (at least 6 h after the previous meal) shows the mucosal cells at the apical part of the villi to be clear and finely vacuolated due to its content of fat (Fig. 7–24); frozen section and staining with oil red O is necessary to demonstrate the intracytoplasmic lipid. In infants, absorbed fat is normally present in the cells of the villi for up to 6 h after a milk feed; care is needed to time the biopsy appropriately.

Abetalipoproteinemia is characterized by steatorrhea, acanthocytosis of peripheral blood erythrocytes, mental retardation, retinitis pigmentosa, and ataxia. Plasma Apo B, cholesterol, and triglyceride levels are very low. A less severe variant of the disease, known as familial hypobetalipoproteinemia, is believed to result from a different mutation involving the gene responsible for synthesis of the Apo B molecule itself.[37] These patients are either asymptomatic or present in later life with steatorrhea; plasma Apo B, cholesterol, and triglyceride levels are only slightly decreased. Mucosal biopsy specimens may show the typical fatty change in the mucosal cells.

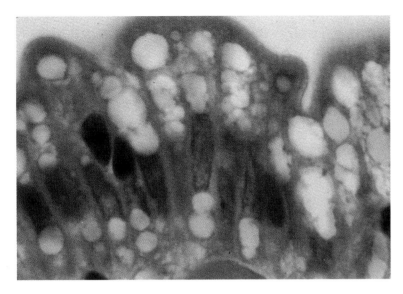

Figure 7–24. Small-intestinal mucosa in abetalipoproteinemia, showing vacuolation of cytoplasm of surface epithelial cells due to lipid accumulation.

Short-Bowel Syndrome

Short-bowel syndrome results from extensive resection of the small intestine, usually as treatment for life-threatening conditions, such as neonatal necrotizing enterocolitis, intestinal infarction secondary to ischemia, and intractable Crohn's disease. Jejunoileal or jejunocolic fistulas of any cause that result in bypassing much of the small intestine have a similar effect.

The total amount of small intestine necessary for normal function depends on which parts remain. When the proximal duodenum, distal ileum, and ileocecal valve are retained, up to 50% of the small-intestinal length can be lost without functional impairment. When the distal ileum and ileocecal valve are removed, however, malabsorption occurs with as little as 30% reduction in small-intestinal length. This information is useful to the pathologist who may rarely be consulted during emergent small-intestinal resections.

The management of short-bowel syndrome involves highly complex dietary adjustments. Total parenteral nutrition is necessary in many patients.

Bacterial Overgrowth

The proximal small intestine is normally bacteriologically sterile. The major factor that prevents bacterial colonization is normal peristalsis, and any cause of stasis will predispose to bacterial overgrowth (see Table 7–1). The bacteria involved are similar to the normal colonic flora, including anaerobes. The bacteria cause deconjugation of bile salts, resulting in failure of micelle formation and fat absorption. In most patients, the intestinal mucosa shows no morphologic abnormality. Rarely, localized bacterial invasion occurs, leading to foci of inflammation and villous atrophy that may resemble celiac disease.

One disease associated with bacterial overgrowth that may be encountered by the surgical pathologist is diverticular disease of the small bowel, usually affecting the duodenum and jejunum (Fig. 7–25). This is a surgically treatable cause of malabsorption; resection of the affected bowel leads to cure.

Radiation Enteritis

Abdominal radiation for malignancy frequently causes acute mucosal damage during therapy, characterized by decreased crypt cell regeneration, resulting in a crypt atrophic type of partial villous atrophy. Radiation doses greater than 60 Gy are usually needed to cause enteritis; simultaneous chemotherapy increases the risk. This causes diarrhea and malabsorption, which is transient, disappearing within 2 weeks of cessation of radiation. The mucosal abnormalities also resolve rapidly.

In a minority of patients who have received abdominal radiation, diarrhea and malabsorption persist after cessation of radiation or develop after several years.[38] Some of these patients have persistent mucosal changes of radiation with villous atro-

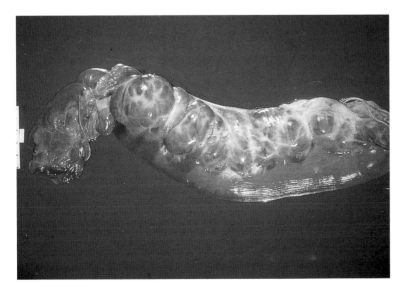

Figure 7–25. Jejunal diverticulosis, showing multiple diverticula in the resected segment of the jejunum. Patient presented with features of malabsorption due to bacterial overgrowth.

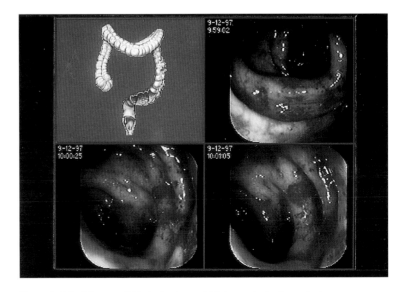

Figure 7–26. Colonic amyloidosis showing multiple hemorrhagic plaques in the mucosa at endoscopy. (Courtesy of Raman Patel, MD, Gastroenterologist, Lancaster, CA).

phy. In some patients other reasons for malabsorption exist, including radiation-induced strictures resulting in bacterial overgrowth and radiation-induced mesenteric fibrosis causing secondary intestinal lymphangiectasia. Chronic diarrhea following radiation is often refractory to treatment.

Common Variable Immunodeficiency

A malabsorptive state often develops in patients with common variable immunodeficiency, a heterogeneous group of diseases characterized by hypogammaglobulinemia and recurrent infections.[39] In most cases, diarrhea and malabsorption have an infectious basis. Giardiasis is the most common infection in these patients, but cryptosporidiosis and *Isospora belli* infection also occur (see Chapter 17). Bacterial overgrowth also occurs in

these patients, and the resulting bile salt deconjugation contributes to malabsorption.

Mucosal biopsies in patients with common variable immunodeficiency may be normal or show severe abnormality. Two types of mucosal abnormality are seen:

1. The mucosa may show varying degrees of villous atrophy, usually short of total villous atrophy. The number of lymphocytes in the lamina propria increases but plasma cell numbers are usually less than normal. When plasma cells are present, they are usually IgG and IgM secreting; IgA-producing plasma cells are consistently decreased.[40] These mucosal changes usually reverse when the associated infections are treated.

2. Nodular lymphoid hyperplasia occurs, which may be so pro-

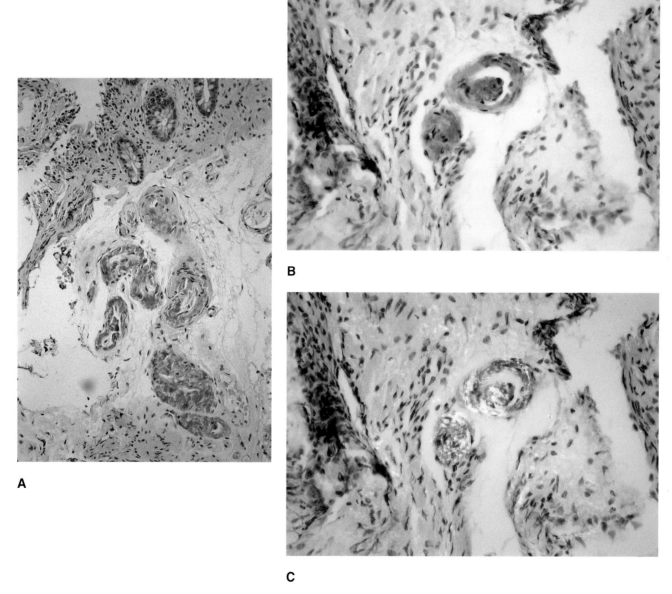

Figure 7–27. A: Amyloidosis, Congo red stain, showing positive staining of amyloid in blood vessels in the submucosa. B: Amyloidosis, Congo red stain, showing positive staining of the wall of a small submucosal blood vessel. This involvement is much more subtle than that seen in part A and would be missed if Congo red stain was not done. C: Same specimen as shown in part A, under polarized light, showing diagnostic apple green birefringence of amyloid.

nounced as to produce multiple nodules at endoscopy. The nodules are composed of hyperplastic lymphoid nodules with prominent germinal centers. The nodular lymphoid hyperplasia usually persists even after infections are treated.

In patients with known common variable immunodeficiency, the diagnosis can be confirmed when hyperplastic lymphoid nodules are found in a small-bowel biopsy. Caution must be exercised, however, when a lymphoid nodule is found in a biopsy in a patient without such a history, because this finding can be normal. The presence of many lymphoid nodules associated with a decrease in plasma cells and abnormal villous architecture permits the diagnosis of common variable immunodeficiency to be suggested on a biopsy.

Amyloidosis

Amyloidosis, a systemic disorder that commonly involves the GI tract, causes malabsorption in two rare clinical settings: (1) In familial Mediterranean fever, diffuse amyloidosis of the small intestine produces malabsorption[41]; (2) Amyloid infiltration of the muscle wall and myenteric plexus rarely causes hypomotility, resulting in bacterial overgrowth and malabsorption.[42] When found in a small-intestinal biopsy, amyloid is usually an incidental finding that may be the first indication of a plasma cell disorder in the individual. Rectal biopsy is a common method of establishing a diagnosis of amyloidosis.

Endoscopically, amyloidosis causes fine granularity, thickening of mucosal folds, and focal erosions with increased friability of the mucosa (Fig. 7–26).[43] Histologically, amyloid is most commonly deposited in the wall of small blood vessels in the mucosa and submucosa (Fig. 7–27), but can also be deposited in the mucosal lamina propria (Fig. 7–28). On routine hematoxylin and eosin (H&E) stains, amyloid appears as an acellular, homogeneous, eosinophilic material, which is difficult to distinguish from collagen. Congo red positivity with apple green birefringence establishes the diagnosis of amyloidosis (Fig. 7–27C). Immunoperoxidase staining can distinguish between AL and AA types of amyloid.

AIDS Enteropathy

Diarrhea is common in patients with acquired immunodeficiency syndrome (AIDS). Although most cases result from infections (see Chapter 17), in some patients chronic diarrhea is associated with partial villous atrophy and an absence of any infection—a condition called AIDS enteropathy.[44]

Waldenström's Macroglobulinemia

Rare patients with Waldenström's macroglobulinemia develop diarrhea and malabsorption. Small-intestinal biopsy samples from these patients show large, globular, homogeneous, eosinophilic, PAS-positive, Congo red-negative, extracellular deposits of monoclonal IgM in the lamina propria. Deposits in

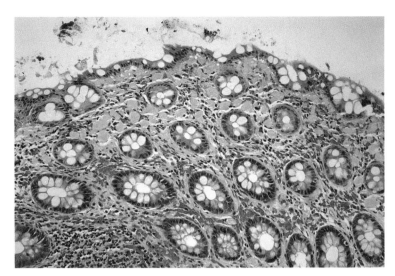

A

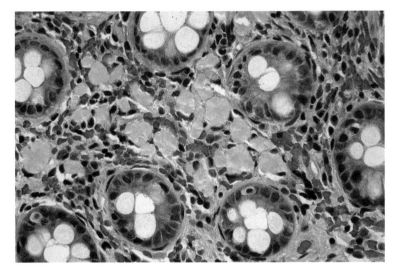

B

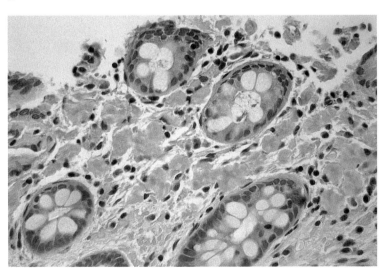

C

Figure 7–28. A: Amyloid in mucosa of rectal biopsy, showing amorphous, eosinophilic, acellular, globular deposits of amyloid under the surface epithelium. This patient had a monoclonal spike on serum immunoelectrophoresis and an increased number of plasma cells in the bone marrow. Presentation was with rectal bleeding (endoscopy shown in Fig. 7–26). B: Higher power micrograph of part A, showing globular amyloid deposits in the lamina propria. C: Congo red stain of rectal mucosa, showing positive staining. With polarized light, this showed apple green birefringence.

the villi cause them to become club-shaped; apart from these deposits, the mucosa is unremarkable. No malignant lymphoid process is evident in the mucosa. The way in which IgM becomes deposited in the mucosa is unknown. In extremely rare cases, Waldenström's macroglobulinemia is associated with intestinal lymphangiectasia; in these cases macroglobulin deposits also occur in the dilated lymphatic channels.[45]

Microvillus Inclusion Disease

Microvillus inclusion disease is a congenital disease presenting with intractable watery diarrhea within a few days of birth. The basic defect is defective assembly and differentiation of the microvilli in the brush border of the enterocyte, probably due to abnormality of cytoskeletal elements. On biopsy, the mucosa is flat with marked atrophy of villi. The surface cells lack a brush border and contain PAS-positive cytoplasmic inclusions. The diagnosis requires electron microscopy, which shows the inclusions in the enterocyte to be composed of a vacuole lined by inwardly facing brush border microvilli.[46] Treatment is ineffective, and the disease is usually fatal shortly after birth.

Congenital X-Linked Agammaglobulinemia

Children with congenital X-linked agammaglobulinemia have a marked paucity or complete absence of plasma cells in the lamina propria. The mucosa is otherwise normal, and patients do not have malabsorption.

References

1. Penna FJ, Hill ID, Kingston D, et al. Jejunal mucosal morphometry in children with and without gut symptoms and in normal adults. *J Clin Pathol.* 1981;34:386–392.
2. Owen RL. And now pathophysiology of M cells—good news and bad news from Peyer's patches. *Gastroenterology.* 1983;85:468–470.
3. Rubin CE, Haggitt RC, Levine DS. Endoscopic mucosal biopsy. *In* Yamada T, Alpers DH, Owyang C, et al (eds): *Textbook of Gastroenterology.* Philadelphia, JB Lippincott, 1991. pp. 2479–2523.
4. Greene HL, Rosensweig NS, Lufkin EG, et al. Biopsy of the small intestine with the Crosby-Kugler capsule: Experience in 3866 peroral biopsies In children and adults. *Am J Dig Dis.* 1974;19: 189–198.
5. Kagnoff MF. Celiac disease. *In* Yamada T, Alpers DH, Owyang C, et al (eds): *Textbook of Gastroenterology.* Philadelphia, JB Lippincott, 1991. pp. 1503–1520.
6. Mearin ML, Biemond I, Pena AS, et al. HLA-DR phenotypes in Spanish coeliac children: Their contribution to the understanding of the genetics of the disease. *Gut.* 1983;24: 532–537.
7. Ellis A, Evans AP, McConnell RB, et al. Liverpool coeliac family study. *In* McConnell RB (ed): *The Genetics of Coelic Disease.* Lancaster, England, MTP Press, 1981. pp. 285–296.
8. Levenson SD, Austin RK, Dietler MD, et al. Specificity of antigliadin antibody in celiac disease. *Gastroenterology.* 1985;89:1–5.
9. Scott BB, Goodall A, Stephenson P, et al. Small intestinal plasma cells in coeliac disease. *Gut.* 1984;25:41–46.
10. Ciclitira PJ, Ellis HJ, Wood GM, et al. Secretion of gliadin antibody by coeliac jejunal mucosal biopsies cultured in vitro. *Clin Exp Immunol.* 1986;64:119–121.
11. Freedman AR, Macartney JC, Nelufer JM, et al. Timing of infiltration of T lymphocytes induced by gluten into the small intestine in coeliac disease. *J Clin Pathol.* 1987;40:741–745.
12. Pietroletti R, Bishop AE, Carlei F, et al. Gut endocrine cell population in coeliac disease estimated by immunocytochemistry using a monoclonal antibody to chromogranin. *Gut.* 1986;27:838–843.
13. Weiss JB, Austin RK, Schanfield MS, et al. Gluten-sensitive enteropathy: Immunoglobulin G heavy chain (Gm) allotypes and the immune response to wheat gliadins. *J Clin Invest.* 1983;72: 96–101.
14. Valdimarsson T, Franzen L, Grodzinsky E, et al. Is small bowel biopsy necessary in adults with suspected celiac disease and IgA anti-endomysium antibodies? 100% positive predictive value for celiac disease in adults. *Dig Dis Sci.* 1996;41:83–87.
15. Talal AH, Murray JA, Goeken JA, et al. Celiac disease in an adult population with insulin dependent diabetes mellitus: Use of endomysial antibody testing. *Am J Gastroenterol.* 1997;92: 1280–1284.
16. Katz SI, Hall RP, Lawley TJ, et al. Dermatitis herpetiformis: The skin and the gut. *Ann Intern Med.* 1980;93:857–874.
17. Ferguson A, Kingstone K. Coeliac disease and malignancies. *Acta Pediatr.* 1996;412:78–81.
18. Baer A, Bayless TM, Yardley JH. Intestinal ulceration and malabsorption syndromes. *Gastroenterology.*1980;79:754–765.
19. Muller AF, Donnelly MT, Smith CM, et al. Neurological complications of celiac disease: A rare but continuing problem. *Am J Gastroenterol.* 1996;91:1430–1435.
20. Weinstein WM, Saunders DR, Tytgat GN, et al. Collagenous sprue—an unrecognized type of malabsorption. *N Engl J Med.* 1970;283:1297–1301.
21. Bossart R, Henry K, Booth CC, et al. Subepithelial collagen in intestinal malabsorption. *Gut.* 1975;16:18–22.
22. Klipstein FA, Holdeman LV, Corcino JJ, et al. Enterotoxigenic intestinal bacteria in tropical sprue. *Ann Intern Med.* 1973;79: 632–641.
23. Schenk EA, Samloff IM, Klipstein FA, et al. Morphologic characteristics of jejunal biopsies in celiac disease and in tropical sprue. *Am J Pathol.* 1965;47:765–774.
24. Ramzan NN, Fredericks DN, Relman DA, et al. Diagnosis and monitoring of Whipple's disease by polymerase chain reaction. *Ann Intern Med.* 1997;126:520–527.
25. Dobbins WO, Klipstein FA. Chronic infections of the small intestine. *In* Yamada T, Alpers DH, Owyang C, et al (eds): *Textbook of Gastroenterology.* Philadelphia, JB Lippincott, 1991. pp. 1472–1485.
26. von Herbay A, Ditton HJ, Schuhmacher F, et al. Whipple's disease: Staging and monitoring by cytology and polymerase chain reaction analysis of cerebrospinal fluid. *Gastroenterology.* 1997;113: 434–441.
27. Cho C, Linscheer WG, Hirschkorn MA, et al. Sarcoid-like granulomas as an early manifestation of Whipple's disease. *Gastroenterology.* 1984;87:941–947.
28. von Herbay A, Maiwald M, Ditton HJ, et al. Histology of intestinal Whipple's disease revisited. A study of 48 patients. *Virchows Arch.* 1996;429:335–343.
29. Waldeman TA, Steinfeld JL, Dutcher TF, et al. The role of the gastrointestinal system in "idiopathic hypoproteinemia." *Gastroenterology.* 1961;41:197–201.
30. Levine C. Primary disorders of the lymphatic vessels—a unified concept. *J Pediatr Surg.* 1989;24:233–240.

31. Duhra PM, Quigley EMM, March MN. Chylous ascites, intestinal lymphangiectasia and the "yellow nail" syndrome. *Gut.* 1985;26:1266–1269.

32. Angle B, Hersh JH. Expansion of the phenotype in Hennekam syndrome: A case with new manifestations. *Am J Med Genet.* 1997;71:211–214.

33. Davis M, Fenoglio-Preiser C, Haque AK. Cavernous lymphangioma of the duodenum. Case report and review of the literature. *Gastrointest Radiol.* 1987;12:10–12.

34. Du EZ, Wang SL, Kayden HJ, et al. Translocation of apolipoprotein B across the endoplasmic reticulum is blocked in abetalipoproteinemia. *J Lipid Res.* 1996;37:1309–1315.

35. Young SG, Hubl ST, Chappell DA, et al. Familial hypolipoproteinemia associated with a mutant species of apolipoprotein B (B46). *N Engl J Med.*1989;320:1604–1610.

36. Hill RE, Herez A, Corey ML, et al. Fecal clearance of alpha-1-antitrypsin: A reliable measure of enteric protein loss in children. *J Pediatr.* 1981;99:416–418.

37. Tift WL, Lloyd JK. Intestinal lymphangiectasia. Long term results with MCT diet. *Arch Dis Child.* 1975;50:269–276.

38. Letschert JG. The prevention of radiation-induced small bowel complications. *Eur J Cancer.* 1995;31A:1361–1365.

39. Cunningham-Rundles C. Clinical and immunologic analysis of 103 patients with common variable immunodeficiency. *J Clin Immunol.* 1989;9:22–33.

40. van den Brande P, Geboes K, Vantrappen G, et al. Intestinal nodular lymphoid hyperplasia in patients with common variable immunodeficiency: Local accumulation of B and CD8(+) lymphocytes. *J Clin Immunol.* 1988;8:296–306.

41. Ravid M, Sohar E. Intestinal malabsorption: First manifestation of amyloidosis in familial Mediterranean fever. *Gastroenterology.* 1974;66:446–449.

42. Battle W, Rubin M, Cohen S, et al. Gastrointestinal motility dysfunction in amyloidosis. *N Engl J Med.* 1979;301:24–25.

43. Tada S, Iida M, Yao T, et al. Endoscopic features in amyloidosis of the small intestine: Clinical and morphologic differences between chemical types of amyloid protein. *Gastrointest Endosc.* 1994;40:45–50.

44. Batman PA, Miller ARO, Foster SM, et al. Jejunal enteropathy associated with human immunodeficiency virus infection: Quantitative histology. *J Clin Pathol.* 1989;42:275–281.

45. Harris M, Burton IE, Scarffe JH. Macroglobulinemia and intestinal lymphangiectasia: A rare association. *J Clin Pathol.* 1983;36:30–36.

46. Cutz E, Rhoads JM, Drumm B, et al. Microvillus inclusion disease: An inherited defect of brush border assembly and differentiation. *N Engl J Med.* 1989;320:646–651.

8

PATHOLOGY OF THE SMALL INTESTINE

Yanling Ma and Parakrama Chandrasoma

▶ CHAPTER OUTLINE

CONGENITAL ABNORMALITIES

Omphalocele and Malrotation

The developing embryonic midgut that gives rise to the jejunum, ileum, and proximal colon protrudes into the embryonic yolk sac (the future umbilical cord). In later fetal life, return of the midgut into the abdominal cavity is associated with a specific counterclockwise rotation that establishes its normal positions.

Omphalocele represents a failure of part of the midgut to return to the abdomen. The infant is born with part of the small intestine, covered by a thin membrane, present at the base of the umbilical cord. This is associated with an abdominal wall defect. Failure to recognize minor forms of omphalocele may result in serious trauma to the intestine at the time of umbilical cord division. Omphalocele requires urgent surgical correction.

Malrotation results in a failure of normal development and attachment of the midgut mesentery. In Kartagener's syndrome, caused by the absence of dynein arms on the cilia (which prevents normal ciliary motility), malrotation is associated with dextrocardia, bronchiectasis, and absent paranasal sinuses. Malrotation is also associated with Down syndrome and trisomy 13 and 18.

In malrotation, the ascending colon and cecum do not become fixed in the retroperitoneum of the right abdomen; rather, they retain a mesocolon and "float" in the abdominal cavity. The cecum commonly gains secondary attachment to the liver by abnormal intraperitoneal fibrous adhesions. These hepatocecal bands may obstruct the second part of the duodenum. The mobile midgut also has a high incidence of twisting on its long, poorly attached mesentery, producing midgut volvulus.

Atresia, Stenosis, and Mucosal Webs

Intestinal atresia, stenoses, and mucosal webs result from varying degrees of failure of development and canalization of the intestine. These conditions occur in 1/5000 live births and repre-

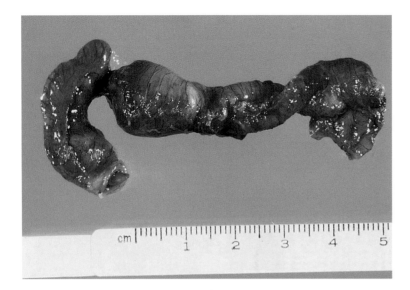

Figure 8–1. Intestinal atresia showing a focal marked narrowing of the small intestine. There was no lumen on dissection.

sent the etiology of about 30% of neonatal intestinal obstruction. The cause of atresia is believed to be intrauterine ischemia. The duodenum is the most common site of involvement, followed by the jejunum and ileum; the colon is rarely affected. In cases of atresia, there is either complete discontinuity of the intestine or the atretic segment is represented by a fibrous cord (Fig. 8–1). Stenosis is characterized by the presence of a pinpoint lumen. Rarely, atresia is associated with absence of the entire ileocecal region including the appendix.[1]

Mucosal webs represent the least severe abnormality. In development, the rapid growth of the mucosal epithelium may transiently outpace the elongation of the intestine, leading to temporary occlusion; rapid recanalization usually occurs, but may result in the presence of mucosal webs, which are frequently multiple. When small, these webs do not cause any obstruction. Rarely, webs are associated with intestinal obstruction in later life and may be encountered in resected segments of obstructed intestine. In these cases, question arises as to whether these webs are congenital or acquired; regular use of nonsteroidal antiinflammatory drugs have been associated with acquired mucosal webs. Histologic examination of webs indicates that they are composed of luminal protrusions of mucosa including muscularis mucosae. The muscularis externa does not participate in the formation of a web.

Intestinal Duplications

Duplications represent a congenital longitudinal division of the developing gut and may occur anywhere from the esophagus to the rectum. The length of duplicated intestine varies. Duplications occur most commonly in the small intestine, followed by duodenum and colon. The duplicated intestinal segment is usually closely apposed to the normal bowel and usually shares the muscularis externa. It may or may not communicate with the normal intestinal lumen. Duplications form cystic structures related to the wall of the bowel. The cysts may be round or elongated and vary in size. They are usually lined by normal mucosa of the region involved, but gastric and squamous metaplasia may occur.

Intestinal duplications are commonly found incidentally. Rarely they undergo infarction, resulting in ulceration and hemorrhage.[2] When gastric mucosa is present, peptic ulceration may occur.[3] Malignant neoplasms have been reported in duplications; these include adenocarcinoma, squamous carcinoma,[4] and carcinoid tumors.[5]

Meckel's Diverticulum

In fetal life, the intestine communicates with the yolk sac via the omphalomesenteric (vitelline) duct. This embryonic structure is usually completely absorbed. Sometimes, resorption is

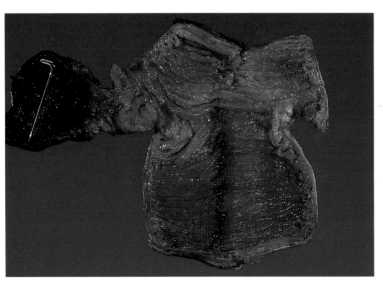

A

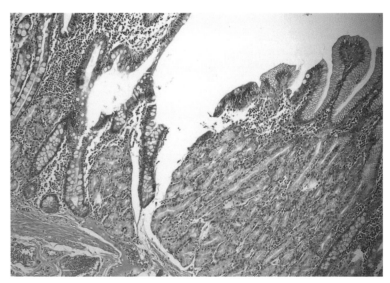

B

Figure 8–2. A: Terminal ileum with a Meckel's diverticulum showing hemorrhagic acute inflammation involving its distal end. B: Mucosal lining of a Meckel's diverticulum showing transition from ileal mucosa to heterotopic gastric mucosa.

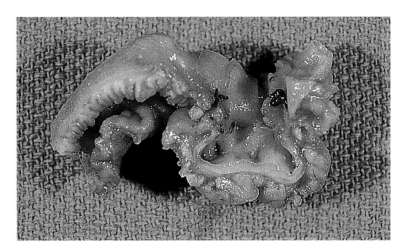

Figure 8–3. Section through the small intestine showing inversion of a Meckel's diverticulum, which forms a polypoid mass protruding into the lumen. Note the invagination of the muscularis externa into the ileal lumen.

incomplete, leading to a fibrous cord that connects the small intestine to the umbilicus, nodular remnants of the duct lined by intestinal epithelium at the umbilicus, or a Meckel's diverticulum. Meckel's diverticulum represents the failure of obliteration of the intestinal end of the omphalomesenteric duct (Fig. 8–2A). Present in 2% of the population, Meckel's diverticulum is usually located in the small intestine within 60 cm (2 ft) from the ileocecal valve, and is approximately 5 cm (2 in) long. It has a lumen that has a wide communication with the small-intestinal lumen. Meckel's diverticulum is a true congenital diverticu-

lum with all the layers of the intestine including muscularis externa; its mucosa is usually lined by ileal-type epithelium with villi; in approximately 30% of cases, heterotopic gastric mucosa or pancreatic tissue is present (Fig. 8–2B). In some cases, the mucosa resembles colonic epithelium; this most likely represents ileal mucosa with flattening of villi due to bacterial overgrowth in the diverticulum.

Meckel's diverticulum is usually asymptomatic throughout life. The risk of complications is significant, however. Complications associated with Meckel's diverticulum include:

1. Acute Meckel's diverticulitis, which clinically resembles acute appendicitis (see Fig. 8–2A). In rare cases, acute inflammation has been attributed to heterotopic pancreatic mucosa, with fat necrosis a prominent feature.[6]
2. Peptic ulceration, in cases associated with heterotopic gastric mucosa, which can be complicated by hemorrhage and perforation.
3. Perforation, due either to acute inflammation or peptic ulceration.
4. Volvulus, which occurs when a fibrous cord is present between the Meckel's diverticulum and the umbilicus as a vestigial remnant of the omphalomesenteric duct.
5. Inversion of the Meckel's diverticulum into the lumen of the small bowel, where it acts as the apex of an intussusception (Fig. 8–3).
6. Endometriosis, which can occur on the serosal aspect (Fig. 8–4).

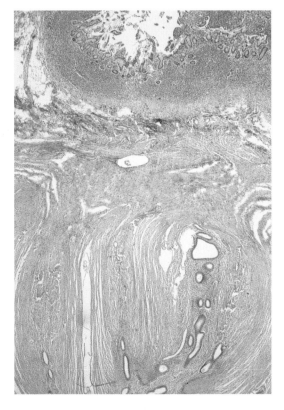

A

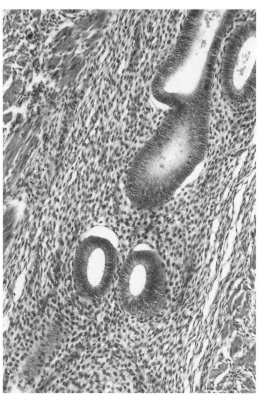

B

Figure 8–4. A: Meckel's diverticulum, showing endometriosis in the muscle wall. B: Endometriosis in the wall of a Meckel's diverticulum, showing endometrial glands and stroma.

7. Neoplasia, which is extremely rare. Carcinoid tumors are the commonest tumor in a Meckel's diverticulum,[9] arising most commonly at the tip. These have a biologic behavior similar to ileal carcinoids and should be considered malignant. Tumors as small as 5 mm have been associated with metastasis. Over 70% of carcinoid tumors in Meckel's diverticula have been metastatic at the time of detection. Adenocarcinomas[10] and gastrointestinal (GI) stromal neoplasms[11] have also arisen in Meckel's diverticula.

MOTILITY DISORDERS

Motility disorders of the intestine typically present with intestinal obstruction in the absence of any anatomic lesion ("intestinal pseudo-obstruction" or functional obstruction). These result from a failure of peristalsis due to abnormalities in neuromuscular function[12] (Table 8–1). Availability of manometric probes that can monitor motor function in the small intestine promises to provide functional insights into these diseases.

Paralytic Ileus

Paralytic ileus is the most common cause of pseudo-obstruction, occurring after abdominal surgery, abdominal trauma, and any cause of peritonitis. Peritoneal irritation evokes an autonomic reflex that suppresses peristalsis. After surgery, paralytic ileus lasts 1–3 days; function returns first in the stomach, then the small intestine, and finally in the colon. Unless controlled with nasogastric suction, curtailment of oral intake, and intravenous fluid management, the paralyzed intestine becomes dilated and distended with fluid and air. Diagnosis is made by the absence of bowel sounds; return of function is best gauged by passage of

TABLE 8–1. CAUSES OF INTESTINAL PSEUDO-OBSTRUCTION

Acute Paralytic Ileus
    Following abdominal surgery
    Acute peritonitis
Acute Colonic Pseudo-Obstruction (Ogilvie's Syndrome)
    May occur in any critically ill patient
Chronic Intestinal Pseudo-Obstruction
    Primary Disorders of Muscle
        Familial visceral myopathy
        Sporadic visceral myopathy
    Primary Disorders of Myenteric Plexus
        Familial visceral neuropathy
        Sporadic visceral neuropathy
        Hirschsprung's disease (see Chapter 10)
        Intestinal neuronal dysplasia (see Chapter 10)
    Secondary Disorders
        Autonomic neuropathy of diabetes mellitus
        Progressive systemic sclerosis
        Amyloidosis
        Hypothyroidism

flatus, which indicates complete return of colonic function. Opiates such as morphine and any drugs with anticholinergic activity aggravate ileus and should be avoided; prokinetic drugs are generally not needed in this transient condition.

Acute Colonic Pseudo-Obstruction

Acute colonic pseudo-obstruction, or Ogilvie's disease, is a rare disorder that occurs in severely ill patients, most commonly in those on respirators.[13] It complicates prolonged severe surgeries, massive infarction, septic shock, and respiratory failure. Presentation is with acute abdominal distension due to massive dilatation of the colon. Recovery from the initiating disease usually results in a return of normal colonic function. In the acute phase, massive cecal dilatation may result in ischemic necrosis of the bowel wall and a likelihood of perforation; decompression by cecostomy is indicated when the colonic diameter exceeds 6 cm. The mortality rate is as high as 30%.

Chronic Intestinal Pseudo-Obstruction

Chronic pseudo-obstruction may result from known diseases such as progressive systemic sclerosis, amyloidosis, hypothyroidism, and the autonomic neuropathy of diabetes mellitus; it may also be idiopathic. Chronic idiopathic intestinal pseudo-obstruction (CIIP) results from a variety of poorly understood and rare familial and acquired diseases involving the smooth muscle (visceral myopathy) or nerves (visceral neuropathy). It is also sometimes associated with neuromuscular dysfunction involving other viscera, such as urinary bladder, biliary tract, uterus, and fallopian tube. A viral etiology has been suggested for some of these cases of CIIP.[14]

Patients with CIIP present with symptoms of intestinal obstruction, including abdominal pain, abdominal distention, constipation, and vomiting. Constipation is more severe when there is colonic involvement. Onset of the familial syndromes usually occurs in childhood. Initially, symptoms tend to be intermittent, but become unremitting as the disease progresses; severe constipation and marked distention of the involved intestine occurs (Fig. 8–5). The hypomotility promotes bacterial overgrowth resulting in bile acid deconjugation and malabsorption in some of these patients.

The diagnosis of chronic intestinal pseudo-obstruction requires an adequately sized full-thickness bowel biopsy specimen that permits evaluation of changes in the muscle wall and myenteric plexus. Changes of visceral myopathy can be evaluated in routine hematoxylin and eosin (H&E) and trichrome stained sections. The diagnosis of visceral neuropathy requires special handling of the tissue. The myenteric plexus is best evaluated by Smith's method,[15] which involves silver impregnation stains done on thick (50 μm) sections cut in the longitudinal plane of the muscle coat. Smith's technique is rarely used except in highly specialized centers. Tissue from full-thickness specimens should also be submitted for electron microscopy; the sample should contain both muscularis externa and myenteric plexus.

The treatment of these diseases is difficult; there are few

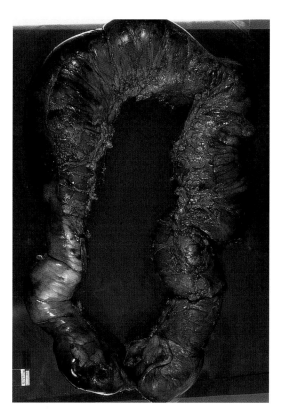

Figure 8–5. Markedly dilated colon in a patient with familial visceral myopathy presenting with chronic constipation.

effective prokinetic agents and surgery to remove the affected segment is often followed by recurrence due to the fact that these diseases can potentially involve the entire bowel.

Primary Visceral Myopathy

Visceral myopathy may be familial or sporadic. Familial visceral myopathy has also been called "hollow visceral myopathy" because of associated neuromuscular abnormalities in other viscera, such as the urinary bladder and biliary tract. Familial cases may have an autosomal-dominant or autosomal-recessive inheritance pattern; some autosomal-recessive cases have had associated involvement of the proximal GI tract with gastroparesis, jejunal diverticula, and ophthalmoplegia.[16] Familial and sporadic cases have identical clinical and morphologic features.[17] The involvement can be patchy or involve the entire GI tract.

The affected bowel is dilated (see Fig. 8–5) and commonly shows diverticula. The muscle may show gross evidence of fibrosis in severe cases, but is usually secondarily thinned out because of the luminal dilatation. Microscopically, degeneration of the smooth muscle of the muscularis externa is evident with replacement fibrosis without inflammation (Fig. 8–6A, B).[18] The degeneration appears to involve the longitudinal muscle preferentially, although this is not a constant feature. The fibrosis is best assessed with a trichrome stain (Fig. 8–6C). The most typical microscopic abnormality is the occurrence of vacuolar degeneration of affected smooth muscle fibers (Fig. 8–7A). Some cases show nuclear atypia and increased numbers of mitotic figures in the muscle cells (Fig. 8–7B).[18] Ultrastructurally, degeneration of the myofibrils in the cytoplasm is evident; in rare cases,

these have aggregated to form cytoplasmic inclusions.[19] The cytoplasmic inclusions are seen in H&E-stained sections as irregular perinuclear eosinophilic inclusions (Fig. 8–7C), or as 2–4 μm, pale, basophilic, ovoid or circular bodies in the cytoplasm (Fig. 8–7A). The inclusions stain positively with periodic acid–Schiff (PAS) stain (Fig. 8–7D), and are seen on electron microscopy to be formed by aggregation of degenerated myofibrils in the muscle cells (Fig. 8–7E).

The muscle degeneration is maximal in the muscularis externa, but changes also occur in the muscle of the muscularis mucosae, vascular media, and other organs such as urinary bladder. Changes in the muscularis mucosae, which include vacuolar degeneration, nuclear atypia, and inclusions,[18,19] are important because they can potentially be seen in endoscopic biopsies. The changes in the muscularis externa can be seen only with full-thickness biopsy specimens. The customary method of diagnosis is to obtain full-thickness wall biopsy samples at open surgery.

The diagnosis of visceral myopathy must be made in the appropriate clinical setting; in some cases, however, the possibility of visceral myopathy has not been appreciated clinically. We have had cases in which the resected intestine was sent to us as "megacolon" and "volvulus" in which histologic examination suggested the correct diagnosis of visceral myopathy. Not all cases of muscle atrophy and fibrosis represent visceral myopathy. Muscle fibrosis occurs in progressive systemic sclerosis and inflammatory mesenteric disorders such as mesenteric fibromatosis.

Primary Visceral Neuropathy

Primary visceral neuropathy may be familial or sporadic. Familial cases may have an autosomal-dominant or autosomal-recessive inheritance pattern. Mental retardation and calcification of the basal ganglia are rarely associated. Clinical presentation is with chronic and often intermittent intestinal obstruction in the absence of a mechanical cause. The affected segment of bowel shows variable degrees of dilatation.

Pathologic examination of routine sections is usually normal without abnormality of the muscle wall. The changes are in the myenteric plexus, but these are usually not detectable in routine sections. One type of visceral neuropathy, characterized by the presence within ganglion cells of large, round, eosinophilic, intranuclear incusions surrounded by a halo, superficially resembling Cowdry A viral inclusions of cytomegalovirus, can be diagnosed in routine H&E sections.[12]

Pathologic diagnosis of cases that do not show changes on routine sections requires silver staining by Smith's technique. These cases show decreased number of neurons, subtle degenerative changes in the neurons, and abnormal dendritic processes.[15] These studies are only done in a few specialized centers.

Progressive Systemic Sclerosis

Involvement of the GI tract is common in progressive systemic sclerosis (scleroderma) and results from vasculopathy leading to progressive ischemic atrophy of the smooth muscle and

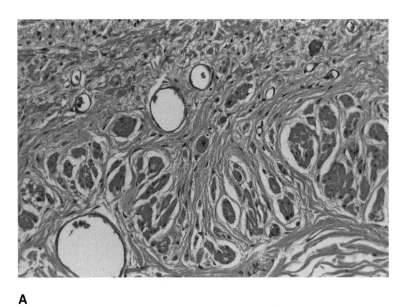

A

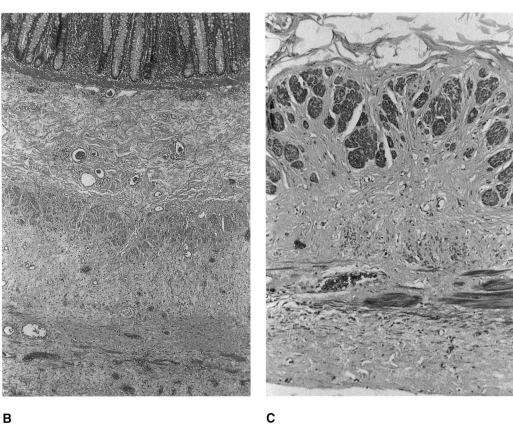

B   C

Figure 8–6. A: Familial visceral myopathy, showing marked degeneration and fibrosis involving the circular muscle layer. Note the absence of inflammation. B: Familial visceral myopathy, showing marked degeneration of the muscle wall of the colon. Both circular and longitudinal muscle layers are affected. C: Trichrome stain showing fibrosis replacing the degenerated muscle.

myenteric plexus followed by fibrous replacement.[20] Most patients have subclinical disease; symptoms occur only in severely affected segments of the bowel.

Atrophy and fibrosis of the gastric wall results in a small shrunken stomach associated with early satiety. In the small intestine and colon, muscle atrophy and fibrosis may result in chronic pseudo-obstruction and the occurrence of diverticula. Chronic pseudo-obstruction is usually mild and intermittent; less commonly, massive dilatation of the affected bowel occurs.

The smooth muscle atrophy and fibrosis resembles the changes of visceral myopathy. Points of distinction are:

1. Progressive systemic sclerosis may be manifested elsewhere in the body and antinuclear antibodies may be present in the serum.
2. The inner circular muscle layer is affected first and more severely than the longitudinal muscle layer in progressive systemic sclerosis.

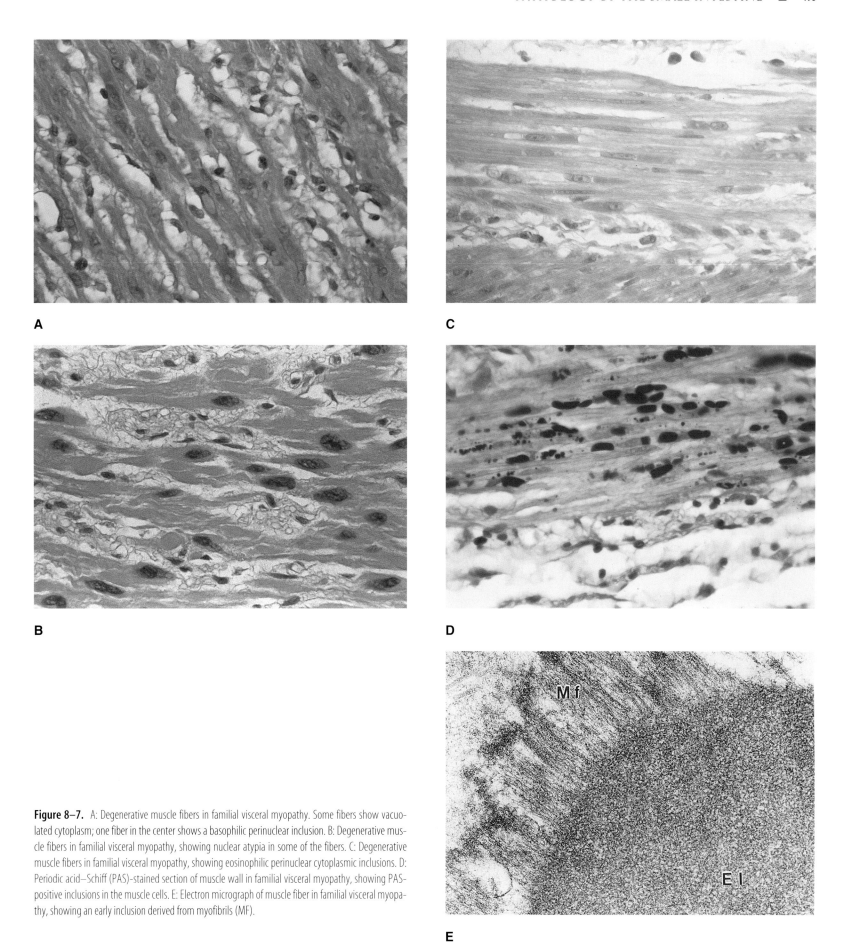

Figure 8–7. A: Degenerative muscle fibers in familial visceral myopathy. Some fibers show vacuolated cytoplasm; one fiber in the center shows a basophilic perinuclear inclusion. B: Degenerative muscle fibers in familial visceral myopathy, showing nuclear atypia in some of the fibers. C: Degenerative muscle fibers in familial visceral myopathy, showing eosinophilic perinuclear cytoplasmic inclusions. D: Periodic acid–Schiff (PAS)-stained section of muscle wall in familial visceral myopathy, showing PAS-positive inclusions in the muscle cells. E: Electron micrograph of muscle fiber in familial visceral myopathy, showing an early inclusion derived from myofibrils (MF).

3. There is no vacuolar degeneration of the muscle fibers, which is characteristic of visceral myopathy.
4. There may be evidence of vasculopathy, characterized by proliferative endarteritis and mucinous change of the media of small vessels.

MECHANICAL INTESTINAL OBSTRUCTION

Acute intestinal obstruction is a common reason for urgent exploratory laparotomy. In many of these cases, a definitive preoperative diagnosis is not possible. Some of these patients have resolution of obstruction during surgery without any resection being performed, for example, freeing of adhesions, correction of a volvulus, reduction of an intussusception, or an obstructed hernia. Resection is necessary when a mural disease is responsible for the obstruction or when the obstruction is associated with strangulative necrosis of the bowel wall.

Clinically, obstructions are of two types: (1) Simple, when there is one point of obstruction. The proximal bowel dilates due to fluid accumulation. Vomiting occurs, resulting in decompression of the bowel. Simple obstruction causes severe colicky abdominal pain and fluid depletion. (2) Closed loop obstruction, when the bowel cannot decompress because there are two points of obstruction, as, for example, in an obstructed hernia (Fig. 8–8). Colonic obstructions act as closed-loop obstructions if the ileocecal valve prevents effective decompression into the small intestine. Closed-loop obstructions carry an increased risk of vascular compromise and gangrene because progressive dilatation of the closed loop results in increased wall pressure.

The pathologist can play a role in the intraoperative diagnosis of obstructive lesions. Although external appearances of the diseased segment of intestine may be diagnostic of a particular entity, for example, creeping fat in Crohn's disease, in most cases, the surgeon who removes the abnormal segment has no definite diagnosis during surgery. In these cases, intraoperative pathologic consultation permits the opening of the intestine during surgery; gross pathologic examination and frozen sections, when indicated, may provide important diagnostic information. For example, the pathologic observations may result in collecting tissue for special diagnostic tests, such as mycobacterial culture and lymphoma markers, which may prove invaluable.

Intraoperative pathologic examination is not helpful in assessing the viability of a segment of ischemic bowel, which is an important consideration in determining the extent of surgical resection. Future viability depends on the absence of necrosis in the muscularis externa; the presence of mucosal necrosis at the margin has no relevance in this regard. Pathologically evident necrosis of the muscle wall is usually obvious at surgery. Segments of intestine with no pathologic evidence of muscle necrosis can be nonviable, most probably because microscopic evidence of muscle necrosis takes several days after its occurrence to develop (a situation that is similar to myocardial infarction). For this reason, the determination of viability must be made by clinical criteria that are presently used by the surgeon.

Mechanical intestinal obstruction results from a large number of diseases (Table 8–2). Pathologic examination provides a diagnosis in most of these cases. In those in which a diagnosis is not made after gross and pathologic examination, the pathologist must obtain clinical and operative findings before reporting, for example, the presence of adhesions or a volvulus.

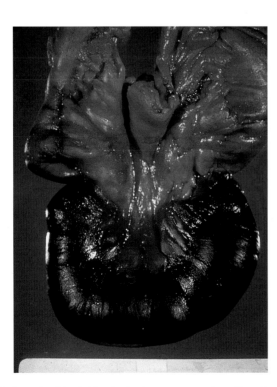

Figure 8–8. Strangulated inguinal hernia, showing a gangrenous loop of bowel in a closed-loop obstruction.

TABLE 8–2. CAUSES OF MECHANICAL INTESTINAL OBSTRUCTION

Intraluminal Causes
    Meconium ileus (in cystic fibrosis)
    Gallstone ileus
    Roundworm infestation
    Bezoars
Intramural Causes
    Congenital atresia and stenosis
    Benign fibrous stricture
    Crohn's disease
    Tuberculosis
    Neoplasms
        Adenocarcinoma
        Carcinoid tumor
        Malignant lymphoma
        GI stromal neoplasms
        Metastatic tumors
Extramural Causes
    Obstructed hernias
    Adhesions
    Mesenteric fibromatosis
    Diverticulitis
    Peritoneal cysts or tumors

Intussusception

Intussusception is an uncommon cause of intestinal obstruction characterized by invagination of one part of the intestine (the intussusceptum) into the lumen of the bowel that is immediately distal (the intussuscepiens) (Fig. 8–9). Once an intussusception begins, it tends to be progressive because of propulsive peristalsis. Intussusception occurs most commonly in children younger than 2 years; the typical site of intussusception is the ileocecal region, with the right colon being the intussuscepiens. Patients present with intestinal obstruction associated with rectal bleeding ("red currant jelly" stool) and a sausage-shaped palpable mass in the abdomen (Fig. 8–9). The intussusceptum is liable to undergo ischemic necrosis because its vascular supply becomes progressively compromised at the neck of the intussusception (see Fig. 8–9B). In adults, intussusception is commonly precipitated by a polypoid lesion, which acts as the apex of the intussusception; hamartomatous polyps of Peutz-Jeghers syndrome, submucosal lipomas, and inflammatory fibroid polyps are associated with intussusception. In children, reactive lymphoid hyperplasia in the ileocecal region is commonly present at the apex of an intussusception. In all cases of intussusception, careful examination of the apex is necessary to establish a cause.

INFLAMMATORY DISEASES

Infectious Diseases

Small-intestinal infections caused by rotaviruses, *Salmonella* spp. other than *S. typhi, Campylobacter jejuni, Yersinia enterocolitica* and *Y. pseudotuberculosis, Vibrio cholerae* and other toxigenic bacterial infections, although extremely common, only rarely come to the attention of the surgical pathologist in a biopsy of the terminal ileum. The biopsy specimen shows nonspecific acute inflammation, sometimes associated with ulceration (Fig. 8–10). Differentiation from Crohn's ileitis is best done with clinical history, but the absence of chronic features, such as villous blunting, chronic inflammation, crypt distortion and fibrosis, as well as the absence of granulomas, are helpful. Acute infectious enteritis is diagnosed by stool and blood culture and serologic testing and effectively treated with antibiotics; complications such as strictures and perforation do not occur, and resections are almost never performed. In rare fatal cases that come to autopsy, and when autolysis has not made pathologic

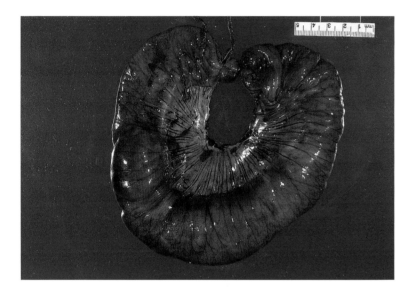

A

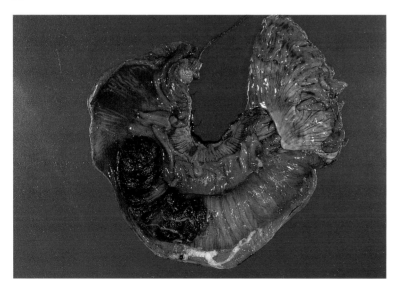

B

Figure 8–9. A: Segment of intestine showing an intussusception. Note the sausage-shaped intussuscepted intestine covered by the intussuscepiens. B: Intussusception, with a intussuscepiens opened to show the intussuscepted loop of bowel. Note the discoloration at the apex resulting from infarction.

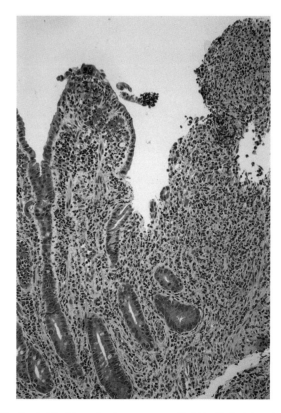

Figure 8–10. Terminal ileal biopsy showing acute nonspecific ileitis with focal ulceration. The villi are long and slender and infiltrated by neutrophils. The ulcer has occurred at the site of a lymphoid follicle.

examination a futile exercise, the small-intestinal mucosa shows the following changes: (1) enterotoxic infections such as cholera do not show any significant abnormality. These cases cause a severe secretory diarrhea resulting from the biochemical effect of toxin attachment to cell receptors. (2) Enteroinvasive infections such as salmonellosis cause an acute inflammation of the mucosa with focal microabscess formation and erosion. A specific diagnosis is not possible without microbiological studies.

We restrict our consideration to those small-intestinal infectious diseases that come to the attention of the surgical pathologist, either in biopsies or resections. It should be noted that appendiceal and colonic infections frequently come to the attention of the surgical pathologist at appendectomy and colonoscopic biopsy; these are considered in Chapters 9 and 10.

Typhoid Fever

Typhoid fever, which is caused by *Salmonella typhi* and *S. paratyphi*, is endemic in parts of Asia and Africa where sanitary conditions do not effectively prevent fecal contamination of food and water. Unlike other forms of *Salmonella* species, which commonly infect animals, *S. typhi* is a human pathogen. Typhoid fever in endemic areas occurs predominantly in young adult males, although both sexes and any age group can be affected.

On ingestion, the organisms enter the mucosa of the small intestine in the region of the lymphoid patches, probably through M cells, and pass to the regional nodes. The bacteria multiply in the intestinal lymphoid patches and lymph nodes for 2–3 weeks (the incubation period), at which time they enter the bloodstream. In the first week, the disease is characterized by bacteremia with fever, severe headache, and splenomegaly. Leukope-

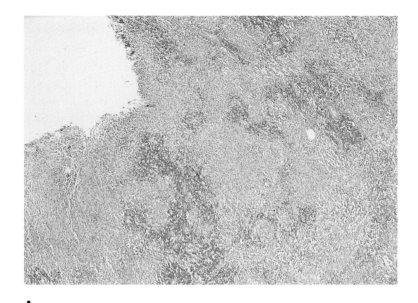

A

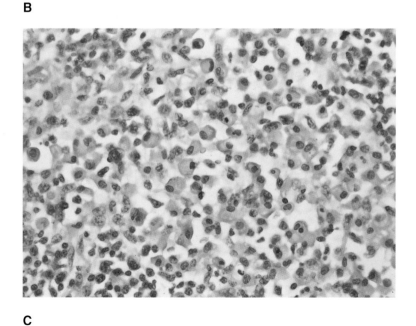

B

C

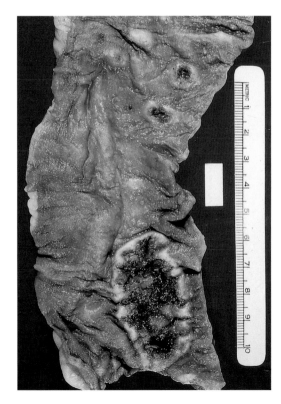

Figure 8–11. Typhoid fever, ileum, showing ulcerated Peyer's patch and smaller lymphoid follicles. The longitudinal ulcers are typical of typhoid fever.

Figure 8–12. A: Typhoid fever, showing mucosal ulceration and extensive necrosis involving a Peyer's patch in the ileum. B: Peyer's patch in acute typhoid fever showing necrosis and inflammation. C: Inflammatory cell reaction in typhoid fever, dominated by macrophages and lacking in neutrophils.

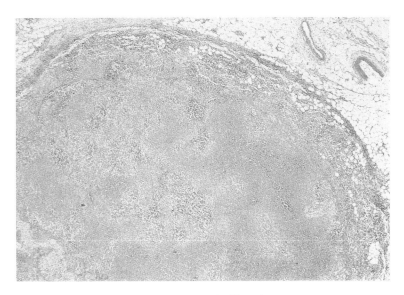

Figure 8–13. Mesenteric lymph node in typhoid fever, showing extensive necrosis.

nia and bradycardia are distinctive features; blood culture is positive. During the second week of illness, the organisms are excreted into the intestine via bile. There they reinfect the Peyer's patches of the small intestine and colonic lymphoid tissue, producing the intestinal phase of the disease, which is characterized by severe diarrhea and dehydration. Diagnosis in this phase is made by culture of blood, stools, and urine. The intestinal lesions are localized to the lymphoid aggregates, taking the longitudinal shape of Peyer's patches in the distal ileum (Fig. 8–11), but smaller and more rounded in the colon. The Peyer's patches are edematous and undergo extensive necrosis and ulceration (Fig. 8–12A, B). The inflammatory infiltrate in the necrotic lymphoid patches consists of macrophages, some of which show erythrophagocytosis; the paucity of neutrophils in this acute inflammatory disease is highly suggestive of typhoid fever (Fig. 8–12C). During the intestinal phase, the mesenteric lymph nodes are also markedly enlarged; histologic examination shows extensive necrosis (Fig. 8–13) and the typical macrophage-dominated, neutrophil-deficient inflammatory response.[21]

Intestinal complications include hemorrhage from the ulcers, which can be life-threatening, and perforation. Perforation usually occurs in a necrotic Peyer's patch in the distal ileum. Multiple perforations may be present.[22] Perforation releases intestinal contents into the peritoneal cavity, resulting in a polymicrobial peritonitis.

Typhoid fever is treated with antibiotics, which are highly effective against *S. typhi*. Medical treatment usually suffices even for complicated cases, although rarely, resection is necessary for perforation and severe hemorrhage.[22] Recovery is associated with a return of the intestine to normal without significant scarring in patients that recover. The longitudinal ulcers of typhoid fever do not produce strictures or intestinal obstruction.

Intestinal Tuberculosis

Intestinal tuberculosis occurs in adults as a manifestation of secondary tuberculosis. In the past, when bovine tuberculosis was common, the intestine was a common site of primary tu-

berculosis; with pasteurization of milk and control of dairy herds, bovine tuberculosis has virtually disappeared. Recently, tuberculosis has increased in incidence in the United States, particularly in immunocompromised patients.

Intestinal tuberculosis in the adult occurs by two different mechanisms: (1) In patients with active pulmonary disease, organisms may be swallowed and cause infection in the intestine.[23] These patients are chronically ill with cough, fever, and weight loss and have a positive chest radiograph. (2) Over 50% of patients who develop intestinal tuberculosis have no active pulmonary disease and have normal chest radiographs.[24] In these patients, intestinal tuberculosis results from reactivation of dormant intestinal foci of infection, which were acquired in the childhood primary phase of lymphohematogenous bacterial dissemination.

Adult intestinal tuberculosis may occur anywhere in the intestine. In the immunocompetent host, the maximum frequency is in the ileum, with colonic involvement being next in frequency. In the immunocompromised host intestinal disease tends to occur in the colon and rectum more frequently.[25] The reactivation occurs in the mucosa and results in granulomatous inflammation with caseous necrosis. Small mucosal ulcers result; in the early stages these are superficial aphthous ulcers (Fig. 8–14). The mucosal infection tends to spread along mucosal and submucosal lymphatics, which are oriented circumferentially in the intestine (Fig. 8–15). The ulcers therefore tend to progress transversely with progressive, caseating, granulomatous inflammation (Fig. 8–16). Involvement of the intestinal wall leads to fibrosis, resulting in strictures and intestinal obstruction, which are typical of intestinal tuberculosis (Fig. 8–17). Strictures are often multiple. Involvement of the serosa

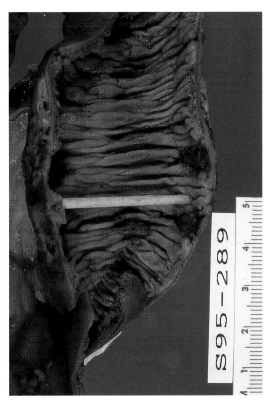

Figure 8–14. Intestinal tuberculosis, showing multiple mucosal ulcers.

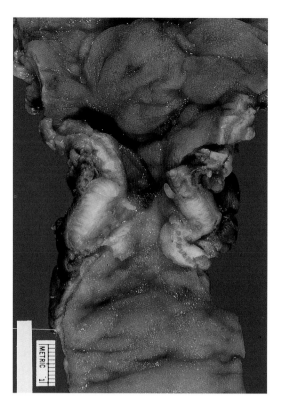

Figure 8–15. Tuberculous enteritis, showing transverse mucosal ulceration and marked thickening of the wall.

leads to tuberculous seeding of the peritoneal cavity, with ascites and multiple tubercles occurring on the peritoneal surface. Peritoneal involvement results in adhesions and fistula formation.

A characteristic hyperplastic form of tuberculosis affects

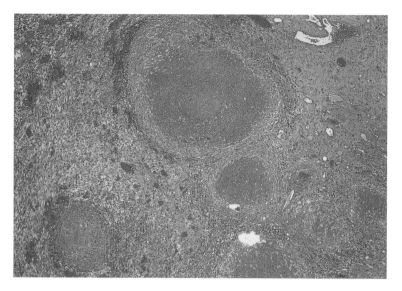

A

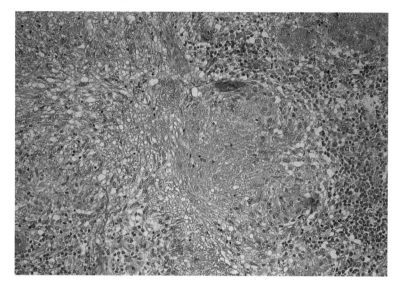

B

Figure 8–16. A: Tuberculous ulcer, showing necrotizing granulomas. B: Tuberculous ulcer, showing central caseous necrosis in a poorly defined epithelioid cell granuloma.

the ileocecal region, presenting as a large exophytic luminal mass with fibrosis of the wall and mesenteric involvement (see Chapter 10).[26] These masses can resemble malignant neoplasms at radiologic and colonoscopic examination.

The diagnosis of intestinal tuberculosis can be made by stool smears for acid-fast bacilli, stool culture, ascitic fluid culture when tuberculous peritonitis coexists, and biopsy when lesions in the terminal ileum are accessible to colonoscopy. Intestinal tuberculosis bears a close resemblance to Crohn's disease, being characterized by ileocolic disease with patchy ulcers, strictures and fistulas, and acute and chronic mucosal inflammation with granulomas on biopsy. On endoscopy, the transverse ulcers of tuberculosis are different from the longitudinal ulcers typical of Crohn's disease. On biopsy, the granulomatous inflammation is more dominant in tuberculosis; the granulomas tend to be more diffuse and associated with caseous necrosis. Acid-fast stains are usually positive and permit definitive differentiation on biopsy. In small specimens

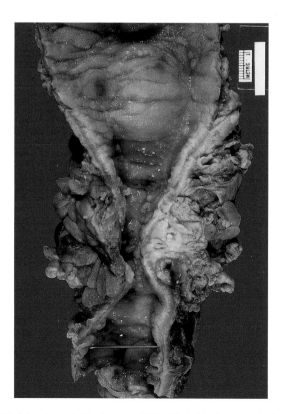

Figure 8–17. Tuberculous enteritis, showing a stricture. Marked luminal narrowing has resulted in intestinal obstruction, evidenced by dilatation of the bowel proximal to the stricture.

with small granulomas in which caseation is not prominent and acid-fast stains are negative, a significant danger of misdiagnosis as Crohn's disease exists. In these cases, the absence of severe crypt distortion and severe chronic inflammation of the background lamina propria in mucosa away from the ulcerated foci should make the pathologist question a diagnosis of Crohn's disease and consider tuberculosis.

In immunocompromised hosts, *Mycobacterium tuberculosis* infection may cause a more diffuse inflammation without distinct granulomas and sometimes without necrosis. Macrophages are prominent and show numerous acid-fast bacilli in specially stained sections. The pathologic picture can be confusing.

Atypical Mycobacterial Enteritis

Mycobacterium avium-intracellulare (MAIC) is also a common cause of intestinal infection in patients with acquired immunodeficiency syndrome (AIDS) (See Chapter 17), producing lesions throughout the gastrointestinal tract. These infections come to the attention of the pathologist when they occur in the gastric, duodenal, terminal ileal, and colonic biopsies. Wherever infection occurs, the organisms cause mucosal disease, with diffuse infiltration of the lamina propria by numerous infected macrophages. The infected macrophages contain huge numbers of organisms, which impart a fibrillary appearance to the cytoplasm in routine sections (Fig. 8–18A). Acid-fast stains show the cytoplasm of these macrophages distended with mycobacteria (Fig. 8–18B; also see Chapter 6).

Yersinia Infection

Infection caused by *Yersinia enterocolitica* and *Y. pseudotuberculosis* commonly manifests as acute terminal ileitis associated with mesenteric lymphadenitis. *Yersinia enterocolitica* tends to produce more intestinal disease, whereas disease due to *Y.*

pseudotuberculosis is dominated by mesentric lymphadenitis. Yersinial infection occurs mainly in children and young adults; males are more commonly affected than females. It is characterized by fever, diarrhea, and right lower quadrant abdominal pain and tenderness, mimicking acute appendicitis. The terminal ileum is acutely inflamed with mucosal ulceration. The inflammation is characterized by necrotizing granulomas with neutrophilic microabscesses in the center of the granuloma (Fig. 8–19). Granulomas are well developed in *Y. pseudotuberculosis* infection; in *Y. enterocolitica* infection, the granulomas are less defined, with palisading histiocytes around large areas of necrosis. Inflammation may be transmural, with neutrophils occurring in the muscularis externa; mural fibrosis and strictures do not occur. The mesenteric lymph nodes are markedly enlarged, particularly in *Y. pseudotuberculosis* infection. In some cases, cervical adenopathy is also present. Lymph nodes show typical stellate granulomas with neutrophils in the center (Fig. 8–20). Yersinial infections can also infect the colon; biopsies usually show features of acute self-limited colitis, with necrotizing granulomas being found only rarely.[27] The diagnosis is made by stool culture.

When laparotomy is performed for suspected acute appendicitis, the appendix appears normal, with swelling, hyperemia and thickening of the terminal ileum, and mesenteric node enlargement. The thickened bowel may have a nodular feel because of the submucosal lymphoid hyperplasia. Most such cases represent *Yersinia* infections.[28] The possibility of acute Crohn's ileitis also exists, however. The usual recommendation for these patients is to perform an appendectomy; if this is done, a swab of the appendix should be submitted to the microbiology department for *Yersinia* culture. The appendix may be normal, but frequently shows the typical granulomas with neutrophils in their center. *Yersinia* ileocolitis and mesenteric adenitis are self-limited diseases with rapid recovery of the patient following surgery and no development of a chronic phase.

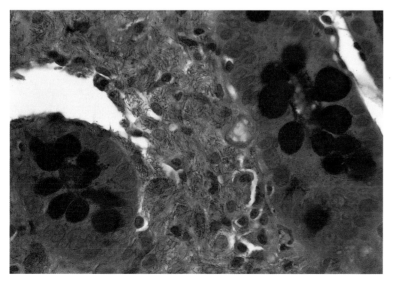

A

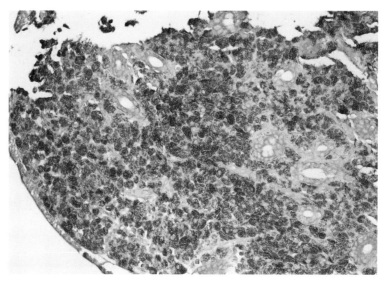

B

Figure 8–18. A: *Mycobacterium avium-intracellulare* infection of small-intestinal mucosa, PAS stain, showing macrophages with numerous bacilli seen faintly as cytoplasmic streaks because of their large numbers. B: *Mycobacterium avium-intracellulare* infection of small-intestinal mucosa, acid-fast stain, showing large numbers of mycobacteria in macrophages.

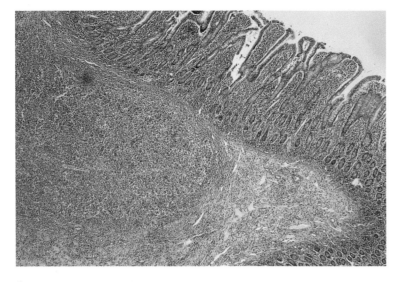

A

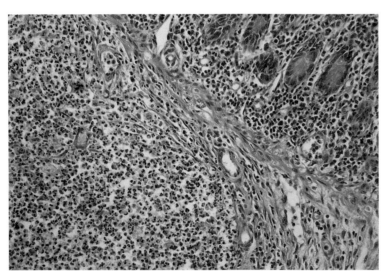

B

Figure 8–19. A: Yersinial enteritis, showing enlarged inflamed lymphoid nodule under the mucosa, which also shows neutrophilic infiltration. B: Higher power micrograph of part A, showing inflammation of lymphoid nodule, consisting mainly of neutrophils.

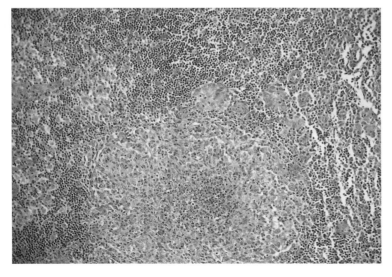

Figure 8–20. *Yersinia pseudotuberculosis* infection in mesenteric lymph node, showing epithelioid cell granuloma in reactive lymphoid tissue. The granuloma shows neutrophils in its center.

Fungal Infections

In endemic areas of the Mississippi River Valley, histoplasmosis causes a granulomatous infection of the intestine that resembles tuberculosis pathologically with maximum involvement in the terminal ileum and ascending colon (see Chapter 10).[29] On microscopy, numerous 2–4 mm yeast forms are seen within macrophages in the lamina propria. These can be accentuated by methenamine silver and PAS stain. The intestine is frequently involved in the disseminated form of the disease. Intestinal histoplasmosis rarely manifests without disease elsewhere in the body. Intestinal histoplasmosis and cryptococcosis

TABLE 8–3. INTESTINAL HELMINTHS AND DISEASES ASSOCIATED WITH THEM

Parasite	Usual Site	Clinical Effects
Nematodes		
Ascaris lumbricoides (roundworm)	Small intestine	Intestinal obstruction with heavy worm loads; Migration up common bile duct and pancreatic duct, causing cholangitis, pancreatitis, and gallstones; Penetration of intestinal wall with peritoneal granulomas; Larval migration to lungs.
Enterobius vermicularis	Cecal region	Anal pruritus; Migration up vagina, urethra; Penetration of intestinal wall.
Trichuris trichiura	Colon	None; bloody diarrhea and rectal prolapse with heavy worm loads.
Ancylostoma duodenale and Necator americanus (hookworms)	Small intestine	Iron deficiency anemia.
Strongyloides stercoralis	Small intestine	Bloody diarrhea; Appendiceal, colonic wall granulomas; Larval migration to lungs; hyperfection in immunocompromised host.
Trichinella spiralis	Small intestine	Abdominal pain, diarrhea; Larval migration causes trichinosis.
Capillaria philippinensis	Small intestine	Malabsorption; protein-losing enteropathy.
Angiostrongylus costaricansis	Terminal ileum, right colon	Inflammatory masses; perforation.
Anisakis larval forms	Stomach	Gastroenteritis with bloody diarrhea;
	Small intestine	Gastric and intestinal granulomas.
Cestodes		
Taenia solium	Small intestine	None Larval migration causes cysticercosis.
Taenia saginata	Small intestine	None
Diphyllobothrium latum	Small intestine	Vitamin B_{12} deficiency.
Trematodes		
Schistosoma mansoni	Colon	Bloody diarrhea; portal hypertension.
Schistosoma japonicum	Small intestine	Diarrhea; portal hypertension.
Fasciolopsis buski	Small intestine	Abdominal pain and diarrhea with heavy worm loads.
Heterophyes heterophyes	Small intestine	Abdominal pain, mild diarrhea.

are seen in the immunocompromised host (see Chapters 10 and 17). Other fungal infections, such as aspergillosis, candidiasis, and mucormycosis,[30] may occur as part of a fungemia; the intestinal lesion in these cases is secondary to a fungal vasculitis, and diagnosis is made by finding the organisms in vascular spaces in the submucosa.

Parasitic Infections

Giardiasis is a common infection throughout the world, mainly affecting the duodenum (see Chapter 6). Helminth infestations of the small intestine and colon are extremely common in developing countries (Table 8–3). The roundworm, *Ascaris lumbricoides,* is estimated to infest 25% of the world's population. Hookworms (*Ancylostoma duodenale* and *Necator americanus*), tapeworms (*Taenia solium* and *T. saginata*), and *Strongyloides stercoralis* are very common small-intestinal helminths. The pinworm (*Enterobius vermicularis*) and whipworm (*Trichuris trichiura*) are not found in the small intestine; they live in the colon. In most cases, these worms exist in the intestinal lumen as commensals and do not cause disease. Whipworms and hookworms normally attach themselves to the intestinal mucosa. Unlike other nematodes that feed on luminal contents, hookworms suck blood from the host, resulting in profound iron deficiency anemia when worm loads are heavy. Hookworm infestation is the commonest cause of iron deficiency anemia in developing countries.

Many helminths can produce clinical disease when worm loads are heavy and when there are abnormal migrations of the worms and its larval forms. Heavy infestations with *Ascaris lumbricoides* is a common cause of intestinal obstruction in endemic countries. The diagnosis of these parasitic infestations is made by examination of stool samples for ova and larval forms. These worms may also be seen at endoscopy and in resected specimens. When encountered in resection specimens, some knowledge of worm identification methods is necessary. In most cases, pathologists are more familiar with the characteristics of worm ova, and the easiest way to make a specific diagnosis is to submit a cross section of the worm for histology; when ova are present, the specific diagnosis is easy.

Strongyloides stercoralis is a relatively common nematode

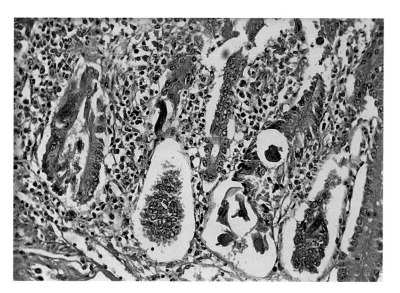

A

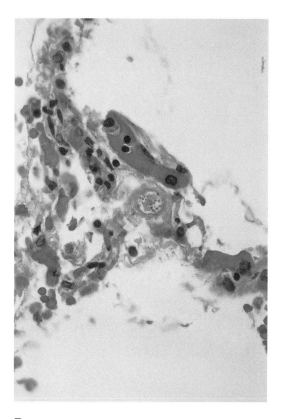

B

Figure 8–22. A: Filariform larvae of *Strongyloides stercoralis* invading colonic mucosa in the autoinfection cycle. B: *Strongyloides stercoralis* larva in pulmonary alveolar capillary in patient who died of overwhelming hyperinfection.

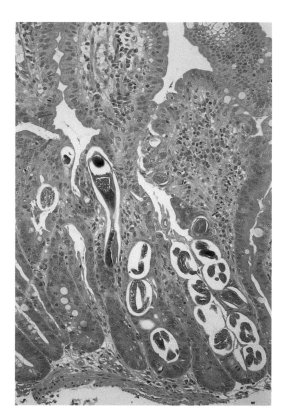

Figure 8–21. *Strongyloides stercoralis,* adult worm with ova in the duodenal mucosa.

parasite in the United States. The adult worms live in the mucosa of the small intestine (Fig. 8–21); with low worm load, the infection is asymptomatic. With high worm loads, diarrhea, malabsorption, and protein-losing enteropathy may occur. The ova hatch in the mucosa into rhabditiform larvae, which are passed in the feces. Some larvae molt in the intestinal lumen into filariform larvae that can penetrate the wall of the intestine, usually in the appendix and colon, causing an eosinophilic colitis characterized by the presence of numerous larval forms in the mucosa (Fig. 8–22A), and eosinophilic granulomas in the wall (see Chapters 9 and 10). The diagnosis is made by identifying the larval forms of this worm in stools or in colonic mucosa. The filariform larvae enter the bloodstream after intestinal mucosal penetration and travel to the lungs. In immunocompromised patients (human immunodeficiency virus [HIV]-positive or patients on cancer chemotherapy), malnourished, and any chronically ill patient, this autoinfective cycle can result in massive and fatal parasitemia, commonly manifesting with pulmonary symptoms. The larvae can be seen in lung capillaries (Fig. 8–22B). *Capillaria phillipinensis* is a nematode found mainly in Southeast Asia. The adult lives in the mucosa of the small intestine, where it resembles *Strongyloides stercoralis* (Fig. 8–23A). Also incidentally found in small-intestinal specimens from patients in endemic areas are ova of *Schistosoma japonicum* (Fig. 8–23B). Ova of *S. japonicum* and its colonic counterpart, *S. mansoni,* may travel to the liver and cause a portal fibrosis with portal hypertension (Fig. 8–23C).

Intestinal parasites also cause disease by virtue of invasion of the intestinal mucosa and unusual migrations. Invasive infections may result from adult worms, such as *Enterobius vermicularis* (see Chapter 10) and *Ascaris lumbricoides,* or from larval stages of animal nematodes such as *Anisakis* (see Table 8–3).[31–33]

Neutropenic Enterocolitis

Neutropenic enterocolitis is a disease seen in patients with severe neutropenia, commonly during treatment for hematopoietic malignancies, but also after organ transplantation. Several infectious agents have been implicated, including cy-

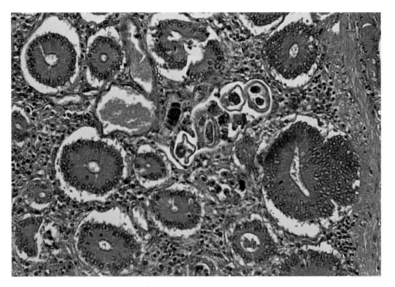

A

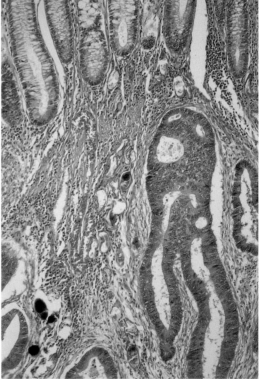

B

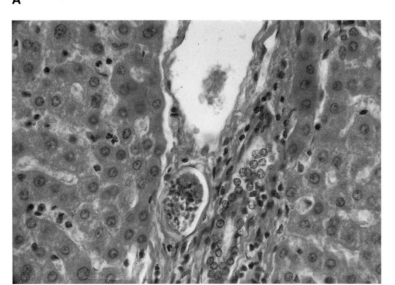

C

Figure 8–23. A: *Capillaria philippinensis,* adult worm in small-bowel mucosa. B: Small-intestinal adenocarcinoma with *Schistosoma* ova found incidentally. Some of the ova are calcified. There is no relationship between schistosomiasis and small-intestine adenocarcinoma. C: Liver showing *Schistosoma* ova in portal area.

tomegalovirus and numerous clostridia. *Clostridium septicum* has been implicated most frequently.[34]

Neutropenic enterocolitis manifests clinically as severe rectal bleeding, often leading to shock. Fever and abdominal pain are common. Perforation may occur. Emergent treatment, which includes withdrawal of immunosuppressive drugs and right hemicolectomy, has resulted in a decrease of the extremely high mortality rate previously associated with this disease.[35]

The terminal ileum, cecum, and ascending colon are usually affected. The mucosal appearance varies from a superficial enterocolitis associated with pseudomembranes to a deeply ulcerative hemorrhagic appearance (Fig. 8–24A). In cases that perforate, ulceration extends into the muscularis externa. Microscopically, necrosis is extensive in severe cases; neutrophils are present, although few in number (Fig. 8–24B, C).

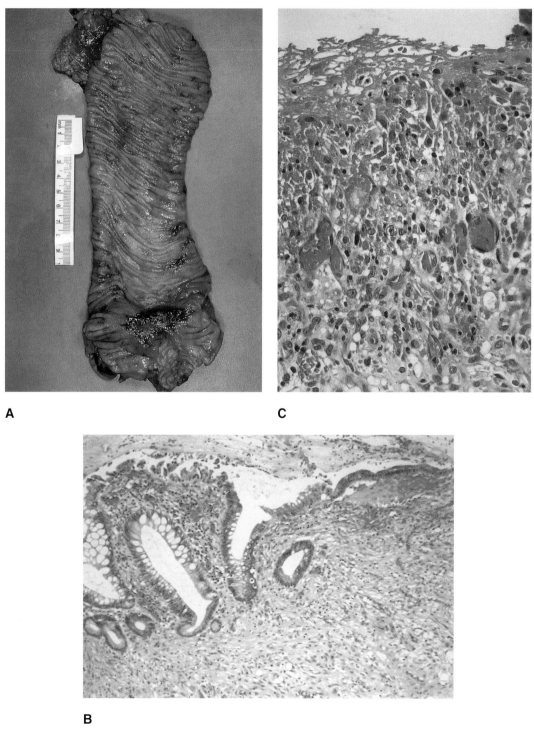

A

C

B

Figure 8–24. A: Neutropenic enterocolitis in patient being treated for acute myeloblastic leukemia complicated by severe gastrointestinal hemorrhage. Specimen shows colon with large hemorrhagic ulcer. B: Neutropenic enterocolitis; edge of mucosal ulcer showing regenerating epithelium with paucity of neutrophils in the lamina propria. C: Neutropenic enterocolitis; ulcer base showing granulation tissue with marked paucity of neutrophils.

Eosinophilic Gastroenteritis

Eosinophilic gastroenteritis is a poorly defined clinicopathological entity characterized by the presence of (1) gastrointestinal symptoms, (2) peripheral blood eosinophilia, and (3) eosinophilic infiltration of the GI tract.[36] Other causes of eosinophilic infiltration of the intestine, such as parasitic infestation and systemic autoimmune diseases, should be excluded. Some authorities do not consider peripheral blood eosinophilia necessary for diagnosis. About half the patients with this condition have a history of allergy, either themselves or in their family.

Eosinophilic gastroenteritis has no known cause. The disease occurs at all ages but is most common in children and young adults. It most commonly affects the gastric antrum and small intestine. Rarely, the entire gastrointestinal tract, including the esophagus and colon can be involved.[37]

The manifestations of eosinophilic gastroenteritis depend on which layer of the gastrointestinal tract is involved.

1. Mucosal involvement causes abdominal pain, vomiting, diarrhea, steatorrhea, and protein-losing enteropathy. Endoscopy shows diffuse and nodular thickening of the mucosal folds, with a "cobblestone" appearance of the antrum. Histologic examination is characterized by marked eosinophilic infiltration of the mucosa of the involved stomach or small intestine. The mucosal involvement is patchy, and multiple biopsy specimens may be necessary to establish the diagnosis. In definitive cases, large numbers of eosinophils are present without other types of inflammatory cells. In less definitive cases, when eosinophils are present in smaller numbers and admixed with many other inflammatory cells, the diagnosis cannot be made on histologic grounds; these cases require the clinical background, particularly the presence of peripheral blood eosinophilia and radiologic evidence of involvement of the muscle layer. It must be remembered that common inflammatory diseases, such as *Helicobacter pylori* gastritis, celiac disease, reflux esophagitis, and ulcerative colitis, frequently shows significant numbers of eosinophils in the inflammatory infiltrate.
2. Muscle layer disease generally shows transmural eosinophilic infiltration of the muscle associated with wall thickening and pyloric and intestinal strictures, leading to obstruction.[38] Mucosal biopsies may not be abnormal in these cases, and the diagnosis is clinical and radiologic.
3. Subserosal involvement is characterized by collections of eosinophils under the peritoneal surface, which can be seen as yellowish plaques at laparotomy. Rarely, this produces eosinophilic ascites, which is diagnosed when ascitic fluid shows numerous leukocytes, the vast majority of which are eosinophils.[39]

Eosinophilic gastroenteritis responds well to steroid therapy. The disease has a chronic course with relapses and remissions, but most patients are well controlled with steroid therapy to control relapses.

Necrotizing Enterocolitis

Necrotizing enterocolitis (NEC) has emerged in the past 30 years as the most common gastrointestinal emergency in neonatal intensive care units, occurring in approximately 2% of all patients in such units.[40] It primarily affects premature neonates, but 5–25% of infants with NEC are full term. The cause of NEC is not yet certain, and the disease is defined by the presence of abdominal distention, hematochezia, and pneumatosis intestinalis in a neonate. Immaturity of the intestinal mucosa predisposing to injury, bacterial overgrowth in the lumen, and formula feeding are the three major pathogenetic factors. Many bacteria are present in NEC, and most of these are normal enteric flora. Strains of toxigenic *Escherichia coli*, staphylococci, and *Clostridium difficile* have been suggested as causing epidemics of NEC in some neonatal units. Intestinal ischemia due to splanchnic vasoconstriction plays a role in the pathogenesis of NEC, but the importance of ischemia as a primary factor may have been overestimated in the past. Many cases develop perforation, which is an indication for surgical resection of the necrotic intestine. The overall survival rate is 60–80%.

The terminal ileum and proximal colon are usually most affected in NEC. In mild cases, involvement is patchy; in severe cases, the entire bowel may be necrotic. Perforations are present in half the patients.[41] On gross examination, the involved bowel is often distended and has a paper-thin, hemorrhagic, friable wall that disintegrates on handling. Pneumatosis, manifesting as large submucosal and subserosal collections of gas, is common. Pneumatosis is believed to result from fermentation by gas-forming microorganisms that enter the intestinal wall from the lumen. Gas can enter the portal venous system. Histologic examination shows extensive coagulative necrosis and inflammation. The necrosis is patchy and involves mainly the mucosa (Fig. 8–25), but areas of transmural necrosis are present at least focally in most patients. Inflammation is usually a mixture of acute and chronic types. It is limited to the mucosa in less affected areas and is transmural in severely affected bowel. Bacterial colonies and gas spaces are commonly found in the intestinal wall. Necrosis usually dominates over the inflammatory reaction. In many cases, changes of repair associated with fibrosis can be seen in areas of older disease, suggesting that NEC is a dynamically evolving disease rather than a one-time injury.

Pneumatosis Intestinalis

Pneumatosis intestinalis (also called pneumatosis cystoides intestinalis) is the presence of gas in the wall of the intestine. Pneumatosis should be regarded as a pathologic abnormality that is associated with several diseases. Its clinical presentation and prognosis is directly related to the underlying disease.[42] Common clinical conditions in which pneumatosis intestinalis occurs are (1) in premature infants with necrotizing enterocolitis, which is a fulminant disease, and (2) in adults with obstructive lung disease, who have a benign course. A large number of other diseases, including peptic ulcer disease, pyloric stenosis, intestinal obstruction, chronic intestinal pseudo-obstruction, ischemic bowel disease, fulminant intestinal infections, and jejunoileal bypass, have also been associated.[42] In a significant number of patients, pneumatosis intestinalis occurs as an incidental finding without an identifiable underlying disease. The cause of pneumatosis intestinalis is unknown.

Three different morphologic types of pneumatosis intestinalis are described:

1. Microvesicular pneumatosis intestinalis refers to the presence of small gas spaces in the superficial lamina propria devoid of any reaction (Fig. 8–26).[43] These resemble fatty infiltration of the mucosa and has been called "pseudolipomatosis." Microvesicular pneumatosis intestinalis occurs mainly in the colon and is seen at colonoscopy as a white

plaque; it rarely occurs in the stomach. It is very likely a change caused by endoscopy in which microscopic surface epithelial breaks permit entry of luminal gas into the mucosa. It has no clinical significance.

2. Cystic pneumatosis intestinalis is the common type of the disease (Fig. 8–27A). It may involve any part of the GI tract from the esophagus to the rectum and affects mainly the submucosa and subserosa. It may be asymptomatic or manifest many gastrointestinal symptoms, including abdominal pain, diarrhea, bloody stools, constipation, and tenesmus when there is rectal involvement. Subserosal cysts can rupture into the peritoneal cavity and cause pneumoperitoneum. When the rectum is involved, tense, gas-filled cysts can be palpated at digital examination. At endoscopy, the submucosal cysts appear as sessile polypoid nodules. Radiol-

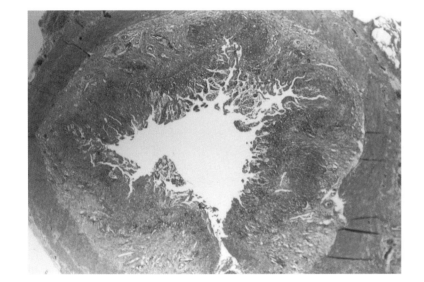

A

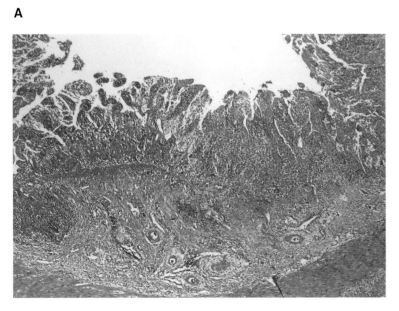

B

Figure 8–25. A: Necrotizing enterocolitis, showing extensive mucosal necrosis in involved small intestine. B: Necrotizing enterocolitis, showing full-thickness mucosal necrosis associated with loss of muscularis mucosae and submucosal and mural inflammation.

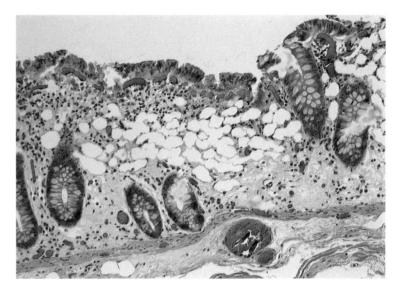

A

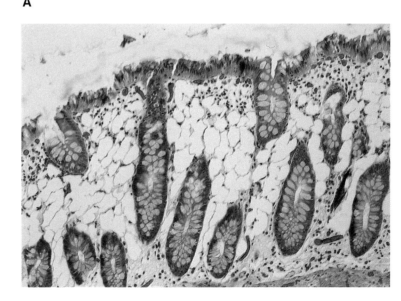

B

Figure 8–26. A: Colonic mucosa showing microvesicular pneumatosis intestinalis. The mucosa contains numerous small air spaces. B: Microvesicular pneumatosis intestinalis of the colon, higher power micrograph of part A, showing resemblance of the air spaces to fat ("pseudolipomatosis").

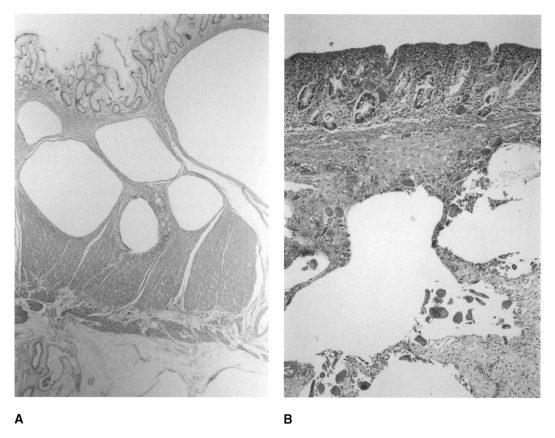

A   **B**

Figure 8–27. A: Small bowel showing pneumatosis intestinalis. Large air spaces are present in the submucosa, muscle wall, and serosa. B: Pneumatosis intestinalis, showing air spaces beneath the mucosa with foreign body-type multinucleated giant cells lining the spaces.

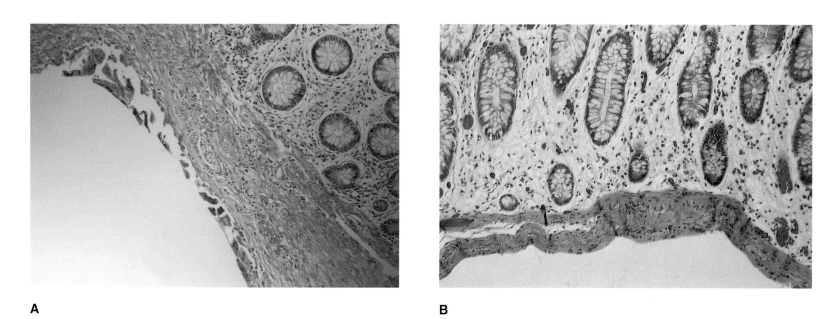

A   **B**

Figure 8–28. A: Pneumatosis intestinalis in a colonic biopsy specimen, showing foreign body-type multinucleated giant cells lining a submucosal air space. B: Colonic biopsy specimen, showing pneumatosis intestinalis. There is an abrupt linear space under the muscularis mucosa that is lined by histiocytes.

ogy is very effective in diagnosing pneumatosis intestinalis; the plain abdominal radiograph shows diagnostic changes in the majority of cases. Subserosal pneumatosis intestinalis can be diagnosed using laparoscopy.[44]

Histologically, biopsies show air spaces lined by macrophages and foreign body-type multinucleated giant cells (Fig. 8–27A, B). Because the cysts are mainly submucosal, endoscopic biopsy specimens, usually colonic, frequently show only the superficial part of the cyst with the macrophage lining occurring immediately beneath the muscularis mucosae (Fig. 8–28). This appearance can be very subtle and is easily overlooked. Sometimes, the cysts are so prominent that a diagnosis of lymphangioma can be considered; in these cases, immunoperoxidase staining for endothelial and histiocyte markers is helpful. The overlying mucosa is either normal or shows mild inflammatory changes; rarely, mucosal granulomas are present apart from the histiocytes around the air-filled cysts.[42]

3. Diffuse pneumatosis intestinalis is characterized by poorly circumscribed gaseous infiltration of the intestinal wall without cyst formation or histiocytic response. This type of pneumatosis intestinalis is associated with necrotizing enterocolitis and ischemic bowel disease.

Treatment of pneumatosis intestinalis is the treatment of the underlying disorder. Oxygen therapy and antibiotics have been helpful in some cases. Surgery is rarely indicated unless the underlying disease requires surgical intervention.

DRUG-INDUCED INTESTINAL PATHOLOGY

A large number of drugs have been reported to cause a myriad of pathologic lesions in the small and large intestines (Table 8–4). Drugs are a common cause of gastrointestinal symptoms, most commonly diarrhea, vomiting, and bleeding. Most of these effects are temporary, however, and reverse when the drug is withdrawn. The pathologist rarely makes specific diagnoses of drug-related intestinal injury, except in gastric biopsies with reactive changes caused by nonsteroidal antiinflammatory drugs (NSAIDs) and in colonic biopsies in which the finding of melanosis coli is drug-induced.

NSAIDs are being increasingly implicated as an important cause of gastrointestinal complications in patients using these agents on a long-term basis.[45] The following changes have been attributed to NSAIDs:

1. Gastric epithelial injury resulting in acute erosive gastropathy and reactive gastropathy.
2. Acute enteritis and colitis, resulting in diarrhea, steatorrhea, and protein-losing enteropathy.
3. Microscopic colitis, causing watery diarrhea.

TABLE 8–4. DRUG-ASSOCIATED INTESTINAL DISEASES

Pseudomembranous Enterocolitis
    Antibiotics
        Clindamycin and lincomycin
        Cephalosporins
        Ampicillin
    Others
        Chlorpropamide
        Mercury-containing laxatives
        NSAIDs
        Gold
Hemorrhage
    Anticoagulants
Arterial or Venous Thrombosis with Ischemia
    Oral contraceptives
    Estrogen
Inflammation (Colitis, Enteritis) or Ulceration
    NSAIDs
    Gold
    Potassium chloride
    Iron
    5-Flucytosine
    Methyldopa
    Clofazimine (granulomatous enteritis)
Melanosis Coli
    Anthraquinone laxatives
Pseudo-Obstruction (myenteric plexus damage)
    Phenothiazines
    Antidepressants

4. Ulcers in the small intestine and cecum, sometimes resulting in significant hemorrhage and perforation.
5. Strictures and mucosal webs, causing intestinal obstruction.

Many of these conditions, when encountered in biopsy or surgical resection specimens, usually receive nonspecific pathologic diagnoses. Careful clinical correlation and the knowledge of dosages and temporal relationships of drug usage is required by the pathologist to even attempt to reach the conclusion that the pathology is caused by drug toxicity. Unfortunately, this information is rarely available to the pathologist.

VASCULAR DISEASES

Ischemia of the small intestine results from inadequate perfusion caused by abnormalities in the superior mesenteric arterial circulation. The majority of cases occur in patients over the age of 60 years with severe generalized atherosclerosis, who become hypovolemic for any reason (eg, myocarcial infarction, dehydration, cardiac dysrhythmia). In these patients, no occlusion of the vessels is evident; hypoperfusion results from the effect of splanchnic vasoconstriction in a compromised mesenteric arterial system. This is called nonocclusive mesenteric ischemia. A smaller number of cases result from superior mesenteric artery thrombosis, embolism, ostial narrowing due to aortic diseases such as aortic aneurysm and Takayasu's arteritis, mesenteric venous occlusion, and vasculitis.

The pathologic changes and clinical manifestations depend on the severity of ischemia. In mild cases, the pathologic abnormalities are minimal and the patient manifests intermittent abdominal pain, usually after meals ("abdominal angina"). In severe cases, intestinal infarction occurs. Infarction causes severe abdominal pain, vomiting, and bloody diarrhea, progressing rapidly to shock and death if not treated emergently. The infarcted bowel is rapidly invaded by luminal bacteria, resulting in gangrene, perforation, and acute peritonitis. Treatment is to resect the infarcted bowel, ideally before perforation, peritonitis, and shock have developed.

At surgery, determining the extent of resection depends on the extent of infarction. If infarction is limited, a generous margin of viable bowel can be removed. When infarction involves a large enough length of intestine to raise questions about the possibility of short-gut syndrome, conservative resection, leaving behind questionably viable intestine, is indicated; in these cases a second-look operation 1–2 days later can be performed to ensure intestinal viability. Intraoperative pathologic assessment of viability of intestine by frozen section has no value; pathologic changes of necrosis of the muscle wall take several days to develop sufficiently to be recognized by light microscopy.

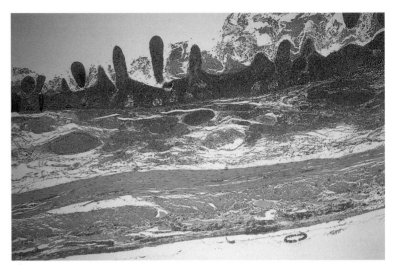

A

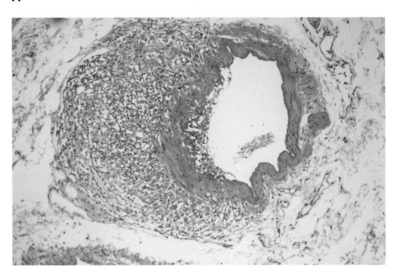

B

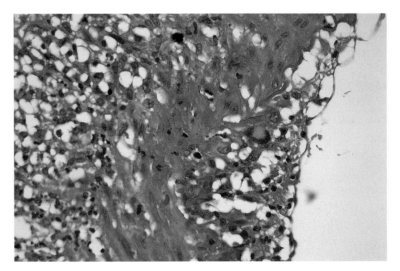

C

Figure 8–30. A: Small-bowel infarction, showing mucosal necrosis and hemorrhage. Note the presence of numerous neutrophils in the wall of the small blood vessel in the submucosa. B: Small artery in submucosa of small bowel in a case of ischemia secondary to vasculitis. Note the absence of inflammation in the submucosa and the uninvolved vein (*bottom*). C: Higher power micrograph of part B, showing fibrinoid necosis of the media and inflammation with histiocytes and a giant cell involving intima and perivascular tissue.

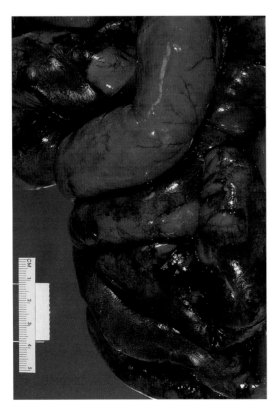

Figure 8–29. Ischemia of the small bowel, showing varying stages of gangrene of the intestine. Some loops are green, others are purple. None has the black color seen in Figure 8–8.

The resected bowel shows variable changes. In severe cases, the necrotic bowel appears blackish green with areas of perforation and peritoneal exudate (Fig. 8–29). More frequently, changes are not severe, and the bowel shows patchy purplish discoloration and a normal shiny peritoneal surface. The mucosa is always more severely affected than the muscle and shows necrosis, edema, hemorrhage, erosions, and linear ulcerations (Fig. 8–30A). In severe cases, extensive mucosal necrosis may cause diffuse pseudomembranous appearance. In most cases, the mesentery is not resected, and it is not possible to dissect the mesenteric vessels in an attempt to identify the cause of ischemia.

Sections are taken from the intestinal surgical margins in all cases to assess viability. This provides clinically significant information only when transmural necrosis is present at the margin. The presence of transmural necrosis at a margin indicates that resection has been through necrotic intestine; these patients are at high risk for developing anastomotic leaks and breakdown. Many cases have mucosal necrosis at the surgical margin (Fig. 8–30A); this has no bearing on intestinal viability. Cases that have no necrosis of the muscle wall at histologic assessment may or may not have nonviable margins because microscopic changes of necrosis often take several days to appear.

Rare cases of intestinal ischemia result from vasculitic diseases such as polyarteritis nodosa and systemic lupus erythematosus. These involve medium- and small-sized vessels and cause a patchy necrosis of the small bowel depending on the severity of vasculitis (Figs. 8–30B and C). Vasculitis should be considered when intestinal ischemia occurs in patients younger than age 40 years and in those who have multifocal ischemia that does not fit into a pattern of involvement of a single artery of supply. Evaluation of resected specimens for vasculitis is difficult because secondary vascular changes are commonly present in relation to ulcers and necrosis (Fig. 8–31). The presence of vasculitis away from inflamed and ulcerated areas should be reported by the pathologist; these cases should be studied clinically for the possibility of a systemic vasculitis.

TUMORS OF THE SMALL INTESTINE (EXCEPT DUODENUM)

Benign Neoplasms

Benign neoplasms are extremely uncommon, except for hamartomas in Peutz-Jeghers syndrome and adenomas in patients with familial adenomatous polyposis. Adenomas occur very rarely distal to the ligament of Treitz and are not detected unless they form the apex of an intussusception or become malignant (Fig. 8–32). The rarity of both these events and the unlikelihood of finding incidental adenomas of the small intestine at autopsy is testimony to the extreme rarity of these tumors.[46] Benign mesenchymal neoplasms, such as lipomas, lymphangiomas, hemangiomas, and neurofibromas, do occur, but also rarely. Benign mesenchymal neoplasms are considered in Chapter 15.

Inflammatory Fibroid Polyp

Inflammatory fibroid polyp (also called inflammatory pseudotumor) is a benign tumor encountered throughout the GI tract. They occur most commonly in the gastric antrum and the small intestine. They can reach a size exceeding 10 cm and cause intestinal obstruction. Intestinal obstruction may also result from intussusception induced by these polyps. The cause of inflam-

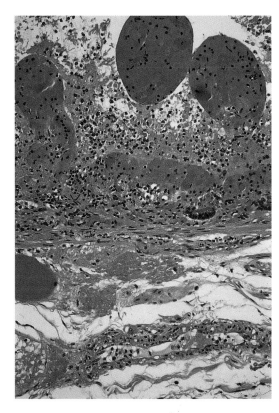

Figure 8–31. Small-bowel infarction, showing hemorrhagic necrosis of the mucosa. Note the small vessel in the submucosa with evidence of acute vasculitis.

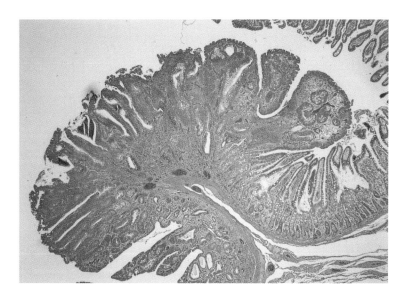

Figure 8–32. Polypoid adenoma of the small intestine. This was found in a patient who had a resection for a nearby adenocarcinoma of the small intestine. There was no history of adenomatous polyposis coli.

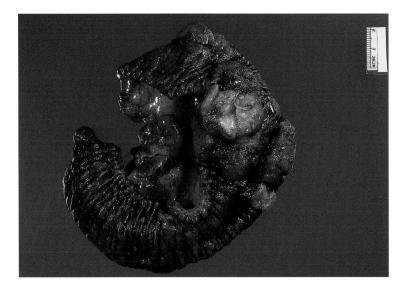

Figure 8–33. Inflammatory fibroid polyp of small intestine, showing an almost sessile mass lesion.

matory fibroid polyps is unknown; the early literature incorrectly suggested that they were polypoid forms of eosinophilic gastroenteritis. A recent report raises the possibility that they may occur as a reaction to damage caused by NSAIDs.[47]

Inflammatory fibroid polyps are sessile or pedunculated masses that project into the lumen of the intestine (Figs. 8–33 and 8–34). The interior of the polyp beneath the surface ulcer is composed of a markedly expanded submucosa made up of loose myxomatous tissue containing a capillary network, stellate stromal cells, and a mixed inflammatory cell infiltrate that is usually dominated by eosinophils (Fig. 8–35). Plasma cells and mast cells can also be prominent. The base of the process frequently extends into the superficial muscularis externa. Some cases show prominent collagen deposition and increased numbers of fibroblasts. The fibroblasts commonly show reactive cytologic atypia. Mitotic figures may be present in the stromal cells. The mucosa covering the polyp frequently shows ulceration and infiltration with numerous eosinophils.

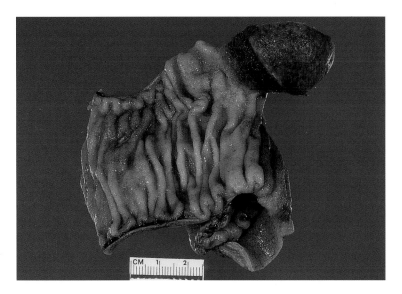

Figure 8–34. Inflammatory fibroid polyp, showing pedunculated polyp with hemorrhage at the tip; this had caused intussusception.

Mesenteric Tumors Involving the Small Intestine

Two unusual mesenteric tumors can secondarily involve the small intestine. These present as mass lesions perceived clinically and radiologically as small-intestinal tumors and are treated by resection of the small intestine.

Mesenteric Fibromatosis

Mesenteric fibromatosis is commonly seen in patients with Gardner's syndrome (Fig. 8–36A).[48] It has features typical of desmoid fibromatosis, consisting of a diffusely infiltrative fibroblastic proliferation of low cellularity. The fibroblasts are uniform, without significant cytologic atypia or mitotic activity, and usually have abundant intercellular collagen, which may have a keloidal appearance (Fig. 8–36B). The fibroblastic proliferation commonly infiltrates the wall of the small intestine and may sometimes reach the mucosal surface. These tumors can reach a large size and cause intestinal obstruction. They should be regarded as low-grade malignant neoplasms and treated with surgical resection with wide margins. Recurrences after surgery are common.

Inflammatory Pseudotumor of the Mesentery

This unusual tumor of the mesentery, also called sclerosing mesenteritis, forms a poorly defined mass lesion that commonly reaches a large size, involves the small-intestinal wall, and causes intestinal obstruction.[49] The terms "mesenteric panniculitis" and "xanthogranuloma" are also used for this lesion. It is composed microscopically of a mixed cellular infiltrate of moderate cellularity. Foamy macrophages and fibroblasts dominate. Lymphocytes, plasma cells, and neutrophils are also present. The tumors frequently show marked fibrosis, resulting in distortion and retraction of the mesentery and small intestine. The cause of this lesion is unknown, but some of these tumors have a locally aggressive behavior with recurrences after surgical excision.

Carcinoid Tumor

Carcinoid tumors are tumors derived from the neuroendocrine cells of the small intestine. The majority have typical histologic features of carcinoid tumor, with an insular pattern, small uniform cells, and serotonin secretion. Tumors producing other hormones are very rare. Small-intestinal carcinoids are multiple in 30% of cases.[50] About half the patients have a second, noncarcinoid, neoplasm of the GI tract.[51]

Classifications

Since the original application of the term "carcinoid tumor" to small-intestinal tumors, similar tumors have been recognized in the rest of the GI tract and the bronchus. The term "carcinoid tumor" is also used for these tumors. Based on their derivation, carcinoid tumors have been classified as foregut, midgut, and hindgut carcinoid tumors (Table 8–5). The value of argyrophil

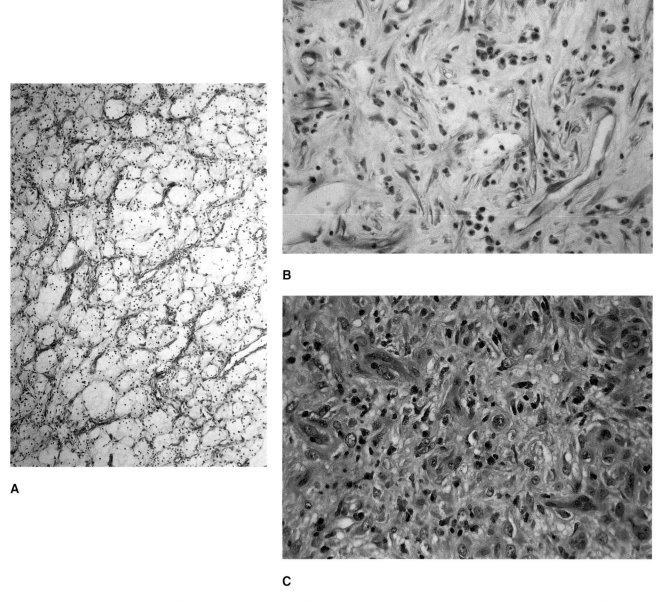

Figure 8–35. A: Inflammatory fibroid polyp, showing cellular proliferation under the flattened mucosa at the surface of the polyp. B: Inflammatory fibroid polyp, showing network of capillaries, myxomatous background, and eosinophils. C: Inflammatory fibroid polyp, showing a more cellular, fibroblastic area with reactive spindle cells, eosinophils, and numerous blood vessels.

TABLE 8–5. CARCINOID TUMORS

	Foregut	Midgut	Hindgut
Location	Stomach, duodenum	Midduodenum to splenic flexure	Splenic flexure to rectum
Histologic pattern	Trabecular and cord-like	Insular	Trabecular and microacinar
Desmoplasia	Negative	Positive	Negative
Argyrophilia*	Majority positive	Majority positive	Majority negative
Argentaffinic*	Negative	Positive	Negative
Secretion	Gastrin, serotonin, nonfunctional	Serotonin	Nonfunctional
Malignancy	Intermediate	Ileal—high Appendix—low	Colon—high Rectum—intermediate

*Argentaffinic cells can reduce silver salts; argyrophilic cells cannot reduce silver salts but can take up silver if exogenous reducing substances were added, as in the Grimelius staining technique.

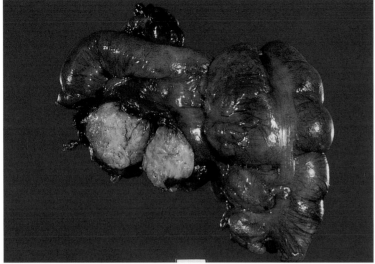

A

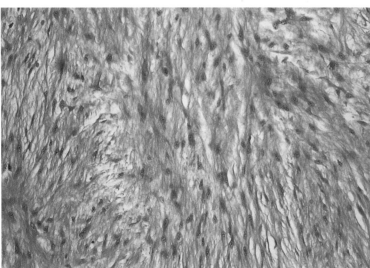

B

Figure 8–36. A: Mesenteric fibromatosis, showing a right hemicolectomy specimen with the mesechymal mesenteric neoplasm sectioned. This tumor showed infiltration through the terminal ileal wall to reach the submucosa. B: Mesenteric fibromatosis, showing the uniform fibroblastic proliferation of low cellularity associated with abundant intercellular collagen.

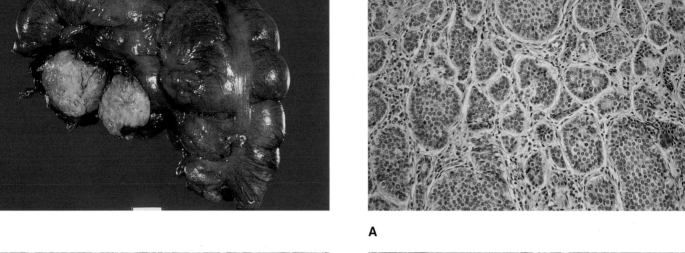

A

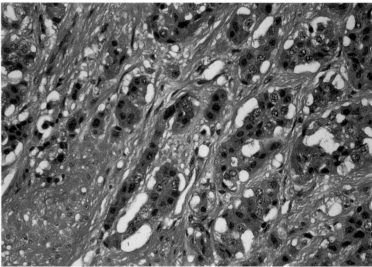

B

Figure 8–37. A: Typical carcinoid tumor, microscopic appearance, showing insular pattern. The small, uniform, round cells are arranged in nests separated by vascular connective tissue. B: Atypical carcinoid tumor of small intestine, showing nuclear pleomorphism and atypia.

and argentaffin staining have decreased with the availability of immunoperoxidase staining for neuroendocrine markers such as chromogranin A, neuron-specific enolase, and synaptophysin. Electron microscopy, which shows cytoplasmic dense core granules in the cells of carcinoid tumors, is rarely necessary.

Carcinoid tumors are also recognized as forming a histologic spectrum from typical carcinoids, which are cytologically uniform (Fig. 8–37A), through atypical carcinoids, which have the typical architecture of carcinoid tumors but show cytologic atypia and increased mitotic activity (Fig. 8–37B), to neuroendocrine carcinomas. The risk of malignancy increases with atypia; neuroendocrine carcinomas are high-grade malignant neoplasms that are rarely differentiated from poorly differentiated carcinomas unless neuroendocrine marker stains are done.

Carcinoid tumors also have varying degrees of admixture with glandular elements. These include (1) composite adenocarcinoma–carcinoid tumors, in which an approximately equal admixture of the two tumor types occurs, and (2) tumors whose individual cells show both neuroendocrine and glandular features, most commonly the presence of mucin secretion (Fig. 8–38)—adenocarcinoid tumors. Carcinoid tumors with glandular admixture occur in the stomach (Chapter 5) and appendix (Chapter 9), but are rarely seen in the small intestine.

Finally, carcinoid tumors can be classified by the hormones they secrete. Foregut carcinoid tumors are either nonfunctional or secrete gastrin or serotonin; midgut tumors secrete serotonin; hindgut carcinoids are nonfunctional. Many nonfunctional carcinoid tumors can be shown by immunostaining to contain hormones in the cytoplasm. Such immuno-

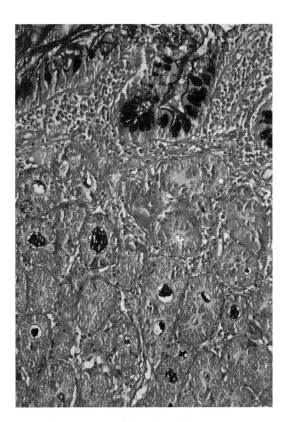

Figure 8–38. Carcinoid tumor, stained with digested PAS, showing mucin in a microacinar component of the tumor.

histochemical demonstration of cytoplasmic hormone does not constitute evidence of function for clinical purposes.

Clinical Features

Small-intestinal carcinoids present with intestinal obstruction, evidence of liver metastases, or functional symptoms resulting from hormonal secretions.

In patients who present with intestinal obstruction, the diagnosis of carcinoid tumor is rarely made preoperatively. At surgery, a tumor, or, more commonly, a distorted piece of thickened small intestine is found at the point of obstruction and resected. Intraoperative pathologic examination is valuable in these cases, because if a diagnosis of carcinoid tumor is made before the abdomen is closed, a careful search can be made for other carcinoid tumors and for evidence of metastasis in lymph nodes and liver. When the diagnosis of carcinoid tumors is known intraoperatively in a patient with obstruction, a cancer resection with removal of regional lymph nodes should be performed. This is indicated even when liver metastases are present.[52]

Liver metastases are not an uncommon mode of presentation of a carcinoid tumor. Fine-needle aspiration of a liver nodule permits specific cytologic diagnosis of carcinoid tumor based on morphologic and immunohistochemical findings (Fig. 8–39).

The carcinoid syndrome is a rare mode of clinical presentation of a small-intestinal carcinoid. Although these tumors secrete serotonin into the portal circulation, this hormone is

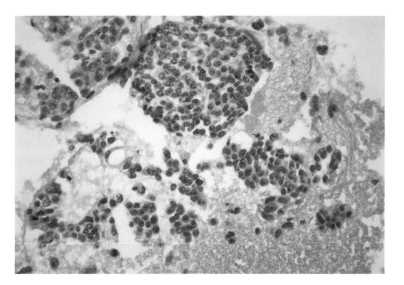

A

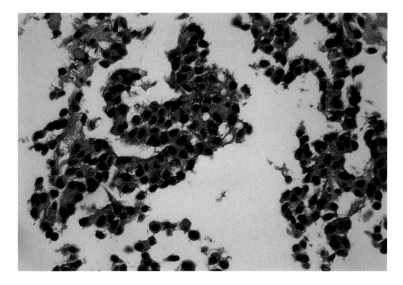

B

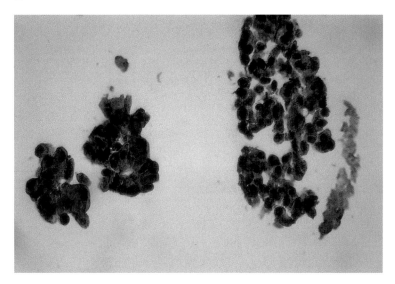

C

Figure 8–39. A: Liver, fine-needle aspiration, showing metastatic carcinoid tumor, characterized by clusters of small, uniform cells. B: Liver, fine-needle aspiration, cell block, showing small cells with round nuclei arranged in cohesive groups. C: Liver, cell block preparation, stained with chromogranin A, showing strong positivity of the neoplastic cells.

rapidly inactivated in the liver and does not enter the systemic circulation. Carcinoid syndrome results from entry of serotonin into the systemic circulation. This usually occurs in patients who have multiple liver metastases that secrete serotonin directly into the hepatic vein. More rarely, patients with cirrhosis who have high-volume porto-systemic venous shunting may develop carcinoid syndrome without liver metastases. Entry of serotonin into the systemic circulation causes cutaneous vasodilatation (episodic cyanotic flushing of the skin of the face) (Fig. 8–40), bronchospasm (asthma), stimulation of intestinal peristalsis (cramping abdominal pain and explosive diarrhea), and cardiac valve fibrosis (pulmonic valve stenosis).

Rare patients with the carcinoid syndrome develop intestinal ischemia, sometimes leading to infarction and death. Intestinal ischemia results from (1) direct involvement of the mesenteric arteries by tumor and desmoplastic response associated with the tumor, and (2) elastic vascular sclerosis in the mesenteric vessels. This is a peculiar obliterative, proliferative vasculopathy that is believed to be caused by serotonin.[53]

Pathologic Features

Grossly, small-intestinal carcinoid tumors have two presentations:

1. They form submucosal nodules that project into the lumen and are covered by normal mucosa. These tumors vary in size; the larger ones infiltrate the muscle wall, often extending into mesenteric fat. On cut section, these tumors have a typical yellow color.

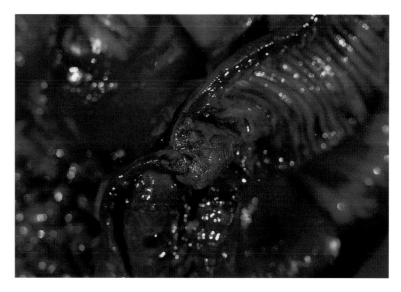

Figure 8–41. Carcinoid tumor, small intestine, showing a small polypoid mass with an indrawing of the intestinal wall due to sclerosis, producing the typical knuckle-like deformity.

2. Desmoplastic carcinoid tumors are associated with dense fibrosis. This causes marked distortion and a localized kinking of the bowel wall (Figs. 8–41 and 8–42); frequently the tumor appears as a knuckle-shaped mass of dense fibrosis, which obstructs the lumen with the entire muscularis externa drawn into the luminal knuckle of tissue. These tumors have a white cut surface and can be extremely hard to cut.

Microscopically, these are typical carcinoid tumors with an insular pattern consisting of nests of small uniform cells with round nuclei that show the typical granular ("salt-and-pepper") chromatin pattern (Fig. 8–43A–B). Desmoplastic tumors show dense fibrosis with distortion of the tumor nests (Fig. 8–43C, D). In some cases, fibrosis dominates to an extent that neoplastic cells are reduced to small insignificant nests of cells amidst the dense collagen (Fig. 8–43D). Lymphovascular invasion is common, even in small carcinoid tumors (Fig. 8–44). The tumor fre-

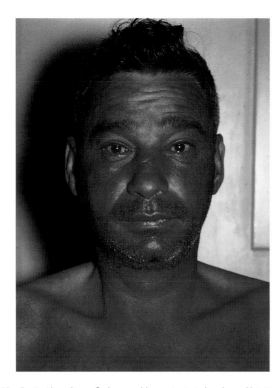

Figure 8–40. Carcinoid syndrome flush, caused by serotonin-induced vasodilatation in cutaneous vessels.

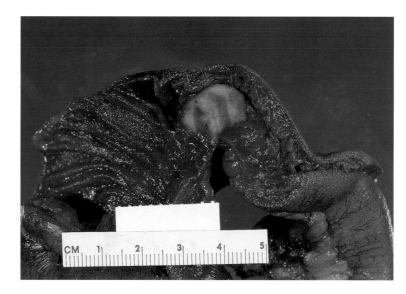

Figure 8–42. Carcinoid tumor, showing the typical knuckle-shaped distortion of the wall of the small intestine resulting from fibrosis associated with the tumor.

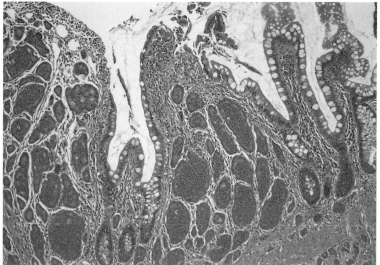

A

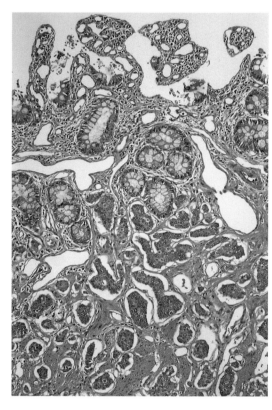

B

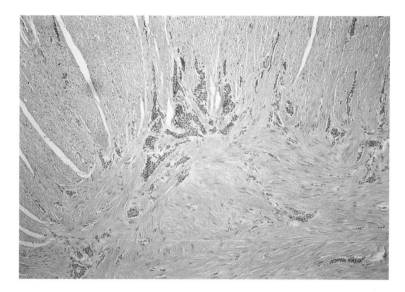

C

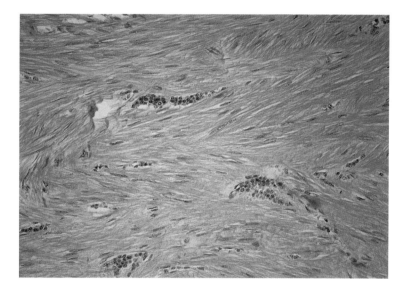

D

Figure 8–43. A: Carcinoid tumor in the small-intestinal mucosa, showing typical insular pattern of midgut carcinoid tumors. B: Small-intestinal carcinoid tumor, showing irregular involvement of the mucosa with carcinoid tumor having an insular architecture. C: Desmoplastic carcinoid tumor, showing dense sclerosis of the serosa beneath the muscularis externa. The tumor is seen in the muscle, but is scanty within the desmoplastic tissue. D: Desmoplastic carcinoid tumor, showing small collection of carcinoid tumor within the dense fibrous tissue.

quently infiltrates the muscle wall in an irregular manner, often extending into the mesenteric fat (Fig. 8–45).

Carcinoid tumors of the small intestine frequently show evidence of metastases, usually to regional lymph nodes. Metastasis to the liver is common. Even with liver metastases, patients with carcinoid tumors have a median length of survival of 3 years because of the slow rate of growth of the tumor.[54]

Prognosis

Small-intestinal carcinoids have a high incidence of malignancy. Tumors that are larger than 0.5 cm have a metastatic potential; the likelihood of metastasis increases with the size of the primary tumor. Ninety-five percent of small intestinal carcinoids larger than 2 cm show metastasis.[54] For these reasons, small-intestinal carcinoids of all sizes are considered malignant. The overall 5-year survival rate of patients with small-intestinal carcinoids is 60%, but many patients surviving 5 years ultimately succumb to the effects of the tumor.

Adenocarcinoma

Although the small intestine comprises 90% of the mucosal surface area of the GI tract, small-intestinal adenocarcinoma accounts for only 1% of gastrointestinal carcinomas. Despite its

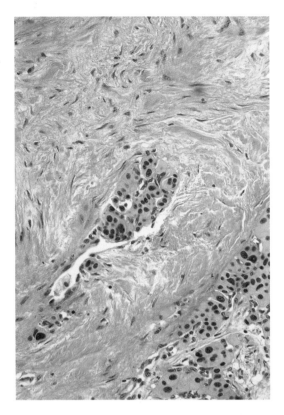

Figure 8–44. Vascular invasion in small-intestinal carcinoid tumor.

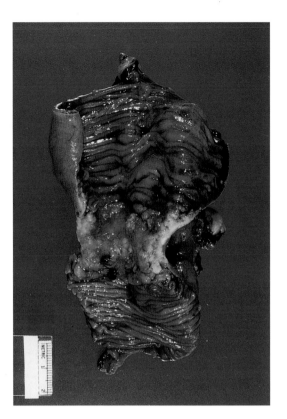

Figure 8–46. Small-intestinal adenocarcinoma, showing a circumferential sclerosing lesion associated with intestinal obstruction.

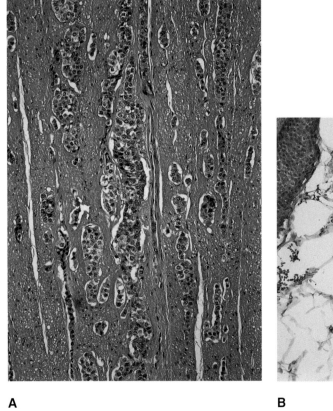

A

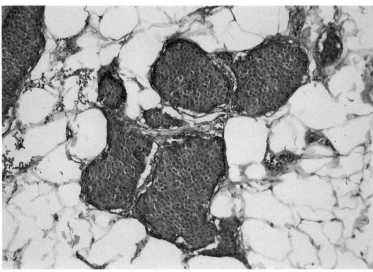

B

Figure 8–45. Invasion of small bowel carcinoid tumor into A: muscularis externa, and B: mesenteric fat.

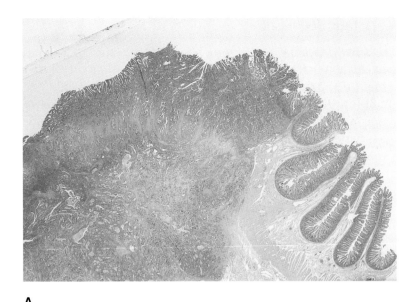

A

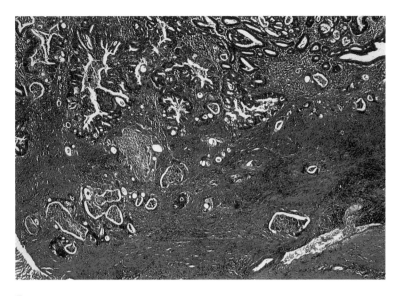

B

Figure 8–47. A: Small-intestinal adenocarcinoma, showing a well-differentiated adenocarcinoma arising in a villous adenoma. B: Small-intestinal adenocarcinoma, moderately differentiated, infiltrating the submucosa and associated with extensive lymphatic invasion.

rarity, adenocarcinoma is the commonest malignancy of the small intestine in most series, being slightly more common than malignant lymphoma, carcinoid tumor, and GI stromal tumor.[55]

The following conditions are associated with an increased risk of small-intestinal adenocarcinoma: familial adenomatous polyposis, celiac disease, Crohn's disease, Peutz-Jeghers syndrome, and ileal conduits.

Small-intestinal adenocarcinoma is rarely diagnosed specifically before surgery. Clinical symptoms are the result of intestinal obstruction and hemorrhage due to mucosal ulceration. In the small intestine, the majority of adenocarcinomas involve the periampullary region (see Chapter 6). Seventy-five percent of tumors in the jejunum and ileum are annular constricting lesions with circumferential mucosal ulceration

(Fig. 8–46); exophytic tumors account for the remainder. Microscopically, most are well-differentiated adenocarcinomas (Fig. 8–47); rarely, poorly differentiated carcinomas, including signet ring cell carcinomas, occur (Fig. 8–48). Small-intestinal adenocarcinoma has an overall resectability rate of 50% and an overall 5-year survival rate of 20%. The poor prognosis of small-intestinal carcinoma is due to the inaccessibility of these tumors, resulting in late-stage presentation. Chemotherapy and radiation offer minimal benefit.

GI Stromal Neoplasm and Malignant Lymphoma

These two small-intestinal tumors are discussed in Chapters 14 and 15, respectively.

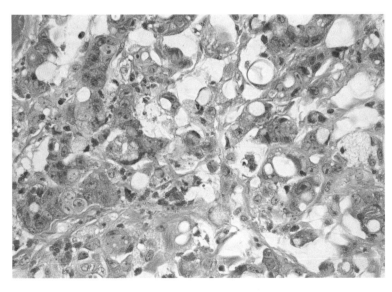

A

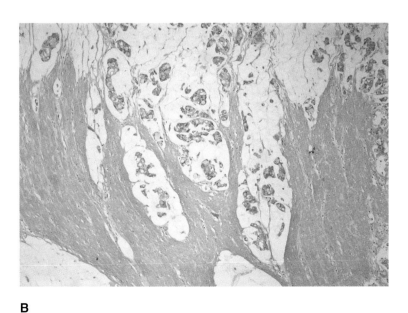

B

Figure 8–48. A: Poorly differentiated adenocarcinoma, small intestine, showing scattered signet ring cells. B: Poorly differentiated adenocarcinoma, small intestine, with signet ring cells and abundant extracellular mucin. The tumor is shown infiltrating the muscularis externa.

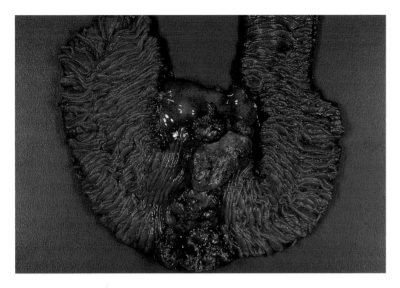

A

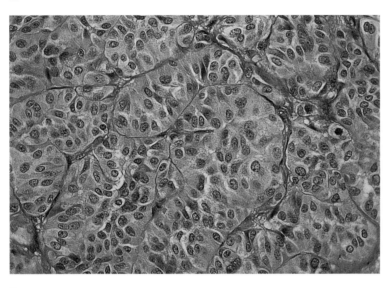

B

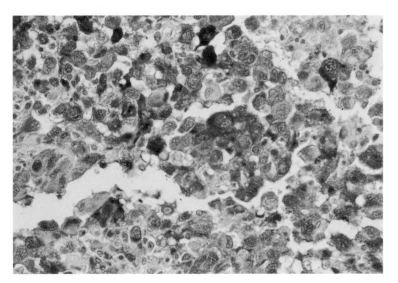

C

Figure 8–49. A: Malignant melanoma, metastatic to the small intestine. B: Poorly differentiated malignant neoplasm in small intestine, characterized by nests of poorly differentiated malignant cells without pigment. C: Immunoperoxidase stain for S100 protein in metastatic malignant melanoma of small intestine, showing positive staining.

Metastatic Neoplasm

The small intestine is a common site of metastasis of malignant melanoma, occurring in over 1% of all patients with malignant melanoma (Fig. 8–49A). In many of these patients, the small-intestinal metastasis represents the only evidence of metastatic disease. In such cases, the solitary, large, tumor mass may be mistaken for a GI stromal neoplasm or poorly differentiated carcinoma when no history of prior melanoma is provided. If the tumor is achromatic, immunoperoxidase staining is necessary for diagnosis (see Fig. 8–49) (see Chapter 14). Surgical resection of solitary metastases of melanoma in the small intestine has been shown to improve survival in these patients.[56]

Metastases to the small intestine from other sites are extremely rare. We have encountered metastases from a squamous carcinoma of the cervix (Fig. 8–50) and testicular germ cell neoplasm with choriocarcinomatous elements (Fig. 8–51). Involvement of the small intestine by disseminated lymphomas and leukemias is more common, but rarely leads to surgical resection. We have seen acute myeloblastic leukemia (granulocytic sarcoma) present as a small-intestinal mass (Fig. 8–52).

Evaluation of a Small-Intestinal Resection for Neoplasm

Resection specimens for small-bowel cancers include the regional lymph nodes. These specimens are handled similarly to colon cancer resection specimens. Staging is by the tumor, node, metastasis (TNM) system adopted for small-bowel carcinomas by the American Joint Committee on Cancer (Table 8–6).[57] Due to the rarity of small-intestinal cancers, the prognostic value of this staging system has not been established.[58]

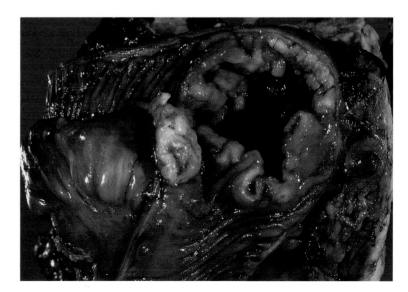

Figure 8–50. Metastatic squamous carcinoma in small intestine, characterized by a large fungating mass. The primary tumor was a carcinoma of the uterine cervix.

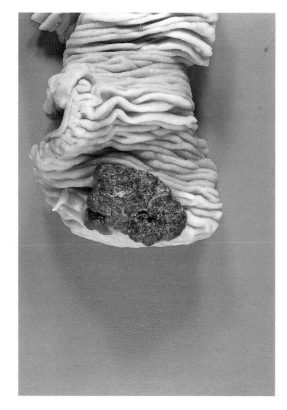

A

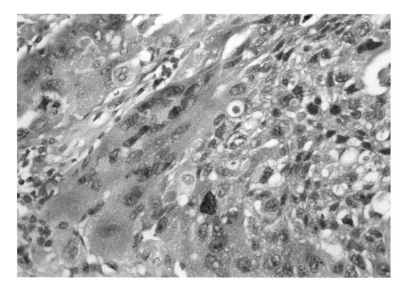

B

Figure 8–51. A: Metastatic germ cell neoplasm from the testis. B: Metastatic germ cell tumor of the testis, showing choriocarcinoma.

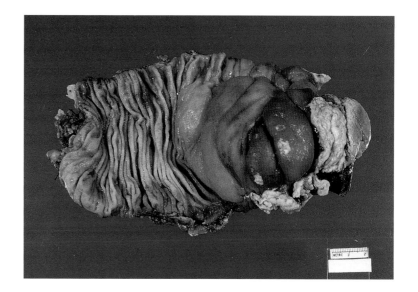

A

B

Figure 8–52. A: Acute myeloblastic leukemia involving the terminal ileum. B: Acute myeloblastic leukemia, showing undifferentiated malignant neoplasm. This showed myeloperoxidase positivity.

References

1. Moore TC. High jejunal atresia with midgut deletion. *J Pediatr Surg.* 1986;21:951–952.
2. Fan ST, Lay WY, Pang SW. Infarction of a duodenal duplication cyst. *Am J Gastroenterol.* 1985;80:337–339.
3. Newmark H. Bleeding peptic ulcer caused by ectopic gastric mucosa in the duplicated segment of jejunum. *Am J Gastroenterol.* 1981;75:158–162.
4. Adair HM, Trowell JE. Squamous cell carcinoma arising in a duplication of the small bowel. *J Pathol.* 1981;133:25–31.
5. Rubin SZ, Mancer JF, Stephens CA. Carcinoid in a rectal duplication: A unique pediatric surgical problem. *Canad J Surg.* 1981;24:351–352.
6. Taylor RH, Owen DA. Acute inflammation of pancreatic tissue in Meckel's diverticulum. *Canad J Surg.* 1982;25:656–657.

TABLE 8–6. STAGING CRITERIA FOR SMALL-INTESTINAL ADENOCARCINOMA

Stage	Staging Criteria
Stage I:	Tumor invades submucosa or partial thickness of the muscularis externa.
Stage II:	Tumor invades through the muscularis externa into mesenteric fat.
Stage III:	Regional lymph nodes are positive.
Stage IV:	Distant metastases are present.

7. Williamson RC, Cooper MJ, Thomas WE. Intussusception of invaginated Meckel's diverticulum. *J Roy Soc Med.* 1984; 77:652–655.

8. Honore LH. Endometriosis of Meckel's diverticulum associated with intestinal obstruction—a case report. *Am J Proctol.* 1980;31:11–12.

9. Nies C, Zielke A, Hasse C, et al. Carcinoid tumors of Meckel's diverticula. Report of two cases and review of the literature. *Dis Colon Rectum.* 1992;35:589–596.

10. Chen KT, Workman RD, Kirkegaard DD. Adenocarcinoma of Meckel's diverticulum. *J Surg Oncol.* 1983;23:41–42.

11. Saadia R, Decker GA. Leiomyosarcoma of Meckel's diverticulum: A case report and review of the literature. *J Surg Oncol.* 1986;32:86–88.

12. Krishnamurthy S, Schuffler MD. Pathology of neuromuscular disorders of the small intestine and colon. *Gastroenterology.* 1987;93:610.

13. Vanek VW, Al-Salti M. Acute pseudo-obstruction of the colon (Ogilvie's syndrome): An analysis of 400 cases. *Dis Colon Rectum.* 1986;29:203–210.

14. Debinski HS, Kamm MA, Talbot IC, et al. DNA viruses in the pathogenesis of sporadic chronic idiopathic intestinal pseudo-obstruction. *Gut.* 1997;41:100–106.

15. Schuffler MD, Jonak Z. Chronic idiopathic intestinal pseudo-obstruction caused by degenerative disorder of the myenteric plexus: The use of Smith's method to define the neuropathology. *Gastroenterology.* 1982;82:476–486.

16. Anuras S, Mitros FA, Nowak TV, et al. A familial visceral myopathy with external ophthalmoplegia and autosomal recessive transmission. *Gastroenterology.* 1983;84:346–353.

17. Mitros FA, Schuffler MD, Teja K, et al. Pathologic features of familial visceral myopathy. *Hum Pathol.* 1982;13:825–833.

18. Fitzgibbons PL, Chandrasoma PT. Familial visceral myopathy. Evidence of diffuse involvement of intestinal smooth muscle. *Am J Surg Pathol.* 1987;11:846–854.

19. Fogel SP, DeTar MW, Shimada H, et al. Sporadic visceral myopathy with inclusion bodies. A light microscopic and ultrastructural study. *Am J Surg Pathol.* 1993;17:473–481.

20. Cohen S, Laufer I, Snape WJ, et al. The gastrointestinal manifestations of scleroderma: Pathogenesis and management. *Gastroenterology.* 1980;79:155–166.

21. Smith JH. Typhoid fever. *In* Binford CH, Connor DH (eds). *Pathology of Tropical and Extraordinary Diseases.* Washington, DC, Armed Forces Institute of Pathology, 1976. pp. 123–129.

22. Badejo OA, Arigbabu AO. Operative treatment of typhoid perforation with peritoneal irrigation: A comparative study. *Gut.* 1980;21:141–145.

23. Mitchell R, Bristol L. Intestinal tuberculosis. Analysis of 346 cases diagnosed by routine intestinal radiography of 5529 admissions for pulmonary tuberculosis, 1924–1949. *Am J Med Sci.* 1954;227:241–249.

24. Schulze K, Warner HA, Murray DA. Intestinal tuberculosis: Experiences at a Canadian teaching institution. *Am J Med.* 1977;63:735–745.

25. Lax JD, Haroutiounian G, Attia A, et al. Tuberculosis of the rectum in a patient with acquired immune deficiency syndrome. Report of a case. *Dis Colon Rectum.* 1988;31:347–349.

26. Anand SS. Hypertrophic ileo-cecal tuberculosis in India with a record of 50 hemicolectomies. *Ann Roy Coll Surg.* 1956;19:687–692.

27. El-Maraghi NRH, Mair NS. The histopathology of enteric infection with *Yersinia pseudotuberculosis. Am J Clin Pathol.* 1979;71:631–639.

28. Jess P. Acute terminal ileitis. *Scand J Gastroenterol.* 1981;16:321–324.

29. Cappell MS, Mandell W, Grimes MM, et al. Gastrointestinal histoplasmosis. *Dig Dis Sci.* 1988;33:353–360.

30. Lyon DT, Schubert TT, Mantia AG, et al. Phycomycosis of the gastrointestinal tract. *Am J Gastroenterol.* 1979;72: 379–394.

31. Chandrasoma PT, de Silva S, Yoganathan M. Roundworm granuloma of the anterior abdominal wall. *Postgrad Med J.* 1978;54:103–107.

32. Chandrasoma PT, Mendis KN. Ectopic Enterobius vermicularis in ectopic sites. *Am J Trop Med Hyg.* 1977;26:644–649.

33. Hulbert TV, Larsen RA, Chandrasoma PT. Abdominal angiostrongyliasis mimicking acute appendicitis and Meckel's diverticulum—Report of a case in the United States with a review of the literature. *Clin Infect Dis.* 1992;14:836–840.

34. Yeing ML, Nicholson GI. *Clostridium septicum* infection in neutropenic enterocolitis. *Pathology.* 1988;20:194–197.

35. Kunkel JM, Rosenthal D. Management of the ileocecal syndrome: Neutropenic enterocolitis. *Dis Colon Rectum.* 1986;29:196–199.

36. Lee M, Hodges WG, Huggins TL, et al. Eosinophilic gastroenteritis. *South Med J.* 1996;89:189–194.

37. Matshushita M, Hajiro K, Morita Y, et al. Eosinophilic gastroenteritis involving the entire digestive tract. *Am J Gastroenterol.* 1995;90:1868–1870.

38. Rumans MC, Lieberman DA. Eosinophilic gastroenteritis presenting with biliary and duodenal obstruction. *Am J Gastroenterol.* 1987;82:775.

39. Kuri K, Lee M. Eosinophilic gastroenteritis manifesting with ascites. *South Med J.* 1994;87:956–957.

40. Foglia RP. Necrotizing enterocolitis. *Curr Probl Surg.* 1995;32:757–823.

41. Balance WA, Dahms BB, Shenker N, et al. Pathology of neonatal enterocolitis: A ten year experience. *Pediatrics.* 1990;117:S6–13.

42. Heng Y, Schuffler MD, Haggitt RC, et al. Pneumatosis intestinalis: A review. *Am J Gastroenterol.* 1995;90:1747–1758.

43. Waring J, Manne R, Wadas D, et al. Mucosal pseudolipomatosis: An air-pressure related colonoscopy complication. *Gastrointest Endosc.* 1980;35:93–94.

44. Mehta SN, Friedman G, Fried GM, et al. Pneumatosis cystoides intestinalis: Laparoscopic features. *Am J Gastroenterol.* 1996;91:2610–2612.

45. Bjarnson I, Hayllar J, MacPherson AJ, et al. Side effects of nonsteroidal anti-inflammatory drugs on the small and large intestine in humans. *Gastroenterology.* 1993;104:1832.

46. Perzin KH, Bridge MF. Adenomas of the small intestine. A clinicopathologic review of 51 cases and a study of their relationship to carcinoma. *Cancer.* 1981;48:799–819.

47. Muniz-Grijalvo O, Reina-Campos F, Borderas F. Could a fibroid polyp be a manifestation of enteropathy induced by nonsteroidal anti-inflammatory drugs? *Am J Gastroenterol.* 1997;92:170–171.

48. Richards RC, Rogers SW, Gardner EJ. Spontaneous mesenteric fibromatosis in Gardner's syndrome. *Cancer.* 1981; 47:597–601.

49. Sheinfeld A, Rubinow A, Steiner A, et al. Retroperitoneal xanthogranuloma. *J Urol* 1982;127:772–774.

50. Norheim I, Oberg K, Theodorsson-Norheim E, et al. Malignant carcinoid tumors: An analysis of 103 patients with regards to tumor localization, hormone production and survival. *Ann Surg.* 1987;206:115–126.

51. Warner TF, O'Reilly G, Power LH. Carcinoid diathesis of the ileum. *Cancer.* 1979;43:1900–1905.

52. Loftus JP, van Heerden JA. Surgical management of gastrointestinal carcinoid tumors. *Adv Surg.* 1995;28:317–336.

53. Strobbe L, Dhondt E, Ramboer C, et al. Ileal carcinoid tumors and intestinal ischemia. *Hepatogastroenterology.* 1994;41:499–502.

54. Moertel CG. An odyssey in the land of small tumors. *J Clin Oncol.* 1987;5:1503–1522.

55. Gore RM. Small bowel cancer. Clinical and pathologic features. *Radiol Clin North Am.* 1997;35:351–360.

56. Ollila DW, Essner R, Wanek LA, et al. Surgical resection for melanoma metastatic to the gastrointestinal tract. *Arch Surg.* 1996;131:975–980.

57. Hermanek P, Sobin LH. *TNM Classification of Malignant Tumours,* 4th ed, 2nd rev. Berlin, Springer-Verlag, 1992.

58. Contant CM, Damhuis RA, van Geel AN, et al. Prognostic value of the TNM classification for small bowel cancer. *Hepatogastroenterology.* 1997;44:430–434.

9

THE APPENDIX

Mark T. Taira and Parakrama Chandrasoma

PATHOLOGIC EXAMINATION OF THE APPENDIX

In most primary care hospitals, the appendix is one of the commonest surgical specimens. In most cases, the appendix is placed in formalin in the operating room and received in the laboratory in the fixed state. This is a disadvantage in cases of infectious diseases for which culture may provide diagnostic information, as well as in rare neoplastic diseases for which special studies such as electron microscopy and gene rearrangement may be required.

The examination of the appendix should include measurement of length and maximum diameter. The length may normally vary from 2 to 15 cm; the normal diameter is approximately 0.5 cm. The external surface and mesoappendix are normally smooth and glistening due to the peritoneal covering. An abnormally located retrocecal appendix may not have a complete peritoneal covering. After recording the external appearance, the appendix is cut by making a midline longitudinal section from the tip extending 2 cm proximally, which is then submitted for microscopy; this is the best method of identifying an incidental microscopic carcinoid tumor of the tip. The appendix is then cross sectioned at 0.3 cm intervals through the proximal part of the organ. Normally, the lumen is empty or contains liquid fecal material; the mucosa is frequently slightly nodular because of the prominent lymphoid tissue in the appendix. Focal obliteration of the lumen is common, particularly at the tip.

It is advisable to mark the proximal surgical margin of the appendix with ink before sectioning. Rarely, a carcinoid tumor is found incidentally at microscopy, and involvement of the basal margin becomes an important question. In these cases, having the base marked makes recognition of this margin much easier in the sectioned appendiceal residual.

The most common reason for appendectomy is a clinical suspicion of acute appendicitis. In cases of acute appendicitis, gross examination shows typical features in 85–90% of cases. In patients who have had an appendectomy for clinical diagnosis of acute appendicitis in whom the appendix is grossly normal, it is important that the entire appendix be submitted for histology; lack of microscopic acute appendicitis should lead to a consideration of other causes for the patient's symptoms.

Numerous things may be found incidentally in the appendiceal lumen. These include fecoliths and parasites. Adult parasites can include *Enterobius vermicularis* (Fig. 9–1A), particu-

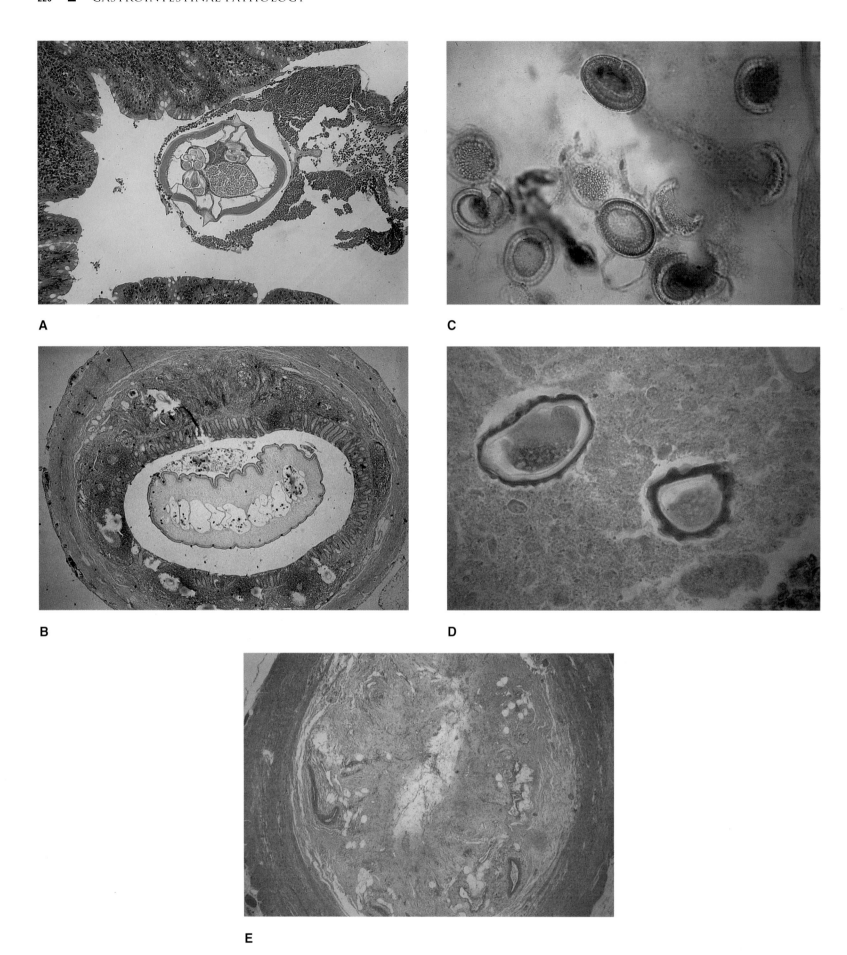

Figure 9–1. A: Appendix with adult *Enterobius vermicularis* in the lumen. Note the lateral spikes that permit identification of this helminth as a pinworm. B: Appendix with a proglottid of *Taenia* species in lumen of appendix. C: Ova of *Taenia* species in lumen of appendix. D: Ova of *Ascaris lumbricoides* in lumen of appendix. E: Fibrous obliteration of the appendiceal lumen.

larly the male worm, which is smaller than the female, proglottides and ova of *Taenia solium* and *T. saginata* (Fig. 9–1B and C), the ova of *Ascaris lumbricoides* (Fig. 9–1D) and *Trichuris trichiura*. In most studies, there is no etiologic relationship between parasitic luminal infestation and fecoliths and acute appendicitis.[1] In a significant number of cases, the lumen of the appendix is obliterated near its tip by fibrous tissue, which frequently contains nerves and adipose tissue (Fig. 9–1E).

ACUTE APPENDICITIS

Acute appendicitis is a common disease, occurring most frequently in children and young adults, but seen in all age groups. When acute appendicitis occurs in the elderly, the possibility of an underlying cause, most importantly carcinoma of the cecum involving the base of the appendix, must be sought.

Clinical Diagnosis

The diagnosis of acute appendicitis remains clinical. No single symptom or sign permits definite diagnosis. The use of scoring systems, such as the Alvarado score, is helpful.[2] The Alvarado score assigns points to the presence of symptoms, signs, and laboratory findings as follows: migratory right iliac fossa pain, anorexia, nausea and vomiting, rebound tenderness in the right iliac fossa, elevated temperature, and left shift of neutrophils in the peripheral blood each count as one point; tenderness in right iliac fossa and leukocytosis each count as two points. Scores greater than 6 have a sensitivity of 100% in children, 93% in men, and 67% in women. Scores 9–10 are an indication for appendectomy; 7–8 are indicative of appendicitis; 5–6 possible appendicitis; 1–4 are unlikely to be appendicitis. Patients with scores of 5–8 are regularly reassessed.

Other diagnostic modalities for appendicitis include plain abdominal radiograph, barium enema, ultrasonography, and computed tomography. Abnormalities can occur with all these modalities in acute appendicitis, but none have a high enough specificity and sensitivity to justify routine use. Fine-catheter peritoneal cytology (FCPC) has a high positive predictive value.[3] In this test, a catheter is introduced into the peritoneal cavity below the umbilicus and directed to the right iliac fossa; the aspirated fluid is smeared and stained by Giemsa stain. The test is positive if more than 50% of the cells are neutrophils. In females, FCPC does not permit differentiation of acute appendicitis from pelvic inflammatory disease, but a positive test is a good indication of the need for laparoscopy.

Laparoscopy is useful not only for visualizing the appendix but also for viewing other intraabdominal organs. Laparoscopic appendectomy has become more frequent in the past decade.[4] In patients with symptoms of appendicitis who appear to have a normal appendix at laparoscopy or open surgery, and no other cause for pain is found in another organ, it is probably wise to perform an appendectomy. A histologically abnormal appendix

is identified by surgeons as grossly normal in approximately 25% of cases.[5] Similarly, appendices described as showing "mild, early, slight, or moderate inflammation" are pathologically normal approximately 15% of the time.[6]

The main aim in the treatment of acute appendicitis is to prevent the occurrence of perforation, which is associated with increased rates of morbidity and mortality. Aggressive appendectomy is recommended in patients with clinical features of acute appendicitis to keep the possibility of perforation to a minimum; this results in a significant number of uninflamed appendices being removed. In most centers, 15–25% of appendices removed with a preoperative diagnosis of acute appendicitis are normal, and 15–25% of appendices show evidence of perforation.[7]

Etiology

The term "acute appendicitis" is restricted to a disease that is confined to the appendix, is characterized by acute inflammation, and has no specific cause. It must be distinguished from acute inflammation of the appendix that may result from specific causes (see discussion in following sections). Specific causes of acute inflammation of the appendix frequently involve other parts of the intestine; their recognition at clinical and pathologic examination is essential because appendectomy is frequently not a curative procedure for many of these diseases. Pathologic examination of the appendix must therefore be directed toward identification of these causes, even though they constitute less than 5% of all cases of acute appendicitis.

Acute appendicitis has no specific cause. It is characterized by acute inflammation that begins in the mucosa and quickly involves the muscle wall and serosa. Culture of appendiceal tissue shows the normal mixed colonic bacterial flora with *Bacteroides fragilis, Escherichia coli,* and streptococcal species predominating in most cases. The bacterial counts are the same in normal and inflamed appendices. The exact role of these bacteria remains uncertain, but it is thought unlikely that they play a primary pathogenic role.[8]

Luminal obstruction is often quoted as being important in the pathogenesis of acute appendicitis since the classical experiments of Wangensteen and Dennis in 1939.[9] The frequency of acute appendicitis in childhood has been attributed partly to the presence of highly reactive lymphoid tissue in the appendix in children; reactive hyperplasia of this lymphoid tissue is believed to cause obstruction. Definite evidence of luminal obstruction is present in as few as 6% of cases of acute appendicitis in some series,[10] and many cases occur in which there is luminal obstruction without inflammation. Fecoliths are more commonly seen incidentally at autopsy in an older population than in appendices surgically removed for acute appendicitis.[11] These findings suggest an unimportant pathogenic role for luminal obstruction.

Pathology

Appendices removed from patients with a preoperative diagnosis of acute appendicitis fall into several pathologic categories.

Pathologically Normal Appendix

A pathologically normal appendix is one that has been submitted completely for microscopy and shows no evidence of acute inflammation. Although the examination does not include serial sectioning of all the tissue, it is reasonable that this degree of sampling is adequate to exclude significant acute appendicitis.

Normal appendices in patients with a clinical diagnosis of acute appendicitis differ from appendices that are removed incidentally at abdominal surgery. Appendices with obvious histologic acute inflammation express tumor necrosis factor alpha (TNT-α) and interleukin-2 (IL-2) in the mucosa; normal appendices that are incidentally removed during abdominal surgery are negative. Approximately 25% of histologically normal appendices removed from patients with a preoperative diagnosis of acute appendicitis show TNF-α and IL-2 similar to that seen in acute appendicitis.[12] The presence of these cytokines suggest early inflammatory changes in these appendices; however, whether these early inflammatory changes could be responsible for clinical symptoms is unknown.

Patients who have pathologically normal appendices should be suspected of having some other cause for their clinical symptoms. For most of these patients no other disease process is found; some continue to have abdominal pain long after appendectomy.[13]

Mucosal Acute Appendicitis

Mucosal acute appendicitis refers to the presence of focal acute inflammation of the mucosa associated with erosion without involvement of the muscle wall of the appendix. It is an uncommon finding in appendices removed for acute appendicitis. The clinical features of patients with mucosal inflammation are similar to those without any inflammation and significantly different from those for patients with inflammation involving the wall.[14] This suggests that acute inflammation restricted to the mucosa is not an adequate criterion for a pathologic diagnosis of acute appendicitis. Acute mucosal appendicitis is also found sometimes in appendices removed incidentally during abdominal surgery and is more common in women.[14,15]

Acute Appendicitis

Typical acute appendicitis causes swelling and hyperemia of the appendix. The smooth, glistening appearance of the serosa is replaced with fibrin and pus (Fig. 9–2). The appendix may be involved diffusely or focally; when focal, the tip is most likely to be inflamed. Focal inflammation may also be localized to an appendiceal diverticulum. Microscopically, mucosal ulceration and suppurative acute inflammation are present, extending to involve the muscle wall and serosa (Fig. 9–3). Involvement of the muscle wall is essential for a diagnosis of acute appendicitis; its presence correlates with the typical clinical symptoms of acute appendicitis.

There is evidence that acute appendicitis is not always a progressive process that invariably leads to perforation. Careful evaluation of past history in patients with acute appendicitis re-

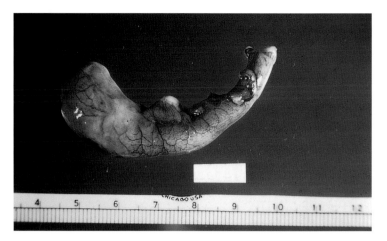

Figure 9–2. Acute appendicitis, gross, showing swollen tip of appendix with serosal purulent exudate.

veal that 5–10% of patients give a history of prior episodes of pain resembling acute appendicitis.[16] The occurrence of fibrous luminal occlusion, which is a common finding in the elderly, may also suggest prior episodes of resolved acute inflammation.

Perforated Acute Appendicitis

Perforation is a common complication of acute appendicitis and is caused by transmural necrosis of the appendiceal wall (Fig. 9–4A). The necrosis is a direct effect of the acute inflammation and ischemia resulting from increased intramural pressure due to swelling and vascular compromise. It is often difficult to demonstrate a gross perforation even in cases of periappendiceal abscess. Rarely, perforation is present without extensive transmural necrosis; these cases most likely represent perforation occurring in an inflamed appendiceal diverticulum that has no muscle wall. When necrosis of the appendiceal tissue has caused complete loss of tissue architecture, the term "gangrenous appendicitis" is used (Fig. 9–4B).

Acute Periappendicitis

Acute periappendicitis is the presence of acute inflammation involving the appendiceal serosa (Fig. 9–5), and sometimes extending to the outer part of the muscle wall in the absence of mucosal inflammation. The pathologist must section the entire appendix before concluding that acute appendicitis does not exist. Acute periappendicitis commonly results from some cause of inflammation in the abdominal cavity secondarily involving the appendiceal serosa. Common causes are pelvic inflammatory disease, ectopic pregnancy, Meckel's and cecal diverticulitis, and ileal Crohn's disease. When pathologic examination of an appendix shows periappendicitis and no cause of extraappendiceal inflammation has been found at surgery, careful reevaluation of the patient must be made for extraappendiceal disease.

Complications of Acute Appendicitis

Spread of acute inflammation outside the appendix results in

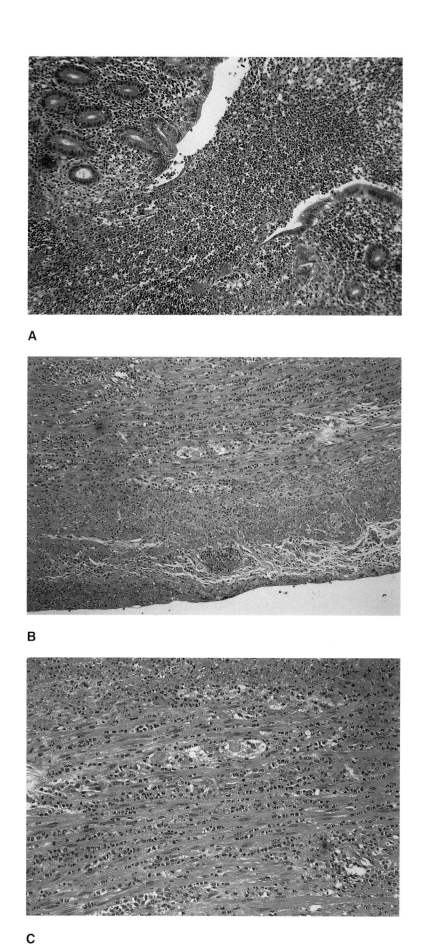

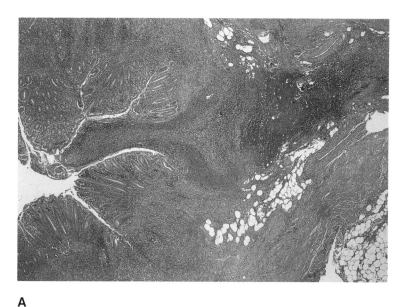

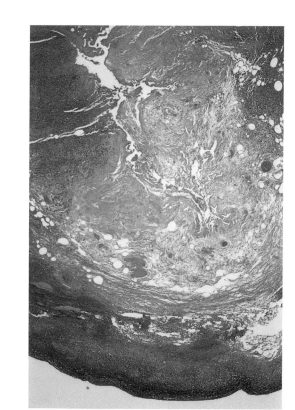

Figure 9–4. A: Microperforation in acute appendicitis, showing a trail of suppuration extending across the full thickness of the wall of the appendix to the serosa, which shows hemorrhagic inflammation. B: Gangrenous acute appendicitis, showing extensive necrosis of the mucosa and wall of the appendix associated with acute inflammation.

1. A phlegmonous inflammatory mass in the right iliac fossa composed of acute inflammation, histiocytes, and fibrosis. The histocytes frequently have foamy cytoplasm and are numerous, giving the appearance of xanthogranulomatous inflammation (Fig. 9–6). This is especially common in patients who have been given antibiotics as treatment for an inflammatory mass prior to the performance of an interval appendectomy.

Figure 9–3. A: Acute appendicitis, showing mucosal ulceration and acute suppurative inflammation. B: Acute appendicitis showing acute inflammation of the wall extending to the serosal surface. C: Acute appendicitis, higher power micrograph of part B, showing marked neutrophil infiltration of the muscle wall.

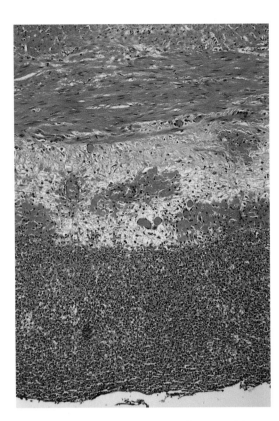

Figure 9–5. Acute periappendicitis showing severe acute inflammation of the serosa of the appendix. The muscle wall shows no evidence of inflammation.

2. Periappendiceal abscess is a common complication. The pus collection is in the right iliac fossa or retroceal area and requires immediate evacuation.
3. Diffuse peritonitis due to free perforation of the appendix is uncommon except in infants.
4. Pylephlebitis suppurativa, which refers to a septic thrombophlebitis extending up the portal venous system and resulting in pyogenic liver abscesses, is rare.
5. Fistula formation between the appendix and the intestine and urinary bladder has been reported.

Specific Types of Appendicitis

Appendiceal Involvement in Ulcerative Colitis

The appendix is involved in 40–50% of cases of ulcerative colitis involving the entire colorectum (Fig. 9–7). Appendiceal involvement may also occur as a "skip lesion" in 15–50% of patients who have sparing of the right colon.[17,18] The changes in the appendix are identical to colonic changes with pathology restricted to the mucosa, with crypt distortion and severe active chronic inflammation (Fig. 9–8).

Granulomatous Appendicitis

The appendix may be involved in several granulomatous diseases, including sarcoidosis,[19] tuberculosis, and Crohn's disease. Patients with sarcoidosis have multiple nonnecrotizing granulomas with minimal inflammation and crypt distortion. Some

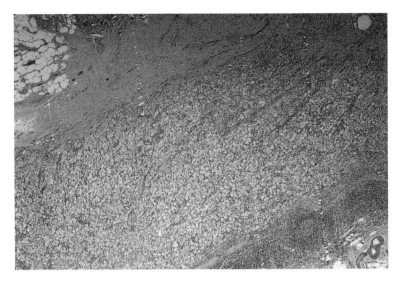

A

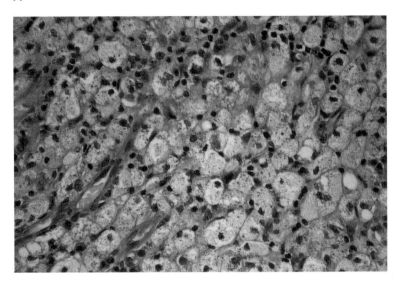

B

Figure 9–6. A: Xanthogranulomatous appendicitis, low power micrograph showing fibrosis and diffuse infiltration of the appendiceal wall with foamy macrophages. B: Xanthogranulomatous appendicitis, high power micrograph of foamy macrophages, PAS stain, showing PAS-positive granularity in the cytoplasm.

patients present with a clinical syndrome resembling acute appendicitis without significant inflammation.[19] Most patients have evidence of sarcoidosis elsewhere. Tuberculous involvement of the appendix is rare except in patients with ileocecal tuberculosis. Caseating granulomas that show acid-fast bacilli are diagnostic. Cases of granulomatous inflammation without much necrosis may occur in immunocompromised patients; the poorly formed granulomas in these cases differ from the tight granulomas that characterize Crohn's disease (Fig. 9–9).

Patients with ileocolic Crohn's disease frequently show appendiceal inflammation characterized by marked thickening of the wall (Fig. 9–10). Crohn's involvement of the appendix is characterized by mucosal acute and chronic inflammation, crypt distortion, transmural inflammation with thickening of the wall, fissure ulcers, and serosal lymphoid aggregates (Fig. 9–10C). Nonnecrotizing epithelioid cell granulomas are seen in

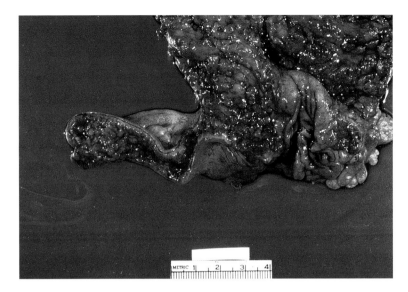

Figure 9–7. Involvement of the appendix in chronic ulcerative colitis. The mucosa of the appendix shows hyperemia and pseudo-polypoid change that is identical to that seen in the cecum.

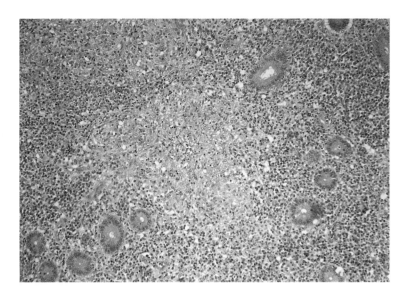

Figure 9–9. Appendiceal tuberculosis, showing a poorly formed granuloma with central necrosis.

about 30% of cases (Fig. 9–10D). Rare cases of Crohn's disease are limited to the appendix.[20] These patients present with symptoms mimicking acute appendicitis, although the course is more prolonged. They also have histologic features identical to Crohn's appendicitis associated with ileocolic Crohn's disease, including the presence of granulomas.[21] Most cases of isolated Crohn's appendicitis do not show Crohn's disease elsewhere

even after long follow-up. Because some patients do go on to develop ileocolic Crohn's disease at a later time, however, it is essential that these patients be kept under surveillance after appendectomy.[21] Appendectomy in isolated Crohn's appendicitis has not been associated with any tendency to fistula formation.[21]

A rare cause of appendiceal inflammation associated with

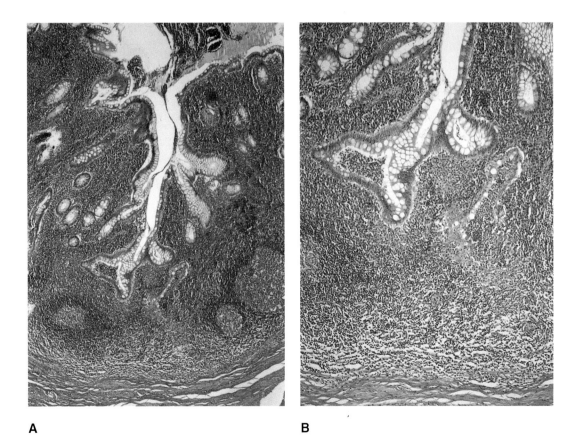

A

B

Figure 9–8. A: Chronic ulcerative colitis involving the appendix, showing mucosal involvement with crypt distortion and chronic inflammation. The muscle wall is normal. B: Chronic ulcerative colitis involving the appendix, higher power micrograph of part A, showing crypt distortion, crypt abscesses, and chronic inflammation.

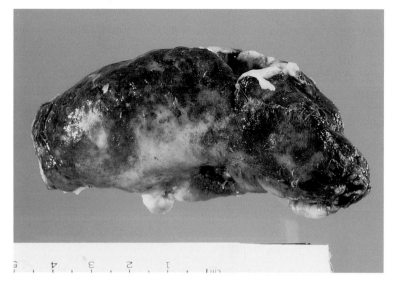

A

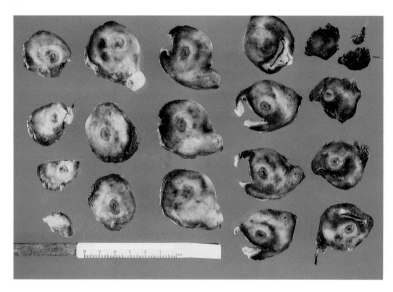

B

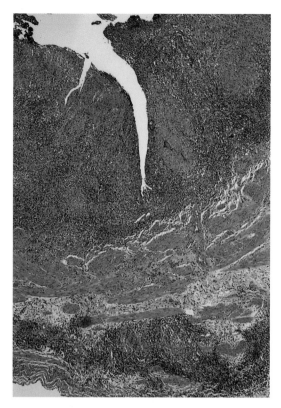

C

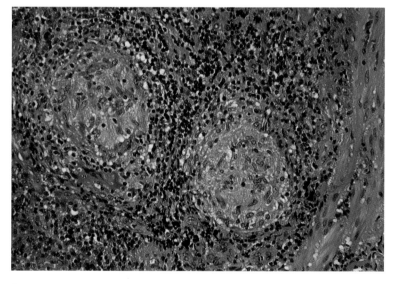

D

Figure 9–10. A: Crohn's disease of the appendix, showing marked enlargement of the appendix with surface congestion and exudate. B: Crohn's disease of the appendix, cut sections of part A, showing marked thickening of the appendiceal wall by fibrosis, luminal narrowing, and severe periappendiceal fibrosis. C: Crohn's disease of the appendix, showing a fissure ulcer and active chronic inflammation of the mucosa. D: Crohn's disease of the appendix, showing nonnecrotizing epithelioid cell granulomas in the submucosa.

histiocytes is malakoplakia. This results in diffuse thickening of the appendiceal wall resulting from an accumulation of histiocytic cells (see Fig. 9–11A). The histiocytes are large with small nuclei, and their cytoplasm is characterized by the presence of numerous rounded, basophilic, mineralized bodies known as Michaelis-Gutmann bodies. These typically have a targetoid appearance with a basophilic rim and a central round basophilic body in a clear interior (see Fig. 9–11B). The appearance resembles a nucleus with a nucleolus. Stains for calcium, iron, and phosphate stain Michaelis-Gutmann bodies positively (Fig. 9–11C).

Amebic Appendicitis

Although uncommon, amebic appendicitis is one of the most important specific types of appendicitis. Patients with amebic appendicitis present very similarly to patients with acute appendicitis.[22] The diagnosis is made by recognizing the typical flask-shaped abscesses with predominantly submucosal involvement and the presence of *Entamoeba histolytica* trophozoites in the necrotic ulcer debris, particularly at the edges of the ulcers (Fig. 9–12). These rounded nucleated structures contain erythrocytes in the cytoplasm. They are readily seen in rou-

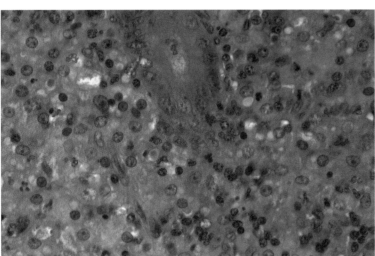

A

B

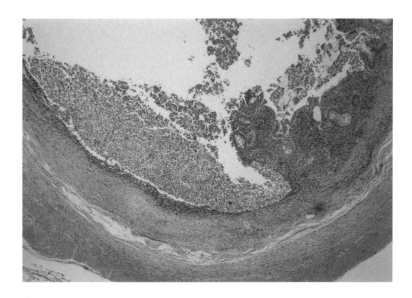

A

B

Figure 9–12. A: Amebic appendicitis, showing the typical focal ulcer with undermining of the mucosa. The ulcer contains necrotic debris. B: Trophozoites of *Entamoeba histolytica*.

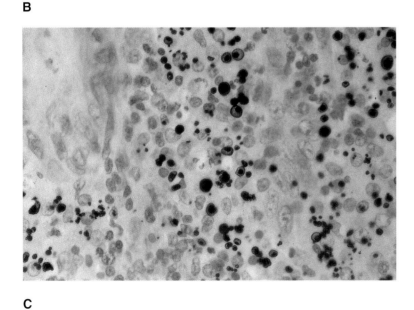

C

Figure 9–11. A: Malakoplakia of the appendix, showing thickened wall resulting from a diffuse histiocytic infiltrate with hardly any other inflammatory cells. B: Malakoplakia of the appendix, higher power micrograph of part A, showing histiocytes with numerous Michaelis-Gutmann bodies in the cytoplasm. These appear as round inclusions of varying size, some resembling nuclei. C: Von Kossa's stain in malakoplakia of the appendix, showing black-staining Michaelis-Gutmann bodies.

tine sections. Patients with amebic appendicitis continue to be symptomatic after appendectomy due to frequent involvement of the adjacent colon; unless the amebae are recognized on pathologic examination of the appendix, these patients can progress to serious infection of the colon.

Actinomycotic Appendicitis

Actinomycosis should always be considered in the differential diagnosis of a periappendiceal abscess, particularly when this condition is associated with a more protracted course than usual and when marked fibrosis and microabscesses are present on histologic examination (Fig. 9–13A). The diagnosis depends on identifying the typical colonies of *Actinomyces* species in routine sections with confirmation by Gram staining and culture (Fig. 9–13B and C).

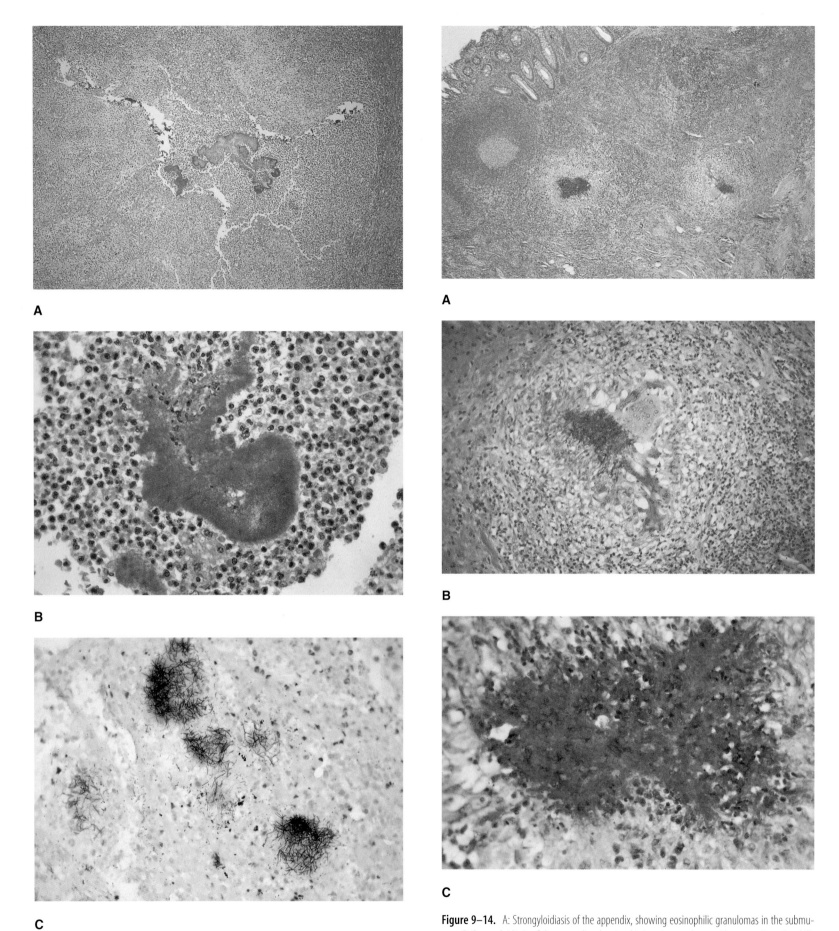

Figure 9–13. A: Actinomycosis involving the periappendiceal region. This was from a large inflammatory mass around the appendix. B: Actinomycosis, showing abscess with a colony of organisms. C: Gram stain showing the typical thin, gram-positive filamentous morphology of *Actinomyces* spp.

Figure 9–14. A: Strongyloidiasis of the appendix, showing eosinophilic granulomas in the submucosa. B: Strongyloidiasis of the appendix, showing histiocytic granuloma with a necrotic eosinophilic center. Numerous eosinophils appear around the granuloma. C: Strongyloidiasis of the appendix, showing the larva of *Strongyloides stercoralis* in the center of the necrotic granuloma, as a small rounded structure containing larval nuclear bodies.

Bacterial Appendicitis

Numerous specific bacterial infections that affect the ileum can involve the appendix. These include infections by *Salmonella enteritidis*[23] and *Vibrio cholerae*.[24] Pathogenic *Yersinia* species and other enteric pathogens have been isolated from the appendix in up to 7% of cases of appendices removed for a diagnosis of acute appendicitis. In most of these patients, there was no evidence of inflammation in the appendix, leading to the suggestion that they represented cases of mesenteric lymphadenitis mimicking acute appendicitis clinically.[25] *Yersinia pseudotuberculosis* is a cause of mesenteric lymphadenitis, but it can also cause acute appendicitis. Histologic examination reveals the presence of granulomas, which can resemble Crohn's disease or be suppurative granulomas that consists of a microabscess in the center of the epithelioid granuloma (see Chapter 8).[26] The diagnosis requires stool culture; the organism cannot be demonstrated specifically in the tissue sections.

Parasitic Appendicitis

Infection of the appendix with larval forms of *Strongyloides stercoralis* produces a distinctive histologic type of appendicitis. This is characterized by the presence of inflammation and multiple eosinophilic granulomas, which consist of a central area of necrosis surrounded by a mass of eosinophils and histiocytes (Fig. 9–14A and B). The *Strongyloides* larva can frequently be identified in the center of the granuloma (Fig. 9–14C); serial sections may be necessary.[27]

Many other helminths and their ova can be seen as incidental findings in the lumen of the appendix (see Fig. 9–1).

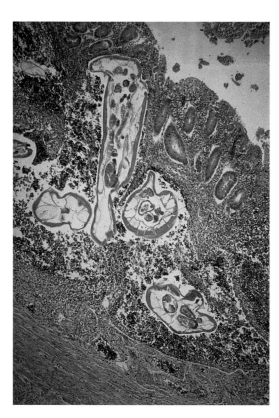

Figure 9–15. Appendix showing invasion of the wall by *Enterobius vermicularis*.

Rarely, *Enterobius vermicularis* penetrates the appendiceal wall and causes inflammation (Fig. 9–15).[28] *Schistosoma mansoni* and its eggs are not uncommonly seen in the submucosa of the appendix in endemic areas.

CARCINOID TUMORS

Typical Carcinoid Tumor

Typical carcinoid tumors occur in 0.3–0.5% of appendices (Table 9–1), but they rarely produce symptoms and are detected in appendices removed for acute appendicitis or incidentally at abdominal surgery.[29] Seventy-five percent of the tumors are at the tip; the rest are distributed throughout the appendix, with the base being involved in 5–10% of cases. The tumor is less than 1 cm in diameter in 75%, and less than 2 cm in 95% of cases. Most of the tumors are restricted to the submucosa and muscle wall of the appendix (Fig. 9–16A); involvement of the serosa occurs in 20% of cases, with half of these demonstrating extension into the mesoappendix. Invasion of the mesoappendix is more common in the larger tumors. Frequently, appendiceal carcinoid tumors are an unexpected microscopic finding, particularly when the tumor is small and restricted to the mucosa and submucosa (Fig. 9–16B).

Appendiceal carcinoids arise from neuroendocrine cells situated at the crypt bases and subepithelial neuroendocrine complexes.[30] Most appendiceal carcinoid tumors are histologically typical and have uniform small cells showing round nuclei with the typical granular ("salt-and-pepper") chromatin pattern (Fig. 9–17A). The vast majority are enterochromaffin (EC) cell argentaffin carcinoid tumors that produce serotonin or substance P; a minority of appendiceal carcinoids are nonargentaf-

TABLE 9–1. CARCINOID TUMORS OF THE APPENDIX

	Typical Carcinoid	Tubular Carcinoid	Goblet Cell Carcinoid	Mixed Carcinoid-Adenocarcinoma
Frequency	Common	Very rare	Rare	Very rare
Pattern	Insular or trabecular	Tubular	Solid or trabecular	Any plus > 50% adenocarcinoma
Mucin	Negative	Positive in lumen	Positive in cells	Positive in cells
Extracellular mucin	Negative	Negative	Positive or negative	Positive or negative
Gross tumor	Positive	Positive	Negative	Positive
Chromogranin	Positive	Positive or negative	Focal	Focal
Serotonin	Positive	Negative	Positive or negative	Positive or negative
Cytokeratin	Positive or negative	Positive	Positive	Positive
5-year survival rate (%)	99	99	80	20

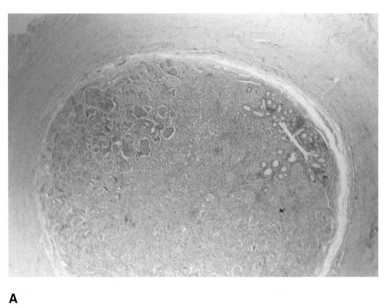

A

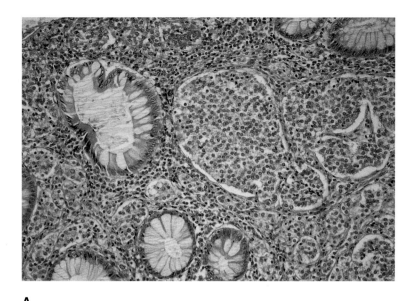

A

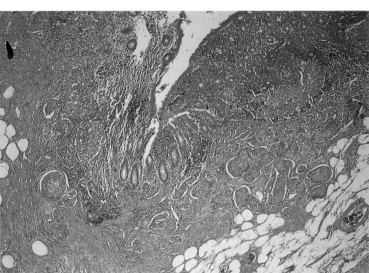

B

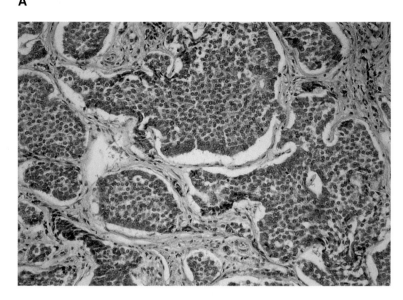

B

Figure 9–16. A: Carcinoid tumor of the appendix, showing circumscribed tumor mass involving the submucosa. The lumen of the appendix is reduced to a slit-like space on one side. The tumor does not infiltrate the muscle wall. B: Appendiceal carcinoid, microscopic, involving mucosa and submucosa.

Figure 9–17. Carcinoid tumor of the appendix. A and B: Insular pattern.

fin L cell tumors producing enteroglucagon-like peptides. The EC-cell-derived, serotonin-producing carcinoid tumors usually have a typical insular or microacinar architecture (Figs. 9–17 and 18). On immunohistochemical staining, they show scattered S100 protein-positive sustentacular cells in addition to the main chromogranin-positive neuron-specific enolase-positive tumor cell nests. The presence of S100 protein-positive sustentacular cells is the main evidence for the origin of these tumors from subepithelial neuroendocrine complexes rather than the crypt bases.[31] Peptide-producing L cell tumors commonly have a trabecular growth pattern.

Appendiceal carcinoid tumors have the lowest overall rate of metastasis among carcinoid tumors. The overall 5-year survival rate is 99%. No tumor smaller than 1 cm in size has

metastasized; as such, all appendiceal carcinoids smaller than 1 cm in size that have been completely excised by appendectomy are adequately treated by the appendectomy. Tumors larger than 2 cm have a significant risk of metastasis, irrespective of any other criterion; these tumors must be treated with a right hemicolectomy with removal of draining lymph nodes.

Tumors between 1 and 2 cm have a low risk of metastasis. Metastasis in these cases is predicted by the following: (1) Infiltration into the mesoappendix, which is a well-established indication for right hemicolectomy; (2) involvement of the base of the appendix; and (3) lymphatic and vascular invasion. The last two criteria are controversial indicators for right hemicolectomy.

Involvement of the base or surgical margin of the appendix

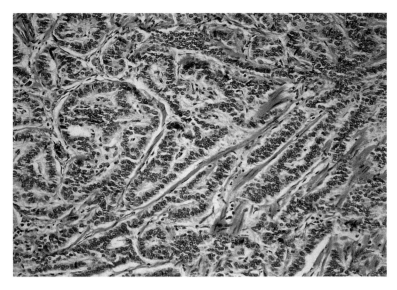

Figure 9–18. Appendiceal carcinoid with microacinar pattern.

is an indication for further surgery. In tumors smaller than 1 cm in size in which the involvement is microscopic without complete transection of the tumor, a local cecectomy usually suffices. In tumors larger than 1 cm with any basal involvement, right hemicolectomy is indicated.

Appendiceal carcinoid tumors are rarely associated with the carcinoid syndrome. Those rare cases with the carcinoid syndrome have widespread metastatic disease in liver or retroperitoneum.[32]

Appendiceal Carcinoid Tumors with Glandular Differentiation

Gladular differentiation occurs in a minority of appendiceal carcinoid tumors. Based on the type of glandular differentiation, three distinct types of tumor can be recognized (see Table 9–1): tubular carcinoid tumor, goblet cell carcinoid tumor, and mixed carcinoid-adenocarcinoma.[33] Although these tumors have some overlap with each other, they have definite criteria for diagnosis that permit practical decisions on how they should be managed.

Tubular Carcinoid Tumor

Tubular carcinoid tumors are composed of compressed tubular structures lined by cuboidal cells, separated by stroma and smooth muscle. The lumina contain small amounts of mucin (positive with digested periodic acid–Schiff (PAS) and Alcian blue stains), but the cells do not have intracytoplasmic mucin. The cells show no significant cytologic atypia, and mitotic activity is either absent or less than 2/10 hpf very focally in the tumor.

Tubular carcinoid tumors are almost always smaller than 1 cm, almost always located in the appendiceal tip, and grow as expansile tumors with minimal infiltrative features. Immuno-

histochemical findings are variable, but tubular carcinoids show weak and sometimes focal chromogranin positivity, negativity for serotonin, and many show positivity for glucagon, carcinoembryonic antigen, and cytokeratin.[33]

Tubular carcinoid tumors are almost always benign, with an overall survival rate of 99%, similar to that for typical carcinoid tumors. They can be managed with the basic principles enumerated for typical carcinoid tumors, that is, right hemicolectomy is indicated only for tumors larger than 2 cm or those tumors that involve the basal margin of the appendectomy.

Goblet Cell Carcinoid Tumor

This distinctive appendiceal tumor is characterized by the presence of tubules or small solid nests of tumor separated by stroma and smooth muscle (Fig. 9–19). The component cells contain large amounts of intracytoplasmic mucin, giving them a distinctive goblet cell appearance, with mucin-distended cytoplasm and an eccentric flattened nucleus (Fig. 9–19B and C). Typical goblet cell carcinoids are composed of solid cell groups. When lumina are present, they resemble normal crypts, frequently containing Paneth cells. Goblet cell carcinoid tumors do not contain large solid glandular structures with cribriform change. Rarely, lakes of extracellular mucin are present, but the cells in these mucin lakes resemble small crypts with small central lumina.

Goblet cell carcinoid has a disputed histogenesis and is known by several synonyms. The designation "goblet cell carcinoid" is used here because it is still the most widely used term for this entity. The main criticism of this term is that the cells show only focal immunoreactivity for neuroendocrine markers; however, most tumors do show focal positivity for chromogranin A and neuron-specific enolase, indicating at least some neuroendocrine differentiation.[34] Mucin production by the cells suggests that the neoplastic cells have gladular characteristics, and Lewin recommends the term "microglandular goblet cell carcinoma."[35] Isaacson, citing the presence of lysozyme-positive Paneth cells in these tumors, coined the term "crypt cell carcinoma."[36] Other descriptive terms, "adenocarcinoid tumor" and "mucinous carcinoid" have also been used, but these clearly have no advantage over "goblet cell carcinoid." It is very likely that this tumor is derived from a mucosal stem cell with the capability to differentiate along glandular, neuroendocrine, and Paneth cell lines. Goblet cell carcinoids frequently show diffuse positivity for carcinoembryonic antigen and cytokeratin.[33]

Goblet cell carcinoids are highly infiltrative tumors that rarely form a defined, grossly recognizable mass lesion. Rather, they produce a diffuse, often circumferential thickening of the appendiceal wall. Although most goblet cell carcinoids occur at the tip, involvement of the entire appendix and basal region are seen in approximately 20%.[33]

Goblet cell carcinoids are biologically more malignant than carcinoid tumors and less malignant than adenocarcinomas.

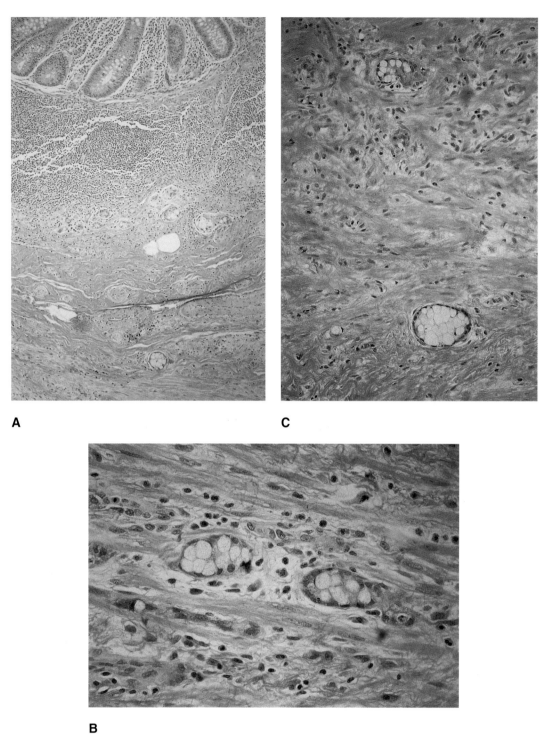

Figure 9–19. Goblet cell carcinoid of the appendix. A: Scattered groups of goblet cell carcinoid tumor in the submucosa and muscle. The tumor is present as scattered cell groups without mass effect. B: Higher power micrograph of part A, showing nests of carcinoid cells with goblet cell features. C: Cell groupings resembling coloic crypts in the muscle wall of the appendix.

Their overall 5-year survival rate is approximately 80%.[34] Size is not a reliable indicator of malignancy, mainly because it has not been assessed by gross examination in many of these tumors. Goblet cell carcinoid tumors that are confined to the appendix, do not extend through the muscle wall, have no severe cytologic atypia, and have a mitotic rate of less than 2/10 hpf are generally adequately treated with appendectomy. Extension to the basal region of the appendix or serosa, the presence of severe cytologic atypia, and a mitotic rate exceeding 2/10 hpf are indications for right hemicolectomy.[37]

Mixed Carcinoid-Adenocarcinoma

Mixed carcinoid-adenocarcinoma of the appendix can be separated from appendiceal adenocarcinomas by the absence of a

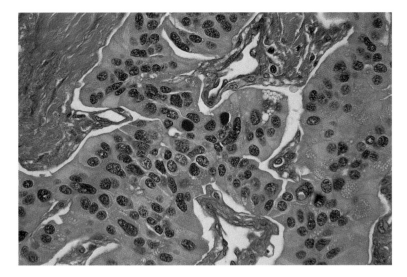

A

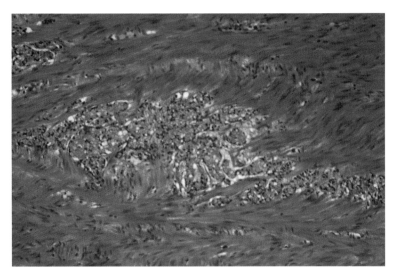

B

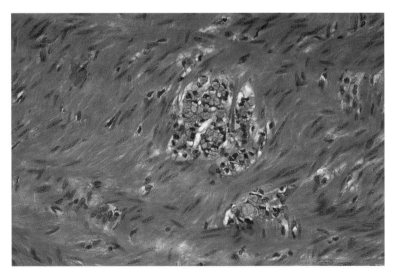

C

Figure 9–20. A: Mixed carcinoid-adenocarcinoma of appendix, showing insular carcinoid pattern with nuclear atypia and focal intracytoplasmic mucin, as shown by positive red globules in this digested PAS-stained section. B and C: Adenocarcinomatous area of mixed carcinoid-adenocarcinoma of the appendix, showing single and groups of cells containing cytoplasmic mucin that resemble goblet cell carcinoid.

mucosal origin and a growth pattern with admixed stroma and smooth muscle typical of appendiceal carcinoid tumors. Most of these tumors have significant components that resemble goblet cell carcinoid tumors, and some have foci of typical insular carcinoid tumors (Fig. 9–20A). Differentiation from goblet cell carcinoid is based on the presence of greater than 50% adenocarcinoma in the tumor. The carcinomatous element consists of signet ring cells with a linear single-cell infiltrative pattern; a mucinous pattern with lakes of mucin-containing signet ring cells; and large, solid groups of malignant cells with cribriform features (Fig. 9–20B and C). The cells comprising mixed carcinoid-adenocarcinoma commonly show malignant cytologic features and high mitotic activity, particularly in the adenocarcinomatous element.

Mixed carcinoid-adenocarcinoma usually forms a grossly apparent mass lesion with evidence of infiltration. Infiltration through the appendiceal wall is common, and involvement of the cecum and lymph nodes occurs. Patients with mixed carcinoid-adenocarcinoma should be treated with right hemicolectomy. This is a highly malignant tumor with a high incidence of metastasis and an overall survival rate of approximately 20%.[33] Metastases occur to lymph nodes, peritoneal cavity, and via the bloodstream to liver and lungs.

EPITHELIAL LESIONS

Epithelial proliferations of the appendix have a spectrum that ranges from retention mucocele and hyperplasia through benign neoplasms to adenocarcinomas. Although the basic features of these lesions are similar to their colonic counterparts, their frequency, appearance, pathologic features, management, and prognosis are very different.

Retention Mucocele

Retention mucocele (simple mucocele) of the appendix is an uncommon condition associated with luminal obstruction and resulting is accumulation of mucin and dilatation of the distal appendix (Fig. 9–21). The mucosa lining the dilated appendix is normal, although flattened. No hyperplastic or dysplastic change occurs, and the lymphoid tissue and muscle are normal. The diameter of the appendix in retention mucocele rarely exceeds 2 cm.

Retention mucocele may rarely be associated with partial rupture, resulting in the mucinal luminal contents dissecting into the wall of the appendix and sometimes into the tissues of the right iliac fossa (Fig. 9–22). The mucin is not associated with epithelial cells and has no adverse prognostic significance when complete examination of the appendix shows the absence of a neoplastic lesion. Mucin extravasation may be associated with a histiocytic response and mesothelial proliferation.

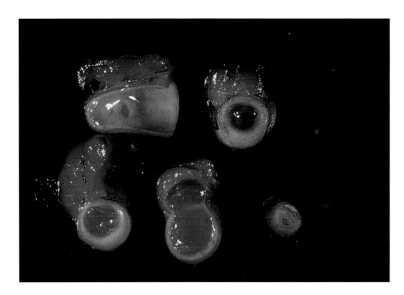

Figure 9–21. Mucocele of the appendix, gross. The dilated appendix is sectioned and shows distension with mucinous material.

Hyperplastic Polyp

Typical hyperplastic polyps, which are identical to those of the colon, occur rarely in the appendix as incidental findings.[38] They are usually small, sessile lesions characterized by hyperplastic crypts with serrated lumina and lined by cells that show no stratification and absolutely normal nuclei. Their appearance is identical to colonic hyperplastic polyps.

In addition to hyperplastic polyps, nonpolypoid diffuse hyperplasia of the appendiceal mucosa occurs more frequently (Fig. 9–23A). These are difficult to distinguish from villous adenomas, which frequently have minimal dysplastic features, resembling serrated adenomas of the colon (Fig. 9–23B).[39] Diffuse hyperplasia has been reported to be associated with colorectal carcinoma, and its finding in an appen-dectomy specimen has been suggested as an indication for colonoscopy.[40]

Mixed Hyperplastic-Adenomatous Polyp

The majority of hyperplastic polyps in the appendix show focal adenomatous change, resulting in their designation as a mixed hyperplastic-adenomatous polyp or serrated adenoma (Fig. 9–23B).

Adenoma

Adenomas (including mucinous cystadenoma) of the appendix are usually sessile, villous adenomas (Fig. 9–24); pedunculated tubular and tubulovillous adenomas are uncommon except in patients with familial adenomatous polyposis. Adenomas are usually found incidentally, but when large, they may produce a palpable mass in the right lower quadrant. Appendiceal adenomas have features similar to colonic adenoma, passing through the same adenoma–carcinoma sequence (Fig. 9–25). A diagnosis of adenoma or mucinous cystadenoma of the appendix indicates a benign lesion that is cured by appendectomy.

Appendiceal adenomas usually begin as sessile villous adenomas that frequently involve the mucosa circumferentially (Fig. 9–26). The lining cells show basal nuclei with minimal stratification and only minimal dysplastic features; they have abundant mucinous cytoplasm that distends the cell. As proliferation proceeds, the villi become shorter and mucin accumulates in the lumen, resulting in dilatation of the appendix to produce a mucocele. The lining epithelium changes from villous to undulating and finally becomes a flat lining to the distended appendix (Fig. 9–27). The lining epithelial cells still retain evidence of mild dysplasia, with enlarged hyperchromatic nuclei and mucin-distended cytoplasm. At this stage, the lesion is

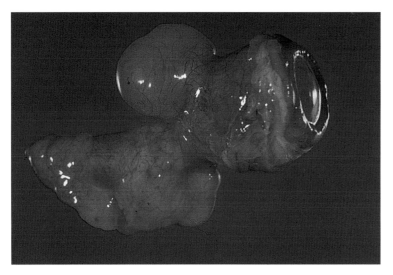

A

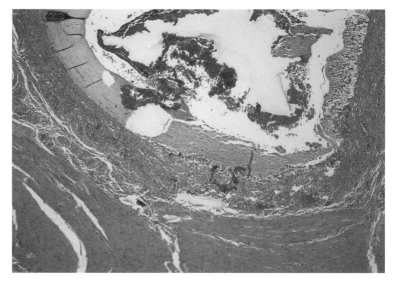

B

Figure 9–22. A: Mucocele of the appendix, gross, showing dissection of mucinous material outside the wall of the appendix. B: Extravasated mucin in the wall of the appendix. There is no associated epithelium; the mucin is surrounded by histiocytes and fibrosis.

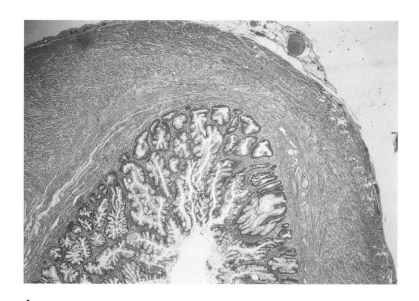

A

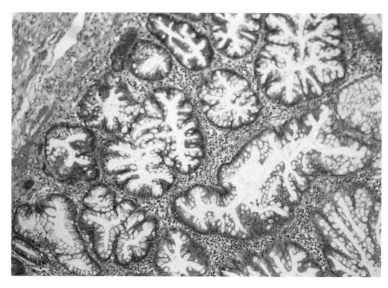

B

Figure 9–23. A: Diffuse hyperplastic polyp of the appendix. B: Papillary proliferation of the appendiceal mucosa that has the architecture of a hyperplastic polyp, but shows adenomatous change. This is a mixed hyperplastic adenomatous polyp or serrated adenoma.

called a "mucinous cystadenoma." Mucinous cystic neoplasms of the appendix have been called "mucoceles" in the past, but this term is now used only descriptively for any dilated appendix filled with mucin rather than as a pathologic entity. The underlying muscularis mucosae is intact in the early stages of this process, but in well-developed cysts, it is replaced by fibrous tissue; the muscularis externa can also undergo attenuation and

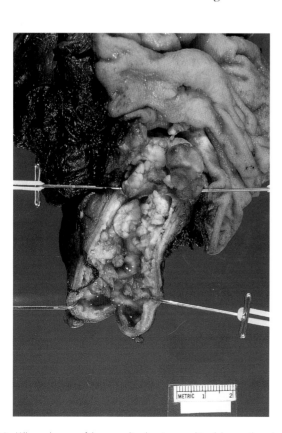

Figure 9–24. Villous adenoma of the appendix, showing a multinodular, sessile, polypoid mass on the mucosal surface.

fibrosis. Lymphoid tissue is usually absent beneath even an early villous adenoma.

The gross appearance of the appendix varies from essentially normal in the early villous adenomatous stage to a large cystic lesion in the mucinous cystadenoma stage. Adenomas of the appendix are treated in a similar manner, whether or not the lesion is associated with cystic dilatation of the appendix. Rarely, the wall of a cystic lesion can undergo calcification and ossification ("porcelain appendix").[41] Rarely, pieces of mucinous material can become detached into the lumen and form small, pearly, luminal spheroids ("myxoglobulosis" or "caviar appendix").[42]

Mucinous Tumor of Uncertain Malignant Potential

In some cases of mucinous cystadenoma, focal leakage of mucin into the muscle wall of the appendix occurs (Fig. 9–28A and B). When these intramural mucin lakes are acellular and when the neoplasm is clearly limited by a normal muscularis mucosae, a diagnosis of adenoma can be made.

In some of these cases, however, focal leakage of mucin into the wall results in marked reactive change, loss and fibrosis of the muscularis mucosae, and distortion of the normal anatomy of the appendix, making the presence of invasion very difficult to evaluate. In many of these cases, distortion results in the presence of histologically benign mucinous epithelium, seemingly deep to the mucosal surface, but when the borders of these epithelial elements have a broad, pushing, rather than an obviously infiltrative, appearance, the term "mucinous tumor of uncertain malignant potential" (UMP) is used.[43]

Cases that show acellular mucin dissection through the wall into the mesoappendiceal connective tissue in which the muscularis mucosa has been lost by fibrosis are also classified

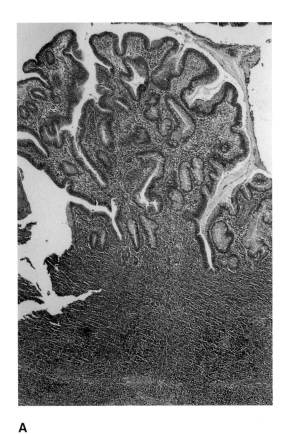

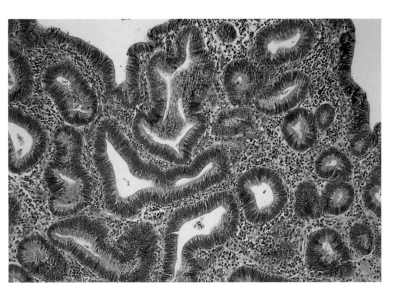

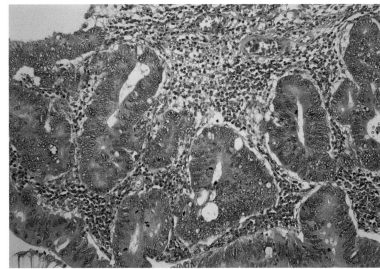

Figure 9–25. A: Adenomatous polyp of appendix. B: Adenomatous polyp of the appendix, showing adenomatous change. C: Adenomatous polyp of the appendix with high-grade dysplasia, characterized by complex glands with severe cytologic atypia, loss of nuclear polarity, and gland complexity.

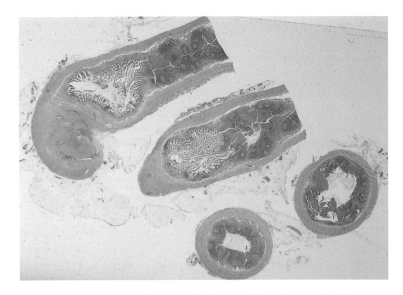

Figure 9–26. Villous adenoma of the appendix, characterized by a villous, sessile proliferation involving the full circumference of the appendiceal wall.

as mucinous tumors of UMP because their invasiveness cannot be clearly excluded.

Mucinous tumors of UMP, when diagnosed in an appendectomy specimen, represent an indication for right hemicolectomy, despite the fact that the risk of residual or metastatic disease in this group is approximately 10%.[43]

Adenocarcinoma of the Appendix

Adenocarcinoma of the appendix is of three distinct types.

Mixed Carcinoid-Adenocarcinoma

This adenocarcinoma arises in association with a carcinoid tumor, usually of goblet cell type. It was discussed earlier with carcinoid tumors.

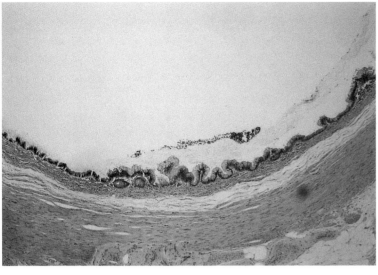

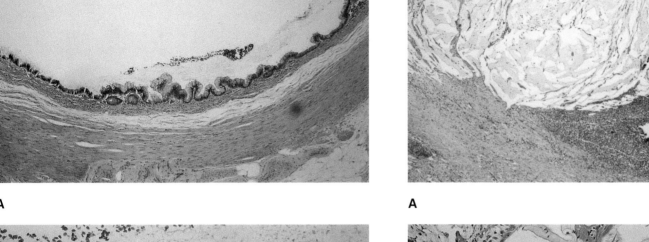

A

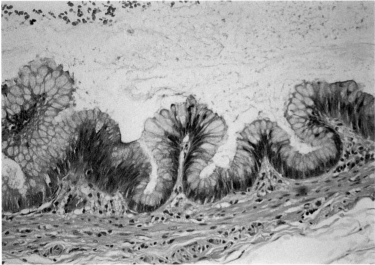

B

Figure 9–27. A: Mucinous cystadenoma of the appendix, showing dilated appendix lined by mucinous epithelium with mild dysplasia. B: Mucinous cystadenoma of appendix, showing slightly infolded mucinous epithelium showing mild dysplasia.

A

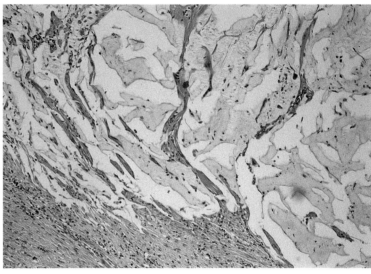

B

Figure 9–28. A: Mucin extravasation into the wall of the appendix in mucinous cystadenoma. The mucin is not associated with malignant epithelial cells; it is surrounded by lymphocytes and fibrosis. B: Higher power micrograph of part A, showing extravasated mucin devoid of epithelial cells and surrounded by fibrosis.

Mucinous Adenocarcinoma

Mucinous adenocarcinoma of the appendix is a malignant counterpart of the mucinous cystadenoma and is the commonest type of appendiceal adenocarcinoma. These tumors have been called "malignant mucocele" in the past. Patients with this tumor commonly present with acute appendicitis. A malignancy is suspected at surgery in about 30% of these cases; in the others, the diagnosis is made during pathologic examination. A minority of patients present with a palpable right lower quadrant mass. Fifty-five percent of appendiceal adenocarcinomas are perforated at presentation, with evidence of disease either localized to the periappendiceal region or present diffusely in the peritoneal cavity.[44] On gross pathologic examination, the majority of mucinous adenocarcinomas are associated with cystic dilatation of the appendix.

Histologically, mucinous adenocarcinoma is extremely well differentiated, with minimal cytologic criteria of malignancy in most cases. They are distinguished from mucinous cystadenoma by the presence of invasive neoplasm below the level of the muscularis mucosae (Fig. 9–29). When the muscularis mucosae cannot be distinguished because of distortion or fibrosis, the diagnosis is made by the finding of infiltrative tongues of tumor or single tumor cells in the wall, as opposed to the broad pushing edge that characterizes mucinous tumor of UMP. The other criterion used to diagnose mucinous adenocarcinoma is the presence of neoplastic epithelial cells in mucin lakes, either in the wall of the appendix or outside the appendix.

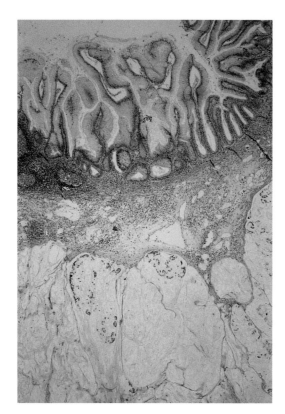

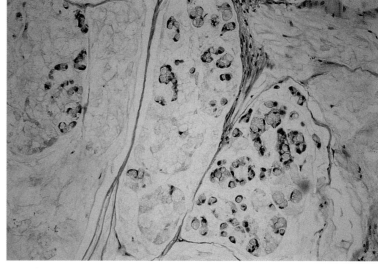

B

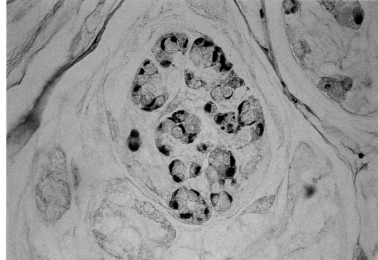

C

Figure 9–29. A: Mucinous carcinoma of the appendix, showing lakes of mucin beneath the mucosa, which shows typical features of mucinous cystadenoma. The lakes of mucin contain malignant cells. B: Mucinous carcinoma of the appendix, showing malignant cells in mucin lakes in the wall of the appendix, higher power micrograph of part A. C: Mucinous carcinoma of the appendix, higher power micrograph of part B, showing signet ring cells in the extracellular mucin.

In most cases, epithelial cells are seen on hematoxylin and eosin (H&E)-stained sections. The use of immunoperoxidase staining is rarely necessary (Fig. 9–30).[43] If keratin-positive cells are found in mucin lakes outside the appendix, the possibility of reactive mesothelial cells must be excluded by further staining for carcinoembryonic antigen (CEA) and BerEp4 (mesothelial cells are CEA-negative and BerEp4-negative, whereas most carcinoma cells show positivity with CEA and BerEp4).

Rarely, appendiceal tumors have two independent pathologic lesions. We have experience with a case of mucinous cystadenoma of the appendix in which glandular elements in the muscle wall resulted from involvement of the appendix by endometriosis (Fig. 9–31A). The diagnosis was simple in this case because of the presence of endometrial stroma around the glands (Fig. 9–31B). In stroma-deficient cases of endometriosis or endosalpingiosis, the differentiation from invasive tumor can be more problematic.

Pathologic staging of mucinous adenocarcinoma is done

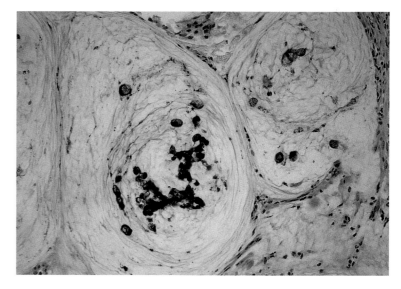

Figure 9–30. Immunoperoxidase stain for keratin, showing positive-staining malignant cells in lakes of mucin in a mucinous deposit in the peritoneal cavity in the right iliac fossa.

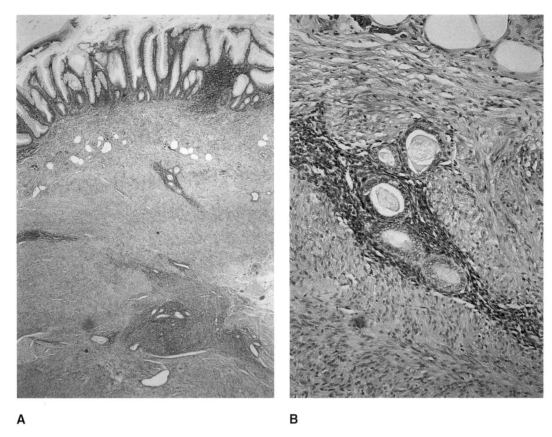

A   **B**

Figure 9–31. A: Endometriosis of the appendix showing multiple foci of endometrial tissue in the wall of the appendix. Note that the mucosa of the appendix shows features of mucinous cystadenoma. B: Endometriosis of the appendix, showing endometrial glands and stroma in the wall of the appendix.

according to tumor, node, metastasis (TNM) criteria, similar to that for colorectal carcinoma. The correct T designation of the tumor is the maximum depth at which tumor cells are seen. The presence of acellular mucin should be disregarded for the purpose of staging; however, its distribution must be carefully recorded in the pathology report.

The overall 5-year survival rate in patients with mucinous adenocarcinoma and mucinous tumor of UMP is approximately 65%.[43] It has been suggested that the overall survival in these patients may be less, because these tumors are noted for their slow growth and potential for late recurrence. The main complication associated with mucinous adenocarcinoma is the occurrence of peritoneal disease, which is discussed separately in the section on pseudo-myxoma peritonei.

Nonmucinous Adenocarcinoma of Colonic Type

Adenocarcinoma with histologic features identical to colorectal adenocarcinoma occur in the appendix, but more rarely than mucinous adenocarcinoma.[45] By definition, these tumors have more than 50% nonmucinous adenocarcinoma of both tubular and solid-cribriform types. Their histologic features are similar to those of appendiceal adenomas (see Fig. 9–25), except for the presence of cytologic features of malignancy, gland complexity, and invasion. They commonly present with acute appendicitis or as solid mass lesions. They have a worse prognosis than mucinous adenocarcinoma. Prognosis varies with TNM stage in a manner that is broadly similar to that for colorectal adenocarcinoma.

Patients with all types of appendiceal adenocarcinoma should be treated with right hemicolectomy if the original surgery was an appendectomy. Right hemicolectomy performed as a second procedure after appendectomy results in an upstaging of the tumor in 38% of patients.[45] The overall survival rate is better after right hemicolectomy than with appendectomy.[45]

PSEUDO-MYXOMA PERITONEI

Pseudo-myxoma peritonei is a loosely used term that has a variety of meanings. As such, it is best to avoid its usage, except as a descriptive term, and to designate the disease by its exact underlying pathology. According to this criterion, pseudo-myxoma peritonei refers to the presence of jelly-like mucinous material on the peritoneal surface.

The presence of mucin in the peritoneal cavity may occur as a result of the rupture of a mucinous cyst or as a result of involvement by a mucin-secreting neoplasm. In the former event, the mucin is progressively removed or becomes organized; the latter represents malignant disease. The presence of mucin in the peritoneal cavity from whatever cause evokes a host response that includes macrophage infiltration, fibrosis, calcification, (rarely) ossification, and mesothelial cellular proliferation. The latter must be distinguished from epithelial malignancy; in particular, it must be remembered that mesothelial cells are strongly positive for cytokeratin by immunoperoxidase.

Several clinical situations of appendiceal lesions associated with peritoneal mucin can be recognized.

1. When the pathology in the appendix indicates a retention mucocele or acute perforated appendicitis. These may be associated with extravasation of small amounts of mucin into the peritoneal cavity. The mucin is localized to the periappendiceal region and does not contain epithelial cells. This is a benign mucin extravasation and has no sinister prognostic significance.
2. When the appendiceal pathology is an adenoma, and the histologic features show an intact muscularis mucosae and clear-cut lack of invasion. When these features are associated with a small amount of mucin without epithelial cells, restricted to the wall of the appendix or the immediate periappendiceal region, a diagnosis of adenoma can be made. Appendectomy is adequate treatment in these cases.
3. When the appendiceal pathology is an adenoma, but invasion cannot be confidently excluded because of distortion or fibrosis. Such cases are diagnosed as mucinous tumor of UMP, and right hemicolectomy is considered.
4. When the appendix shows a mucinous adenocarcinoma with invasion. The extraappendiceal mucin associated with appendiceal mucinous adenocarcinoma may or may not contain malignant epithelial cells. Irrespective of its location, the presence of malignant epithelial cells in mucin collections outside the visceral peritoneal lining of the appendix is associated with progressive disease and a low likelihood of survival. Patients with mucinous adenocarcinoma associated with acellular mucin restricted to the periappendiceal region have a good prognosis. Patients with acellular mucin in the peritoneal cavity away from the right lower quadrant, however, have a poor prognosis.[43]

Patients with diffuse pseudo-myxoma peritonei with extensive mucinous deposits in the peritoneal cavity associated with malignant epithelial cells, often present clinically with abdominal distension. This syndrome of peritoneal mucinous carcinomatosis is most commonly associated with appendiceal mucinous neoplasms, but has also been associated with ovarian mucinous tumors and, more rarely, with low-grade mucinous carcinomas of the gallbladder and pancreas.[39] In some cases, a primary tumor is never found, even at autopsy, leading to the suggestion that a primary peritoneal mucinous carcinoma must exist.[46] There has also been a suggestion that ovarian neoplasms seen in these patients are metastasis from a frequently associated appendiceal primary.[47] Most authorities now believe, however, that primary ovarian mucinous neoplasms can produce diffuse pseudo-myxoma peritonei.[48] The rate of progression of the peritoneal disease may depend on the primary tumor; appendiceal neoplasms are generally the most slow-growing among the various primary sites.

Patients with diffuse mucinous carcinomatosis of the peritoneal cavity have a slowly progressive illness with increasing abdominal distension and progressive compression of abdominal structures. Patients survive many years, and although the 5-

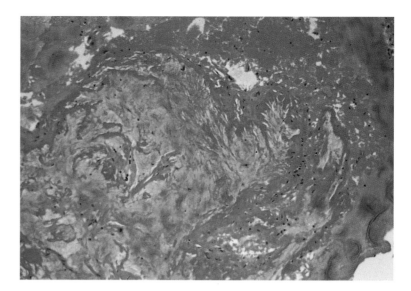

Figure 9–32. Cell block preparation of ascitic fluid in a patient with pseudo-myxoma peritonei. Although no epithelial cells are seen, the presence of a large amount of mucin should suggest this diagnosis.

year survival rate is 65%, the ultimate prognosis is poor. Recent aggressive treatment modalities, which include extensive surgical resection of involved peritoneum, frequently with involved organs, followed by intraperitoneal chemotherapy, have improved survival. In some series, patients treated in this aggressive manner have a 10-year survival rate approaching 80%.[49]

The finding of mucin in the peritoneal cavity on a percutaneous biopsy specimen or peritoneal lavage in a patient without any apparent lesion is highly suggestive of a low-grade mucinous adenocarcinoma of the abdominal cavity (Fig. 9–32). Many of these cases show no evidence of epithelial cells associated with the mucin.[50] If an ovarian or pancreaticobiliary lesion is excluded on computed tomography (CT) scan, an appendectomy should be considered to exclude a mucinous tumor. A similar indication for appendectomy is suggested when pools of acellular mucin are found within a hernia sac.

MISCELLANEOUS CONDITIONS

Endometriosis

The appendix is a rare but well-recognized site of endometriosis. It is most commonly associated with extensive pelvic endometriosis, but it may be found incidentally in an appendix removed for acute appendicitis or tumor (see Fig. 9–31). Endometriosis appears as glands surrounded by endometrial stroma, frequently associated with hemorrhage and hemosiderin pigment. The serosa is maximally involved, but the endometriosis may on occasion extend into the outer part of the muscle wall.

Appendiceal Intussusception

Appendiceal intussusception is a rare cause of right lower quadrant pain. Intussusception is usually precipitated by a le-

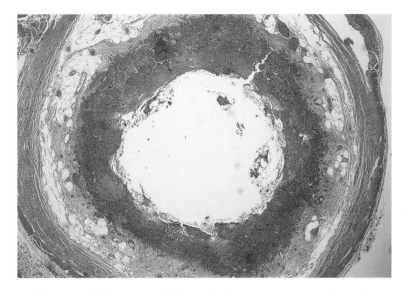

Figure 9–33. Ischemic necrosis of the appendiceal mucosa in an intussuscepted appendix.

sion such as adenoma, adenocarcinoma, carcinoid tumor, or endometriosis.[51] Appendiceal intussusception may be restricted to the appendix, with a more distal segment telescoping into the proximal appendix without involvement of the cecum. More commonly, the base of the appendix protrudes into the cecum, presenting as a cecal polyp at endoscopy. Some cases have been reported in which endoscopic polypectomy of a cecal mass resulting from appendiceal intussusception led to peritonitis.[52] The most extreme form of appendiceal intussusception is a complete invagination of the appendix into the cecum. In these cases, a cross section of the intussuscepted appendix shows an "inside-out" appearance, with a mucosa being on the outside and the muscle wall and serosa being inside. Ischemic necrosis may occur in the intussusceptum (Fig. 9–33).

Appendiceal Diverticula

Pulsion diverticula of the appendix are not widely reported in the literature, but they are reported in up to 1% of appendices.[53] They appear mainly in the distal part of the appendix as a small mucosal herniation through the muscle wall (Fig. 9–34). The mucosal diverticulum is covered only by muscularis mucosae and periappendiceal connective tissue. Diverticula of the appendix may be a site of acute inflammation. This results in a localized acute inflammation outside the muscle wall of the appendix. The exact nature of this lesion can be recognized only when residual glandular mucosa is present in the inflamed diverticulum. When the mucosa has been completely destroyed, the lesion appears as a periappendiceal abscess, sometimes without associated acute appendicitis.

References

1. Dorfman S, Talbot IC, Torres R, et al. Parasitic infestation in acute appendicitis. *Ann Trop Med Hyg.* 1995;89:1:99–101.
2. Calder JDF, Gajraj H. Recent advances in the diagnosis and treatment of acute appendicitis. *Br J Hosp Med.* 1995;54: 129–133.
3. Caldwell M, Watson R. Peritoneal aspiration cytology as a diagnostic aid in acute appendicitis. *Br J Surg.* 1994;81: 276–278.
4. McAnena OJ, Wilson PD. Laparoscopic appendicectomy: Diagnosis and resection of acute and perforated appendices. *Baillieres Clin Gastroenterol.* 1993;7:851–866.
5. Grunewald B, Keating J. Should the "normal" appendix be removed at operation for appendicitis? *J Roy Coll Surg Edinb.* 1993;38:158–160.
6. Jones MW, Paterson AG. The correlation between gross appearance of the appendix at appendicectomy and histological examination. *Ann R Coll Surg Engl.* 1988;70:93–94.
7. Butler C. Surgical pathology of acute appendicitis. *Hum Pathol.* 1981;12:870–878.
8. Roberts JP. Quantitative bacterial flora of acute appendicitis. *Arch Dis Childhood.* 1988;63:536–540.
9. Wangensteen OH, Dennis C. Experimental proof of the obstructive origin of appendicitis in man. *Ann Surg.* 1939;110:629.
10. Chang AR. An analysis of the pathology of 3003 appendices. *Aust NZ J Surg.* 1981;51:169.
11. Andreou P, Blain S, Du Boulay CE. A histopathological study of the appendix at autopsy and after surgical resection. *Histopathology.* 1990;17:427–431.
12. Wang Y, Reen DJ, Puri P. Is a histologically normal appendix following emergency appendicectomy always normal? *Lancet.* 1996;347:1076–1079.
13. Walker SJ, West CR, Colmer MR. Acute appendicitis: Does removal of a normal appendix matter, what is the value of diagnostic accuracy and is surgical delay important? *Ann R Coll Surg Engl.* 1995;77:358–363.
14. Pieper R, Kager L, Nasman P. Clinical significance of mucosal inflammation of the appendix. *Ann Surg.* 1983;197: 368–374.
15. Onuigbo WI, Chukudebelu WO. Appendices removed at Cesarean section: Histopathology. *Dis Colon Rectum.* 1981;24: 507–509.
16. Barber MD, McLaren J, Rainey JB. Recurrent appendicitis. *Br J Surg.* 1997;84:110–112.
17. Kroft SH, Stryker SJ, Rao MS. Appendiceal involvement as a skip lesion in ulcerative colitis. *Modern Pathol.* 1994;7: 912–914.

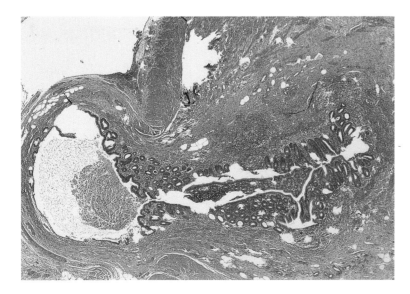

Figure 9–34. Diverticulum of the appendix, showing mucosal outpouching from the lumen extending across the wall of the appendix into the mesocolon.

18. Groisman GM, George J, Harpaz N. Ulcerative appendicitis in universal and nonuniversal ulcerative colitis. *Modern Pathol.* 1994;7: 322–325.

19. Cullinane DC, Schultz SC, Zellos L, et al. Sarcoidosis manifesting as acute appendicitis. *Dis Colon Rectum.* 1997;40: 109–111.

20. Ruiz V, Unger SW, Morgan J, et al. Crohn's disease of the appendix. *Surgery.* 1990;107:113–117.

21. Timmcke AE. Granulomatous appendicitis: Is it Crohn's disease? Report of a case and review of the literature. *Am J Gastroenterol.* 1986;81:283–287.

22. Malik AK, Hanum N, Yip CH. Acute isolated amoebic appendicitis. *Histopathology.* 1994;24:87–88.

23. Deutsch A, Wasserman D, Ruchelli E, et al. An uncommon presentation of *Salmonella. Pediatr Emer Care.* 1996;12: 285–287.

24. Cook MA, Nedunchezian D, Manfredi OL. Acute appendicitis secondary to non-O group 1 *Vibrio cholerae. J Am Osteopath Assn.* 1996;96:432–433.

25. Van Noyen R, Selderslaghs R, Bekaert J, et al. Causative role of *Yersinia* and other enteric pathogens in the appendicular syndrome. *Eur J Clin Microbiol Infect Dis.* 1991;10:735–741.

26. El-Maraghi NR, Mair NS. The histopathology of enteric infection with *Yersinia pseudotuberculosis. Am J Clin Pathol.* 1979;71:631.

27. Stemmermann GN. Eosinophilic granuloma of the appendix. *Am J Clin Pathol.* 1961;36:524.

28. Chandrasoma PT, Mendis KN. Ectopic *Enterobius vermicularis* in ectopic sites. *Am J Trop Med Hyg.* 1977;26:644–649.

29. Roggo A, Wood WC, Ottinger LW. Carcinoid tumors of the appendix. *Ann Surg.* 1993;217:385–390.

30. Capella C, Heitz PU, Hofler H, et al. Revised classification of neuroendocrine tumors of the lung, pancreas and gut. *Digestion.* 1994;55:11–23.

31. Lundqvist M, Wilander E. A study of the histopathogenesis of carcinoid tumors of the small intestine and appendix. *Cancer.* 1987;60:201–206.

32. Thirlby RC, Kasper CS, Jones RC. Metastatic carcinoid tumor of the appendix: Report of a case and review of the literature. *Dis Colon Rectum.* 1984;27:42–46.

33. Burke AP, Sobin LH, Federspiel BH, et al. Goblet cell carcinoids and related tumors of the vermiform appendix. *Am J Clin Pathol.* 1990;94:27–35.

34. Anderson NH, Somerville JE, Johnston CF, et al. Appendiceal goblet cell carcinoids: A clinicopathological and immunohistochemical study. *Histopathology.* 1991;18:61–65.

35. Lewin KJ, Riddell RH, Weinstein WM. Gastrointestinal pathology and its clinical implications. Igaku-Shoin, New York, 1992. pp. 238–246.

36. Isaacson P. Crypt cell carcinoma of the appendix (so called adenocarcinoid tumor). *Am J Surg Pathol.* 1981;5:213–224.

37. Bak M, Asschenfeldt P. Adenocarcinoid of the vermiform appendix. A clinicopathologic study of 20 cases. *Dis Colon Rectum.* 1988;31:605–612.

38. Blair NP, Bugis SP, Turner LJ, et al. Review of the pathologic diagnoses of 2216 appendectomy specimens. *Am J Surg.* 1993;165: 618–620.

39. Carr NJ, Sobin LH. Unusual tumors of the appendix and pseudomyxoma peritonei. *Semin Diag Pathol.* 1996;13: 314–325.

40. Younes M, Katikaneni PR, Lechago J. Association between mucosal hyperplasia of the appendix and adenocarcinoma of the colon. *Histopathology.* 1995;26:33–37.

41. Skaane P. Radiological features of mucocele of the appendix. *Fortschr Rontgenstr.* 1988;149:624–628.

42. Gonzalez JE, Hann SE, Trujillo YP. Myxoglobulosis of the appendix. *Am J Surg Pathol.* 1988;12:962–966.

43. Carr NJ, McCarthy WF, Sobin LH. Epithelial noncarcinoid tumors and tumor-like lesions of the appendix. *Cancer.* 1995;75: 757–768.

44. Cerame MA. A 25-year review of adenocarcinoma of the appendix. *Dis Colon Rectum.* 1988;31:145–150.

45. Nitecki SS, Wolff BG, Schlinkert R, et al. The natural history of surgically treated primary adenocarcinoma of the appendix. *Ann Surg.* 1994;219:51–57.

46. Banerjee R, Gough J. Cystic mucinous tumors of the mesentery and retroperitoneum: Report of three cases. *Histopathology.* 1998;12:527–532.

47. Prayson RA, Hart WR, Petras RE. Pseudomyxoma peritonei. A clinicopathologic study of 19 cases with emphasis on site of origin and nature of associated ovarian tumors. *Am J Surg Pathol.* 1994;18:591–603.

48. Seidman JD, Elsayed AM, Sobin LH, et al. Association of mucinous tumors of the ovary and appendix. A clinicopathologic study of 25 cases. *Am J Surg Pathol.* 1993; 17:22–34.

49. Sugarbaker PH. Pseudomyxoma peritonei. *Cancer Treat Rev.* 1996;81:105–119.

50. Costa M, Oertel YC. Cytology of pseudomyxoma peritonei: Report of two cases arising from appendiceal cystadenomas. *Diagn Cytopathol.* 1990;6:201–203.

51. Sakaguchi N, Ito M, Sano K, et al. Intussusception of the appendix: A report of three cases with different clinical and pathologic features. *Pathol Int.* 1995;45:757–761.

52. Fazio RA, Wickremasinghe PC, Arsura EL, et al. Endoscopic removal of an intussuscepted appendix mimicking a polyp: An endoscopic hazard. *Am J Gastroenterol.* 1982;77: 556–558.

53. Deschenes L, Couture J, Garneau R. Diverticulitis of the appendix: Report of sixty-one cases. *Am J Surg.* 1971;121:706.

10

NONNEOPLASTIC DISEASES OF THE COLON

Greg Kobayashi and Parakrama Chandrasoma

▶ CHAPTER OUTLINE

MOTILITY DISORDERS

Generalized motility disorders that involve both the small and large intestine were considered in Chapter 8. Motility disorders that are largely restricted to the colorectum are considered in this chapter.

Hirschsprung's Disease

Hirschsprung's disease (HD) is a common congenital disorder affecting 1/5000 newborns. Characterized by a lack of propulsive peristalsis in the distal colon, it results from an absence of ganglion cells in the wall. Both submucosal and myenteric plexi are affected in the aganglionic segment. An increase in adrenergic and cholinergic nerves is associated in the aganglionic segment.[1] In addition to a lack of peristalsis in HD, colonic smooth muscle relaxation is deficient due to disturbed function of non-adreneregic, noncholinergic (NANC) inhibitory nerves.[2] Vasoactive intestinal polypeptide (VIP) and nitrous oxide are important mediators of NANC inhibitory nerves; a marked decrease in VIP and nitric oxide synthase are seen in the aganglionic segment of HD.

As a rule, the aganglionic segment begins in the distal rectum and extends proximally (Fig. 10–1B). Eighty percent to 90% of cases are characterized by a short (< 40 cm) aganglionic segment involving the rectum and distal sigmoid colon. Up to 25% of this group is a subset of the disease known as ultrashort-segment HD, which is characterized by an aganglionic segment restricted to the low anorectal region (Fig. 10–1C). Long-segment HD, sometimes affecting the entire colon and extending into the small intestine, is rare. Zonal aganglionosis in which aganglionosis is patchy rather than continuous is a very rare variant of HD (Fig. 10–1D). In these cases, an area of aganglionosis may occur above an area shown by biopsy to have ganglion cells, leading to failure of surgical correction.

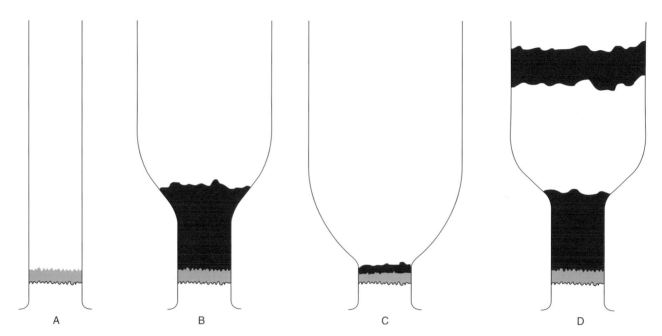

A   B   C   D

Figure 10–1. Hirschsprung's disease. A: Normal. There is an approximately 2-cm segment of rectum above the pectinate line that has a paucity of ganglion cells in the submucosa. B: Typical pathologic findings in Hirschsprung's disease, with a narrow distal aganglionic segment of varying length and a proximal dilated segment composed of normal colon. C: Ultrashort-segment Hirschsprung's disease; this is difficult to distinguish pathologically from normal. D: Zonal Hirschsprung's disease, in which a skip occurs in the aganglionic segment; this is very uncommon. (Orange = 2 cm of lowest rectum above pectinate line where there is normally a paucity of ganglion cells. White = normal ganglionic zone. Red = aganglionic zone.)

The disease is more common in males. Although most cases are sporadic, 10% are familial. Several different abnormal genes have been identified in both familial and sporadic cases[4]: (1) the *RET* protooncogene on chromosome 10 in 50% of familial and 15% of sporadic cases; (2) the endothelin β receptor gene on chromosome 13. Ten percent of patients have Down syndrome; 5% of cases are associated with other neurologic abnormalities.

Ninety percent of patients present in early infancy with constipation and abdominal distension. Presentation in older infancy and early childhood may occur. The most serious complication is the occurrence of Hirschsprung's-associated enterocolitis (HAEC). This is of unknown cause; defects in IgA secretion and infection by toxigenic bacteria have been suggested.[5] HAEC is characterized by fever and diarrhea associated with an acute colitis with pseudo-membranes; this condition can be life-threatening. Histologic features progress through mild cryptitis, crypt abscesses, mucosal necrosis, and transmural necrotizing inflammation with perforation. HAEC tends to occur more commonly in HD associated with Down syndrome.

Preoperative Pathologic Diagnosis

The aperistaltic tonic segment of affected colon is typically a distal narrow segment. Proximal to the aganglionic area, the colon shows marked dilatation due to the obstruction (congenital megacolon is an alternative name for HD). The diagnosis is best established by acquiring an adequate suction biopsy specimen of the rectum that contains submucosa. An adequate biopsy sample is one taken at 2 cm or above the pectinate line and containing a thickness of submucosa equal to that of the overlying mucosa. The 2 cm of rectum immediately above the

pectinate line normally has a paucity of ganglion cells and prominent nerve trunks, which may lead to false positive diagnosis in normals, if biopsied (Fig. 10–1A).

Absence of ganglion cells in the submucosa of the rectum 2 cm or greater above the pectinate line is diagnostic of HD. Most cases also show nerve hypertrophy in the submucosa, but this finding is more variable than aganglionosis. Normally, one to five ganglion cells are found in clusters for every 1 mm of normal rectal mucosa.[1] Ganglion cells are typically seen as large cells with abundant eosinophilic cytoplasm and eccentric round nuclei that contain prominent nucleoli (Fig. 10–2). In the first year of life, ganglion cells may be immature, appearing as small neuroblast-like cells with scanty cytoplasm and nuclei that do not contain nucleoli. Their arrangement in clusters often associated with nerve elements permits recognition. In difficult cases, neuron-specific enolase positivity by immunoperoxidase establishes their ganglionic nature.

Intraoperative Pathologic Diagnosis

Intraoperative determination of the extent of the aganglionic segment is crucial for surgical correction. Usually, ganglion cells are present proximal to the narrow aganglionic segment. Sometimes, though, the aganglionic segment extends to a variable distance into the dilated proximal colon. It is therefore important to confirm the presence of myenteric plexus ganglion cells at the site of intended surgical correction by submitting seromuscular biopsies for intraoperative frozen sections. Hematoxylin and eosin (H&E)-stained serial frozen sections are generally adequate for this purpose (Fig. 10–3). Rapid intraoperative immunoperoxidase staining for synaptophysin[6] has

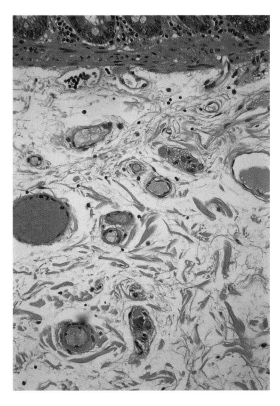

Figure 10–2. Normal rectal submucosa, showing a cluster of ganglion cells.

been reported to show results that are superior to intraoperative frozen sections stained with H&E for identification of ganglion cells. The coexistence of intestinal neuronal dysplasia (see following section) above the aganglionic segment of HD can complicate interpretation of intraoperative biopsies in HD.

Intestinal Neuronal Dysplasia

Intestinal neuronal dysplasia (IND) commonly occurs as a sporadic disorder; it may also be associated with neurofibromatosis or multiple endocrine neoplasia type IIb or III and may be found

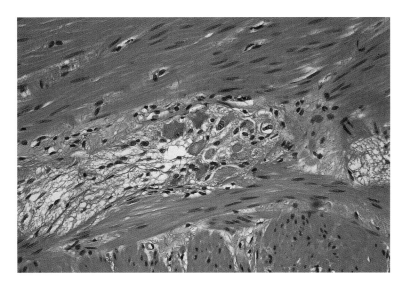

Figure 10–3. Ganglion cells in myenteric plexus of colon, as evaluated in an intraoperative full-thickness biopsy specimen of the colonic muscle wall.

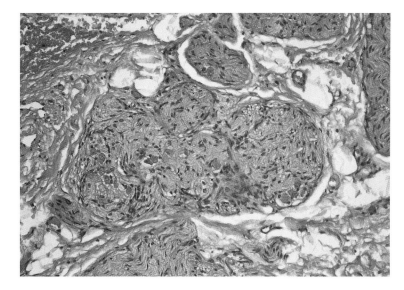

Figure 10–4. Intestinal neuronal dysplasia, showing neural hypertrophy associated with increased numbers of ganglion cells.

proximal to the aganglionic segment of HD. In sporadic cases, IND clinically mimics HD. In rectal biopsies, IND is characterized by marked neural hypertrophy and the presence of increased numbers of large ganglion cells. Clusters of more than seven ganglion cells establishes the diagnosis of IND[7] (Fig. 10–4).

Irritable Bowel Syndrome

Irritable bowel syndrome is a common disorder mainly affecting adult females with symptoms that include any combination of diarrhea, constipation, bloating, and abdominal pain, often of several years duration. There is an association with interstitial cystitis. It is believed to be caused by a disturbance of intestinal motility and enhanced visceral sensitivity. The diagnosis can be made by symptom-based criteria (Manning and Rome systems). Colonoscopy is normal, and biopsies are not necessary for diagnosis. When biopsies are done, they show no pathologic abnormality. One study reports an increased number of mast cells associated with substance P-positive nerves in the mucosa.[8]

Toxic Megacolon

Toxic megacolon is a fulminant colitis characterized by marked dilatation of the colon associated with features of toxicity, such as high fever, tachycardia, and neutrophil leukocytosis. Radiologic demonstration of colonic dilatation greater than 6 cm, which is the upper limit of normal, is the diagnostic criterion used. Megacolon cannot be accurately documented pathologically in a resected specimen because of postoperative collapse of the dilated colon. The circumference of the colon is commonly increased (Fig. 10–5), but not necessarily so (Fig. 10–6).

The majority of cases of toxic megacolon occur as a complication of ulcerative colitis (see also Chapter 11), in which the incidence of toxic megacolon is 6%.[9] Crohn's disease is less frequently associated. Most patients who develop toxic megacolon

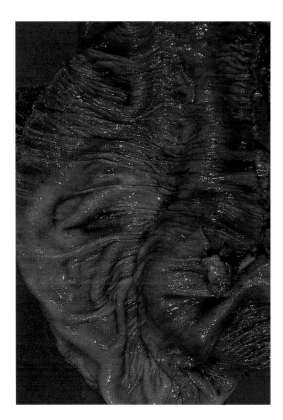

Figure 10–5. Colon resected for toxic megacolon, showing increased circumference of longitudinally opened colon.

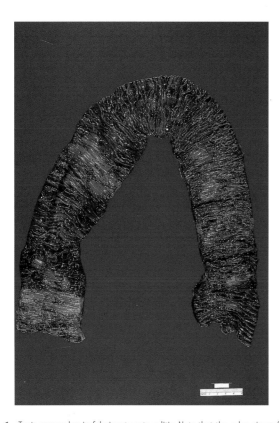

Figure 10–6. Toxic megacolon in fulminant acute colitis. Note that the colon circumference is not increased; this was a markedly dilated colon at radiologic examination; collapse of the dilated colon after removal makes pathologic diagnosis of megacolon by measurement of circumference unreliable.

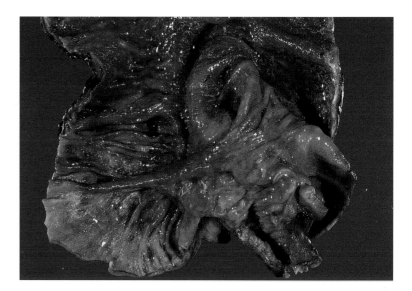

Figure 10–7. Toxic megacolon complicating ulcerative colitis, showing dilatation, thinning of the wall, and greenish discoloration of the mucosa due to necrosis.

have a known history of chronic inflammatory bowel disease; some develop it during the initial presentation. Numerous other colitides may be complicated by toxic megacolon: *Salmonella* colitis and *Shigella* colitis, *Clostridium difficile*-induced pseudo-membranous colitis, ischemic colitis, and amebic colitis. In HIV-positive individuals, cytomegalovirus (CMV) colitis is a common cause of toxic megacolon; some of these patients have an endoscopic and histologic appearance that resembles pseudo-membranous colitis[10]; others have ulceration. Laboratory studies helpful in identifying a cause include stool culture,

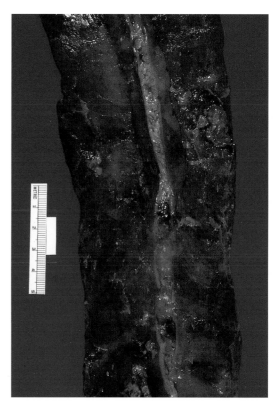

Figure 10–8. Serosal aspect of the colon in toxic megacolon, showing serosal exudate resulting from peritonitis secondary to colonic perforation.

stool for *Clostridium difficile* toxin, and endoscopic biopsy. A biopsy may show diagnostic features of ulcerative colitis, Crohn's disease, acute nonspecific colitis, ischemic colitis, pseudo-membranous colitis, and CMV and amebic colitis.

In toxic megacolon, the acute inflammation involves the muscle wall and myenteric plexus (see Chapter 11, Figs. 11–22B), resulting in paralysis of the muscle leading to failure of peristalsis and dilatation. Dilatation increases wall tension, leading to ischemic necrosis (Fig. 10–7) and perforation with acute peritonitis (Fig. 10–8). Toxic megacolon requires emergency treatment. The likelihood of death resulting from this condition increases when surgery is undertaken after free perforation has occurred.

COLONIC DIVERTICULAR DISEASE

Left-sided Diverticular Disease

The common form of colonic diverticular disease that affects the left colon is a disease prevalent in industrialized countries. It is relatively uncommon in Africa and Asia. The rapid increase in incidence of diverticular disease coincided with the beginning of grain milling in the early part of the twentieth century. The presence of asymptomatic diverticula is known as diverticulosis; when inflammation is superimposed, the disease is called diverticulitis.

Diverticulosis has a less than 5% incidence before age 40 years, but increases to 30% at age 50 years, 50% at age 70 years, and over 65% at ages over 80 years. Both incidence and number of diverticula increase with age. The diverticula are pulsion diverticula (mucosal herniations through the muscle wall) that occur at points of entry of the perforating muscular arteries of the sigmoid colon, usually in two longitudinal rows between the mesocolic and antimesocolic taenia coli (Figs. 10–9 and 10–10). Diverticulosis is strongly associated with low fiber in the diet. A low-fiber diet causes hard, low-volume feces, which result in the development of higher intraluminal pressures during evacuation, predisposing to pulsion diverticula. The association with age is believed to be the result of aging-related degeneration in collagen and elastin in the wall.

Diverticulosis is usually asymptomatic; 80% of cases never present clinically. It can, however, be associated with left-sided abdominal pain, often colicky and related to meals and passage of flatus. Although this is termed "painful diverticular disease,"[11] no pathologic alteration occurs in the diverticula and the pain is as likely to be related to heightened motor activity in the left colon.

The diverticula are usually small and multiple. Rarely, giant diverticula occur[12]; these have a higher rate of complications and represent an indication for elective surgical removal.

Clinical Features

Diverticulitis, the common cause of symptoms in diverticular disease, occur in 10–20% of patients with diverticulosis, almost always affecting the sigmoid colon. It is characterized by acute

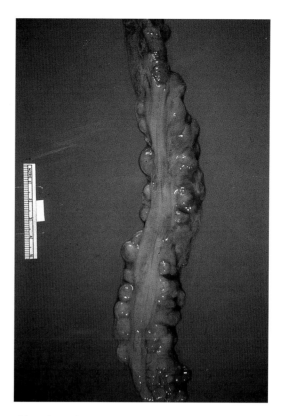

Figure 10–9. Colonic diverticulosis, showing two rows of diverticula along the antimesocolic taenia coli.

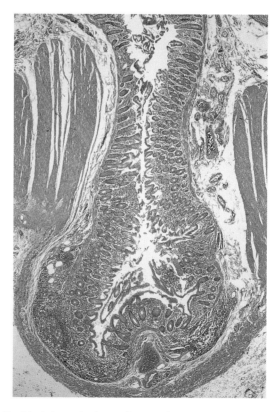

Figure 10–10. Colonic diverticula, showing the mucosal protrusion through the muscle wall of the colon. The diverticulum has a thin layer of muscularis mucosae separating it from pericolic fat.

left lower quadrant abdominal pain associated with fever and leukocytosis. In its mildest form, the acute inflammation involves the mucosa and the immediate pericolic connective tissue (Fig. 10–11). Inflammation may be associated with mucin extravasation into the pericolic fat, resulting in a mucus escape reaction (Fig. 10–12). With more severe disease, pericolic abscess formation occurs (Fig. 10–13). Severe diverticulitis may result in free perforation into the peritoneal cavity. In the chronic phase, severe pericolic fibrosis is associated with the inflammation, causing strictures, adhesions, and fistula formation with adjacent structures such as the ileum, urinary bladder, and vagina (Fig. 10–14).

Diverticular disease is the most common cause of major lower gastrointestinal (GI) bleeding in the elderly. Bleeding commonly occurs as an isolated event in a previously asymptomatic patient. It results from erosion and rupture of an adja-

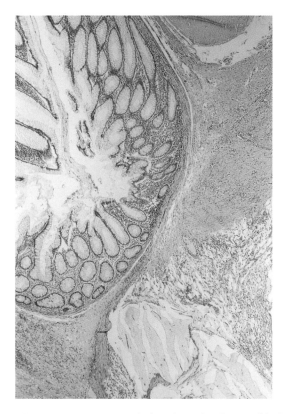

Figure 10–12. Mucin extravasation into pericolic fat in diverticulitis. The apex of the diverticulum is shown surrounded by pericolic fat. A lake of mucin is present outside the diverticulum in the pericolic fat.

cent penetrating muscular artery; the cause of arterial rupture is unknown, but it is rarely associated with significant diverticulitis.

Pathologic Features

The colonic mucosa in the area of diverticulosis is commonly normal; prominent mucosal folds around the ostia of the diverticula resulting from submucosal tissue excess is a common finding (Fig. 10–15).[13] Mucosal biopsy samples taken from

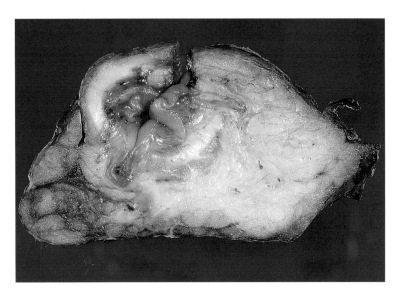

A

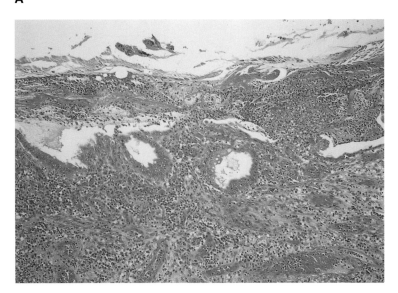

B

Figure 10–11. A: Colonic diverticulum, showing protrusion of the mucosa through the colonic wall. Focal discoloration is present in one area of the diverticulum, indicating early acute diverticulitis. B: Acute inflammation in a colonic diverticulum with pericolic extension.

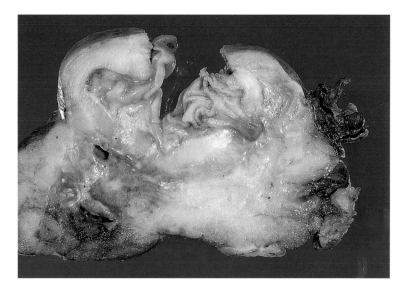

Figure 10–13. Acute diverticulitis with a pericolic abscess.

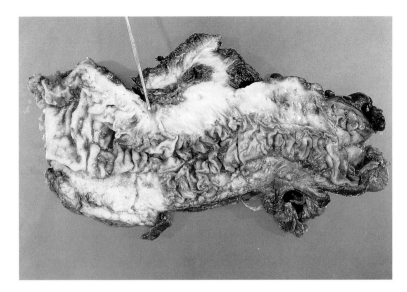

Figure 10–14. Chronic diverticulitis with marked fibrosis of the colonic wall, adherence to the urinary bladder, and resulting colovesical fistula.

around the ostia of diverticula are usually normal. They may, however, show mild crypt changes and a slight increase in the number of lymphocytes and plasma cells in the lamina propria, sometimes associated with small numbers of neutrophils (Fig. 10–16). Changes resembling mucosal prolapse, including lamina propria smooth muscle hypertrophy and fibrosis, and crypt elongation, may also occur.

Diverticula are often collapsed and difficult to demonstrate in resected specimens, particularly if they have been submitted after formalin fixation. Careful examination of the mucosal surface to identify the ostia followed by deep dissection in that vicinity permits recognition of the muscle wall defect and mucosal protrusion. In cases of diverticulitis, acute inflammation of the mucosa, pericolic suppuration, and pericolic fibrosis are present.

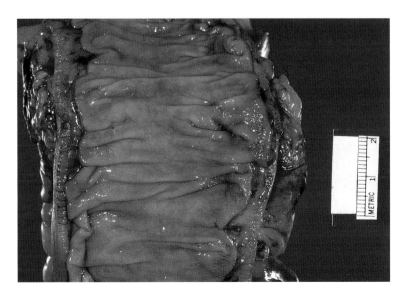

Figure 10–15. Mucosal surface of diverticulosis, showing the normal appearance of the mucosa except for the slight prominence of the ostia of the diverticula.

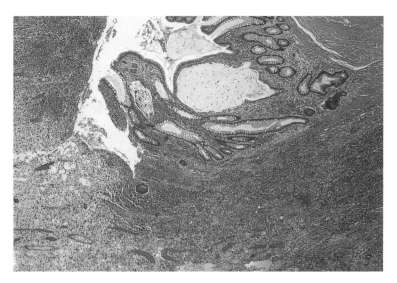

A

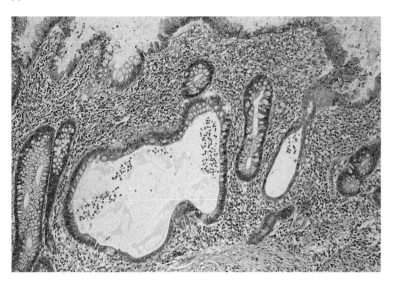

B

Figure 10–16. A: Diverticulitis, showing mild changes in the mucosa at the ostium of the diverticulum. These can be seen in a biopsy specimen from the ostium of a diverticulum. B: Mucosal changes at the ostium of a diverticulum (higher power micrograph of part A), showing crypt distortion and acute and chronic inflammation. These changes can simulate idiopathic inflammatory bowel disease.

Diverticular Disease-Associated Chronic Colitis

Chronic colitis clinically resembling idiopathic inflammatory bowel disease but restricted to the sigmoid colon may rarely complicate diverticular disease.[14] Patients present with abdominal pain and diarrhea with blood and mucus. Endoscopically, mucosal granularity and friability occur around the diverticular ostia (Fig. 10–17). The colon proximal and distal to the sigmoid colon are normal. The mucosa within the diverticula may be affected, leading to marked acute and chronic inflammation with crypt distortion and pericolic fibrosis. Mucosal biopsies show all the features of idiopathic inflammatory bowel disease, including surface erosion, increased lymphocytes, plasma cells and eosinophils, cryptitis with crypt abscesses, basal plasmacytosis, basal lymphoid aggregates, distorted crypt architecture, and Paneth cell metaplasia (see Chapter 11). The combination

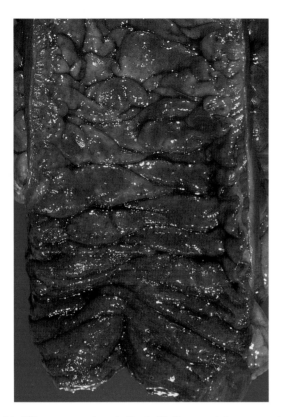

Figure 10–17. Diffuse mucosa erythema in diverticulitis. The mucosal changes were similar to mild ulcerative colitis. The mucosal abnormality was restricted to the part of the left colon involved with diverticulitis.

of mucosal changes of idopathic inflammatory bowel disease, rectal sparing, and thickening of the wall of the affected colon mimics Crohn's colitis.

Right-sided Diverticular Disease

Right-sided diverticular disease of the colon is much less common than left-sided in the United States. It has a male predominance and tends to occur more frequently in Asians. In Singapore, over half the patients with colonic diverticular disease have right-sided disease.[15] In 30% of cases of right-sided diverticular disease, left-sided diverticula are also present. Patients commonly have a presentation that mimics acute appendicitis, and the diagnosis is usually made intraoperatively when the appendix is found to be normal. Right-sided diverticular disease usually presents with severe lower GI hemorrhage, which is more common than in left-sided diverticular disease. Diverticulitis and fistula formation also occur, but less frequently than in left-sided disease.

COLITIDES (EXCLUDING IDIOPATHIC INFLAMMATORY BOWEL DISEASE)

Colitides are a group of diseases of diverse etiology that are characterized by inflammation of the colonic mucosa. The term "idiopathic inflammatory bowel disease" is used for ulcerative

colitis and Crohn's disease, which are considered in Chapter 11. Colitides that have specific clinical relevance are considered in this section.

Colitides must be interpreted by viewing the colon as a whole rather than through individual biopsy specimens. To do this, correlation of the endoscopic findings with biopsy samples that represent an adequate sampling of the observed changes is necessary. When colitis is patchy, distinguishing which areas are involved from those that are not is important. Endoscopic evaluation of colitis is more accurate than for gastritis, but minor endoscopic changes such as hyperemia and a perceived erosion frequently do not manifest histologically as colitis. When multiple specimens are taken from different parts of the colon, each site sampled must be submitted as a separate specimen, with its location denoted accurately on the request form. Ideally diagrams of the colon can be used to mark the biopsy sites.

Normal Colonic Mucosa

Normal colonic mucosa is composed of a flat surface from which the crypts extend vertically down to the level of the muscularis mucosae (Fig. 10–18A). The crypts are straight, tubular structures without any bending or branching. The surface epithelium and crypts are lined by columnar cells of colonic type with numerous goblet cells.

The crypts are separated by a small amount of lamina propria that normally contains small numbers of lymphocytes, plasma cells, and eosinophils (see Fig. 10–18A). Eosinophils occur in greater numbers in the right colon than in the left colon. Normal colonic mucosa does not have any extravascular neutrophils in the lamina propria or crypts. No inflammatory cells occur between the crypt base and muscularis mucosae in normal mucosa. Intraepithelial lymphocytes are present in the surface epithelium; normally 6 or fewer lymphocytes are present for every 100 epithelial cells (Fig. 10–18B). The nuclei of the surface epithelial cells are ovoid, with their longitudinal axis perpendicular to the basement membrane. The nuclei are seen as a row in the basal region of the cell, separated from the basement membrane by a thin layer of subnuclear eosinophilic cytoplasm (see Fig. 10–18B). A thin layer of collagen is normally associated with the basement membrane; this is seen in trichrome stains as a uniform layer less than 5 μm thick (Fig. 10–18C). Frequently, capillaries are present immediately below the basement membrane. Macrophages with abundant foamy cytoplasm are sometimes seen in otherwise normal colonic mucosa; these are called muciphages and are of no significance.

Apoptosis, manifested by the presence of cellular nuclear debris immediately beneath the surface epithelium, is sometimes seen in colon biopsies that are otherwise normal (Fig. 10–19). Normal apoptosis is the mechanism of programmed cell death at the surface; in normal apoptosis, nuclear debris does not accumulate in the mucosa. The presence of apoptotic material in the mucosa most likely indicates increased surface cell death. Its clinical significance is unknown; when seen, the pos-

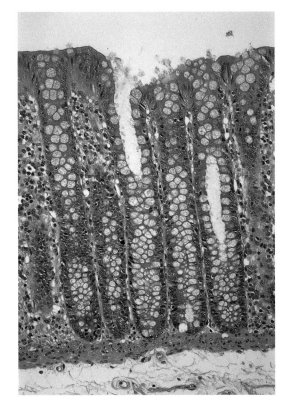

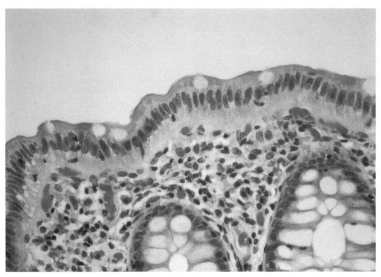

B

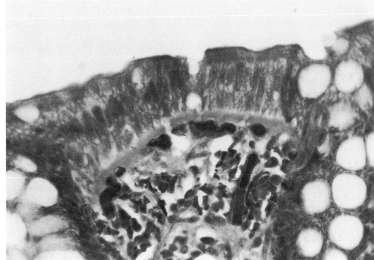

C

Figure 10–18. A: Normal colonic mucosa showing vertical crypts extending down to the muscularis mucosae and very little lamina propria cellularity. B: Normal colonic mucosa, showing the normal surface epithelium, which has its nucleus separated from the basement membrane by subnuclear cytoplasm. The lamina propria cellularity is normal. C: Normal colonic mucosa, trichrome stain showing a thin layer of basement membrane collagen. Note the smooth uniform appearance of the layer and the capillaries immediately below the collagen.

A

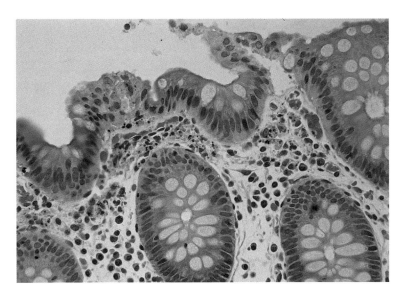

Figure 10–19. Colonic mucosa showing increased apoptosis with nuclear debris and a focus of disorganization of the surface epithelium, most likely representing minimal surface epithelial damage.

sibility of mild injury to colonic mucosa, such as that produced by nonsteroidal antiinflammatory drugs, should be considered. The highest amounts of apoptotic material is seen in patients being treated with chemotherapeutic agents such as 5-fluorouracil.[16] Increased apoptosis is associated with melanosis coli (see following section).

The lamina propria contains capillaries. Lymphatics, however, are restricted to the deepest region of the mucosa. The paucity of lymphatics in colonic mucosa explains the absence of risk for metastasis in intramucosal carcinoma of the colon. Lymphoid nodules are normally present in the deep mucosa and submucosa. These are usually small and widely scattered; they frequently show reactive centers. Sometimes, the crypts are associated intimately with the lymphoid tissue forming lymphoglandular structures (Fig. 10–20). In these foci, the crypts frequently show mild distortion and extend below the muscularis mucosae to come into intimate relationship with the underlying lymphoid tissue. The epithelium associated with lym-

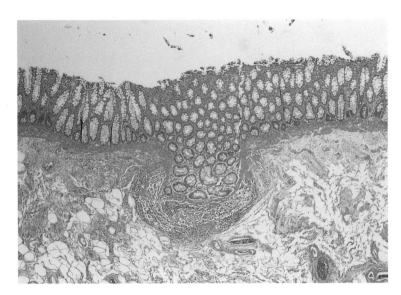

Figure 10–20. Normal colonic mucosa showing a lymphoglandular structure. The crypts are somewhat distorted and dip down below the muscularis mucosae to come into intimate relationship with the underlying lymphoid follicle.

phoid follicles contains specialized membranous epithelial cells (M cells), which take up antigens from the lumen and transfer them to the associated lymphoid tissue.

Melanosis Coli

Melanosis coli refers to a black discoloration of the colonic mucosa. It affects the entire colon and rectum with a coloration that ranges from a brownish tinge to deep black depending on the amount of pigment deposition. Melanosis does not produce any clinical symptoms. Histologically, varying numbers of macrophages occur in the lamina propria that contain brown pigment granules (Fig. 10–21). Ultrastructural studies have shown that the pigment is lipofuscin, which is produced by residual bodies resulting from cellular material digested in autolysosomes. Melanosis coli is associated with increased colonic epithelial apoptosis (see Fig. 10–21).[17]

Melanosis coli has a strong association with chronic constipation and the chronic use of laxatives of the anthracene group (cascara, senna, aloes, rhubarb). These anthracene laxatives produce melanosis by causing epithelial cell damage, visible as increased apoptosis. The damaged cellular organelles are digested in autolysosomes, resulting in residual bodies containing lipofuscin pigment. Any cause of toxic epithelial cell damage leading to increased apoptosis can result in melanosis coli, providing an explanation for those cases not associated with chronic laxative intake.

Acute Nonspecific Colitis

Acute nonspecific colitis (also called acute self-limited colitis) is a clinicopathologic entity in which patients present with fever and acute-onset diarrhea, sometimes associated with blood and mucus, and the colonic mucosa shows acute inflammation characterized by the presence of extravascular neutrophils in

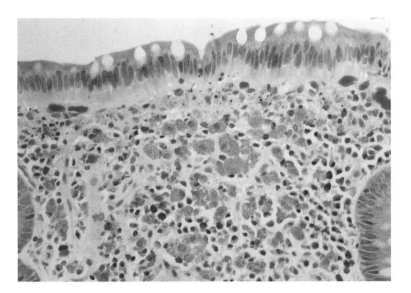

A

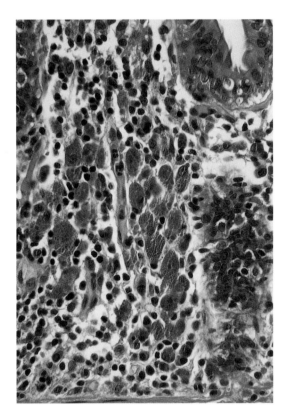

B

Figure 10–21. A: Melanosis coli, showing macrophages containing brown pigment in the colonic mucosa. Apoptosis is increased as shown by increased nuclear debris under the surface epithelium. B: Melanosis coli showing numerous pigment-laden macrophages in the lamina propria.

the lamina propria (Fig. 10–22). Acute cryptitis and crypt abscesses may occur, but these are less prominent than in idiopathic inflammatory bowel disease. Even a small number of extravascular neutrophils in the colonic lamina propria is abnormal; it is important, however, to recognize that extravascular neutrophils are present whenever lamina propria hemorrhage occurs without signifying acute inflammation. The presence of marginated neutrophils within capillaries in the mucosa does not constitute acute inflammation. Acute nonspecific coli-

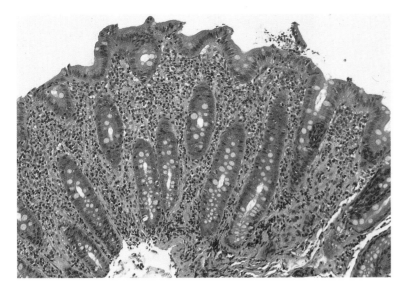

A

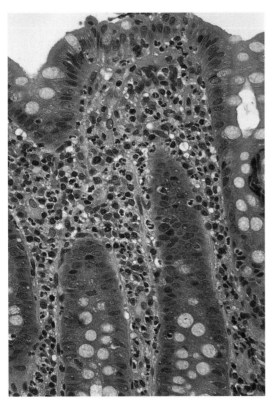

B

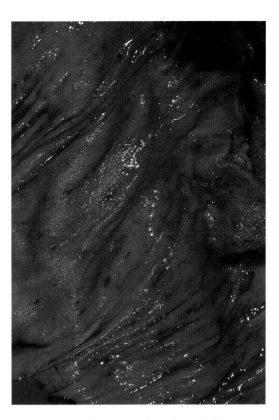

Figure 10–23. Acute colitis with multiple, small, superficial mucosal erosions.

Figure 10–22. A: Acute nonspecific colitis, showing normal crypt architecture and increased numbers of inflammatory cells in the lamina propria, including extravascular neutrophils. B: Acute nonspecific colitis, showing neutrophils in the lamina propria.

tis may involve the colon diffusely or it may be patchy. When surface erosion is present, the term "acute erosive colitis" may be used (Fig. 10–23). Acute colitis must be distinguished from cases of chronic colitis (idiopathic inflammatory bowel disease) in a phase of activity.

In most cases of acute colitis, a cause is not found on histologic examination. Many of these cases have an infectious etiology, proven by stool culture or culture of a biopsy specimen; commonly responsible organisms are *Salmonella, Campylobac-*

ter, Yersinia, and *Shigella* species among bacteria and rotavirus. Cases in which an infectious cause is found on stool culture can be specifically named after the agent, for example, acute *Salmonella* colitis. In at least 30% of cases of acute colitis, no infectious agent is found; these cases are called acute nonspecific colitis. Acute nonspecific colitis has a self-limited clinical course, with spontaneous resolution of symptoms and absence of recurrence. For this reason, the term "acute self-limited colitis" is often used for these cases.

At the time of biopsy reporting in a patient with acute colitis, results of stool culture are unknown to the surgical pathologist. Because some cases reported as acute nonspecific (or self-limited) colitis may represent specific infections identified by stool culture, it is the gastroenterologist's responsibility to identify these cases and treat them accordingly.

Diffuse Acute Nonspecific Colitis

Diffuse acute nonspecific colitis represents an important clinicopathologic entity. Typically, endoscopy and biopsy samples have shown acute colitis involving the whole colorectum or a large contiguous area of it. Cultures have been negative, excluding an infectious agent. The patient is still symptomatic 3–4 days after presentation when the study results have returned. Further treatment of this patient depends on whether he or she has acute self-limited colitis, which requires no treatment and will resolve spontaneously, or this is the first episode of an idiopathic inflammatory bowel disease, which requires aggressive treatment and presents a lifelong problem to the patient.

Evaluation of endoscopic biopsies is a highly reliable method of distinguishing between acute self-limited colitis and idiopathic inflammatory bowel disease (Table 10–1).[18] Endoscopic features such as diffuse or focal friability, erythema, and edema have no discriminating value. Acute self-limited colitis is characterized by normal crypt architecture associated with acute inflammation of the lamina propria (see Fig. 10–22). These changes are present even when the initial biopsy is delayed by up to 4 days. Idiopathic inflammatory bowel disease is characterized by diffusely abnormal crypt architecture and mixed acute and chronic inflammation, changes that are present as early as 7 days after the primary onset of illness.

In most cases, the biopsy distinction between acute self-limited colitis and idiopathic inflammatory bowel disease is clear-cut and definite. A small gray area exists, however, where differentiting between them is difficult; in these cases, biopsy specimens show mild, focal crypt distortion and a slight increase of chronic inflammatory cells, both of which occur in acute self-limited colitis. (see Table 10–1). In Surawicz and colleagues' original study,[18] 8% of patients with acute self-limited

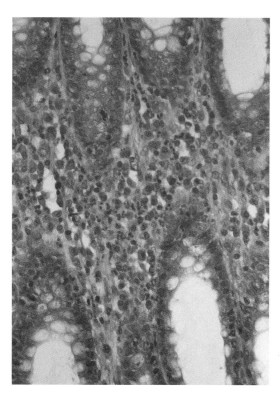

Figure 10–24. Focal acute colitis, showing focal infiltration of the lamina propria by neutrophils. This was an incidental finding in a random section of a colon removed for familial adenomatous polyposis.

TABLE 10–1. SIGNIFICANT HISTOLOGIC FEATURES IN DIFFERENTIATING ACUTE SELF-LIMITED COLITIS FROM ACUTE-ONSET IDIOPATHIC INFLAMMATORY BOWEL DISEASE

	Acute Self-Limited Colitis	Acute-Onset IIBD
Crypt Architecture		
Normal	Yes	Rare
Marked, diffuse distortion	No	Yes
Focal or slight diffuse changes	Possible	Possible
Branched glands	Rare	Yes
Villiform surface	No	Rare
Crypt atrophy	Rare	Possible
Lamina propria inflammation		
Acute only	Yes	No
Acute and chronic	Possible	Yes
Crypt abscesses	Common	Yes
Cryptitis without abscesses	Possible	Rare
Basal plasmacytosis	Rare	Yes
Basal lymphoid aggregates	Rare	Yes
Basal lymphoid hyperplasia	Rare	Common
Isolated giant cells	Rare	Rare
Epithelioid granuloma	Rare	Rare
Granulomatous crypt abscess	Possible	Possible
Other		
Goblet cell mucin depletion	Yes	Yes*
Reactive epithelial hyperplasia	Yes	Yes*

Abbreviation: IIBD = idiopathic inflammatory bowel disease.
Source: Surawicz CM, Haggitt RC, Husseman M, et al. Mucosal biopsy diagnosis of colitis: acute self-limited colitis and idiopathic inflammatory bowel disease. Gastroenterology. 1994;107:755–763.
Yes = found in >50% of cases; Common = found in 25–50% of cases; Possible = found in 10–25% of cases; Rare = found in <10% of cases; No = not found.
*These features, although usually found in both, are significantly more common in acute IBD.

colitis were diagnosed with idiopathic inflammatory bowel disease, and rare patients with idiopathic inflammatory bowel disease had specimens interpreted as acute self-limited colitis. Therkildsen and colleagues[19] followed a group of 32 patients with acute diarrhea who had normal crypt architecture and

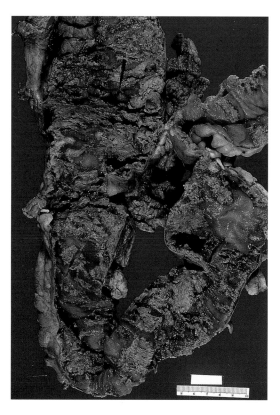

Figure 10–25. Acute amebic colitis with toxic megacolon. The mucosa shows diffuse confluent ulcers with relatively normal intervening colonic mucosa.

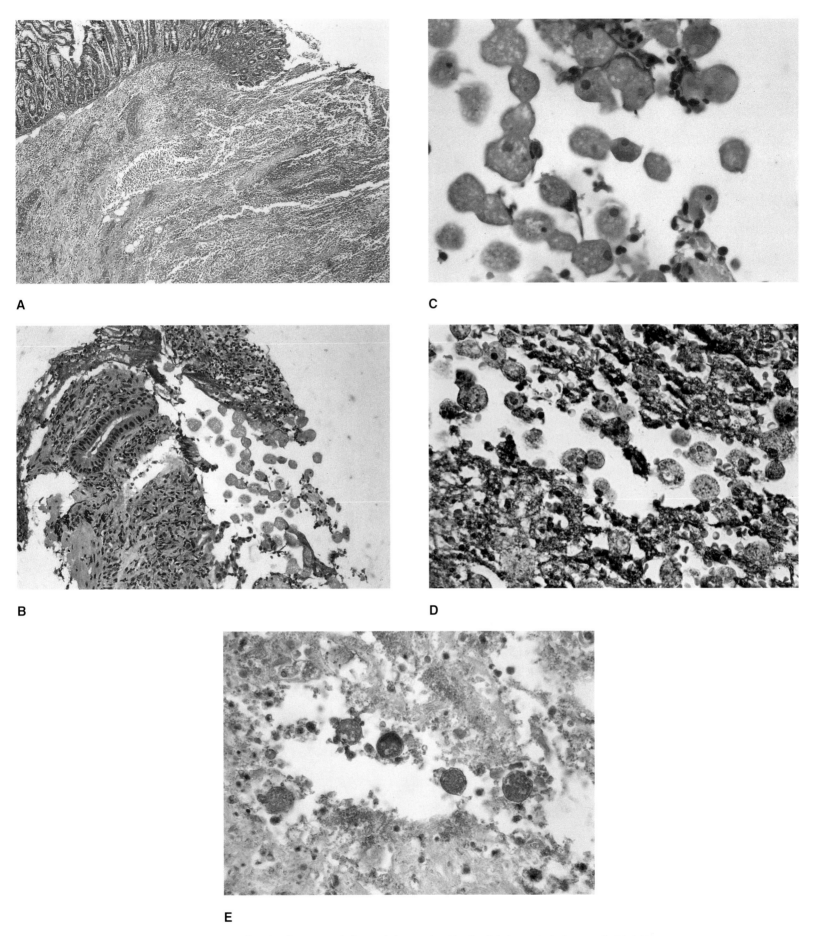

Figure 10–26. A: Acute amebic colitis, showing typical submucosal abscess undermining the relatively normal colonic mucosa. B: Colonic biopsy specimen in amebic colitis, showing mucosal inflammation, reactive atypia in the crypts, and a collection of amebic trophozoites on the surface. C: Amebic trophozoites in colonic biopsy specimen. D: Amebic trophozoites in necrotic debris, trichrome stain. Note the presence of intracytoplasmic erythrocytes in the trophozoites. E: Immunoperoxidase stain for *Entamoeba histolytica*, showing positive staining in trophozoites.

nonspecific inflammation in the initial biopsy specimen; after several years, 30% of these patients had developed idiopathic inflammatory bowel disease. In practice, it is advisable to make a diagnosis of acute self-limited colitis in all specimens with borderline features and to recommend follow-up with repeat biopsy if symptoms persist or relapse. In this way, the pathologist makes use of the final criterion for diagnosis of acute self-limited colitis, that is, the fact that these patients recover spontaneously and do not recur.

Focal Active Colitis

Focal active colitis is a common abnormality encountered in mucosal biopsy samples of the colon, both in patients with acute diarrhea as well as an isolated finding in patients undergoing screening colonscopy to exclude neoplasia. This condition is defined by the presence of cryptitis and crypt abscesses associated with neutrophils in the lamina propria in a small area of the mucosa with the rest of the mucosa being normal (Fig. 10–24).[20]

Focal active colitis is commonly seen in patients with a history of Crohn's disease, representing patchy colonic involvement, or partially treated ulcerative colitis. When there is no history of chronic idiopathic inflammatory bowel disease, and focal active colitis is encountered in a patient with acute diarrhea, most cases are due to acute self-limited colitis or infectious colitis, with rare cases due to ischemic colitis. The risk that these patients will progress to idiopathic inflammatory bowel disease in the future is minimal. Focal active colitis found in an asymptomatic patient without diarrhea when the endoscopy is a screening procedure is not clinically significant.[20]

Specific Infectious Colitides

Rarely, a specific infectious agent is identified in a biopsy showing colitis. In these cases, a specific diagnosis is possible by histologic examination; although most of these cases also have positive stool examinations, it is imperative that the pathologist makes the diagnosis based on the biopsy specimen. Many of these infections are not self-limited and can progress to severe acute life-threatening disease as well as chronic disease.

Amebic colitis and tuberculosis of the colon progress into a chronic phase in which chronic inflammation and significant regenerative changes, including mild crypt distortion, may occur in the colonic mucosa. Differentiation from idiopathic inflammatory bowel disease may be difficult in these cases unless the specific agent is identified.

Amebic Colitis

Amebic colitis is characterized by acute onset of diarrhea, often with blood and mucus. Any part of the colon can be affected; the disease is commonly focal, but diffuse involvement occurs in severe cases. Amebic colitis is characterized by flask-shaped ulcers that are mainly submucosal with a small mucosal ulcer. Endoscopically, small mucosal ulcers are separated by normal-appearing mucosa; this normal-appearing mucosa is undermined by the submucosal abscess. With increasing severity, the undermined mucosa sloughs off, leading to large areas of confluent ulceration (Fig. 10–25). Specimens should be taken from the normal-appearing mucosa at the ulcer's edge and from the necrotic ulcer's base. Microscopically, the submucosal ulcer is composed of necrotic tissue surrounded by inflammatory cells (Fig. 10–26A). Biopsy samples from the center of the ulcer show necrotic debris in which *Entamoeba histolytica* trophozoites can be seen. These are large, rounded structures with granular cytoplasm and a small, round, eccentric nucleus (Figs. 10–26B and C). They may contain ingested erythrocytes in the cytoplasm. *Entamoeba histolytica* trophozoites are easily visible in routine H&E-stained sections. Special stains, such as periodic acid–Schiff (PAS), trichrome stain (Fig. 10–26D), and immunoperoxidase stain (Fig. 10–26E), can be useful when organisms are few in number. The intact mucosa shows acute and chronic inflammation, with mild crypt distortion and regenerative change that can mimic mild idiopathic inflammatory bowel disease (Fig. 10–27). Amebae are generally not present in the mucosal part of the biopsy sample, except when a biopsy is performed on a very early lesion (Fig. 10–28). In severe cases, the colon shows features of a fulminant colitis with severe hemorrhage or toxic megacolon with multiple perforations (see Fig. 10–25). A diagnosis of amebic colitis is liable to be missed because most pathologists do not focus on the necrotic tissue where the diagnostic trophozoites are present.

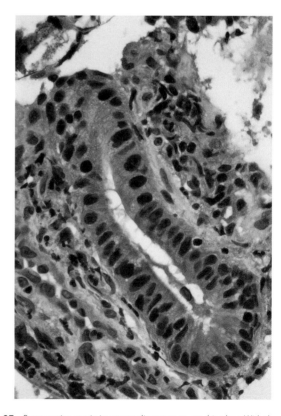

Figure 10–27. Regenerative atypia in crypts adjacent to an amebic ulcer. With the crypt atrophy and severe inflammation, this has the potential to be misinterpreted as low-grade dysplasia in ulcerative colitis if the amebic trophozoites are not identified.

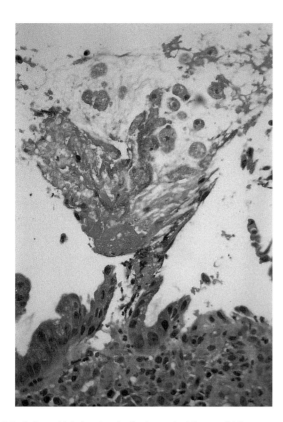

Figure 10–28. Early amebic lesion, showing focal necrosis of the superficial mucosa associated with a necrotic exudate containing *E. histolytica* trophozoites.

The chronic phase of amebic colitis may result in localized mass lesions that contain necrosis, disorganized mucosal regeneration, and fibrosis (Fig. 10–29). These so-called amebomas occur most commonly in the cecum and rectum and can mimic malignant neoplasms and cause intestinal obstruction.

Colonic Tuberculosis

Colonic tuberculosis can involve any part of the colorectum. In the acute phase, localized ulceration of the mucosa occurs; the ulcers tend to be transverse. In the early acute stage of tubercu-

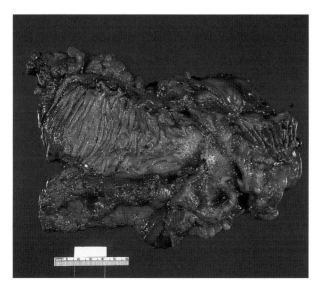

Figure 10–29. Chronic amebic colitis, showing mass effect and luminal narrowing.

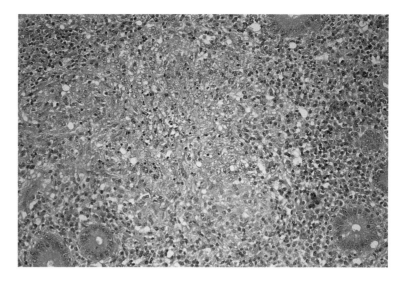

A

B

C

Figure 10–30. A: Colonic biopsy specimen in tuberculosis, showing necrotizing granulomatous inflammation. The epithelioid cell granuloma has a central area of necrosis. B: Colonic biopsy sample, showing poorly defined granulomatous inflammation with diffuse macrophage infiltration in between colonic crypts. C: Acid-fast stain in colonic tuberculosis, showing numerous mycobacteria in macrophages in the colonic mucosa.

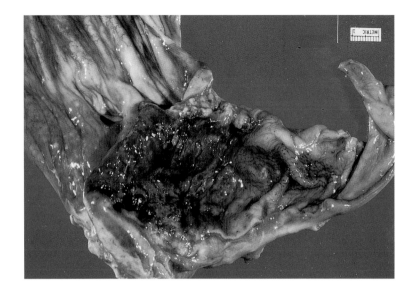

Figure 10–31. Hyperplastic cecal tuberculosis, showing a necrotic mass lesion.

losis, the small ulcers scattered in a mildly inflamed segment of the mucosa can resemble Crohn's colitis. Biopsy specimens, which show acute and chronic inflammation, surface erosion, mild crypt distortion, and epithelioid granulomas, can also mimic Crohn's disease. The diagnosis is obvious when caseous necrosis is present in the center of the granuloma (Fig. 10–30A). When ceseation is not obvious, tuberculosis should be suspected when the granulomatous inflammation is somewhat diffuse (Fig. 10–30B), as opposed to the tightly circumscribed sarcoid-like granulomas of Crohn's disease. Nongranulomatous inflammation with numerous macrophages is typical of tuber-

culosis occurring in immunocompromised patients, particularly those who are human immunodeficiency virus (HIV)-positive. Staining for acid-fast bacilli is usually positive and permits diagnosis, especially in lesions without well-formed necrotizing granulomas, where organisms are usually plentiful (Fig. 10–30C).

In the more chronic phase of colonic tuberculosis, extensive caseation and fibrosis may result in a mass lesion; this occurs mainly in the ileocecal region (hyperplastic cecal tuberculosis) (Fig. 10–31). Chronic colonic tuberculosis may also be associated with fibrous thickening of the wall with obstruction (Fig. 10–32). These cases are frequently mistaken for malignant neoplasms clinically. Tuberculous strictures are much more common in the small intestine than in the colon (see Chapter 8).

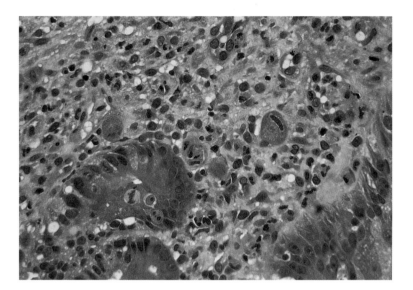

A

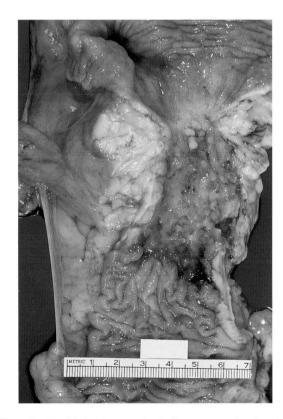

Figure 10–32. Colonic stricture associated with a transverse tuberculous ulcer.

B

Figure 10–33. A: Cytomegalovirus colitis showing CMV-infected cells with typical cell enlargement and inclusions in a mucosal biopsy. B: Cytomegalovirus colitis showing inclusions in enlarged vascular endothelial cells in granulation tissue in the base of a mucosal ulcer.

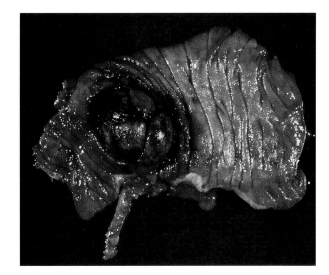

A

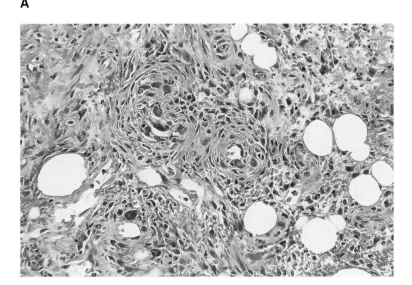

B

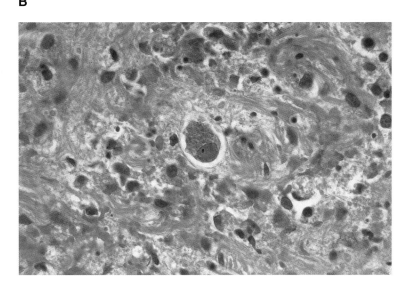

C

Figure 10–34. A: Hemorrhagic cecal mass lesion secondary to cytomegalovirus infection. B: Vascular proliferation and inflammation in the submucosa in the lesion illustrated in part A. Note the numerous CMV-infected enlarged cells with hyperchromatic nuclei lining some of the vascular spaces. C: Cytomegalovirus inclusion in stromal cell in the colonic mass lesion shown in part A, showing cell enlargement, Cowdry A intranuclear inclusion, and granular intracytoplasmic inclusions.

Cytomegaloviral Colitis

Cytomegalovirus proctocolitis may result in an acute colitis with multiple ulcers; the typical virally infected cells are seen in both the glandular epithelial cells and vascular endothelial cells in the lamina propria (Fig. 10–33). Rarely, the vascular proliferation associated with this infection results in a mass-like effect that grossly resembles a hemorrhagic malignant neoplasm (Fig. 10–34A). Microscopically, this is characterized by a vascular proliferation that superficially resembles Kaposi's sarcoma, necrosis, hemorrhage, and inflammation (Fig. 10–34B). Cytomegaloviral inclusions are present in the endothelial cells and stromal cells (Fig. 10–34C). Some cases resemble pseudo-membranous colitis[10]; rarely, toxic megacolon may occur.

Colonic Histoplasmosis

Histoplasma capsulatum infection may involve both the small and large intestine, ordinarily in disseminated disease. This occurs commonly in endemic areas such as the Ohio and Mississippi River valleys, affecting both immunocompetent and immunocompromised individuals. In nonendemic areas, the disease is usually only seen in immunocompromised patients, particularly those who are HIV-positive.

In both the small and large intestine, the lesions resemble tuberculosis with ulcers, mass-like lesions, and strictures (Fig. 10–35). In biopsy specimens from colonic lesions, acute and chronic inflammation is evident, with macrophages containing the organisms. The macrophages may form granulomas or appear as a diffuse infiltrate in the lamina propria (Fig. 10–36A). *Histoplasma capsulatum* is 2–4 mm, round, and intracellular. They can be seen clearly in routine H&E sections (Fig. 10–36B), but are accentuated with fungal stains such as PAS and methenamine silver (Fig. 10–36C). When organisms are few in number in a biopsy sample from a patient not known to have histoplasmosis, careful examination and considerable diagnostic acumen is required for diagnosis.

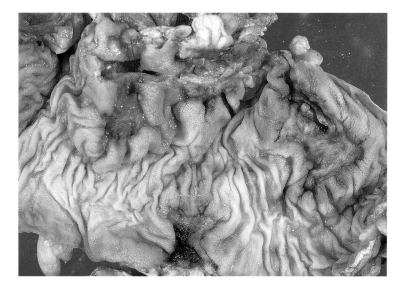

Figure 10–35. Histoplasmosis, showing two large ulcers in the ascending colon. These resemble malignant ulcers grossly.

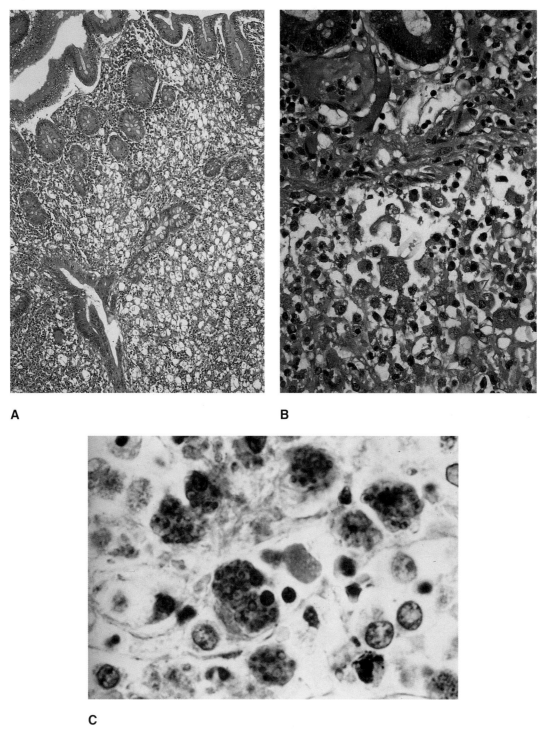

Figure 10–36. A: Colonic histoplasmosis, showing diffuse infiltration of the lamina propria by foamy macrophages. B: Colonic macrophages, showing multiple, small, intracellular yeast forms in the cytoplasm of macrophages. C: Methenamine silver stain, showing yeasts in the macrophages.

Other Specific Colitides

Intestinal spirochetosis is seen commonly in colonic samples from patients with acquired immunodeficiency syndrome (AIDS); this appears as a layer of basophilic bacilli lining the surface epithelium, giving the surface a "hair-like" appearance (Fig. 10–37). This is discussed in more detail in Chapter 17.

Balantidium coli, the only ciliated protozoan parasite that infects humans, causes a very rare disease similar to amebic col-

itis with submucosal abscesses. Patients are usually asymptomatic, but may have a mild diarrhea. The organism can be found in stool samples or in biopsy specimens of the ulcer base; it is a very large trophozoite or cyst with a characteristic large V-shaped nucleus (Fig. 10–38).

Nematode parasites that exist in the lumen of the colon in infested individuals include *Trichuris trichiura* (whipworm) and *Enterobius vermicularis* (pinworm). Sometimes, these worms are encountered during surgery or gross examination of a re-

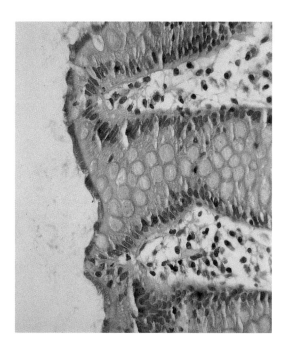

Figure 10–37. Intestinal spirochetosis, showing the basophilic hair-like surface infestation of spirochetes on the surface epithelium.

sected colon. Whipworms are long, thin worms with a whip-like narrowing at one end; the mature female worm has the typical barrel-shaped ova with a plug at either end (Fig. 10–39). *Enterobius vermicularis* is most commonly seen in the appendiceal lumen (see Chapter 9). Rarely, *Enterobius* penetrates the wall of the colon, forming eosinophilic abscesses in the wall with marked fibrosis; the abscesses contain adult worms (Fig. 10–40).

Schistosoma mansoni infection is common in endemic parts the world, usually the Middle East. Adult worms and ova can be found in the mucosa of colonic biopsy specimens from

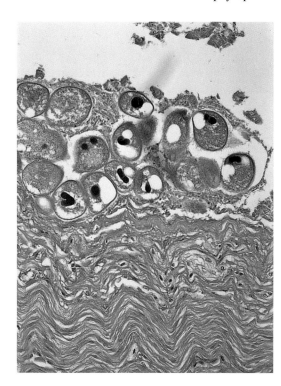

Figure 10–38. *Balantidium coli* infection of the colon, showing the base of an ulcer with numerous large organisms with the typical V-shaped nucleus.

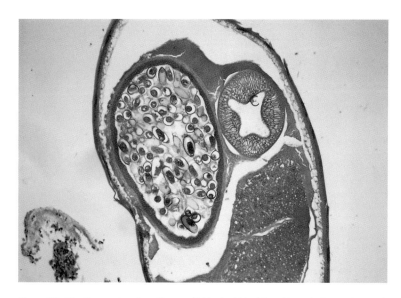

Figure 10–39. Cross section of a whipworm (*Trichuris trichiura*) found in a colonic resection specimen showing the typical barrel-shaped ova in the worm's uterus.

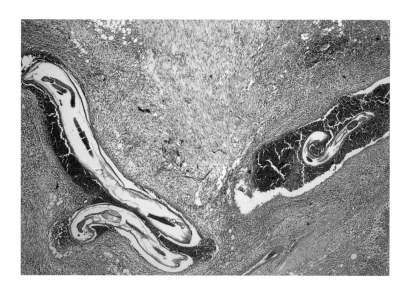

A

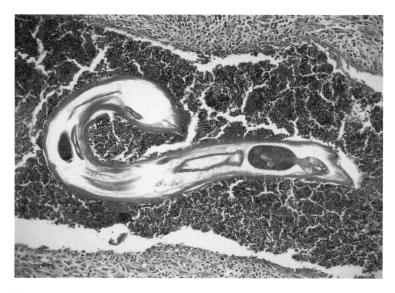

B

Figure 10–40. A: Fibrosis and eosinophilic abscesses in colonic wall containing several adult *Enterobius vermicularis*. B: Eosinophilic abscess in colonic wall containing *E. vermicularis* adult.

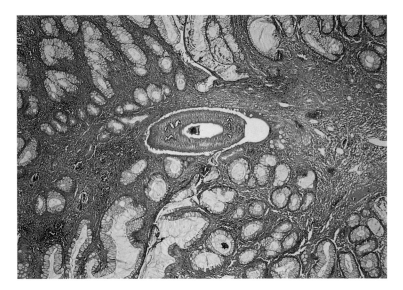

Figure 10–41. *Schistosoma mansoni* adult worm in a venule in the colonic mucosa.

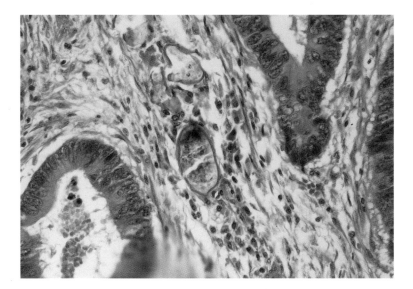

Figure 10–43. *Schistosoma mansoni* ovum in relation to an adenocarcinoma of the colon.

patients from endemic areas (Figs. 10–41 and 10–42). Schistosomiasis is usually an incidental finding and is not associated with colitis; presence of this organism should not divert the pathologist's search for other pathology. We have encountered a case of colonic adenocarcinoma with *Schistosoma* ova (Fig. 10–43); there is no known causal relationship between schistosomiasis and colorectal cancer.

Lymphocytic, Microscopic, and Collagenous Colitis

Lymphocytic and collagenous colitis are uncommon diseases of unknown cause that have been grouped together under the

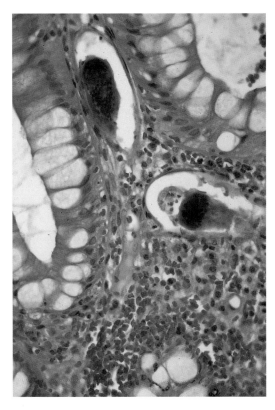

Figure 10–42. *Schistosoma mansoni* ovum in colonic mucosa.

term "microscopic colitis" because they are defined by microscopic abnormalities alone.[21] Lymphocytic and collagenous colitis frequently coexist in the same biopsy specimen or in different specimens in the same patient. Evolution of one form of disease to the other has also been reported. There is no evidence that these diseases are in any way related to idiopathic inflammatory bowel disease. Patients with celiac disease frequently show changes similar to lymphocytic colitis in the colonic mucosa. There is an association between these colitides and (1) the regular intake of nonsteroidal antiinflammatory drugs and (2) autoimmune diseases.

Patients are predominantly female and, although the disease can be seen in a wide age range, the majority of cases are in the 40–70-year group. The dominant symptom is high-volume watery diarrhea. Mucus is rarely present, and bleeding does not occur. Colicky abdominal pain, fecal incontinence particularly at night, and mild weight loss are common. Colonoscopy and radiologic studies are normal. The natural history of the disease is benign, with remissions and relapses. A few patients have debilitating diarrhea.

The diagnosis is made by histologic changes in mucosal specimens. Lymphocytic colitis is characterized by:

1. An increased number of intraepithelial lymphocytes in the surface and crypt epithelium (Fig. 10–44). Normally there are 6 or fewer lymphocytes/100 epithelial cells. In lymphocytic colitis, this increases greatly, often to over 25/100 epithelial cells. The intraepithelial lymphocytes are predominantly CD8+ suppressor/cytotoxic T cells (Fig. 10–44D).
2. An increased number of lymphocytes, plasma cells, eosinophils, and mast cells in the lamina propria (Fig. 10–44B). The lamina propria lymphocytes are mainly CD4+ helper T cells (Fig. 10–44D). The inflammatory cells often cluster at the crypt base, but are present throughout the mucosa. Neutrophils are rarely present, and then in very small numbers.
3. Evidence of surface epithelial damage with decreased cell height and mucin depletion (Fig. 10–44B and C). This is often

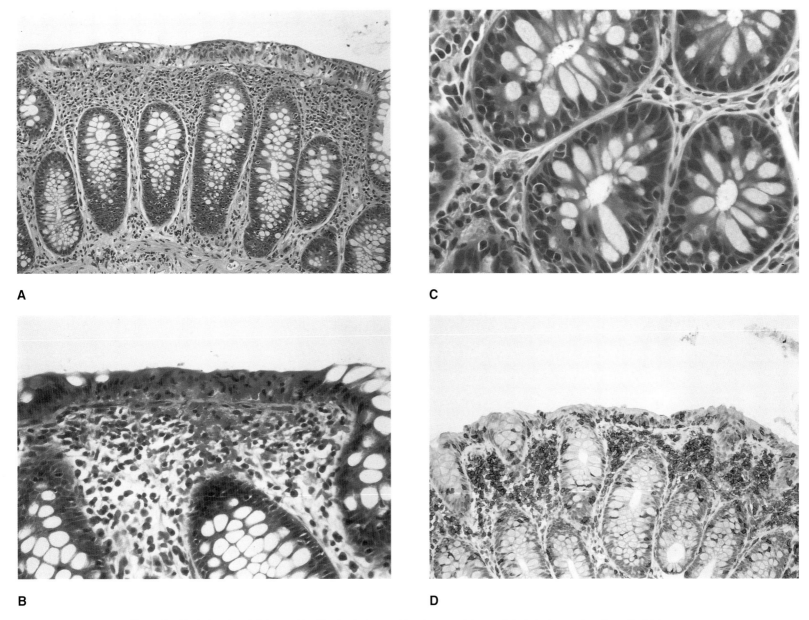

Figure 10–44. A: Lymphocytic (microscopic) colitis, showing increased lymphocytes and plasma cells in the lamina propria, surface epithelial damage, and an increased number of intraepithelial lymphocytes. B: Lymphocytic (microscopic) colitis, showing surface epithelial damage and inflammatory cells in the lamina propria and surface epithelial. In this trichrome-stained section, the collagen layer is of normal thickness. C: Lymphocytic (microscopic) colitis, showing infiltration of crypts by lymphocytes. D: Lymphocytic colitis, immunoperoxidase stain for the pan-T-cell marker CD3, showing increased T lymphocytes in both the surface epithelium and the lamina propria.

associated with surface epithelial detachment in biopsy samples.

4. Crypts that are normal in length and architecture. Lymphocytic colitis may or may not be associated with features of collagenous colitis (Fig. 10–45A).

Collagenous colitis is characterized by:

1. A subepithelial collagen band that is thicker than 10 μm (a band >15μm makes the diagnosis less sensitive and more specific) and sometimes reaches over 50 μm (Fig. 10–45B and C). The "normal" thickness of collagen in the basement membrane is less than 7 μm, but slight thickening without inflammation may be seen in hyperplastic polyps, diverticu-

lar disease, and megacolon. In routine sections, care must be taken not to mistake the layer of subnuclear eosinophilic cytoplasm normally present in the colonic epithelial cell for the basement membrane. Collagen deposition is visible in H&E sections, but is better seen in trichrome-stained sections (see Fig. 10–45C). The thickness of the collagen layer must be measured in a vertically oriented part of the mucosa. The basement membrane collagen deposition is frequently patchy and tends to favor the right side of the colon. However, the rectosigmoid area that is accessible to a flexible sigmoidoscope has a 90% probability of providing diagnostic tissue, particularly when multiple specimens are taken.

2. The collagen layer has an irregular lower edge due to exten-

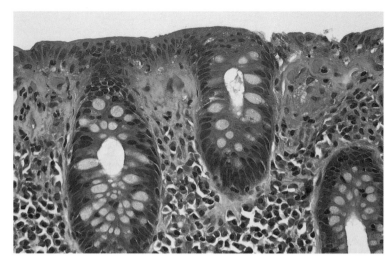

A

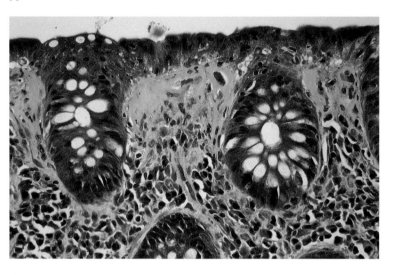

B

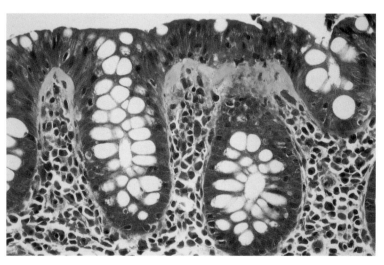

C

Figure 10–45. A: Collagenous colitis, showing a thick, irregular layer of collagen beneath the basement membrane. B: Collagenous colitis, trichrome stain, showing entrapped capillaries in the thickened collagen layer under the basement membrane. This degree of collagen deposition satisfies minimal criteria for collagenous colitis. C: Collagenous colitis, showing thickened collagen layer under the basement membrane. This has an irregular lower edge. Again, the degree of collagen thickening shown here satisfies minimal criteria for a diagnosis of collagenous colitis. Most cases have more collagen deposition than shown here.

sion of collagen into the lamina propria in contrast with the sharp and distinct lower edge of the normal basement membrane (Fig. 10–45C).

3. Superficial capillaries are entrapped within the thickened collagen layer (see Fig. 10–45B). The majority of cases of collagenous colitis have features of lymphocytic colitis. The diagnosis of collagenous colitis should be made with caution when changes of lymphocytic colitis are not present. It is particularly important in these cases to ensure that tangential sectioning is not the cause for a thickened collagen layer (Fig. 10–46); the section must show the entire longitudinal extent of the crypt in the affected area.

Diarrhea in collagenous colitis is a secretory diarrhea, the severity of which is more closely related to surface epithelial damage and the degree of lamina propria inflammation than to the thickness of the collagen band.[22] Treatment with sulfasalazine and other 5-ASA derivatives has been reported to be beneficial.

Eosinophilic Colitis

Eosinophils are normally present in the colonic lamina propria in variable numbers and are more numerous in the right colon than in the left. Eosinophils accompany other inflammatory cells in ulcerative colitis, Crohn's colitis, lymphocytic colitis, parasitic infestations of the colon, and allergy to drugs like nonsteroidal antiinflammatories. In patients with quiescent ulcerative colitis, eosinophils may be the dominant inflammatory cell in the mucosa.

When prominent eosinophils are an isolated finding in colonic mucosa, they merit description, but no clinical significance is usually ascribed to their presence. Their presence in large numbers (Fig. 10–47) or as local eosinophilic microabscesses should prompt a search for parasitic agents such as

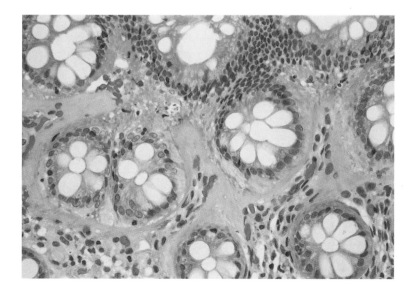

Figure 10–46. Normal colonic mucosa, tangentially cut (note the horizontally cut crypts), giving a spurious impression of a thickened collagen layer. Note the absence of abnormality in the surface and crypt epithelium.

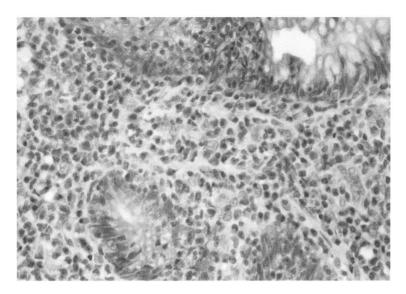

Figure 10–47. Eosinophilic colitis, showing lamina propria and crypts infiltrated by numerous eosinophils.

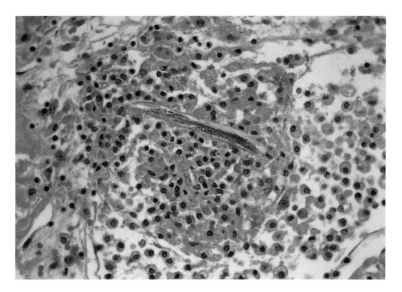

Figure 10–49. Section showing *Strongyloides stercoralis* larvae in an eosinophilic abscess in the colonic wall.

Strongyloides stercoralis, a small intestine helminth that produces larval forms that pass through the colon. Rarely, the larvae penetrate the mucosa to form eosinophilic abscesses in the wall (Figs. 10–48 and 10–49).

In young children with an allergy to cow's milk and soybean protein, a marked eosinophil infiltration of the rectal mucosa unassociated with crypt distortion suggests a diagnosis of eosinophilic proctitis. Eosinophilic colitis may also accompany eosinophilic gastroenteritis when diffuse mucosal eosinophilic infiltration occurs throughout the GI tract and is associated

with peripheral eosinophilia and a good response to treatment with steroids.

Radiation Proctocolitis

Radiation of the pelvis to treat malignant tumors may cause radiation proctocolitis. Acute radiation proctocolitis results when higher radiation doses are given over shorter intervals and produces clinical effects during or immediately after treatment.[23] It is characterized by abdominal pain, diarrhea, and tenesmus and may occur in up to 50% of patients undergoing pelvic radiation therapy. Symptoms usually resolve within 6 months. The diagnosis is clinical and does not usually lead to endoscopy and biopsy. If biopsy specimens are taken, they show depletion of actively proliferating crypt cells, resulting in decreased crypt length, edema, and neutrophil infiltration. The degree of change corresponds with the amount of acute radiation injury.

More important, and more unpredictable, is the occurrence of chronic radiation proctocolitis, which usually manifests 6–24 months after cessation of radiation therapy with chronic abdominal pain, constipation, diarrhea, blood loss, or intestinal obstruction. It occurs in 2–5% of patients undergoing pelvic radiation therapy; its occurrence is related to the total dose of radiation given and the volume of rectum included in the radiation field. Chronic radiation proctocolitis is characterized by a progressive obliterative arteritis with hyaline change in the vessel wall and submucosal and intramural fibrosis. The arteritis may cause ischemic changes in the mucosa with ulceration and hemorrhage, and even perforation may result. The radiation-induced mural fibrosis results in strictures and fistula formation. Biopsy samples show crypt atrophy and mild distortion, edema, infiltration with acute and chronic inflammatory cells, superficial mucosal telangiectasia, and submucosal fibrosis with thick-walled hyalinized vessels (Fig. 10–50). Radiation-induced cytologic atypia may be present in crypt epithelium and submucosal fibroblasts. These changes are usually not very

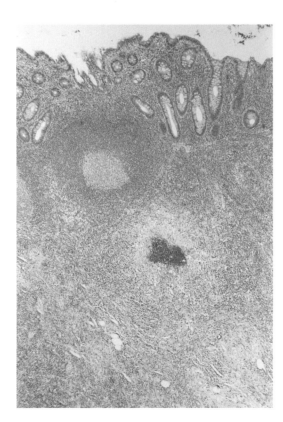

Figure 10–48. Lower power micrograph of Figure 10–49, showing an eosinophilic abscess in the colonic wall. This was proven secondary to *Strongyloides stercoralis.*

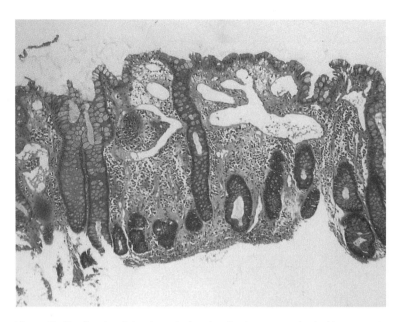

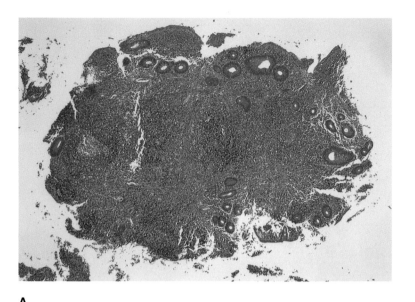

A

Figure 10–50. Chronic radiation change in the colon, showing crypt atrophy, focal lamina propria fibrosis and inflammation, marked superficial mucosal telangiectasia, and atypia of lining epithelium.

impressive, and diagnosis without the appropriate history of radiation can be difficult.

Chronic radiation injury may rarely be complicated by post-irradiation colitis cystica profunda; this commonly occurs several years after cessation of radiation therapy. This most likely results from repeated ischemic ulceration and fibrosis of the rectal wall, resulting in gland displacement. When associated with radiation-induced cytologic atypia, the displaced glands of colitis cystica profunda may mimic adenocarcinoma.[24]

Diversion Colitis

Diversion colitis is an almost invariable result of exclusion of a segment of colorectum from the normal fecal stream when a diverting colostomy is performed. The reason for diverting colostomy is irrelevant; diversion colitis complicates colostomy performed for ulcerative colitis, Hirschsprung's disease, diverticulosis, cancer, and even after spinal injury. The cause of diversion colitis is unknown; lack of luminal nutrients such as short-chain fatty acids and an alteration of the normal bacterial flora in the diverted colorectum have been suggested as causes.

Most patients have mild disease without symptoms. In the more severe cases, symptoms may begin 1–2 weeks after colostomy and include pain, tenesmus, and rectal discharge that may contain blood and mucus. Ulceration, fissures, and strictures may occur.

Pathologically, the mucosal changes closely resemble those of mild idiopathic inflammatory bowel disease with erosion, acute and chronic inflammation with cryptitis and crypt abscesses, and distorted crypt architecture with crypt branching (Fig. 10–51A). Pseudo-membranes may be present. Marked nodular lymphoid hyperplasia is an invariable and dominant feature (Fig. 10–51A and B). Inflammation and lymphoid nodules extend into the submucosa and sometimes the full thick-

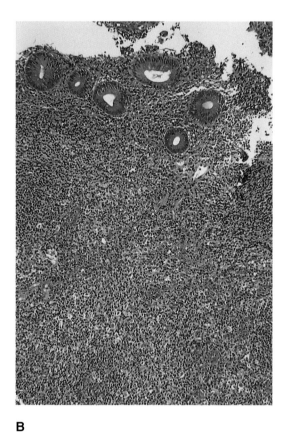

B

Figure 10–51. A: Diversion colitis, showing marked acute and chronic inflammation associated with crypt distortion and crypt atrophy. B: Diversion colitis showing marked crypt atrophy and severe lymphocytic infiltration.

ness of the wall and are associated with fibrous thickening. Poorly formed granulomas may be present at all levels. When transmural inflammation and granulomas are present, Crohn's disease is mimicked exactly.

When these changes occur in patients with a prior colectomy done for ulcerative colitis, question arises as to whether the original diagnosis was in reality Crohn's disease. Reexamination of the original colectomy in these cases shows features of ulcerative colitis, suggesting that the changes of diversion colitis have no relationship with Crohn's disease, despite their morphologic similarity.[25] Follow-up of patients with diversion colitis shows that the changes are restricted to the diverted segment, and no patients have progressed to Crohn's disease elsewhere.

Treatment of diversion colitis with short-chain fatty acid enemas and 5-ASA derivatives are only partly successful. Reanastomosis of the colon results in rapid reversal of the pathologic changes of diversion colitis.

Pouchitis

Rectal pouches (Koch pouch, J pouch, S pouch) are fashioned out of a segment of small bowel in patients who undergo total colectomy and mucosal proctectomy with ileoanal anastomosis for the treatment of familial adenomatous polyposis and chronic ulcerative colitis. Inflammation in these pouches (pouchitis) is common. Anaerobic bacterial overgrowth[26] and damage resulting from oxygen-based free radicals[27] have been implicated in the etiology. Pouchitis is usually mild and asymptomatic; severe cases cause pain, discharge, and, rarely, form strictures.

Mucosal changes consistently present include atrophy of villi associated with crypt elongation and acute and chronic inflammation (Fig. 10–52). Mucosal changes do not correlate well with either symptoms or pouch function. Metronidazole is reported as being effective treatment. Rare cases develop granulomas and transmural inflammation resembling Crohn's disease, requiring resection of the pouch. The significance of this is unknown, but when the reason for colectomy was ulcerative colitis, the possibility of misdiagnosis of Crohn's disease should be excluded by reexamination of the original colectomy specimen.

Pseudo-membranous Colitis

Pseudo-membranous colitis is a clinicopathologic diagnosis made when any type of colitis is associated with pseudo-membrane formation. A pseudo-membrane is a plaque of necrotic cells and acute inflammatory exudate that adheres to the surface of the mucosa (Figs. 10–53 and 10–54). Pseudo-membranes may be diffuse, involving large areas of necrotic mucosa (Fig. 10–55) or, more typically, appear as multiple, small 2–5-mm yellow plaques on the mucosal surface (Fig. 10–56).

Causes of Pseudo-membranous Colitis

The term "pseudo-membranous colitis" should not be equated with the specific entity of antibiotic-induced *Clostridium difficile* toxic colitis. Pseudo-membranous colitis can occur in: (1) ischemic colitis, in which pseudo-membranes are associated with atrophic microcrypts, lamina propria hemorrhage, full-thickness mucosal necrosis with large pseudo-membranes, and inflammatory polyps;[28] (2) diversion colitis; and (3) idiopathic inflammatory bowel disease, in which microscopic changes typical of these diseases coexist with pseudo-membrane formation.

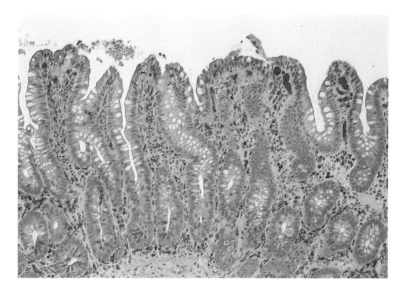

Figure 10–52. Chronic pouchitis in an ileal rectal pouch. There is moderate villous atrophy and crypt hyperplasia.

In cases of ischemic colitis, diversion colitis, and idiopathic inflammatory bowel disease, in which pseudo-membranes are seen endoscopically, testing for *Clostridium difficile* toxin should be done to exclude the possibility that *C. difficile* toxic damage is superimposed on the primary colitis.

Clostridium difficile *colitis*

Clostridium difficile is present in the normal colonic luminal flora in 40% of newborns, but only 1–5% of healthy adults.[29] Administration of almost any antibiotic can favor *C. difficile* overgrowth, but colitis has been reported most frequently with clindamycin, lincomycin, ampicillin, and cephalosporins. Both oral and intravenous antibiotics have been implicated. Rarely, *C. difficile* colitis occurs in patients who undergo gastrointestinal tract surgery or are on chemotherapy without a history of an-

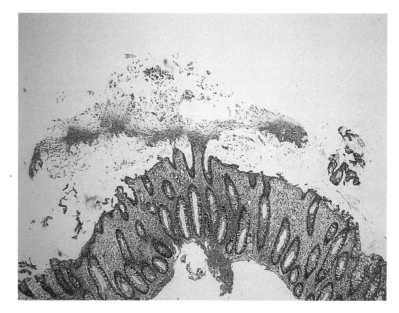

Figure 10–53. Pseudo-membranous colitis, showing the typical mushroom-shaped membrane consisting of acutely inflamed necrotic tissue. The superficial part of the mucosa shows focal necrosis.

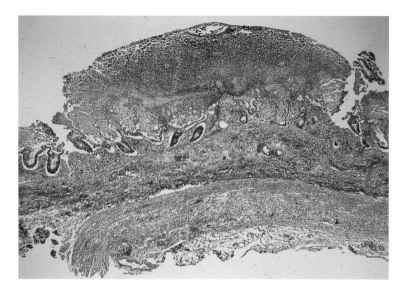

Figure 10–54. Pseudo-membranous colitis, showing a larger membrane composed of necrotic tissue and acute inflammation.

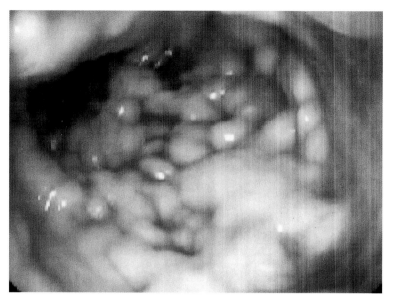

A

tibiotic use. *Clostridium difficile* produces enterotoxin (toxin A), which causes cell damage and inflammation; cytotoxin (toxin B), which causes cell death; and a third toxin, which stimulates colonic motor activity.

Clostridium difficile colitis manifests as watery diarrhea, often associated with fever, colicky abdominal pain, and leukocytosis. Bleeding and rebound tenderness are uncommon. Toxic megacolon and perforation are rare complications associ-

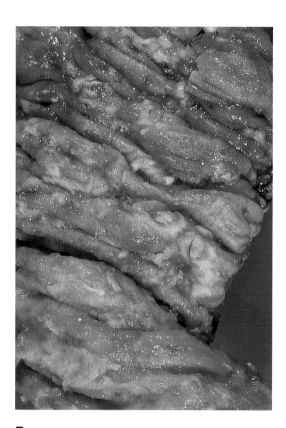

B

Figure 10–56. Pseudo-membranous colitis. A: Endoscopic appearance showing multiple yellow plaques on the mucosa. B: Small yellowish pieces of membrane on the colonic mucosa. (Part A: Courtesy of Aslam Godil, MD, Dept. of Gastroenterology, Loma Linda University, CA).

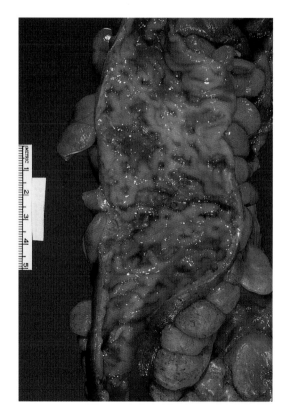

Figure 10–55. Pseudo-membranous colitis, showing the diffuse membrane-like material on the mucosal surface.

ated with a high mortality rate that necessitate emergent colectomy.

The finding of multiple 2–5-mm yellow raised plaques in an otherwise unremarkable mucosa is a typical endoscopic appearance (see Fig. 10–56). The disease may affect the entire colon or be patchy; some patients have disease only in the right colon that may be missed with flexible sigmoidoscopy. Mild *C. difficile* colitis may not show pseudo-membranes. Biopsy specimens of the smaller plaques show a mushroom-like architecture with a small focus of superficial mucosal inflammation and necrosis from which the pseudo-membranous inflammatory exudate radiates out on the surface (see Fig. 10–53).

The diagnosis is established by testing for *C. difficile* toxin, which is present in 97% of cases of pseudo-membranous colitis and 27% of patients with antibiotic-associated diarrhea.[29] The toxin assay takes 48 h; endoscopic and biopsy diagnosis therefore have practical value in initiating treatment. A newer rapid test to detect *C. difficile* antigen is available. Treatment with vancomycin or metronidazole is highly effective.

Solitary Cecal Ulcer

Solitary cecal ulcer is an uncommon clinical entity characterized by the presence of an ulcer in the cecum without any evidence of disease elsewhere in the gastrointestinal tract (Fig. 10–57). The ulcer may be acute or chronic and cause abdominal pain and severe lower GI bleeding. Chronic ulcers may be associated with marked thickening of the wall, rarely causing obstruction. Endoscopy shows ulceration; when biopsies fail to provide an etiology, some of these patients undergo right hemicolectomy to exclude malignancy.

Solitary ulcers of the cecum occur in two main clinical situations: (1) Patients who are immunocompromised; in these cases, the association between cecal ulcer and cytomegalovirus infection is high. Careful examination of biopsy specimens or resected tissue for CMV-infected cells is indicated. (2) As a complication of regular use of nonsteroidal antiinflammatory drugs.[30] The natural history of this disease is unknown because the diagnosis is usually made after resection.

Other Specific Colitides

Acute colitis may occur in graft-versus-host disease (see Chapter 17) and Stevens-Johnson syndrome (bullous erythema multiforme). In Stevens-Johnson syndrome, colonic involvement may be associated with diarrhea.[31] Endoscopy shows patchy colonic inflammation with ulcers. Biopsy specimens show mucosa with focal, acute, and chronic inflammation and necrosis of crypts (Fig. 10–58A). The crypts show necrotic cells in their lumina and are lined by a flattened epithelium; regenerative changes are present in some of the crypts (Fig. 10–58B).

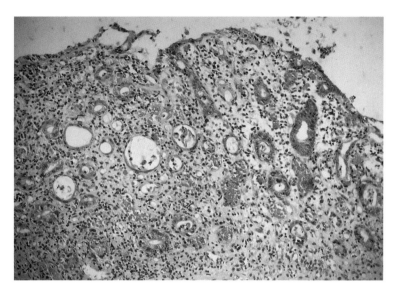

A

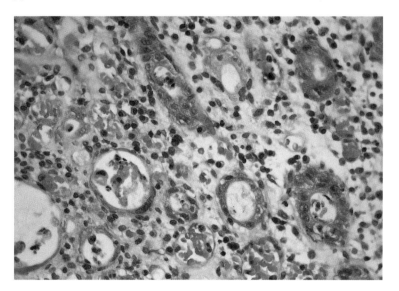

B

Figure 10–58. A: Colitis in a patient with Stevens-Johnson syndrome, showing inflammation and crypt necrosis. B: Colitis in a patient with Stevens-Johnson syndrome, showing crypt necrosis with the necrotic debris being found in damaged crypts lined by a flat or regenerating epithelium.

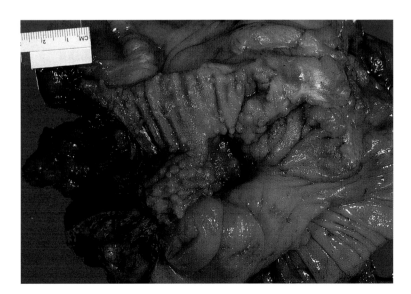

Figure 10–57. Solitary cecal ulcer with an appearance that mimics a punched-out peptic ulcer in the stomach.

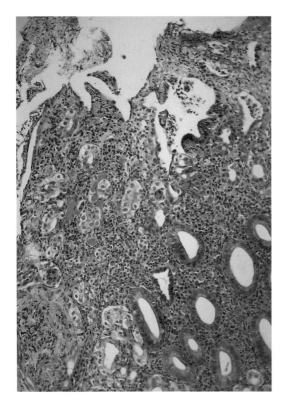

Figure 10–59. Focal erosive colitis associated with heterotopic gastric mucosa containing parietal cells.

Gastric heterotopia in flat colonic mucosa is another rare cause of an appearance at endoscopy that resembles colitis. The heterotopic gastric mucosa consists of glands containing parietal cells, often associated with inflammation and mucosal ulceration (Fig. 10–59).

Colonic Fistulae

Colonic fistulae occur in a variety of colonic diseases, including Crohn's disease (see Chapter 11), tuberculosis, diverticulitis,

and colorectal malignant neoplasms. In addition to these colonic causes of fistulae, extracolonic diseases occur that open into the colon via a fistulous tract. The commonest cause of these is benign gastric ulcers, especially the gastrojejunocolic fistula that complicates Billroth II surgery for benign gastric ulcer. Rarer extracolonic diseases associated with colonic fistulae are (1) malignant neoplasms of other abdominal viscera, such as the urinary bladder, stomach, and gallbladder; (2) pancreatic pseudocyst, which may open into the colon (Fig. 10–60), an event that results in severe rectal bleeding; and (3) xanthogranulomatous pyelonephritis, in which the chronic inflammatory process in the kidney can rarely produce a fistula between the renal pelvicalyceal system and the colon (Fig. 10–61).

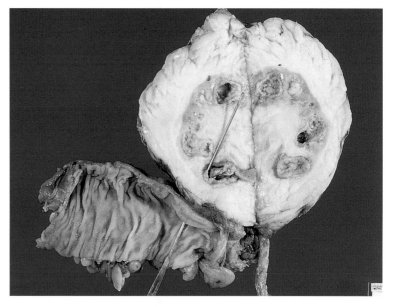

A

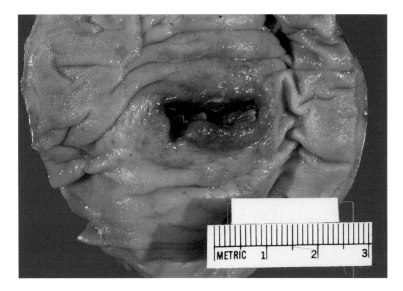

Figure 10–60. Ulcer in the descending colon, showing the colonic opening of a fistula between the colon and a pancreatic pseudocyst. This was found in a colon removed emergently for acute rectal bleeding.

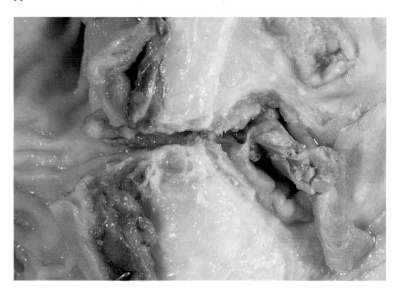

B

Figure 10–61. A: Xanthogranulomatous pyelonephritis, showing the renal lesion and adherent colon. B: Fistulous track passing from the renal pelvicalyceal system to the colon.

SOLITARY RECTAL ULCER SYNDROME

Solitary rectal ulcer syndrome is a pathologically defined entity of the rectum. Physiologic testing (which includes evacuation proctography, wherein evacuation of semisolid contrast material from the rectum is monitored radiologically; anorectal manometry; and electromyography of the pelvic floor muscles) has shown that most cases result from abnormal motility associated with defecation. Almost all patients with solitary rectal ulcer syndrome have abnormal contraction of the puborectalis muscle of the pelvic floor, increased external sphincter tone, increased intrarectal pressure during evacuation, and overt or occult prolapse of the rectal mucosa.[32] Because of its association with rectal mucosal prolapse, the etiologic term "mucosal prolapse syndrome" has been suggested as an alternative to the somewhat unsatisfactory "solitary rectal ulcer syndrome." The etiologic relationship, however, is not absolute. Cases of solitary rectal ulcer syndrome have been reported secondary to trauma associated with rectal digitation.[33] Because the etiology may be multifactorial, it is preferable at this time to retain the term "solitary rectal ulcer syndrome" for this condition.

Clinically, most patients are healthy adults between 20 and 40 years old. Rectal bleeding during defecation is the most common symptom, followed by mucus discharge, anorectal pain and tenesmus, and lower abdominal pain. Most patients have had symptoms for several years. Patients may have regular bowel habits or complain of chronic constipation. Demonstrable overt rectal prolapse is present in less than 20% of cases. Rarely, bleeding may be severe enough to require transfusion. Solitary rectal ulcer syndrome remains localized to the rectum; there is no increase in the incidence of idiopathic inflammatory bowel disease or malignancy. The disease may remain stable, regress, or progress to become disabling. In severe cases, surgery is required; this usually consists of a rectopexy, and only rarely is proctectomy needed.

Endoscopic examination shows the classical solitary ulcer in the anterior or anterolateral wall of the rectum in only 40% of cases. The ulcer is commonly located 6–8 cm from the anal verge (range 3–15 cm) and may be of any shape; its size can vary between 0.5–5 cm. Multiple ulcers are present in 20% of cases, and many patients do not have any ulceration. In early cases, the rectal mucosa is granular and erythematous; in other cases, a cystic mass, polyp, or a sessile villous lesion may be seen.

Solitary rectal ulcer syndrome is diagnosed by pathologic examination. In the acute phase, ulceration occurs (Fig. 10–62A and B). In the chronic, nonulcerated phase of the disease, the following occur: (1) Crypt hyperplasia is evident with elongation and serration of the lumen, a villiform surface and enlargement of the lining cells, an appearance that resembles hyperplastic polyp (Fig. 10–62C and D). (2) Fibromuscular replacement of the lamina propria is the most characteristic feature (Fig. 10–62E). This is associated with smooth muscle ingrowth into the lamina propria from a thickened muscularis mucosae. The muscle fibers are oriented perpendicular to the basement membrane and may be present in bundles. Fibrosis accompanies the muscle and in some cases is the dominant change. (3) The number of inflammatory cells is scanty.

Erosion and ulceration of the surface is common and produces reactive atypia of the crypts, inflammatory cell infiltration of the lamina propria, and increasing fibrosis. The fibrosis often results in crypt distortion and displacement of crypts downward, sometimes into the submucosa (Fig. 10–63). The deeper crypts frequently become dilated due to accumulation of inspissated mucin, forming cystic structures. Reactive atypia of the crypt cells in the regenerative phase can produce a disturbing cytologic appearance. The surface epithelium rarely shows metaplasia to squamous or transitional-type epithelium that typifies the anorectal junctional region.

Based on which particular histologic feature is prominent, solitary rectal ulcer syndrome has been referred to by many names: localized colitis cystica profunda of the rectum and enterogenous cyst of the rectum when the mucin-distended deep crypts are prominent; hamartomatous inverted polyp of the rectum and inflammatory cloacogenic polyp when the crypt distortion, hyperplasia, and inflammation are prominent. Inflammatory cloacogenic polyp was defined by its surface lining of transitional-type epithelium, but this is now believed to occur as a metaplastic change in solitary rectal ulcer syndrome.

The array of histologic features may mimic many other pathologic diseases.

1. Idiopathic inflammatory bowel disease because of the market crypt distortion. The crypt hyperplasia and elongation in solitary rectal ulcer syndrome contrasts with the crypt atrophy that usually occurs in idiopathic inflammatory bowel disease. Inflammation is usually not prominent in solitary rectal ulcer syndrome. Fibromuscular replacement of the lamina propria is not seen in ulcerative colitis, although considerable fibrosis may occur in Crohn's disease.
2. Villous adenoma may be closely mimicked in the phase of crypt hyperplasia when reactive changes resulting from a healing erosion are superimposed. The regenerative atypia in such cases can closely mimic the adenomatous change of a villous adenoma. Again, recognition of the associated fibromuscular replacement of the lamina propria permits diagnosis.
3. Well-differentiated mucinous adenocarcinoma is mimicked when a combination of distorted submucosal-displaced crypts are associated with fibrosis. Sometimes, lakes of extravasated mucin may be present in these cases of colitis cystica profunda-type solitary rectal ulcer syndrome. The displaced crypts are lined by benign epithelium or epithelium showing inflammatory atypia; absence of malignant cytologic features permits carcinoma to be excluded.

COLITIS CYSTICA PROFUNDA

Colitis cystica profunda is an unusual cause of polypoid lesions in the colon. A regenerative change that results from any cause of deep ulceration of the colon, it occurs most commonly in the

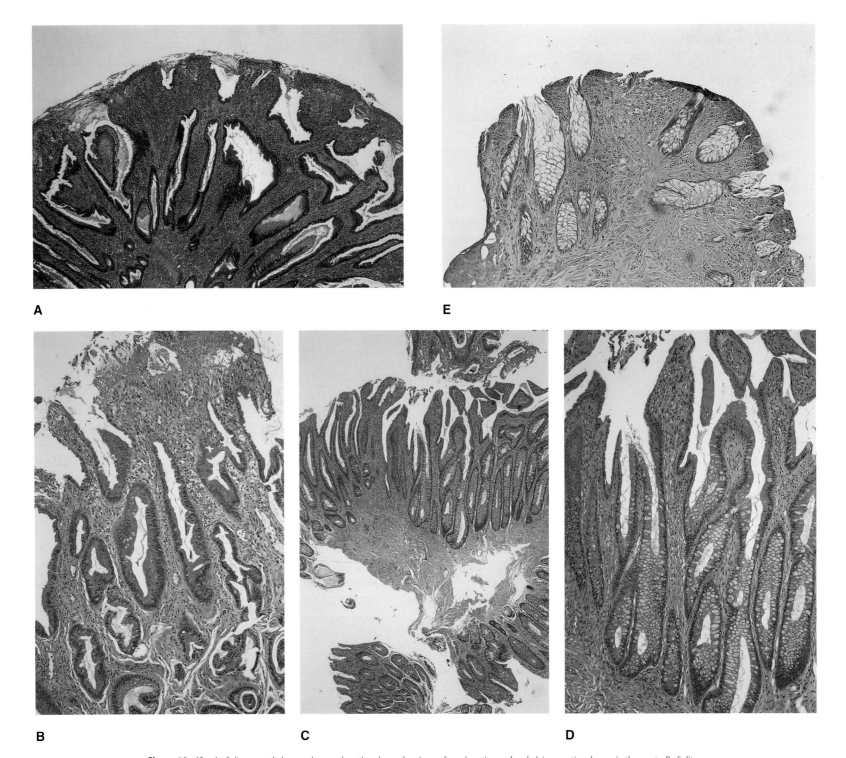

Figure 10–62. A: Solitary rectal ulcer syndrome, ulcerative phase, showing surface ulceration and underlying reactive change in the crypts. B: Solitary rectal ulcer syndrome, showing healing ulcer with greater reactive hyperplasia of the crypts. C: Solitary rectal ulcer syndrome, ulcerative phase, showing a villous architecture to the surface mucosa. There is no evidence of ulceration. D: Solitary rectal ulcer syndrome, showing hyperplastic polyp-like changes in the crypts. E: Solitary rectal ulcer syndrome, showing fibromuscular replacement of the mucosa.

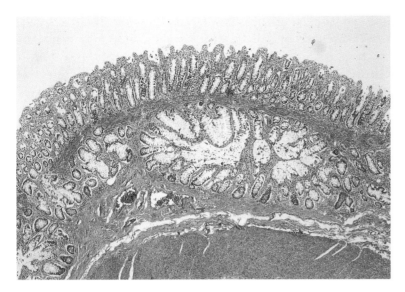

Figure 10–63. Colitis cystica profunda, showing a large focus of submucosal glands separated from the colonic mucosa by the muscularis mucosae.

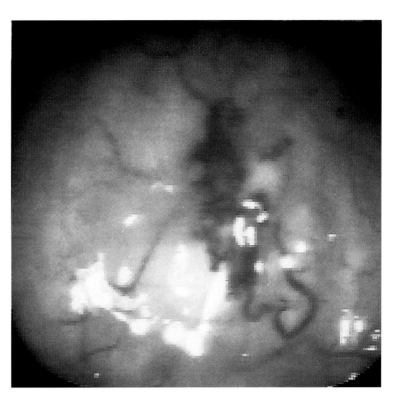

Figure 10–64. Colonic mucosa at endoscopy, showing abnormal vascular lesion with hemorrhage typical of angiodysplasia (arteriovenous malformation).

rectum as part of solitary rectal ulcer syndrome (see Fig. 10–63). Colitis cystica profunda may also occur in the rest of the colon in idiopathic inflammatory bowel disease (see Chapter 11), after an attack of infectious colitis, and following radiation therapy.[34]

Endoscopically, colitis cystica profunda presents most commonly as a polypoid mass. Rarely, stenosis is associated with it, and colonic obstruction may occur. Histologic examination shows marked distortion of the crypts, which are displaced below the musuclaris mucosae into the submucosa (see Fig. 10–63). Microcystic change with dilated crypts distended with mucin is common. Inflammation is not usually prominent; fibrosis is common. Not uncommonly, the displaced crypts extend into the muscularis externa, being surrounded by smooth muscle. The architectural pattern can result in a false-positive diagnosis of well-differentiated adenocarcinoma. Colitis cystica profunda shows only regenerative and hyperplastic cytologic changes, however, which are not difficult to distinguish from the malignant cytology of an adenocarcinoma.

Colitis cystic profunda is a benign condition, which has no increased risk of malignancy.

VASCULAR DISEASES

Angiodysplasia

Angiodysplasia (also called vascular ectasia and arteriovenous malformation) is a common cause of severe lower GI bleeding and is responsible for approximately 20% of such cases.[24] It occurs in elderly patients and is most likely a degenerative vascular disease. The right colon is most commonly affected, and the lesions are often multiple. In most cases, the diagnosis is made at colonoscopy by demonstrating a bleeding site associated with abnormal vessels (Fig. 10–64). Treatment by endoscopic

injection therapy, monopolar electrocoagulation, contact probes, or the yttrium aluminum garnet (YAG) laser is effective. In rare cases, when there is continued bleeding with no endoscopically visible lesion, angiography identifies the bleeding site. In severe, uncontrolled bleeding, colectomy to remove the segment of colon containing the angiographically defined bleeding site is indicated.

It is extremely difficult for the pathologist to identify angiodysplasia in a resected specimen because the vessels collapse on removal of the colon. The best technique for visualizing angiodysplasia is by intravascular injection of a silicone rubber compound immediately after the colon has been removed. Unfortunately, this technique is both time-consuming and expensive and is therefore rarely undertaken. A simpler method of demonstrating angiodysplasia is by intraluminal formalin fixation in the distended state followed by dissection of the mucosa from the muscle wall. In these preparations, angiodysplastic lesions can be recognized as engorged tortuous submucosal veins, often more than three times the caliber of adjacent arterioles. These are accompanied by ectatic veins in the mucosal lamina propria and muscularis mucosae. Congested pericryptal capillaries are also seen.[24]

In common practice, the diagnosis of vascular lesions of the colon is an inexact science. Examination of a colonic segment that is shown by angiography to harbor a bleeding point frequently shows no convincing pathologic lesion. Diffuse submucosal microscopic vascular ectasia is sometimes present in these cases,[35] but it is difficult to diagnose this as abnormal because the limits of normal submucosal vascularity are not clearly established.

Ischemic Colitis

Normal Blood Supply

The right colon and the right half of the transverse colon receive their blood supply from branches of the superior mesenteric artery. The left half of the transverse colon, descending colon, and sigmoid colon are supplied by branches of the inferior mesenteric artery. The upper rectum is supplied by the superior hemorrhoidal artery, which is the termination of the inferior mesenteric artery. The lower rectum is supplied by branches of the internal iliac artery. The maximum area of susceptibility to ischemia is the region of the splenic flexure (Griffith's point) because of frequent inadequate collaterals between the superior and inferior mesenteric arterial branches in this area.

The major arteries form a marginal artery near the colonic wall. End arteries, called vasa recta, supply the colon from the marginal artery. The vasa recta are better developed in the left colon than the right; nonocclusive ischemic changes occur commonly in the right colon.

Etiology of Colonic Ischemia

Colonic ischemia may be occlusive or nonocclusive. Atherosclerosis involving the mesenteric arteries is the commonest cause, resulting in ischemic colitis being predominently a disease of older people. Occlusive plaques, thrombi, emboli, and ostial occlusion by aortic atherosclerosis are all important causes. Less common causes of mesenteric occlusion include ligation of the inferior mesenteric artery during abdominal surgery and extrinsic occlusion by tumors and aortic aneurysms. Ischemic colitis has been reported after coronary artery bypass surgery and aortic reconstruction.[36]

More rarely, ischemic colitis results from small-vessel disease involving the vasa recta. These tend to affect a different age group and tend to be more patchy because of the less regional nature of the end-artery involvement. Diabetic microangiopathy, vasculitis associated with polyarteritis nodosa, Churg-Strauss angiitis, small-vessel vasculitis,[37] and radiation-induced vascular changes may all cause ischemic colitis. Small-vessel vasculitis associated with systemic lupus erythematosus has been reported to cause ischemic proctitis[38]; the rectum is otherwise rarely involved in ischemic colitis because of its dual blood supply. Vasculitis may be localized to the colon[37] or be part of a systemic vasculitis; approximately 30% of cases with systemic vasculitis show involvement of the gastrointestinal tract.

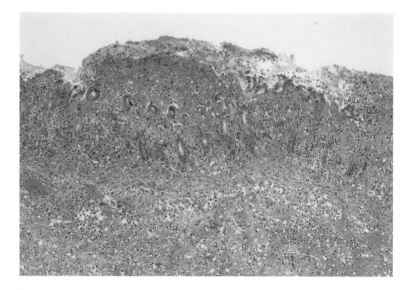

A

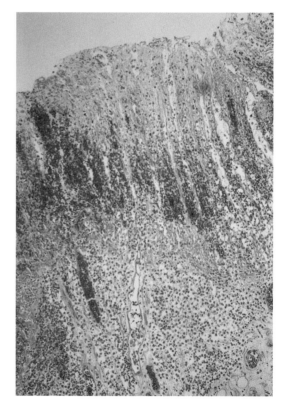

B

Figure 10–66. Acute ischemic colitis. A: Surface erosion, marked crypt necrosis. B: Hemorrhagic necrosis of the full thickness of the mucosa with acute inflammation in the deep mucosa and submucosa.

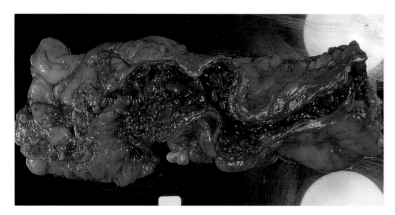

Figure 10–65. Ischemic colitis. Resected left colon showing marked brownish discoloration of mucosa with ulceration and pseudo-polypoid change. The lumen appears narrowed.

Nonocclusive causes include any cause of shock or hypotension in which severe and prolonged splanchnic vasoconstriction may occur. Drugs such as digoxin, catecholamines, diuretics, and antihypertensives may cause a similar splanchnic vasoconstriction.

Clinicopathologic Features

Ischemic colitis commonly affects elderly patients; presentation is usually insidious with abdominal pain, distension, and diarrhea. Bleeding occurs in the more severe cases. A subset of young patients have a more acute onset with rectal bleeding. Most patients tend to have mild disease with remissions and relapses. In more severe chronic cases, strictures occur in the affected colon. Acute infarction of the colon occurs in 10–20% of cases, resulting in an acute illness with severe bleeding, colonic perforation, and peritonitis.

Mild cases show pathologic features restricted to the mucosa and submucosa. Endoscopic findings in the acute phase include mucosal pallor with focal hemorrhage in mild disease. With increasing severity, the likelihood of hemorrhage increases and the mucosa becomes dark with focal erosions; extensive ulceration is present in severe cases (Fig. 10–65). The endoscopic appearance mimics idiopathic inflammatory bowel disease. Biopsy specimens show erosion of the surface epithelium, crypt necrosis and loss, lamina propria edema and hemorrhage, associated with a mild inflammatory cell infiltrate (Fig. 10–66). Mucosal biopsy does not permit evaluation of submucosal and intramural fibrosis, which is present in chronic cases associated with strictures.

Thrombosis may be present in small vessels in the mucosa irrespective of the etiology of ischemia (Fig. 10–67). Rarely, in cases associated with vasculitis, deep mucosal and submucosal vessels may show involvement. Care must be taken, however, to interpret inflammation in vessels as vasculitis; secondary inflammation may occur in relation to ulcers in ischemic colitis.

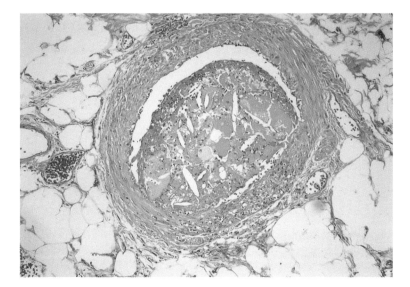

Figure 10–67. Thrombosis in a small artery in the resected specimen. There is a suggestion of cholesterol clefts in the thrombus indicating the possibility of embolized material from a more proximal atherosclerotic plaque.

References

1. Qualman SJ, Murray R. Aganglionosis and related disorders. *Hum Pathol.* 1994;25:1141–1149.
2. Larsson LT. Hirschsprung's disease—immunohistochemical findings. *Histol Histopathol.* 1994;9:615–629.
3. Weinberg AG. Hirschsprung's disease—a pathologist's overview. *Perspect Pediatr Pathol.* 1975;2:207–239.
4. Attie T, Salomon R, Amiel J, et al. Genetics of Hirschsprung's disease. *C R Soc Biol.* 1996;190:549–556 (in French).
5. Teitelbaum DH, Caniano DA, Qualman SJ. The pathophysiology of Hirschsprung's associated enterocolitis: Importance of histologic correlates. *J Pediatr Surg.* 1989;24: 1271–1277.
6. Kobayashi H, Miyano T, Yamataka A, et al. Use of synaptophysin polyclonal antibody for the rapid intraoperative immunohistochemical evaluation of functional bowel disorders. *J Pediatr Surg.* 1997;32:38–40.
7. Meier-Ruge WA, Bronimann PB, Gambazzi F, et al. Histopathological criteria for intestinal neuronal dysplasia of the submucosal plexus (type B). *Virchows Arch.* 1995;426:549–556.
8. Pang X, Boucher W, Triadafilopoulos G, et al. Mast cell and substance P-positive nerve involvement in a patient with both irritable bowel syndrome and interstitial cystitis. *Urology.* 1996;47: 436–438.
9. Present DH. Toxic megacolon. *Med Clin North Am.* 1993;77: 1129–1148.
10. Beaugerie L, Ngo Y, Goujard F, et al. Etiology and management of toxic megacolon in patients with human immunodeficiency virus infection. *Gastroenterology.* 1994;107: 858–863.
11. Cheskin LJ, Bohlman M, Schuster MM. Diverticular disease in the elderly. *Gastoenterol Clin North Am.* 1990;19:391–403.
12. Carlas-de-Oliveira N, Welch JP. Giant diverticula of the colon: A clinical assessment. *Am J Gastroenterol.* 1997;92:1092–1096.
13. Goldstein NS, Ahmad E. Histology of the mucosa in sigmoid colon specimens with diverticular disease: Observations for the interpretation of sigmoid colonoscopic biopsy specimens. *Am J Clin Pathol.* 1197;107:438–444.
14. Makapugay LM, Dean PJ. Diverticular disease-associated chronic colitis. *Am J Surg Pathol.* 1996;20:94–102.
15. Wong SK, Ho YH, Leong AP, et al. Clinical behavior of complicated right-sided and left-sided diverticulosis. *Dis Colon Rectum.* 1997;40:344–348.
16. Lee FD. Importance of apoptosis in the histopathology of drug related lesions in the large intestine. *J Clin Pathol.* 1993;46:118.
17. Byers RJ, Marsh P, Parkinson D, et al. Melanosis coli is associated with an increase in colonic epithelial apoptosis and not with laxative use. *Histopathology.* 1997;30:160–164.
18. Surawicz CM, Haggitt RC, Husseman M, et al. Mucosal biopsy diagnosis of colitis: Acute self-limited colitis and idiopathic inflammatory bowel disease. *Gastroenterology.* 1994;107:755–763.
19. Therkildsen MH, Jensen BN, Teglbjaerg PS, et al. The final outcome of patients presenting with their first episode of acute diarrhoea and an inflamed rectal mucosa with preserved crypt architecture. A clinicopathologic study. *Scand J Gastroenterol.* 1989;24: 158–164.
20. Greenson JK, Stern RA, Carpenter SL, et al. The clinical significance of focal active colitis. *Hum Pathol.* 1997;28:729–733.

21. Jawhari A, Talbot IC. Microscopic, lymphocytic and collagenous colitis. *Histopathology.* 1996;29:101–110.

22. Lee E, Schiller LR, Vendrell D, et al. Subepithelial collagen table thickness in colon specimens from patients with microscopic colitis and collagenous colitis. *Gastroenterology.* 1992;103:1790–1796.

23. Nussbaum ML, Campana TJ, Weese JL. Radiation-induced intestinal injury. *Clin Plastic Surg.* 1993;20:573–580.

24. Ng WK, Chan KW. Postirradiation colitis cystica profunda. Case report and literature review. *Arch Pathol Lab Med.* 1995;119:1170–1173.

25. Warren BF, Shepherd NA. Diversion proctocolitis. *Histopathology.* 1992;21:91.

26. Santavirta J, et al. Mucosal morphology and faecal bacteriology after ileoanal anastomosis. *Int J Colorectal Dis.* 1991;6:38.

27. Levin KE, Pemberton JH, Phillips SF, et al. Role of oxygen free radicals in the etiology of pouchitis. *Dis Colon Rectum.* 1992;35:452–456.

28. Dignan CR, Greenson JK. Can ischemic colitis be differentiated from *C. difficile* colitis in biopsy specimens? *Am J Surg Pathol.* 1997;21:706–710.

29. Counihan TC, Roberts PL. Pseudomembranous colitis. *Surg Clin North Am.* 1993;73:1063–1074.

30. Kaufman HL, Fischer AH, Carroll M, et al. Colonic ulceration associated with nonsteroidal anti-inflammatory drugs. Report of three cases. *Dis Colon Rectum.* 1996;39:705–710.

31. Zweiban B, Cohen H, Chandrasoma P. Gastrointestinal involvement complicating Stevens-Johnson's syndrome. *Gastroenterology.* 1986;91:469–474.

32. Bogomoletz WV. Solitary rectal ulcer syndrome; mucosal prolapse syndrome. *Pathol Annu.* 1992;27:75–86.

33. Contractor TQ, Contractor QQ. Traumatic solitary rectal ulcer in Saudi Arabia. A distinct entity? *J Clin Gastroenterol.* 1995;21:298–300.

34. Thelmo WL, Vetrano JA, Wibowo A, et al. Angiodysplasia of the colon revisited: Pathologic demonstration without the use of intravascular injection technique. *Hum Pathol.* 1992;23:37–40.

35. Weinstock LB, Larson RS, Stahl DJ, et al. Diffuse microscopic angiodysplasia—a previously unreported variant of angiodysplasia. *Dis Colon Rectum.* 1995;38:428–432.

36. Bower TC. Ischemic colitis. *Surg Clin North Am.* 1993; 73:1037–1053.

37. Burke AP, Sobin LH, Virmani R. Localized vasculitis of the gastrointestinal tract. *Am J Surg Pathol.* 1995;19:338–349.

38. Reissman P, Weiss EG, Teoh TA, et al. Gangrenous ischemic colitis of the rectum: A rare complication of systemic lupus erythematosus. *Am J Gastroenterol.* 1994; 89:2234–2236.

11

IDIOPATHIC INFLAMMATORY BOWEL DISEASES

Rashida Soni and Parakrama Chandrasoma

▶ CHAPTER OUTLINE

DEFINITIONS

"Inflammatory bowel disease" is a general term that includes all inflammatory diseases of the intestine and colorectum. Idiopathic inflammatory bowel disease (IIBD) is a restrictive term used for ulcerative colitis, Crohn's disease, and cases with features of both these entities that are termed indeterminate IIBD. Although these strict definitions are without controversy, it is not uncommon for the term "inflammatory bowel disease" to be used synonymously with IIBD by clinicians. Pathologists must strenuously avoid this loose terminology and adhere to strict terminology in their reporting so as to avoid confusion.

Although a clear distinction exists between IIBD and other types of inflammatory diseases, the differentiation of IIBD from acute infectious diseases, ischemic colitis, microscopic colitis, and solitary rectal ulcer syndrome can sometimes be difficult. The diagnosis of IIBD depends on clinical and pathologic criteria, and the exclusion of other etiologies for inflammatory disease; there is no specific test based on the etiology of IIBD because the etiology is not known with certainty. When in doubt, the diagnosis of IIBD must be made with great caution, because both ulcerative colitis and Crohn's disease carry with them the prospect of lifelong chronic disease with significant morbidity and life-style adjustment.

In cases of definitive IIBD, every attempt must be made to differentiate between ulcerative colitis and Crohn's disease because these two conditions are managed differently and have different consequences. One of most important methods of differentiating between ulcerative colitis and Crohn's disease is evaluating the distribution of disease. For this purpose, multiple labeled biopsy specimens from different parts of the colorectum must be supplied. When skip areas are seen endoscopically, a biopsy must be performed on these areas to document that they are also histologically uninvolved. It is not uncommon for endoscopic skip areas to show microscopic involvement, a fact that may significantly affect differential diagnosis.

ULCERATIVE COLITIS

Etiology and Epidemiology

Ulcerative colitis has an incidence of 2–5/100,000 population and a prevalence of 0.1%. It occurs slightly more frequently in females. All ages are affected, with maximum incidence between 15–40 years. Childhood onset and onset after age 40 are not rare. Ulcerative colitis has a tendency to affect city dwellers at the higher socioeconomic levels; there is a slight familial tendency.

The etiology of ulcerative colitis is unknown. Dietary factors, bile acid metabolites, psychological stress, microbes, and genetic and immunologic factors have been suggested. An immunologic, possibly autoimmune, basis is considered the most likely etiology. None of the reported etiologic or immunologic associations are consistent enough to permit rational disease prevention or to be useful as a diagnostic test, however.

Distribution of Lesions

Ulcerative colitis is a disease restricted to the colorectum, excepting for backwash ileitis, which affects the terminal ileum in 15% of patients with pancolitis. The disease almost always begins in the rectum and extends proximally into the colon in a contiguous manner without skip areas (Figs. 11–1, 11–2, and 11–3). The diseased area gradually transitions into normal colon without a sharp demarcation (Fig. 11–4). Based on the amount of colorectal involvement, three types of disease distribution are recognized: (1) ulcerative proctitis, which is restricted to the rectum; (2) left-sided ulcerative colitis, which involves rectum, sigmoid colon, and descending colon (see Fig. 11–1); and (3) pancolitis, which affects the entire colon (see Fig. 11–3). The appendix is involved in 40% of cases of pancolitis. In

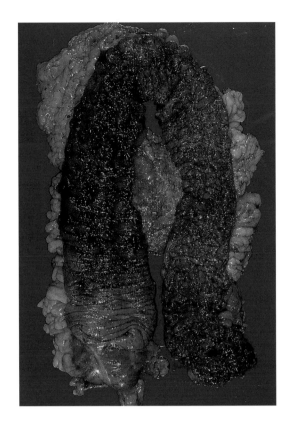

Figure 11–2. Severe ulcerative colitis, acute phase, involving almost the entire colon. Grossly, the disease appears to spare the cecal region.

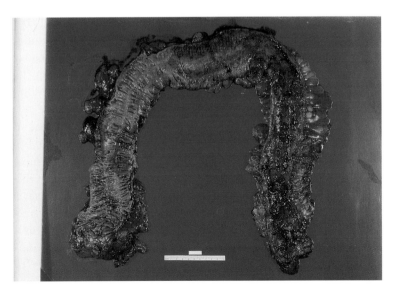

Figure 11–1. Ulcerative colitis, acute phase, showing involvement of the left side of the colon. A lesser degree of change is also evident in the transverse and ascending colon; this is possibly pancolitis on microscopic examination.

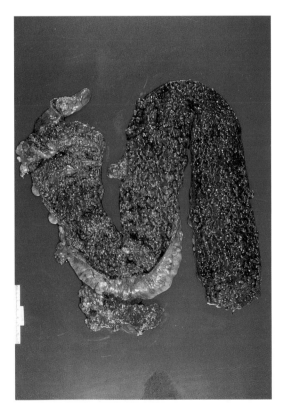

Figure 11–3. Ulcerative pancolitis, acute phase, involving the entire colon including the appendix. The severity of mucosal disease is macroscopically greater in the distal colon.

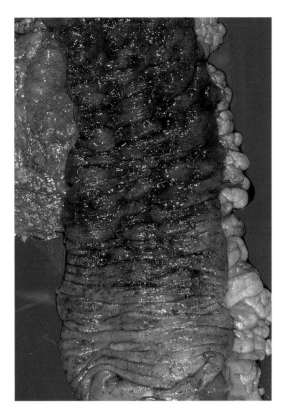

Figure 11–4. Transition from grossly normal to involved mucosa in ulcerative colitis, acute phase, showing the gradual nature of the transition in ulcerative colitis. Compare with Figures 11–41 through 11–46 (Crohn's disease), in which the transition between involved and uninvolved mucosa is sharp.

Figure 11–5. Ulcerative colitis, acute phase, showing mucosal edema, congestion, hemorrhage, and superficial ulceration.

10% of cases, the rectal involvement is less severe and somewhat patchy compared with more proximal disease, both at endoscopy and histologic examination ("rectal sparing"). In a patient with typical features of ulcerative colitis, rectal sparing does not preclude the diagnosis.

Clinical Features

Rectal bleeding, which is present in 90% of patients at the onset of disease, is the common presenting symptom. This is accompanied by diarrhea, the severity of which increases as the extent of colonic involvement increases. In patients with ulcerative proctitis, bleeding may be associated with constipation. Fever and abdominal pain occur in a minority of patients at onset; the presence of high fever, tachycardia, elevated erythrocyte sedimentation rate (>30 mm/h), and anemia may indicate fulminant disease.

Endoscopic examination shows mucosal edema, loss of the normal vascular pattern, and friability with bleeding on minor trauma. With increasing severity, the mucosa becomes granular, hemorrhagic, eroded, and covered with a purulent exudate, and bleeds spontaneously (Figs. 11–5, 11–6, and 11–7). Leukocytes are present in large numbers in the stool.

The outcome of the first attack depends on disease severity, which in turn is determined by disease extent.[1] Mild disease carries no increase in mortality and has a 91% remission rate with medical treatment and almost no necessity for surgery.

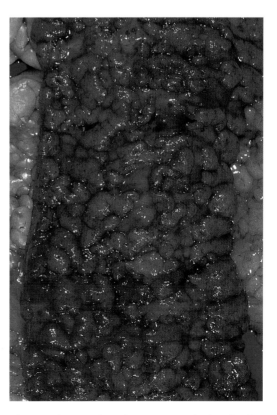

Figure 11–6. Ulcerative colitis, acute phase. The mucosa is acutely inflamed and has a pseudo-polypoid appearance due to edema of surviving mucosa between ulcers that are hidden under the edematous mucosa.

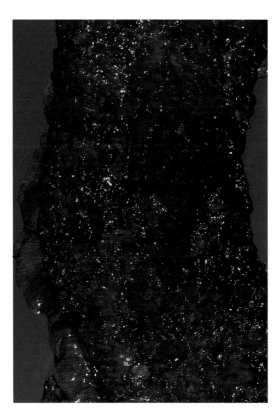

Figure 11–7. Ulcerative colitis, acute phase, showing extensive ulceration and the presence of exudate on the surface. Pseudo-polypoid islands of residual mucosa are present.

With severe disease, failure of medical treatment results in colectomy in 28% of cases; mortality is 23% for patients needing colectomy in the acute phase. These figures represent a tremendous improvement from the presteroid era when the overall mortality rate for patients suffering first attacks was 14% and that for severe disease was 43%.[2]

Ulcerative colitis is a chronic, lifelong disease. Less than 10% of patients do not relapse within 10 years after the first attack. Seventy percent of patients have a chronic intermittent course with relapses and remissions. The others have continuous symptoms of varying severity without achieving complete remission. The severity of the first attack has no predictive value in determining the long-term outcome of the disease.

The fact that ulcerative colitis is a disease restricted to the colorectum makes it potentially curable by total proctocolectomy. Surgical treatment rates vary; in northern Scotland and Stockholm, 11% and 28% of patients who survive the first attack without surgery have a colectomy within 10 years.[1]

Pathologic Changes

The primary pathologic changes of ulcerative colitis are limited to the mucosa, which is diffusely affected (Fig. 11–8A). There is rarely involvement of the muscularis externa; typically, the colorectal wall is not thickened. On radiologic study, the normal haustrations are frequently lost. The mucosal changes (these share many features with Crohn's disease; when a given feature is seen in both diseases, it will be termed an IIBD feature) include:

1. Chronic inflammation: IIBD is characterized by the presence of markedly increased numbers of chronic inflammatory cells in the lamina propria (Fig. 11–8B). These include lymphocytes, plasma cells, and eosinophils (Fig. 11–8C). Eosinophils may be present in large numbers. The chronic inflammatory cells separate the crypts from one another and separate the crypt base from the muscularis mucosae (Fig. 11–8D). The chronic inflammation in ulcerative colitis is restricted to the mucosa, but may extend down into the superficial part of the submucosa immediately beneath the muscularis mucosae. When it extends into the submucosa, it has a band-like appearance with a relatively sharp lower border that demarcates it from the more normal underlying submucosal tissue (Fig. 11–8E). Chronic inflammation is frequently accompanied by lymphoid aggregates and reactive lymphoid follicles in the deep mucosa. In inactive disease, in clinical remission, and in treated ulcerative colitis, the inflammation subsides and ulceration heals (Fig. 11–9A), and the number of chronic inflammatory cells decreases, sometimes to within normal levels (Fig. 11–9B and C),

2. Acute inflammation: Acute inflammation, characterized by neutrophil infiltration of the lamina propria and crypts, is present in the active phase of IIBD (Fig. 11–10A). The neutrophil infiltration of the crypts is commonly associated with the formation of crypt abscesses, which are crypts that contain neutrophils in the lumen (Fig. 11–10B). The typical crypt abscess is a distended crypt with a flat epithelial lining. Crypt abscesses are not specific for IIBD, being also seen frequently in acute infectious colitis. Acute inflammation is associated with lamina propria edema, congestion, hemorrhage, and surface erosion and ulceration (Fig. 11–11A). Ulcers appear as necrotic, acutely inflamed debris or inflamed granulation tissue (Fig. 11–11B). The degree of acute inflammation and ulceration correlate best with the severity of clinical symptoms.

3. Crypt destruction and regeneration: The inflammatory process in IIBD results in progressive crypt destruction. This is associated with ongoing attempts at regeneration. The combination of these two processes results in distortion of normal crypt architecture (Fig. 11–12A). The crypts, normally vertical, show evidence of horizontal and vertical branching (Fig. 11–12B and C). Although crypt distortion is best evaluated in vertically oriented specimens, it can be recognized even in tangential sections. In general, the number of crypts per unit area of colonic mucosa is reduced (crypt atrophy) (Fig. 11–13). This atrophy may be difficult to evaluate accurately in some specimens when edema has caused separation of crypts. More rarely, the regenerative process results in elongation of crypts, resulting in an abnormal villous surface (Fig. 11–14). Even more rarely, the crypt abnormality may result in crypts being displaced underneath the muscularis mucosae into the superficial submucosa, resulting in colitis cystica profunda (Fig. 11–15). Active ongoing crypt regeneration often produces cytologic features of repair in the crypt cells. These include mucin depletion, enlarged and hyperchromatic nuclei with prominent nucleoli, increased nuclear:cytoplasmic (N:C) ratio, and increased mitotic activity.

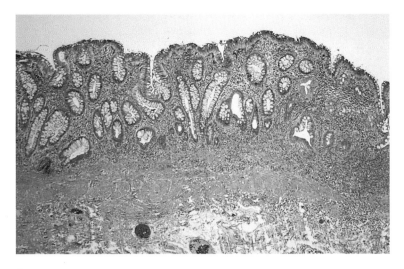

A

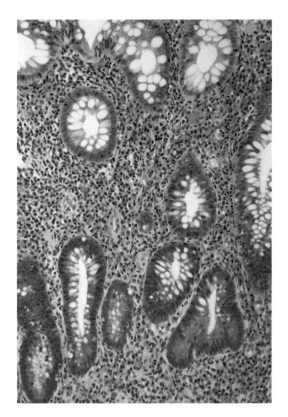

B

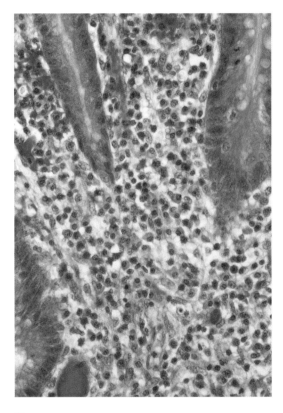

C

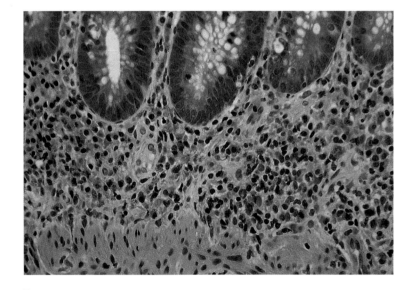

D

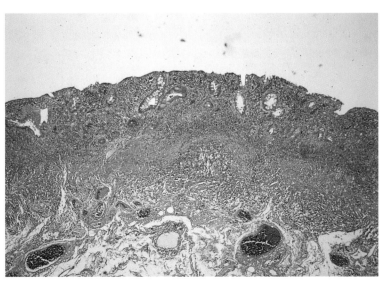

E

Figure 11–8. A: Chronic ulcerative colitis, showing marked crypt distortion and inflammation re-stricted to the mucosa. Note the somewhat thickened muscularis mucosae and the normal submucosa. B: Chronic ulcerative colitis, showing marked increase in chronic inflammatory cells in the lamina pro-pria. C: Chronic ulcerative colitis, higher power micrograph of part B, showing lymphocytes, plasma cells, and eosinophils. D: Chronic ulcerative colitis, showing a band of lymphocytes, plasma cells, and eosinophils separating the base of the crypts from the muscularis mucosae. E: Chronic ulcerative colitis, showing extension of the inflammatory process across the muscularis mucosae to involve the superfi-cial part of the submucosa. The base of the infiltrate has a band-like appearance with a sharp demarca-tion from the deep submucosa, which is normal.

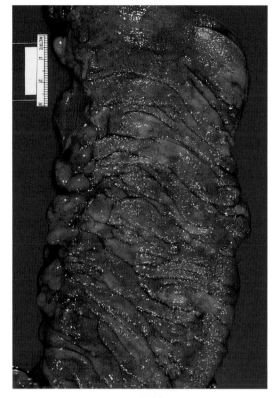

A

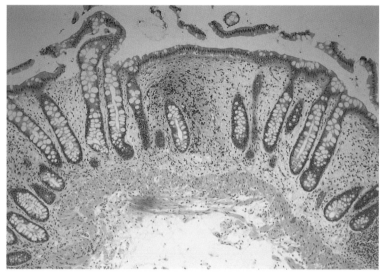

B

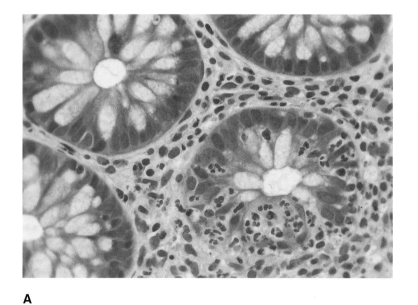

Figure 11–9. A: Ulcerative colitis, inactive phase. The mucosa shows loss of normal folds and a granularity with only mild focal hyperemia and no evidence of ulceration. B: Chronic ulcerative colitis, treated and in remission, showing atrophic mucosa with distorted crypts and moderate chronic inflammation in the lamina propria. C: Chronic ulcerative colitis, treated and in remission, showing return of mucosa to essentially normal. The crypt architecture is normal as is the amount of chronic inflammatory cells in the lamina propria. The base of the crypt is separated from the muscularis mucosae by a band of fibrosis. The diagnosis of ulcerative colitis in remission can only be made by examining prior biopsy material.

C

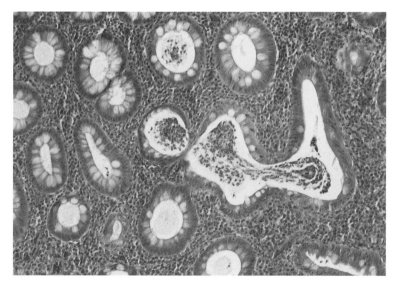

A

B

Figure 11–10. A: Active inflammation in lamina propria and crypts (cryptitis) in ulcerative colitis, active phase. B: Crypt abscess formation in ulcerative colitis, acute phase. The involved crypts show dilatation and luminal neutrophils.

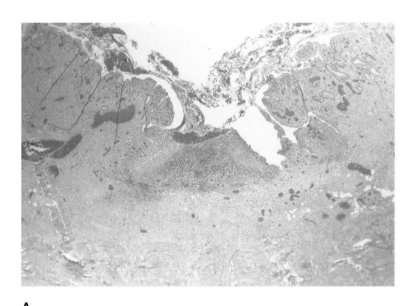

A

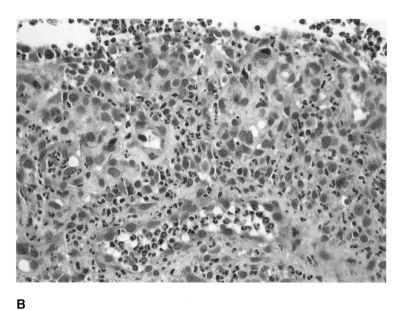

B

Figure 11–11. A: Surface ulceration in ulcerative colitis, active phase, showing acutely inflamed necrotic debris on the denuded mucosal surface surrounded by inflamed mucosa. B: Ulcer base in active ulcerative colitis, showing inflamed granulation tissue. Note the enlarged, active-appearing endothelial cells lining the neovascular spaces.

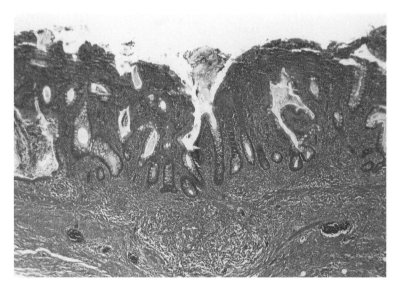

A

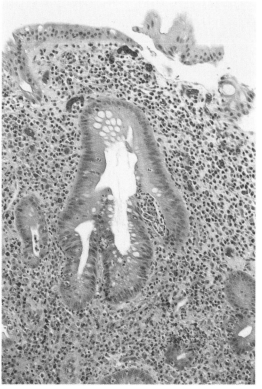

C

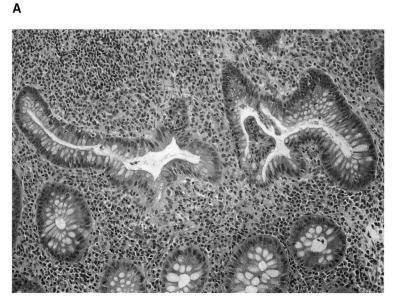

B

Figure 11–12. A: Chronic ulcerative colitis, showing severe crypt distortion and a marked increase in chronic inflammatory cells in the lamina propria. B: Horizontal branching of crypts in chronic ulcerative colitis. C: Vertical branching of crypts in chronic ulcerative colitis.

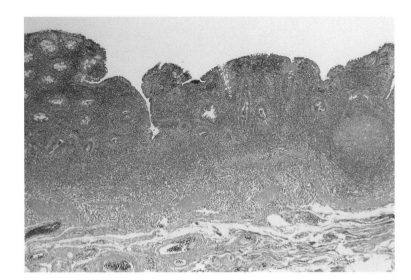

Figure 11–13. Marked crypt loss due to destruction by the inflammatory process. The number of crypts per unit area of colonic mucosa is greatly reduced.

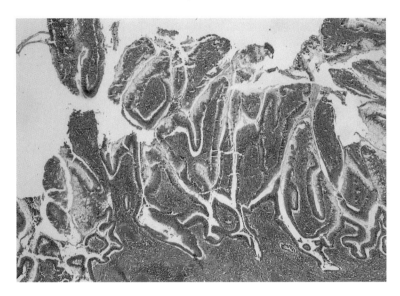

Figure 11–14. Abnormal villous surface of the mucosa in chronic ulcerative colitis. The appearance mimics villous adenoma microscopically. One difference between the two is that this sample is taken from a flat mucosa unlike in villous adenoma, which is a macroscopically polypoid lesion.

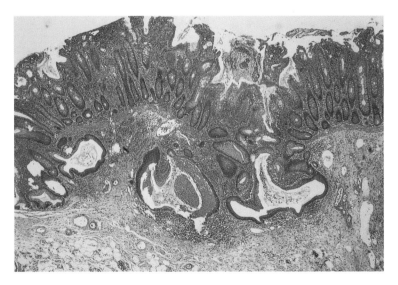

Figure 11–15. Colitis cystica profunda in the active phase of acute ulcerative colitis, showing displacement of distorted crypts beneath the muscularis mucosa into the superficial submucosa.

Crypt destruction in the acute phase may lead to crypt rupture and mucin extravasation into the lamina propria, resulting in histiocytic collections (Fig. 11–16A). When part of the crypt is present, crypt granulomas are obvious; when the crypt epithelium has disappeared, crypt granulomas may resemble epithelioid cell granulomas, leading to potential misdiagnosis as Crohn's disease (Fig. 11–16B). Well-defined epithelioid granulomas do not occur in ulcerative colitis. In

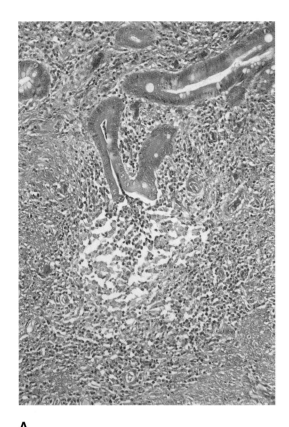

A

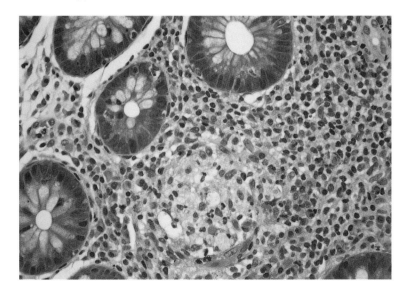

B

Figure 11–16. A: Chronic ulcerative colitis, active phase, showing destruction of a crypt by the inflammatory process. The partially disrupted crypt is surrounded by a collection of histiocytes ("crypt granuloma"). B: Small focus of mucosal histiocytes in chronic ulcerative colitis, most likely representing a resolving crypt granuloma. Note the resemblance to an epithelioid cell granuloma.

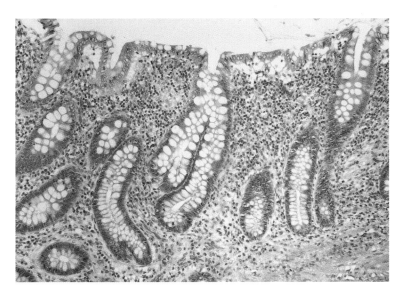

Figure 11–17. Chronic ulcerative colitis, in clinical remission, showing mild crypt distortion and residual chronic inflammation.

inactive and treated ulcerative colitis, the crypt distortion often decreases, but in most cases, mild crypt architectural distortion remains, permitting recognition of inactive disease (Fig. 11–17); rarely, the crypts return to an essentially normal appearance (see Fig. 11–9C).
4. Cellular changes in crypt epithelium in IIBD: Goblet cell mucin depletion is a typical feature (Fig. 11–18), but this can be seen in any form of inflammatory disease. Its severity is related to the amount of inflammation present. Paneth cell

metaplasia is another common feature of IIBD (Fig. 11–19). Normally, Paneth cells are rarely seen distal to the ascending colon. Increased numbers of Paneth cells are not specific for IIBD and should not be considered a reliable diagnostic criterion. Increased numbers of neuroendocrine cells have also been reported in IIBD; this is also not of proven specificity for diagnosis.

Complications

Fulminant Ulcerative Colitis

Fulminant ulcerative colitis is a severe attack of ulcerative colitis, with massive diarrhea and hemorrhage that cannot be controlled by medical therapy. It occurs in approximately 8–15% of patients with ulcerative colitis.[1,3] Emergency colectomy is needed. Fulminant ulcerative colitis may occur at any stage of the disease, although it tends to be more common in the early stages.

The resected specimen shows severe mucosal inflammation. The mucosa is dark red to purple and shows extensive ulceration and mucosal necrosis (Fig. 11–20). The residual mucosa between confluent ulcers is markedly edematous, forming red, elevated islands (pseudo-polyps) (Fig. 11–21). The nonulcerated mucosa shows severe inflammation restricted to the mucosa, with marked cryptitis and hemorrhage. Ulceration often extends below the mucosa to involve submucosa and the muscularis externa (Fig. 11–22A). Severe inflammation around the ulcers can extend deep into the muscle, but this does not represent true transmural inflammation. Vascular inflamma-

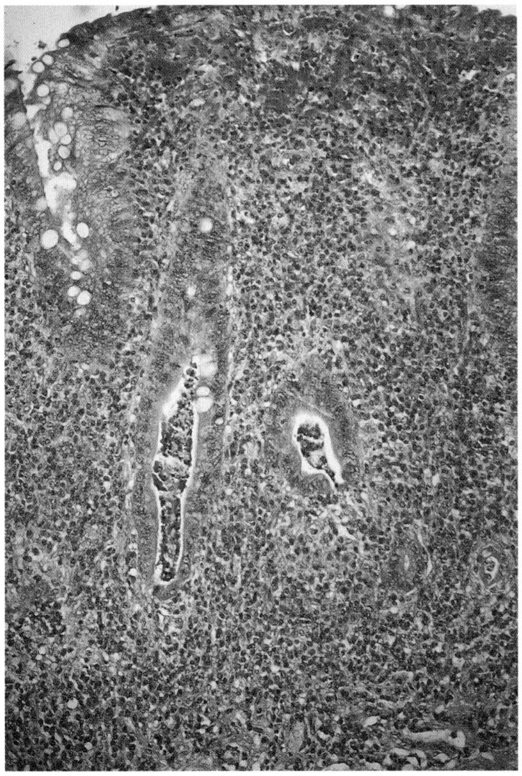

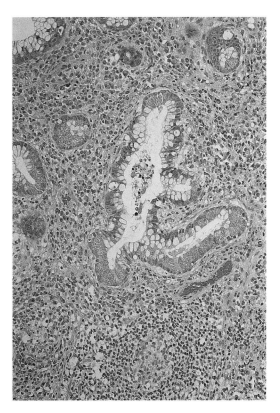

Figure 11–18. Chronic ulcerative colitis, active phase, showing reactive changes in the crypt epithelium characterized by nuclear enlargement and hyperchromasia and cytoplasmic mucin depletion.

Figure 11–19. Paneth cell metaplasia in a rectal biopsy specimen from a patient with ulcerative colitis, showing Paneth cells with eosinophilic cytoplasm lining the base of a crypt.

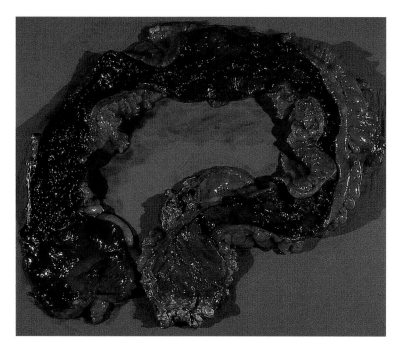

Figure 11–20. Fulminant colitis in a case of histologically proven ulcerative colitis. The mucosa shows severe hemorrhagic necrosis.

tion and thrombosis may be seen in relation to the ulcers. Foreign body granulomas may be present in relation to the deeper ulcers. Perforation is rare.

Toxic Megacolon

Toxic megacolon is the complication of ulcerative colitis that has the maximum risk of mortality. It occurs in 2–4% of patients with ulcerative colitis and tends to be more frequent early

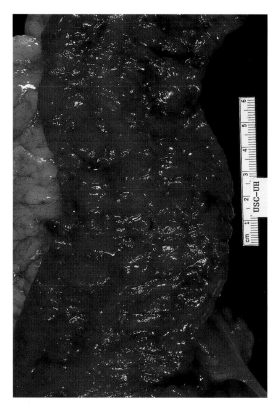

Figure 11–21. Fulminant colitis, showing severe mucosal hemorrhagic inflammation.

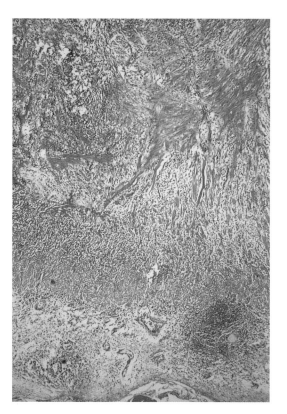

A

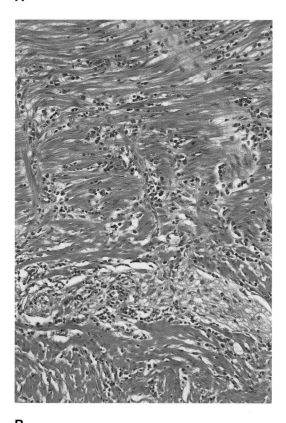

B

Figure 11–22. A: Fulminant colitis in ulcerative colitis, showing extensive and deep surface ulceration extending deep into the submucosa, associated with transmural inflammation. B: Fulminant colitis with toxic megacolon, showing involvement of the muscle wall and myenteric plexus by severe inflammation under a deep ulcer. This was associated with focal colonic perforation.

in the course of the disease. Toxic megacolon is a radiologic diagnosis, made when the diameter of the colon, measured at the transverse colon, exceeds 6 cm. Dilatation is maximal in the transverse colon, but may involve the entire colon. Perforation is common and associated with a 50% mortality rate. When emergency colectomy is performed for toxic megacolon prior to perforation, the mortality rate is less than 10%.

Toxic megacolon cannot be diagnosed accurately by examination of the resection specimen because the colon collapses on removal. The pathologic features of toxic megacolon complicating ulcerative colitis are commonly those of fulminant colitis with severe hemorrhagic mucosal inflammation with deep ulcers and pseudo-polyps. The circumference of the colon may be increased, but this is not a constant finding. The inflammation involves the entire thickness of the colonic wall, including the myenteric plexus (Fig. 11–22B). The muscle wall becomes thin and friable, tending to undergo spontaneous perforation with any handling at surgery. The serosal surface is opaque and frequently covered by exudate.

Secondary Infections

The role played by infectious diseases in acute exacerbations of ulcerative colitis is controversial. Among the infectious agents that have been cultured from stools in acute exacerbations of ulcerative colitis are *Clostridium difficile*,[4] *Campylobacter jejuni*,[5] and *Salmonella* spp.[6] Histologic examination does not permit differentiation of an acute exacerbation of ulcerative colitis from acute infectious colitis superimposed on chronic ulcerative colitis. The addition of the appropriate antibiotic to the standard treatment for a relapse of ulcerative colitis is advisable when the culture is positive.

Strictures

Strictures occur in approximately 5% of patients with ulcerative colitis; 75% are benign and 25% are malignant.[7] Most benign strictures are nonobstructive and asymptomatic, resulting from segmental narrowing caused by hyperplasia of the muscularis mucosae and submucosal fibrosis (Fig. 11–23). Rarely, severe strictures associated with mural fibrosis may occur; these most likely represent scarring associated with deep ulcers that occur in more severe episodes of ulcerative colitis.

Benign strictures can be managed with endoscopic dilatation in most cases. It is essential in these cases to exclude a carcinomatous stricture by performing adequate biopsies. Resection is indicated anytime the stricture precludes adequate biopsy evaluation. Cases have been reported in which unsus-

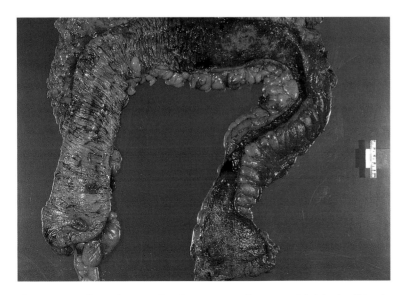

Figure 11–23. Chronic ulcerative colitis, showing an area of narrowing of the left colon. This stricture was due to submucosal fibrosis and edema without transmural inflammation.

TABLE 11–1. EXTRAINTESTINAL MANIFESTATIONS OF IDIOPATHIC INFLAMMATORY BOWEL DISEASE

Hepatobiliary

Fatty liver (on biopsy)	Present in 50% of liver biopsies in both CUC and CD.
Cholelithiasis	Common in CD; due to effect of terminal ileal disease on bile salt metabolism.
Primary sclerosing cholangitis	Occurs in 1–5% of patients with IIBD; is more common in males and in CUC.
Pericholangitis	Present in 30% of IIBD patients, commonly as a biopsy finding without clinical symptoms.
Bile duct adenocarcinoma	Occurs in 0.5–1% of patients with CUC.
Cryptogenic cirrhosis	Occurs in 20% of both CUC and CD; complication of pericholangitis (?).
Other rare complications	Hepatic amyloidosis, granulomatous hepatitis, liver abscess.

Rheumatologic

Peripheral arthritis	Develops in 15–20% of IIBD patients; more common in CD.
Ankylosing spondylitis	Occurs in 15–20% of IIBD patients; more common in CD.
Sacroiliitis	Common; occurs in both CUC and CD.
Other rare complications	Granulomatous synovitis in CD, hypertrophic osteoarthropathy, relapsing perichondritis.

Skin

Erythema nodosum	Occurs in 15% of CD and 10% of CUC patients.
Pyoderma gangrenosum	Occurs mainly in CUC; uncommon but fairly specific for CUC.
Vesiculopustular eruption of UC	Rare; in CUC.
Perianal skin tags	In 75% of CD.
Aphthous stomatitis	Common in CD.

Eye

Uveitis, episcleritis	Common in both CUC and CD.
Other rare complications	Chorioretinopathy, retinal vasculitis.

Other Complications

Hyperoxaluria with nephrolithiasis	Seen in 10% of CD with terminal ileal disease/resection.
Thromboembolic phenomena	Occurs in 1–5% of patients with IIBD.
Pleuropericarditis	Common in CUC.
Osteoporosis	Common in CUC and CD.
Cerebral microangiopathy	Rare; in CUC.

Abbreviations: CUC = chronic ulcerative colitis; CD = Crohn's disease; IIBD = idiopathic inflammatory bowel disease; UC = ulcerative colitis.

pected advanced carcinomas were found in colons resected for benign stricture.[8]

Backwash Ileitis

Backwash ileitis occurs in approximately 15% of patients with pancolitis. It is usually associated with an incompetent ileocecal valve, leading to the suggestion that ileal involvement is secondary to regurgitation of colonic contents. Ileal inflammation is restricted to the mucosa and is not associated with thickening or strictures; it is clinically of no significance. Its only importance is that its presence should not lead to a misdiagnosis of Crohn's disease.

Extraintestinal Complications

Extraintestinal complications occur in a minority of patients with IIBD.[9,10] The particular complications occur with different frequency in patients with ulcerative colitis and Crohn's disease (Table 11–1). In ulcerative colitis, the common complications are polyarthritis, pericholangitis and primary sclerosing cholangitis, erythema nodosum and pyoderma gangrenosum, and uveitis. The incidence of bile duct adenocarcinoma is increased in patients with chronic ulcerative colitis.

Polyps in Ulcerative Colitis

Polyps occurring in ulcerative colitis may be inflammatory polyps, adenomas, and dysplasia-associated lesions or masses.

Inflammatory Polyps. Inflammatory polyps occur in both ulcerative colitis and Crohn's disease. They are seen in the acute phase as edematous, acutely inflamed polyps with ulceration and granulation tissue in addition to cryptitis (Fig. 11–24). Inflammatory polyps may also be seen in the chronic stage of the disease (Fig. 11–25A), and consist of a combination of reactive distorted crypts and inflammation (Fig. 11–25B). They vary in size, but are usually less than 1 cm in diameter; frequently they are long and finger-like and may form mucosal bridges (Fig. 11–26). Most small inflammatory polyps can be recognized as

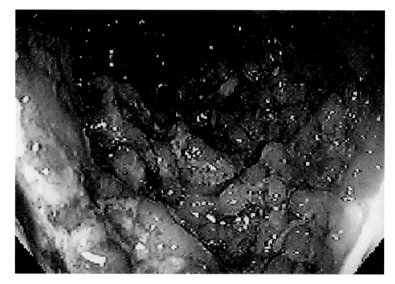

A

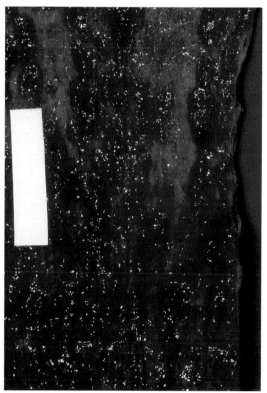

B

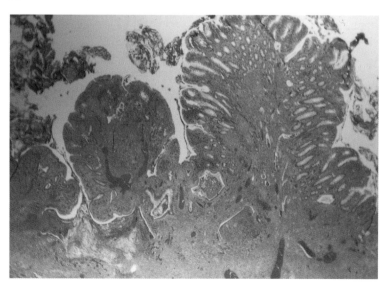

C

Figure 11–24. A: Colonoscopy showing multiple inflammatory pseudo-polyps in chronic ulcerative colitis. B: Chronic ulcerative colitis, in relapse, showing inflammation with inflammatory polyps superimposed on a flat, atrophic mucosa. C: Pseudo-polyps in active phase of ulcerative colitis, showing polypoid islands of mucosa with marked crypt distortion and inflammation separated by mucosal ulcers. (Part A: Courtesy of Aslam Godil, MD, Loma Linda University, CA).

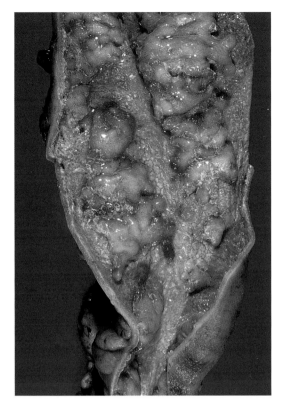

A

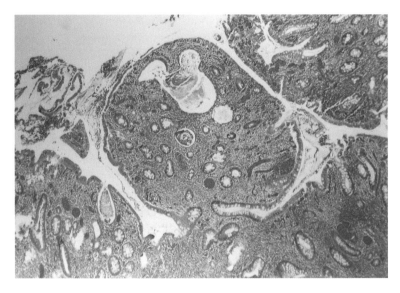

B

Figure 11–25. A: Chronic ulcerative colitis, in remission, showing inflammatory polyps on a flat atrophic mucosa. B: Pseudo-polyp in chronic ulcerative colitis, showing marked crypt distortion, crypt dilatation, and inflammation. The lining epithelium of the crypts does not show hyperplastic or adenomatous changes.

such at endoscopy. They have no malignant potential and a biopsy does not need to be performed on them nor do they need to be removed unless they are causing bleeding or if they have features that are suggestive of malignancy (larger than 1 cm or have an irregular color or surface appearance).

Two rare variants of inflammatory polyps occur: (1) Sometimes, large numbers of inflammatory polyps cover the entire mucosa; this is sometimes called colitis polyposa (Figs. 11–26

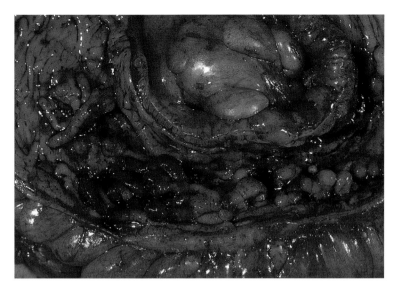

Figure 11–26. Crohn's disease with inflammatory polyps, showing a mass of polyps in an area of narrowing of the colon ("colitis polyposa"). The polyps have the typical elongated, finger-like appearance typical of inflammatory polyps. Mucosal bridges caused by fusion of these inflammatory polyps are also present.

and 11–27A). (2) Giant inflammatory polyps occur; these can reach a size larger than 10 cm and have an exophytic villous appearance (see Fig. 11–27). They may cause intussusception and obstruct the lumen. Giant inflammatory polyps are composed of distorted crypts that commonly show cystic dilatation and mucin distention, and acute and chronic inflammation. They are usually associated with active colitis in the surrounding mucosa. Rarely, they occur as solitary mass lesions in an otherwise normal colon; in such cases, they bear a strong endoscopic resemblance to villous adenoma and carcinoma.

Adenoma and Dysplasia-Associated Lesion or Mass. Adenoma and dysplasia-associated lesion or mass (DALM) represent polypoid lesions that may resemble usual pedunculated adenomas that occur in patients who do not have colitis (Fig. 11–28A), or they may be mistaken at endoscopy for inflammatory polyps and a biopsy may be done because they present some unusual feature. Both are characterized by the presence of adenomatous change (ie, low-grade dysplasia) on histologic examination (Fig. 11–28B and C). Care must be taken not to mistake regenerative or inflammatory atypia in an inflammatory polyp as adenomatous change.

When polypoid lesions are removed in patients with ulcerative colitis, it is very important to take specimens of the mucosa immediately surrounding the base of the stalk; these should be submitted as separately labeled specimens.

Adenomas occurring in ulcerative colitis are generally regarded as being identical to adenomas occurring in the general population. DALM has been reported to be associated with a high risk of malignancy, however, even when the dysplasia is low grade and therefore represents an indication for colectomy.[12]

The differentiation of adenoma from DALM is unclear. The following factors should be taken into account:

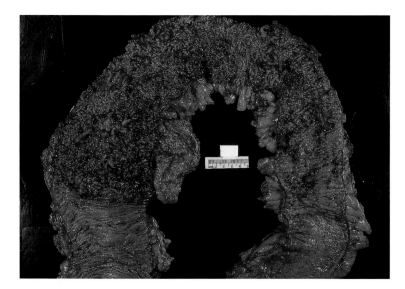

A

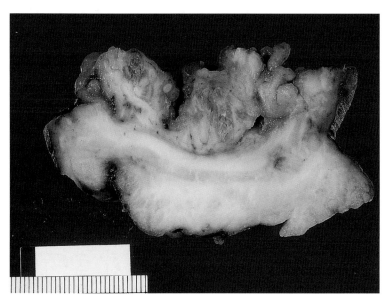

B

Figure 11–27. A: Giant inflammatory polyp in chronic ulcerative colitis. Coalescence of inflammatory polyps has resulted in a large polypoid structure in the midst of a mass of smaller polypoid structures. B: Giant inflammatory polyp, cross section through the wall of a fixed specimen showing the large exophytic inflammatory polyp. This had an appearance simulating a villous adenoma, but microscopically showed changes of inflammatory polyp, with distended and distorted crypts showing marked inflammation.

1. If the lesion had the typical endoscopic appearance of a pedunculated polyp, it is more likely to be an adenoma.
2. If the lesion occurs in patients younger than age 40, it is more likely to be DALM.
3. If the adenomatous change is restricted to the head of the polyp, and the stalk base region and biopsies of adjacent colonic mucosa are negative for dysplasia, adenoma is favored.
4. If the lesion occurs in an area of colon not affected by ulcerative colitis at any stage of the disease (established by evaluation of the initial diagnostic specimens from the patient), adenoma is favored.

Dysplasia and Carcinoma

Malignant transformation in ulcerative colitis represents the most important complication of ulcerative colitis because it is the commonest cause of death and because it is preventable. Cancer risk is greatest in patients with pancolitis and in those who have disease onset in childhood. The risk begins to rise at 8–10 years after onset, after which there is a 2% per year additive risk, giving a cancer rate of 20% per decade.[13] The risk does not depend on the degree of activity of ulcerative colitis; patients with continuous chronic symptoms have an equal risk to those with intermittent disease.

Ulcerative colitis is associated with increasing genetic abnormalities that are similar to those seen in noncolitis colorectal carcinoma. The morphologic expression of the genetic sequence, however, commonly lacks the adenoma phase in patients with ulcerative colitis. Instead the progression is from colitis to low-grade dysplasia to high-grade dysplasia and invasive carcinoma. Both low-grade dysplasia and high-grade dysplasia commonly occur in mucosa that appears endoscopically normal. Less commonly, dysplasia may be associated with a visible lesion (Fig. 11–29).

The genetic abnormalities described in carcinomas associated with ulcerative colitis include adenomatous polyposis coli (*APC*) gene mutation, microsatellite instability associated with mutations in DNA mismatch repair genes, *p53* mutations and loss of heterozygosity. K-*ras* mutations are less common than in noncolitis colorectal carcinomas. The most consistent change is *p53* loss of heterozygosity; this is found in a majority of carcinomas, but also in a significant number of high- and even low-grade dysplasias.[14] This suggests that *p53* loss occurs at an earlier stage in the sequence in carcinomas associated with ulcerative colitis than in noncolitis colorectal carcinoma.

Aneuploidy has been reported to be present in mucosal biopsies of ulcerative colitis and correlates with *p53* loss of heterozygosity.[14] Its correlation with dysplasia is poor, but a suggestion has been made that aneuploidy precedes dysplasia and therefore may be an independent marker of high risk in patients with ulcerative colitis.[15] Flow cytometry is presently not routinely recommended for biopsies in ulcerative colitis.

Carcinomas occurring in ulcerative colitis occur in the 30–50 year age group, earlier than usual sporadic colorectal carcinoma. They tend to be evenly distributed throughout the colon. Grossly and endoscopically, carcinomas can be nodular, ulcerative, and plaque-like and may be associated with strictures. Flat, plaque-like infiltrative carcinomas tend to be common. These are commonly associated with deep infiltration and stricture formation at a stage when the intraluminal tumor is still difficult to detect endoscopically or radiologically and tend to present at a later stage.[8] Biopsy specimens may be negative in the flat infiltrative carcinomas, and endoscopically suggestive strictures with negative biopsies should be resected.[16] Stage for stage, carcinoma in ulcerative colitis has a prognosis equal to that for noncolitis colorectal carcinoma; the overall 5-year survival rate ranges from 33–55%.[17]

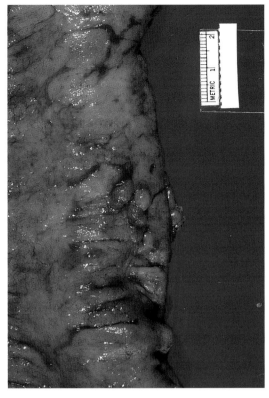

A

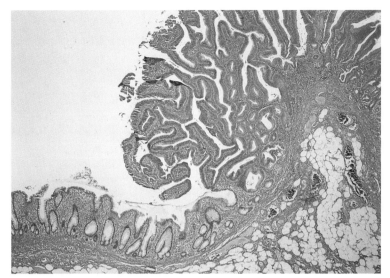

B

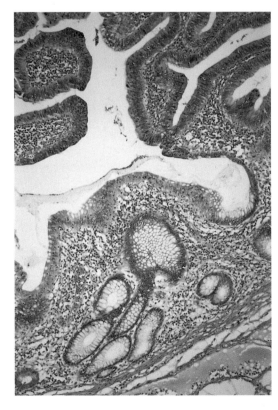

C

Figure 11–28. A: Chronic ulcerative colitis, showing two small polyps in flat mucosa. This was a colectomy done in a 39-year-old male. B: Microscopic appearance of one of the polyps in part A, showing a polypoid mass with low-grade dysplasia. Note the adjacent mucosa, which shows features of ulcerative colitis in remission. This lesion was interpreted as low-grade dysplasia in a mass lesion. C: Higher magnification micrograph of part B, showing adjacent mucosa with crypt distortion indictive of inactive chronic ulcerative colitis. A part of the polypoid lesions is shown with an appearance morphologically identical to adenoma.

The vast majority of carcinomas that occur in ulcerative colitis are adenocarcinomas. The flat infiltrative growth pattern tends to have an unusual histologic appearance, with a villous surface lined by highly dysplastic cells (Fig. 11–30), and relatively bland-appearing, small, malignant glands infiltrating deeply into the wall, sometimes without much desmoplasia (Fig. 11–31). Other types of carcinoma, such as squamous and adenosquamous carcinoma,[18] small-cell undifferentiated carcinoma,[19] and carcinoid tumors, have also been described in patients with ulcerative colitis.

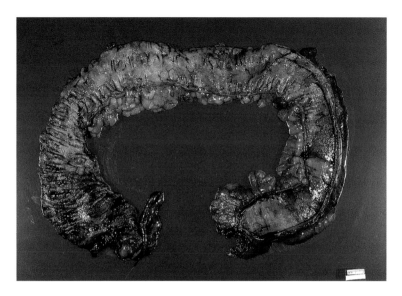

Figure 11–29. Colectomy specimen illustrated in Figure 11–28, showing chronic ulcerative colitis in an inactive phase. High-grade dysplasia was found in the flat mucosa in the rectosigmoid region in addition to the dysplasia-associated polypoid mass.

Surveillance for Carcinoma

The high risk of colorectal carcinoma mandates some method of prevention. The most certain method of prevention is to perform a proctocolectomy after 8–10 years of disease, which is when the risk of carcinoma begins. As the surgical techniques of mucosal proctectomy and creation of artificial ileal reservoirs to replace the rectum improve, this may well become a more viable option in the future.

At present, annual endoscopic surveillance is undertaken after 8–10 years of ulcerative colitis. If no lesions are seen at endoscopy, four biopsy specimens are taken randomly at every 10 cm of the colon; even this "extensive" sampling examines less than 1% of the total colonic mucosal surface. The aim of surveillance is to detect premalignant lesions before cancer develops. The presence of high-grade dysplasia or low-grade dysplasia in a DALM are indicators of high risk for malignancy and are presently indications for proctocolectomy. The recognition of low-grade dysplasia in the absence of DALM is a signal to heighten surveillance by increasing the frequency of colonscopy from annually to every 3–6 months. Some authorities recommend colectomy for low grade dysplasia.

This surveillance protocol has many flaws: (1) Up to 50% of patients with resected carcinomas do not show high-grade dysplasia in the surrounding mucosa.[20] This indicates either that the dysplasia was very focal or that carcinoma occurred de novo without a dysplastic phase. (2) Dysplasia does not usually produce an endoscopic abnormality. It must be detected in random biopsies of the colon. The risk of false-negative diagnosis due to sampling error is very high.

In 1983, a group of gastrointestinal pathology experts developed a detailed pathologic classification of dysplasia (Table 11–2). Such a detailed classification has limited practical value because of its complexity. Subtle differences in dysplasia grades such as those proposed are difficult to achieve even among ex-

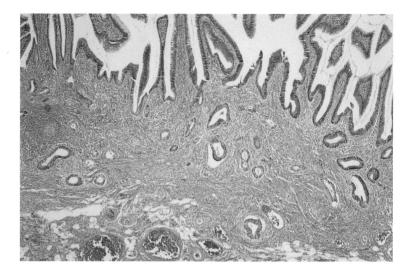

A

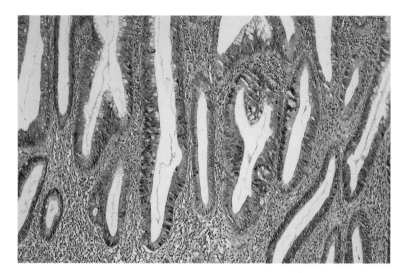

B

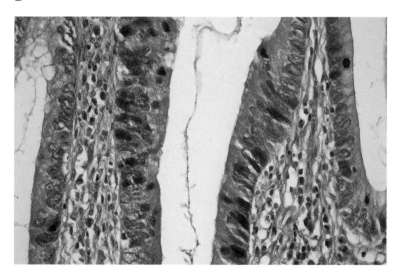

C

Figure 11–30. A: Adenocarcinoma in chronic ulcerative colitis, showing a microscopically villous surface with small glands infiltrating the muscularis mucosae. This specimen was from a flat mucosal lesion that had wall thickening. B: Villous surface in adenocarcinoma occurring in ulcerative colitis. Note the similarity to a villous adenoma; the distinction is made by the fact that this section was taken from flat mucosa rather than from a grossly visible sessile polyp. C: Higher power micrograph of part B, showing severe cytologic abnormality and loss of nuclear polarity indicative of high-grade dysplasia.

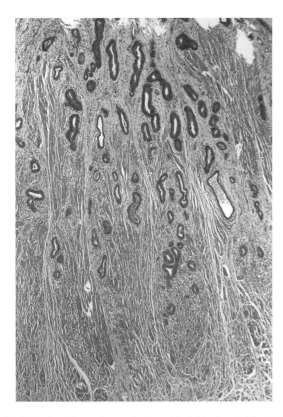

Figure 11–31. Infiltrating adenocarcinoma, showing relatively bland, well-differentiated adenocarcinomatous glands infiltrating muscularis externa with only minimal desmoplastic response.

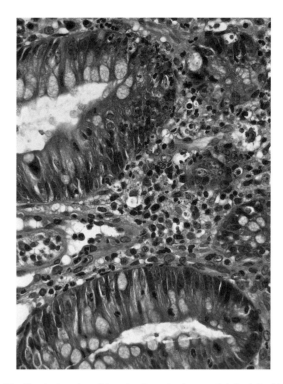

Figure 11–32. Chronic ulcerative colitis, active phase, showing crowded glands lined by cells showing marked cytologic atypia and mucin depletion. This was classified as reactive atypia because of the presence of active inflammation. This type of appearance is frequently classified as "indefinite for dysplasia."

perts, as shown by the considerable intraobserver and interobserver variation in the intermediate grades of dysplasia.[21] A recent study[22] that attempted to evaluate gastroenterologists' understanding of the meaning of dysplasia in ulcerative colitis found that only 19%, 16%, and 48% correctly identified the basic definitions of dysplasia, low-grade dysplasia, and high-grade dysplasia, respectively. Only 69% of gastroenterologists in this study recommended colectomy when high-grade dysplasia was present in a biopsy specimen.

It is not surprising that the proposed classification has not gained wide usage except in academic practice. Even if it is used by the pathologist, it is not likely, except in extraordinary circumstances, that its subtleties are appreciated or understood by the gastroenterologist making the clinical decisions. In practice, diagnosis such as "indefinite for dysplasia, probably negative," "indefinite for dysplasia, unknown," and "indefinite for dysplasia, probably positive" serve more to alienate pathologists from their clinical counterparts than to provide any useful information.

TABLE 11–2. PATHOLOGIC CLASSIFICATION OF DYSPLASIA

Standard designation	Implication for management	Suggested designation
Negative for Dysplasia		
Normal mucosa	Regular surveillance	Negative for dysplasia
Inactive colitis	Regular surveillance	Negative for dysplasia
Active colitis	Regular surveillance	Negative for dysplasia
Indefinite for Dysplasia		
Probably negative	Regular surveillance	Negative for dysplasia
Unknown	Decrease surveillance interval	Indefinite for dysplasia
Probably positive	Decrease surveillance interval	Low-grade dysplasia
Positive for Dysplasia		
Low grade in flat mucosa	Decrease surveillance interval	Low-grade dysplasia
Low grade in DALM	Consider colectomy	Low-grade dysplasia in DALM
High grade	Consider colectomy	High-grade dysplasia

Abbreviations: DALM = dysplasia-associated lesion or mass.

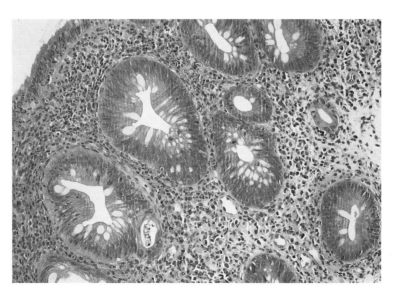

Figure 11–33. Cytologic abnormality resembling low-grade dysplasia in ulcerative colitis. The lamina propria contains neutrophils indicating active disease, leading to a diagnosis of indefinite for dysplasia.

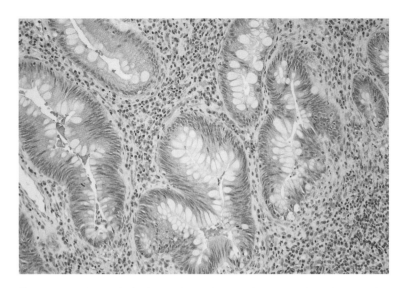

Figure 11–34. Low-grade dysplasia in chronic ulcerative colitis, inactive phase, showing nuclear stratification and atypia. The polarity of the cells is maintained, and the glands do not show complexity.

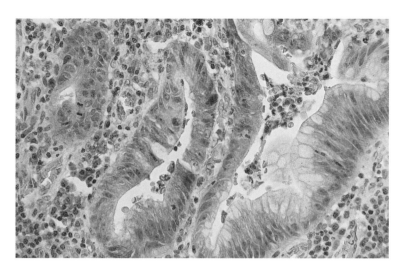

Figure 11–36. Transition from low-grade dysplasia to high-grade dysplasia in chronic ulcerative colitis, showing one crypt lined by cells with severe cytologic abnormality associated with loss of nuclear polarity adjacent to a crypt with features of low-grade dysplasia.

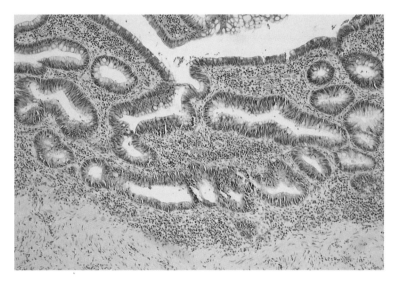

A

B

Figure 11–35. A. Extensive low-grade dysplasia in chronic ulcerative colitis. B: Higher power micrograph of part A, showing a greater degree of cytologic atypia in the cells lining the crypts, but the crypts are still simple and nuclear polarity is retained.

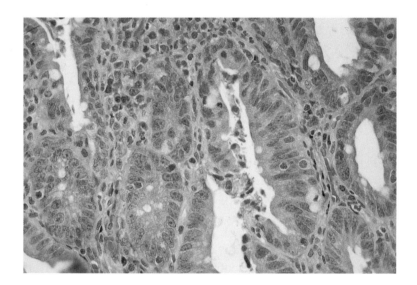

A

B

Figure 11–37. A: High-grade dysplasia in chronic ulcerative colitis, showing severe cytologic abnormality and loss of nuclear polarity. B: High-grade dysplasia in chronic ulcerative colitis, showing extreme cytologic abnormality and loss of nuclear polarity.

At the University of Southern California (USC), we use a much simpler and more practical classification of dysplasia (see Table 11–2) that is more in line with general usage among most pathologists. We make every attempt to make a clear-cut decision as to whether true dysplasia is present or not (Fig. 11–32). When true dysplasia is present (Figs. 11–33 through 11–37), the classification as high-grade dysplasia is based on the presence of severe cytologic abnormality plus either complete loss of nuclear polarity in the cells lining the crypt or the presence of gland complexity manifested by luminal bridging and cribriform change. All other cases of true dysplasia are classified as low-grade dysplasia.

Cytologic changes associated with active inflammation and regeneration can mimic the changes of low-grade dysplasia (see Figs. 11–18 and 11–32). In most cases when active inflammation or ulceration accompanies mild to moderate cytologic atypia of the crypt epithelium, true dysplasia is therefore considered absent. These cases are all reported as negative for dysplasia. High-grade dysplasia can be diagnosed in the presence of inflammation and ulceration because the criteria for its diagnosis are not seen in reactive akypia (Fig. 11–38).

The number of cases classified as indefinite for dysplasia should be kept as low as possible because it is unlikely that anyone reading the report will know what significance it has (the pathologist who reports it included!). The only instance for using this diagnosis is when the biopsy shows active inflammation or ulceration and the pathologist is concerned that the cytologic changes, although not satisfying criteria for high-grade dysplasia, are too severe for reactive atypia. Pathologists experienced in cytopathology know that reactive changes in epithelial cells frequently show cytologic features that are highly atypical. The more a pathologist recognizes this fact, the fewer diagnoses of "indefinite for dysplasia" he or she will make; most of these cases will be classified as negative for dysplasia. In a recent report, cases diagnosed as "indefinite for dysplasia" did not have value in predicting malignancy.[23]

The end-point of surveillance is the finding of high-grade dysplasia in a random biopsy or low-grade dysplasia in a DALM. These have a 30–50% risk that an invasive carcinoma is present elsewhere in the colon; this is a sufficient reason for colectomy.[24] Even if no malignancy is found, the risk of developing a carcinoma in the near future is much higher in a patient with high-grade dysplasia in a biopsy than for a similar patient without dysplasia in a surveillance biopsy.

CROHN'S DISEASE

Etiology and Epidemiology

Crohn's disease has an incidence of 2–5/100,000 population and a prevalence of slightly less than 0.1%, very similar to the statistics for ulcerative colitis. It has a definite female predominance. The maximum age incidence is between 15–40 years; Crohn's disease is rare under the age of 10 years; onset after age 40 years is not unusual. Jews have a higher incidence of Crohn's disease than the general population; there is a slight familial tendency.

The cause of Crohn's disease is unknown. The earliest lesion in Crohn's disease is a minute aphthous ulcer that develops over a mucosal lymphoid patch (Figs. 11–39 and 11–40).

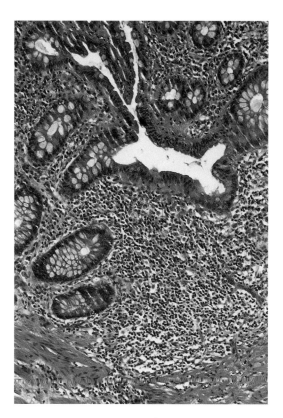

Figure 11–39. Normal colonic mucosa showing an area of close association between lymphoid tissue and crypt epithelium. In these lymphoglandular foci, the crypt frequently becomes focally distorted as it relates to the lymphoid tissue. Note also that the cells in the horizontal part of the crypt base are not goblet cells; this is the region where M cells are found, representing the area of antigen uptake from lumen to the lymphoid aggregate.

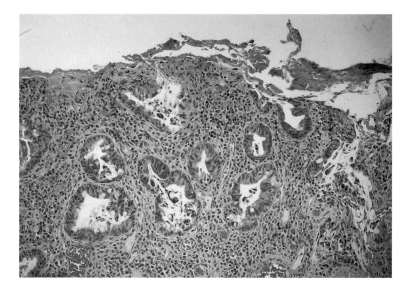

Figure 11–38. High-grade dysplasia in ulcerated mucosa in ulcerative colitis, showing glands with severe cytologic abnormality and loss of nuclear polarity. These changes are not consistent with reactive atypia.

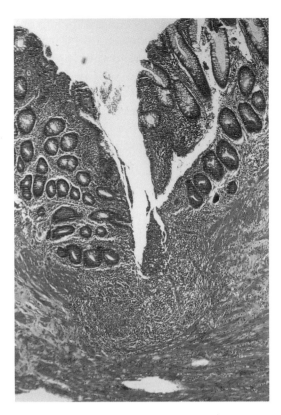

Figure 11–40. Earliest lesion of Crohn's disease showing a small aphthous ulcer overlying a small lymphoid aggregate.

The epithelium overlying lymphoid patches have interspersed membranous epithelial cells (M cells), which are specialized epithelial cells that transport antigens, including microorganisms from the lumen into the lamina propria.[25] M cells have short, fat microvilli, which permit their differentiation from absorptive cells on electron microscopy. The occurrence of the early aphthous ulcer in Crohn's disease at the location of M cells suggests the possibility of an immune reaction against a luminal antigen that has been taken up by the M cell. Many antigens, mostly microbial, have been suggested as the agent evoking the abnormal immune response in Crohn's disease. Although of considerable theoretical interest, these concepts have no practical use as yet.

Distribution of Lesions

Crohn's disease can affect the entire gastrointestinal tract from mouth to anus. At presentation, 40% of patients show involvement of the ileocecal region, 30% have small-bowel disease, and 25% colonic disease; involvement of esophagus, stomach, and duodenum are rare. Involvement of the anal region is common. Patchy and regional disease involving the full thickness of the bowel wall is typical and permits differentiation from ulcerative colitis in most cases (Figs. 11–41, 11–42, and 11–43). The presence of gastrointestinal disease proximal to the colon in excess of what is acceptable for "backlash ileitis" in a patient with IIBD indicates a diagnosis of Crohn's disease (Fig. 11–44).

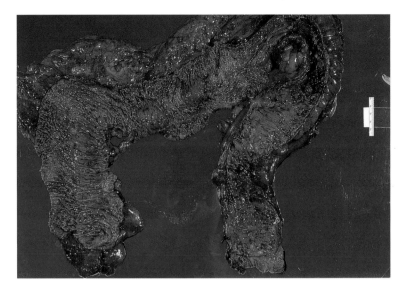

Figure 11–41. Colon in Crohn's disease, showing sparing of the distal rectal mucosa, a localized area of gross mucosal disease in the sigmoid colon, a skip area, and an area of strictured involvement in the distal transverse colon.

Clinical Features

Diarrhea, colicky abdominal pain, and low-grade fever are the common presenting symptoms. In patients with colonic disease, overt rectal bleeding occurs in about 40%; the amount of bleeding is generally less than in ulcerative colitis. In patients with ileocolic disease, a mass can sometimes be felt in the right lower abdomen. Perianal lesions, which include anal fistulae, anal strictures, perianal abscesses, and skin tags, are common (see Fig. 11–42). Some patients present with complications

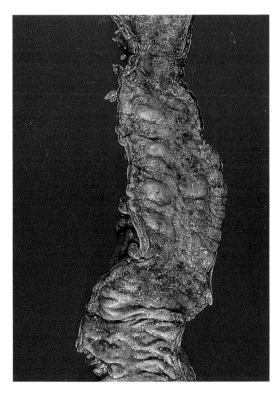

Figure 11–42. Crohn's colitis, showing patchy involvement of the colon associated with a stricture in the anal canal.

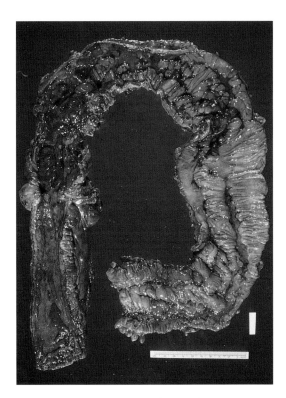

Figure 11–43. Crohn's colitis, showing patchy involvement of the colonic mucosa with extensive areas of ulceration alternating with intact mucosa. A long serpiginous ulcer is evident in the descending colon.

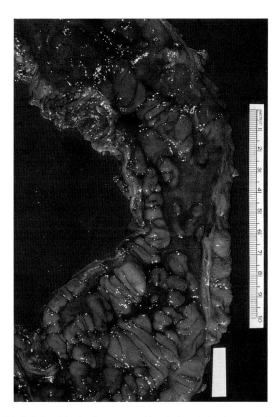

Figure 11–45. Crohn's colitis, showing mucosa with typical patchy involvement, with flat, ulcerated areas alternating with residual islands of normal-appearing mucosa.

such as intestinal obstruction and fistulae. The commonest fistula, which occurs in 10% of female patients, is a rectovaginal fistula.

Endoscopy permits visualization of colonic (and gastroduodenal) involvement. Colonic involvement appears as scattered aphthous ulcers and larger, linear, often longitudinal, serpiginous ulcers in regionally inflamed mucosa (Fig. 11–45).

Even in an area of involvement, mucosal changes are patchy with sharp demarcation between involved and uninvolved mucosa (Figs. 11–45 and 11–46). Rectal sparing, skip lesions, and strictures are typical (see Fig. 11–41). Endoscopic evaluation does not permit adequate evaluation of submucosal changes. Endoscopic ultrasound examination is an excellent method for evaluating wall thickness.

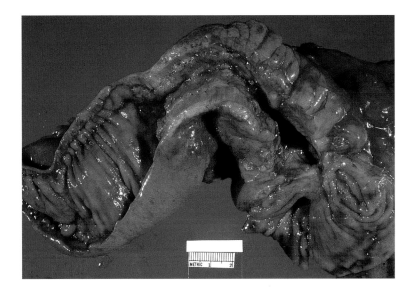

Figure 11–44. Crohn's disease of the ileum, showing the typical "lead pipe," or "garden hose," appearance. The area of involvement shows mucosal ulceration, marked wall thickening associated with luminal narrowing, and mesenteric creeping fat. This is sharply demarcated from uninvolved small intestine, which shows a normal mucosal pattern, normal wall thickness, and absence of serosal fat overgrowth.

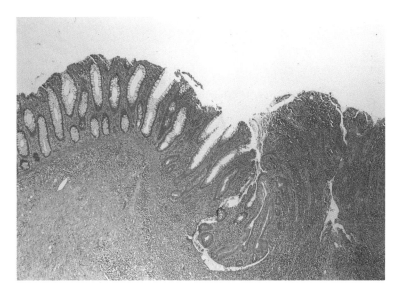

Figure 11–46. Crohn's colitis, showing the relatively sharp demarcation between severely involved and less involved mucosa. This focal colitis pattern is typical of Crohn's disease and is a useful criterion for distinguishing it from ulcerative colitis, where the involvement is diffuse.

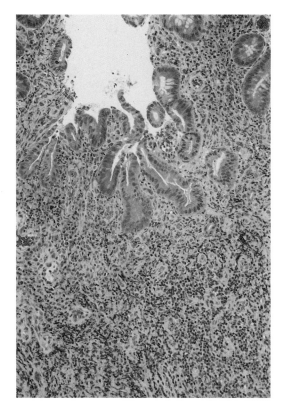

A

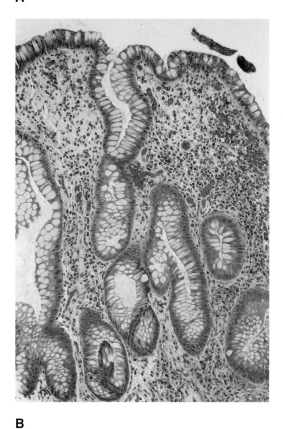

B

Figure 11–47. A: Terminal ileal biopsy specimen from a patient with no colonic disease. This shows focal erosion, acute and chronic inflammation, and reactive changes in the crypts. In the absence of granulomas, this appearance is not specific for Crohn's ileitis. B: Terminal ileal biopsy specimen, showing blunting of villi, inflammation, and crypt distortion. These features suggest chronic ileitis, but are not specific for Crohn's disease in the absence of granulomas.

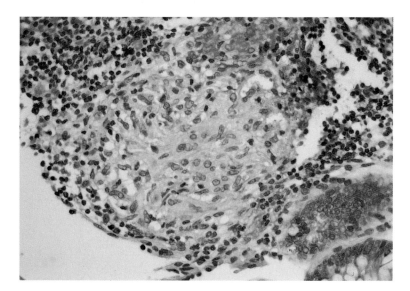

Figure 11–48. Crohn's disease, showing a well-formed nonnecrotizing epithelioid cell granuloma in a mucosal biopsy.

The small bowel cannot be directly visualized at endoscopy. Terminal ileal biopsy samples can be taken at colonoscopy and may show evidence of ileal involvement (Fig. 11–47). Because this part of the terminal ileum may be affected in ulcerative colitis, however, such biopsy samples are not very helpful in patients with colonic disease, unless the changes are severe with ulceration or they are associated with epithelioid granulomas. If no colonic disease is evident, the presence of terminal ileal changes are very helpful in establishing a diagnosis of Crohn's disease (see Fig. 11–47).

Radiologic study is much more important in the diagnosis of Crohn's disease than it is in ulcerative colitis. It permits evaluation of the entire small intestine and provides information about colonic wall thickening and the presence of fistulae, sinus tracts, and strictures.

Crohn's disease is a chronic, lifelong disease with remis-

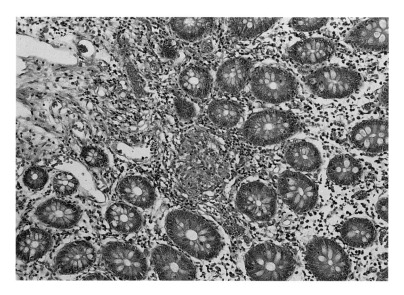

Figure 11–49. Small mucosal nonnecrotizing epithelioid cell granuloma in a patient with chlamydial proctitis. Note the absence of crypt distortion and significant chronic inflammation.

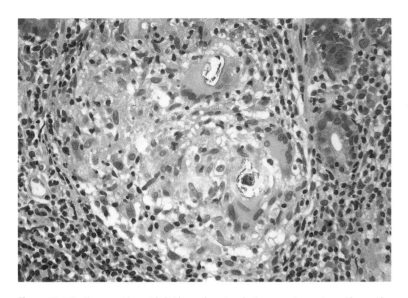

Figure 11–50. Nonnecrotizing epithelioid granuloma in colonic mucosa in a patient with sarcoidosis. No associated inflammation or crypt distortion is present. Note the calcified Schaumann body.

sions and relapses at varying intervals. Relapses are linked to cigarette smoking, which should be avoided in all patients with Crohn's disease.

Unlike ulcerative colitis, Crohn's disease cannot be cured surgically. The emphasis in the management of Crohn's disease is to minimize surgical excision of bowel. Severe disease with complications is helped considerably by surgery, however, which is often needed. Patients requiring surgery have a 75% incidence of recurrence, usually immediately proximal to the anastomosis,[26] and a 50% chance that a second surgery will be needed in their lifetime.

Pathologic Features

The earliest recognizable mucosal lesion of Crohn's disease is the aphthous ulcer (see Fig. 11–40). This is a shallow irregular ulcer commonly located over a mucosal lymphoid aggregate. Progression of the aphthous ulcer by enlargement and coalescence results in serpiginous ulcers that surround islands of uninvolved mucosa (see Fig. 11–45). The mucosal islands show variable, often focal inflammation and marked edema involving both mucosa and submucosa; this results in the typical "cobblestone" pattern of Crohn's disease. In the ileum, the villi in the intact mucosa are blunted, the crypts are distorted, and marked acute and chronic inflammation is evident with infiltration of the crypt and villous epithelium (see Fig. 11–47). The ileal crypts frequently show metaplasia of the crypts to pyloric-type glands. Ulceration and granulomas may be seen. In colonic involvement, the mucosal changes are identical to those seen in ulcerative colitis, except that the involvement tends to be more focal. Epithelioid granulomas are present in mucosal biopsies in approximately 10% of patients with Crohn's disease (Fig.

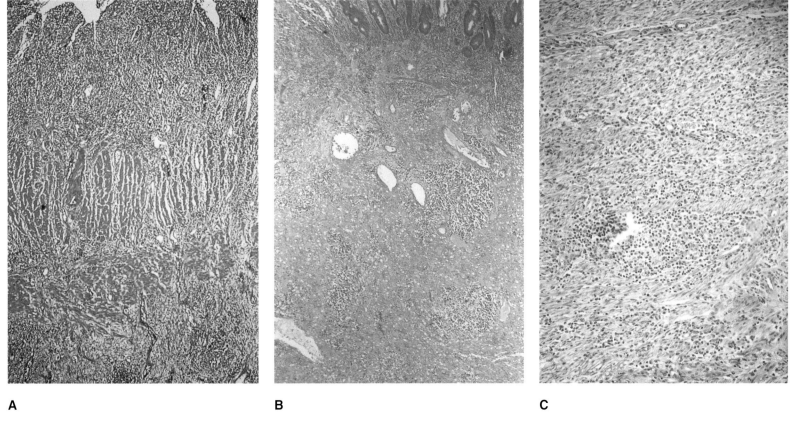

A   B   C

Figure 11–51. A: Transmural inflammation in Crohn's disease, showing mucosal, submucosal, and full-thickness inflammation of the muscularis externa. Note the lymphoid aggregate in the subserosa. B: Crohn's colitis, showing marked submucosal expansion, fibrosis, and lymphoid aggregation. C: Transmural inflammation in Crohn's colitis. Note the lymphoid aggregates on the submucosal and serosal sides of the muscularis externa.

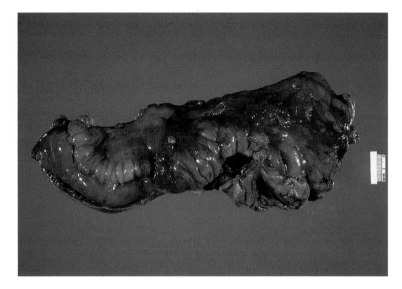

Figure 11–52. Crohn's disease of the ileum, showing "fat-wrapping," or "creeping fat." The involved segment of the bowel is completely wrapped by mesenteric fat, which has extended over the entire antimesenteric surface, compared with the uninvolved bowel, which has a smooth serosal surface.

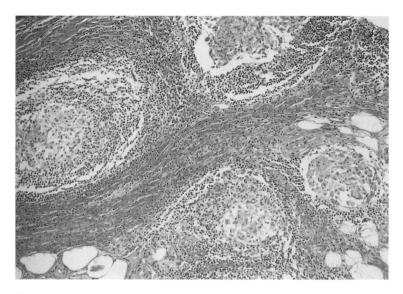

Figure 11–54. Crohn's colitis, showing numerous, large, nonnecrotizing epithelioid cell granulomas in the muscularis externa.

11–48). Epithelioid granulomas in colorectal mucosa are diagnostic for Crohn's disease only when they occur in mucosa that shows diagnostic histologic features of idiopathic inflammatory bowel disease, such as crypt distortion and severe chronic inflammation. When present in mucosa that does not show changes of IIBD, other possibilities of granulomas, such as infection (Fig. 11–49) and sarcoidosis (Fig. 11–50), should be considered.

Inflammation in Crohn's disease involves the full thickness of the bowel wall (Fig. 11–51A). The submucosa is edematous and shows lymphangiectasia in the acute phase; in the chronic phase the submucosa is markedly expanded and shows marked fibrosis and numerous lymphoid aggregates in the interphase between submucosa and muscularis externa (Fig. 11–51B). Deep submucosal lymphoid aggregates at the interphase be-

tween submucosa and muscularis externa are a typical feature of Crohn's disease (Fig. 11–51C). The muscularis externa shows diffuse lymphocytic infiltration, lymphoid aggregates, and fibrosis. Hyperplastic lymphoid nodules are also present on the serosal side of the muscularis externa (see Fig. 11–51C). The serosa shows "creeping fat," or "fat-wrapping," consisting of overgrowth of mesenteric fat over the peritoneal surface of the bowel wall (Figs. 11–52 and 11–53). Epithelioid granulomas are present in 60% of cases when the resected bowel is available for examination (Fig. 11–54). Granulomas can also be found in the enlarged, reactive lymph nodes in the mesentery (Fig. 11–55). True granulomas must be differentiated from foreign body-type granulomas that occur around luminal contents in fistulous tracts (Fig. 11–56), and foreign body type reactions around mucin extravasated from damaged crypts (Fig. 11–57). The lat-

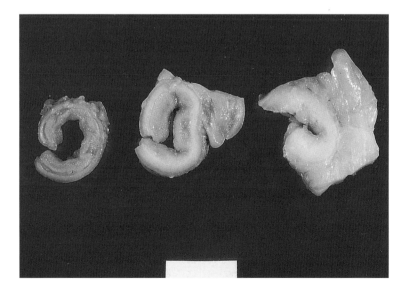

Figure 11–53. Cross section of the ileum in Crohn's ileitis, showing uninvolved intestine on the left; mildly involved intestine in the middle with wall thickening but no appreciable fat wrapping; and severely involved bowel on the right with severe wall thickening, luminal narrowing, and almost complete fat wrapping.

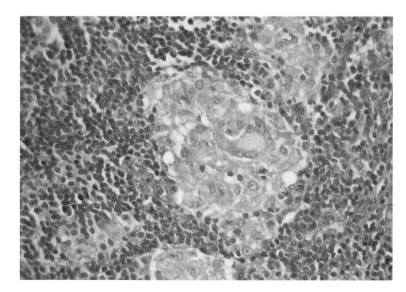

Figure 11–55. Mesenteric lymph node in the patient with Crohn's colitis, showing a nonnecrotizing epithelioid cell granuloma.

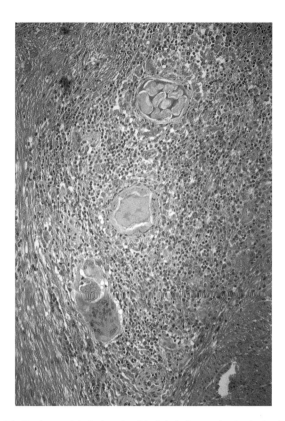

Figure 11–56. Fistulous track in the bowel wall in Crohn's disease, showing foreign body granulomatous response against food particles in the fistula track.

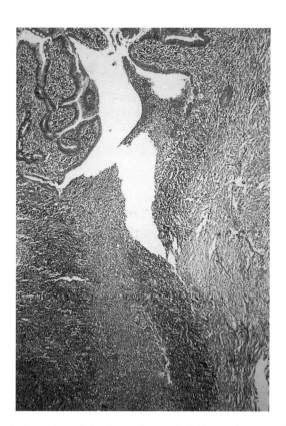

Figure 11–58. Fissure ulcer in Crohn's disease showing a knife-like vertical extension of the surface aphthous ulcer extending into the submucosa.

ter resemble mucous escape reactions ("mucoceles") that are commonly seen in the floor of the mouth.

Fissures and fistulae are typical of Crohn's disease. Fissures are knife-like ulcers that extend downward into the wall from the edge of an aphthous ulcer (Fig. 11–58). Fissure ulcers are lined by neutrophils and can extend deep into the muscle wall; rarely, they are transmural and cause pinpoint perforations. Fistulae are communications between the lumen of the affected bowel and an adjacent epithelium-lined organ, such as the vagina, another loop of bowel, skin, or the urinary bladder (Figs. 11–59 and 11–60). Fistula formation is preceded by adherence of the thickened bowel wall to an adjacent structure. Deep ulceration and abscess formation in the area of the adherence ultimately results in a mucosal connection. Crohn's disease commonly causes marked mural fibrosis, resulting in luminal narrowing and strictures (Fig. 11–61).

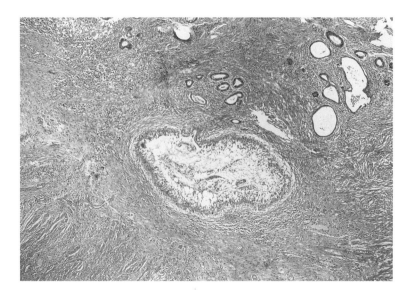

A

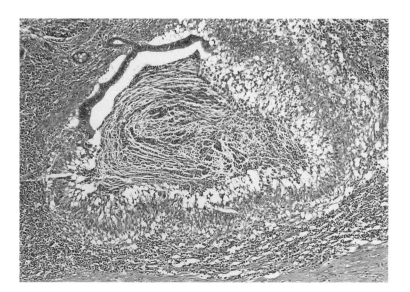

B

Figure 11–57. A: Ruptured crypt in the deep mucosa in Crohn's disease, producing a rounded histiocyte response against the extravasated mucin ("mucus escape reaction," or "mucocele," appearance): B: Higher power micrograph of part A, showing residual crypt lining and palisading histiocytes around the extravasated mucin.

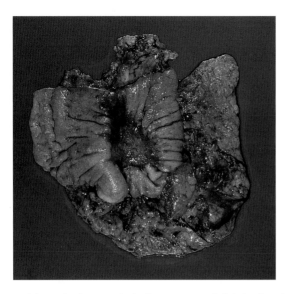

Figure 11–59. Colonic side of a gastrocolic fistula in a patient with Crohn's colitis, showing deep ulcer in the region of the colonic end of the fistula. The fistula itself cannot be seen.

Rare cases of Crohn's disease are associated with a granulomatous vasculitis involving the submucosal and intramural arterioles. This finding does not usually indicate a systemic vasculitis such as Wegener's granulomatosis or polyarteritis nodosum.

Complications

Intestinal Complications

Intestinal complications such as strictures, fissure ulcers, fistulae, and perianal lesions are part of the usual pathology of Crohn's disease. Inflammatory polyps, including giant inflammatory polyps, occur commonly in Crohn's disease and are identical to those seen in ulcerative colitis (see Fig. 11–26). Toxic megacolon and free perforation occur, but much less commonly than in ulcerative colitis.

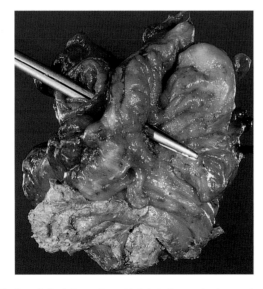

Figure 11–60. Ileocolic fistula in a patient with Crohn's disease, showing a probe passed through the fistulous track.

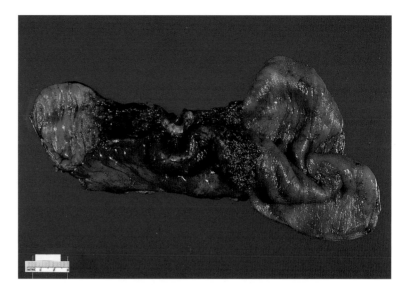

Figure 11–61. Stricture in Crohn's disease associated with intestinal obstruction. Note the marked distension of the intestine proximal to the obstruction.

Extraintestinal Complications

Many of the extraintestinal complications of ulcerative colitis (see Table 11–1) also occur in Crohn's disease. Ankylosing spondylitis, erythema nodosum, uveitis, and pericholangitis are common in Crohn's disease.

In addition, Crohn's disease involving the terminal ileum, with or without resection, leads to metabolic abnormalities resulting from the absence of the terminal ileum. These include (1) vitamin B_{12} malabsorption; (2) cholelithiasis due to interference of bile salt metabolism; and (3) hyperoxaluria, which is associated with fat malabsorption, leading to nephrolithiasis.

Dysplasia and Carcinoma

Patients with Crohn's disease have an increased incidence of adenocarcinoma of the colon and small intestine compared with the general population. Small-bowel adenocarcinomas are rare. The risk of colon cancer is considered to be much less than that seen in ulcerative colitis, although this has been questioned.[27] Colon carcinoma in Crohn's disease is associated with colonic involvement, disease duration longer than 10 years and the presence of strictures, fistulae, and bypassed loops of bowel.[24] Cancer is preceded by low- and high-grade dysplasia in a manner similar to that for ulcerative colitis. Surveillance for Crohn's disease has been suggested, but is not widely practiced at the present time.

INDETERMINATE COLITIS

Indeterminate colitis is a diagnosis that was originally applied when the resected colon has overlapping pathologic features of ulcerative colitis and Crohn's disease.[28] Some of these features represent a failure to recognize a given pathologic abnormality accurately. The following problematic pathologic changes are worthy of review:

1. The presence of inflammation extending into the muscularis externa in ulcerative colitis does not represent transmural inflammation if it is localized to areas of deep ulceration that may be seen in severe cases.
2. Granulomas occurring in ulcerative colitis are of two types: (a) Ill-defined histiocyte collections in the mucosa formed in response to mucin extravasation from a disrupted crypt. (b) Deeper foreign body-type granulomas associated with fulminant colitis. Well-formed epithelioid cells granulomas do not occur in ulcerative colitis; in the setting of idiopathic inflammatory bowel disease, their presence indicates Crohn's colitis.
3. Diffuse wall inflammation and fissure ulcers occur in fulminant ulcerative colitis; their presence does not indicate indeterminate colitis.
4. Rectal sparing and skip lesions that are defined by macroscopic or endoscopic examination may result in a false impression of Crohn's colitis. In many of these cases, microscopic involvement is present in these areas when the diagnosis is ulcerative colitis.
5. Wall thickening may be associated with inflamed diverticula in cases of ulcerative colitis coexisting with diverticular disease. This may mimic Crohn's disease. Diverticular disease-associated chronic colitis[29] is a specific entity in which changes similar to those of ulcerative colitis are restricted to the segment with diverticulosis (see Chapter 10).

In most cases, careful study of the resected specimen permits classification as Crohn's disease or ulcerative colitis. In our experience, the diagnosis of indeterminate colitis is rare, with a prevalence much lower than the 15% of cases of IIBD quoted in the literature. The majority of cases diagnosed as indeterminate colitis commonly become reclassified as ulcerative colitis at a later examination; reclassification as Crohn's disease is less common.[30,31]

PATHOLOGIC DIAGNOSTIC PROBLEMS IN IIBD

Initial Presentation to a Gastroenterologist

Histologic examination of endoscopic biopsy samples is the best method for establishing the diagnosis of IIBD in a patient with symptoms of colitis. Features in the biopsy specimen permit accurate differentiation of acute self-limited colitis from IIBD in the majority of cases[32] (also see Chapter 10).

When a diagnosis of IIBD has been made on a biopsy specimen, every attempt must be made to characterize the patient as having ulcerative colitis or Crohn's disease. This requires clinical, radiologic, and endoscopic findings as well as the features observed in colonic specimens from multiple sites. Features helpful in this differential diagnosis are listed in Table 11–3.

If the clinical information about a patient is inadequate or multiple, labeled specimens are not supplied, the pathologist will have serious difficulty differentiating ulcerative colitis from Crohn's colitis. The biopsy sample features that distinguish ul-

TABLE 11–3. DIFFERENTIAL DIAGNOSIS OF ULCERATIVE COLITIS AND CROHN'S DISEASE

	Ulcerative colitis	Crohn's disease
Clinical and Laboratory		
Perianal disease	Rare	75%
Aphthous stomatitis	No	Common
Smoking history	No	Yes
Serum ANCA	75%	Rare
Radiology		
Proximal small-bowel disease	No	Yes
Terminal ileal disease	15%, mild	Common, narrowing +
Colonic wall thickening	No	Yes
Fistulae	No	Yes
Endoscopy		
Rectal sparing	10%	50%
Skip areas	No	Yes
Mucosal involvement	Diffuse	Patchy
Granularity, friability	Yes	Rare
Aphthous ulcers	Rare	Yes
Longitudinal ulcers	Rare	Yes
Cobblestone appearance	No	Yes
Biopsy		
Epithelioid granulomas	No	Yes (10%)
Focal mucosal involvement	No	Yes

Abbreviations: ANCA = Anti-neutrophil cytoplasmic autoantibody

cerative colitis from Crohn's disease (epithelioid granulomas and focal active colitis) are not present in most cases, particularly when only a few specimens have been submitted. The presence of submucosal inflammation, which is said to be a biopsy criterion for diagnosing Crohn's disease, is unreliable in small endoscopic biopsy samples.

When lack of communication precludes the pathologist from differentiating between ulcerative colitis and Crohn's disease, the pathologic diagnosis is commonly IIBD. In such cases, it is imperative that the gastroenterologist makes the differential diagnosis between ulcerative colitis and Crohn's disease, using the clinical information available.

It is also important to recognize that a diagnosis of IIBD should not be made without histologic confirmation. Even when clinical and endoscopic features are highly suggestive of IIBD, specific treatment should not be undertaken for IIBD if the biopsy sample is not diagnostic for IIBD. Unfortunately, this rule is frequently broken by gastroenterologists. What then happens is that a patient carries a clinical, non-biopsy-proven diagnosis of ulcerative colitis or Crohn's disease for life. After symptoms have subsided with treatment, this patient is deemed to have all the risks of future disease and malignancy associated with IIBD.

Treatment for ulcerative colitis causes reversal of histologic features. The acute inflammation and erosions subside quickly. Chronic inflammation decreases, but commonly remains slightly increased and associated with mild lamina propria fibrosis even in patients who are in clinical remission. In particular, the crypt base remains separated from the muscularis mucosae by fibrosis and mild chronic inflammation. Crypt distortion also decreases, but mild abnormalities frequently remain (see Figs. 11–9B and C and 11–17). In cases of mild disease, almost complete return to normal may occur (Fig. 11–62).

Interpretation of biopsy samples from a patient in remission with or without treatment is best done by comparing the present specimen with the previous ones on which the diagnosis of IIBD was made. This permits accurate conclusions regarding reversal of pathologic changes. When posttreatment biopsy specimens are received on patients with "a clinical history of ulcerative colitis" for whom no prior diagnostic samples exist, biopsy interpretation is difficult. When the samples show no diagnostic criteria for IIBD, there is no way of knowing whether these patients have had ulcerative colitis in the past with complete histologic reversal or they never had the disease.

Examination of temporally sequential specimens is important in patients with IIBD because in approximately 10% of cases the diagnosis changes from ulcerative colitis to Crohn's disease and vice versa.[31] The change from ulcerative colitis to Crohn's disease is more common and is easy to understand. If, for example, a patient with ulcerative colitis develops an ileal lesion, it is likely that the diagnosis will change to Crohn's disease, as would the finding of an epithelioid granuloma in a subsequent biopsy of a patient with ulcerative colitis.

Presentation at Surgery with Complicated IIBD

The pathologist is frequently asked to provide intraoperative assistance when a patient without a prior diagnosis of IIBD has presented with a complication that required urgent surgery. Two situations are encountered within this category:

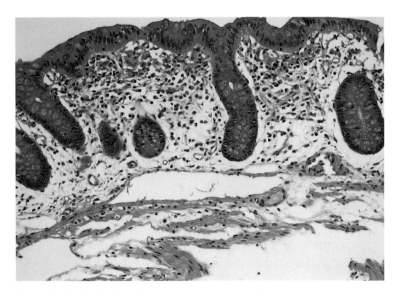

Figure 11–62. Inactive idiopathic inflammatory bowel disease. The crypts are separated by edema, suggesting atrophy, but have a normal architecture. The number of chronic inflammatory cells is within normal limits and no ulceration or acute inflammation are evident. This patient gave a 16-year history of ulcerative colitis with severe histologic abnormalities during relapses.

1. Patients presenting with small-bowel obstruction secondary to Crohn's disease: Small-bowel narrowing in Crohn's disease is commonly associated with palpable thickening of the bowel and the presence of creeping fat from the mesentery, which envelops the involved bowel (or fat wrapping). Creeping fat is highly specific for Crohn's disease (see Figs. 11–52 and 11–53).[33] Creeping fat correlates with transmural involvement, and for this reason, surgeons use its presence, along with palpable wall thickening, to determine the limit of resection. The aim of surgical resection in Crohn's disease is to remove gross disease and make an anastomosis at grossly normal bowel. Unfortunately, the presence of creeping fat frequently underestimates the extent of gross mucosal ulcerative disease. Opening the specimen during surgery is imperative to ensure clear gross margins. The use of intraoperative endoscopy has been shown to increase the precision of surgical excision in these cases.[34] It should also be recognized that microscopic involvement of margins does not have any value in predicting recurrence; frozen sections of margins are therefore not indicated in Crohn's disease resections.

2. In patients with fulminant colitis and toxic megacolon (see Figs. 11–20 and 11–21), colon resection is urgently undertaken. There is usually no need for an immediate intraoperative diagnosis in these cases. Many cases of toxic megacolon have so many secondary changes in the wall consequent to dilatation and ischemia that it is difficult to evaluate diagnostic criteria with accuracy. In many cases, the most appropriate diagnosis for these cases is "fulminant colitis or toxic megacolon of undetermined etiology."

At Elective Proctocolectomy for Ulcerative Colitis

Patients with a preoperative diagnosis of chronic ulcerative colitis may have a total proctocolectomy for many reasons. Intraoperatively, three questions may face the pathologist:

1. Is there cancer? This question arises when the indication for surgery is a prior diagnosis of high-grade dysplasia or carcinoma. Carcinomas are usually obvious, but in cases of a flat infiltrative tumor, close mucosal examination and careful palpation of the wall for infiltration may be necessary. This question need not be answered at the time of surgery unless the tumor is close to a surgical margin.

2. Is the rectum completely removed? Mucosal proctectomy, when performed, involves removing the rectal mucosa in one piece in the plane of the submucosa (Fig. 11–63). Totality of removal requires that the distal margin be composed of squamous or transitional epithelium of the anal canal and that the specimen be intact. When tears or holes are present in the rectal specimen, the pathologist cannot guarantee that small islands of rectal mucosa have not been left behind. This is not a common problem for the pathologist to encounter.

3. Is the diagnosis of ulcerative colitis confirmed? This is a very relevant question because proctocolectomy is generally followed by creation of an ileal pouch/anal anastomosis. The

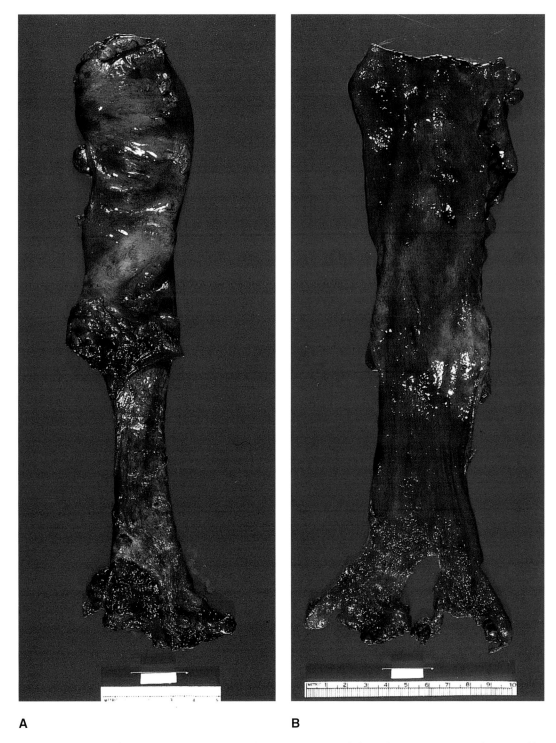

A   B

Figure 11–63. A: Specimen from a colectomy with rectal mucosal resection in a patient with chronic ulcerative colitis. B: Mucosal resection of the rectum in ulcerative colitis, showing difficulty in assessing completeness of the mucosal removal, particularly at the distal end where a mucosal defect is evident.

rate of complications is greater if the pouch is created to treat Crohn's disease rather than ulcerative colitis. To answer this question with certainty intraoperatively is impossible because examination of the permanent sections the next day may show some manifestation of Crohn's disease, such as a granuloma. A reasonable approach, however, is to carefully examine the colon for any evidence of Crohn's disease, such as wall thickening, and to take two or three random frozen sections in a search for granulomas. In the absence of gross evidence of Crohn's disease, and absent granulomas in the frozen sections, a diagnosis of ulcerative colitis is made, usually with a word of caution to the surgeon about lack of certainty. This method permits the surgeon to progress with the ileal pouch/anal anastomosis. In large series, ileal pouch/anal anastomoses are sometimes created in patients who actually have Crohn's disease rather than ulcerative colitis. Some of these patients have no pouch dysfunction; others need removal and revision.[35] Approximately 30% of patients with ulcerative colitis develop pouchitis[36]; this condition, which may resemble Crohn's disease, is discussed in Chapter 10.

References

1. Singleton JW. Clinical features, course, and laboratory findings in ulcerative colitis. *In* Kirsner JB, Shorter RG (eds.): *Inflammatory Bowel Disease,* 4th ed. Baltimore, Williams & Wilkins, 1995. pp. 335–343.

2. Edwards EC, Truelove SC. The course and prognosis of ulcerative colitis. *Gut.* 1963;4:299–312.

3. Riddell RH. Pathology of idiopathic inflammatory bowel disease. *In* Kirsner JB, Shorter RG (eds.): *Inflammatory Bowel Disease,* 4th ed. Baltimore, Williams & Wilkins, 1995. pp. 517–552.

4. Bolton RP, Sheriff RJ, Read AD. *Clostridium difficile* associated diarrhoea: A role in inflammatory bowel disease. *Lancet.* 1980; 1:383–384.

5. Newman A, Lambert JR. *Campylobacter jejuni* causing flare-up in inflammatory bowel disease. *Lancet.* 1980;2:919.

6. Dronfield MW, Fletcher J, Langman MJS. Coincident *Salmonella* infections and ulcerative colitis: Problems of recognition and management. *Br Med J.* 1974;1:99–100.

7. Gumaste V, Sachar DB, Greenstein AJ. Benign and malignant strictures in ulcerative colitis. *Gut.* 1992;33:938–941.

8. Reiser JR, Waye JD, Janowitz HD, et al. Adenocarcinoma in strictures of ulcerative colitis without antecedent dysplasia by colonoscopy. *Am J Gastroenterol.* 1994;89:119–122.

9. Retsky JE, Kraft SC. The extraintestinal manifestations of inflammatory bowel disease. *In* Kirsner JB, Shorter RG (eds.): *Inflammatory Bowel Disease,* 4th ed. Baltimore, Williams & Wilkins, 1995. pp. 474–491.

10. Dejaco C, Fertl E, Prayer D, et al. Symptomatic cerebral microangiopathy preceding initial manifestation of ulcerative colitis. *Dig Dis Sci.* 1996;41:1807–1810.

11. Kelly JK, Langevin JM, Price LM et al. Giant and symptomatic inflammatory polyps of the colon in idiopathic inflammatory bowel disease. *Am J Surg Pathol.* 1986;10: 420–428.

12. Blackstone MO, Riddell RH, Rogers BHG, et al. Dysplasia associated lesion or mass (DALM) detected by colonoscopy in long-standing ulcerative colitis: An indication for colectomy. *Gastroenterology.* 1981;80:366–374.

13. Kewenter J, Ahlman H, Hulten L. Cancer risk in extensive ulcerative colitis. *Ann Surg.* 1978;188:824–828.

14. Burmer GC, Rabinovitch PS, Haggitt RC. Neoplastic progression in ulcerative colitis: Histology, DNA content and loss of a *p53* allele. *Gastroenterology.* 1992;103:1602–1610.

15. Befrits R, Hammarberg C, Rubio C, et al. DNA aneuploidy and histologic dysplasia in long-standing ulcerative colitis. A 10 year follow up study. *Dis Colon Rectum.* 1994;37: 313–319.

16. Hughes RG, Hall TJ, Block GE, et al. The prognosis of carcinoma of the colon and rectum in complicating ulcerative colitis. *Surg Gynecol Obstet.* 1978:146:46–48.

17. Lynch DAF, Lobo AJ, Sobala GM, et al. Failure of colonoscopic surveillance in ulcerative colitis. *Gut.* 1993;34:1075–1080.

18. Kulaylat MN, Doerr R, Butler B, et al. Squamous cell carcinoma complicating idiopathic inflammatory bowel disease. *J Surg Oncol.* 1995;59:48–55.

19. Yaziji H, Broghamer WL, Jr. Primary small cell undifferentiated carcinoma of the rectum associated with ulcerative colitis. *South Med J.* 1996;89:921–924.

20. Ransohoff D, Riddell RH, Levin B. Ulcerative colitis and colonic cancer: Problems in assessing the diagnostic usefulness of mucosal dysplasia. *Dis Colon Rectum.* 1985;28: 383–388.

21. Riddell RH, Goldman H, Ranschoff DF, et al. Dysplasia in inflammatory bowel disease: Standardized classification with provisional clinical applications. *Hum Pathol.* 1983;14:931–966.

22. Bernstein CN, Weinstein WM, Levine DS, et al. Physician's perceptions of dysplasia and approaches to surveillance colonscopy in ulcerative colitis. *Am J Gastroenterol.* 1995;90:2106–2114.

23. Rozen P, Baratz M, Fefer F, et al. Low incidence of significant dysplasia in a successful endoscopic surveillance program of patients with ulcerative colitis. *Gastroenterology.* 1995;108:1361–1370.

24. Levin B. Gastrointestinal neoplasia in inflammatory bowel disease. *In* Kirsner JB, Shorter RG (eds.): *Inflammatory Bowel Disease,* 4th ed. Baltimore, Williams & Wilkins, 1995. pp. 461–473.

25. Owen RL. And now pathophysiology of M cells—good news and bad news from Peyer's patches. *Gastroenterology.* 1983;85: 468–470.

26. Lashner BA. Clinical features, laboratory findings, and course of Crohn's disease. *In* Kirsner JB, Shorter RG (eds.): *Inflammatory Bowel Disease,* 4th ed. Baltimore, Williams & Wilkins, 1995. pp. 344–354.

27. Choi PM, Zelig MP. Surveillance of colorectal cancer in Crohn's disease and ulcerative colitis. *Gastroenterology.* 1993;104:A628.

28. Price AB. Overlap in the spectrum of nonspecific inflammatory bowel disease—"colitis indeterminate." *J Clin Pathol.* 1978;31: 567–577.

29. Makapugay LM, Dean PJ. Diverticular disease-associated chronic colitis. *Am J Surg Pathol.* 1996;20:94–102.

30. Wells AD, McMillan I, Price AB et al. Natural history of indeterminate colitis. *Br J Surg.* 1991;78:179–181.

31. Moum B, Ekbom A, Vatn MH, et al. Inflammatory bowel disease: Reevaluation of the diagnosis in a prospective population based study in south eastern Norway. *Gut.* 1997;40:328–332.

32. Surawicz CM, Haggitt RC, Husseman M, et al. Mucosal biopsy diagnosis of colitis: Acute self-limited colitis and idiopathic inflammatory bowel disease. *Gastroenterology.* 1994;107:755–763.

33. Kotanagi H, Kramer K, Fazio UM et al. Do microscopic abnormalities at resection margins correlate with increased anastomotic recurrence in Crohn's disease? Retrospective analysis of 100 cases. *Dis Colon Rectum.* 1991;34:909–916.

34. Sheehan AL, Warren BF, Gear MW, et al. Fat-wrapping in Crohn's disease: Pathological basis and relevance to surgical practice. *Br J Surg.* 1992;79:955–958.

35. Deutsch AA, McLeod RS, Cullen J, et al. Results of the pelvic-pouch procedure in patients with Crohn's disease. *Dis Colon Rectum.* 1991;34:475–477.

36. Lohmuller JL, Pemberton JH, Dozois RR, et al. Pouchitis and extraintestinal manifestations of inflammatory bowel disease after ileal pouch-anal anastomosis. *Ann Surg.* 1990;211:622–627.

12

COLORECTAL POLYPS AND POLYPOSIS SYNDROMES

Yanling Ma and Parakrama Chandrasoma

▶ CHAPTER OUTLINE

COLORECTAL POLYPS

Colorectal polyps are among the commonest lesions encountered by the surgical pathologist. The reason for this, apart from the fact that they are very common lesions, is that colonoscopy and flexible sigmoidoscopy are recommended for all people over the age of 40 years in the United States as a population screening method for colorectal carcinoma. A polyp is any projection above the surface of the mucosa. Most colorectal polyps occur as isolated lesions in an otherwise normal colorectal mucosa. Polyps may also occur in the setting of diffuse inflammatory diseases of the colon. When the pathologist encounters a specimen submitted as a polyp, it is important to know whether the lesion is an isolated one or one associated with inflammatory bowel disease, because pathologic interpretation can be different.

Polyps result from many pathologic processes (Table 12–1). Over 90% of polyps encountered in colonoscopic specimens are tubular adenomas and hyperplastic polyps. Multiple polyps are common, particularly in older people. Most small polyps are asymptomatic. Larger polyps may develop surface erosions that result in bleeding. The bleeding is commonly occult, but may rarely be symptomatic.

TABLE 12–1. PATHOLOGIC TYPES OF COLONIC POLYPS

Common
  1. Adenoma
  2. Hyperplastic polyp
  3. Mixed adenomatous-hyperplastic polyp (ie, serrated adenoma)
  4. Retention polyp (juvenile retention polyp)
Uncommon
  5. Carcinoid tumor (Chapter 13)
  6. Mesenchymal neoplasms—lipoma, GI stromal neoplasm, neurofibroma (Chapter 14)
  7. Inflammatory pseudo-polyps in idiopathic inflammatory bowel disease, including giant inflammatory polyps (Chapter 11)
  8. Colitis cystica profunda and solitary rectal ulcer syndrome (Chapter 10)
  9. Lymphoid polyps (Chapter 15)
  10. Pneumatosis intestinalis (Chapter 8)
Very Rare
  11. Malakoplakia
  12. Gastric heterotopia

Note: Polyps 1–4, 11, and 12 are discussed in this chapter; 5–10 are considered in the designated chapters.

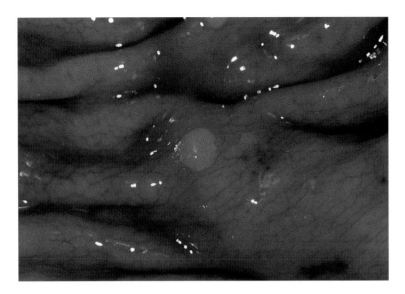

Figure 12–1. Colonic mucosa showing a diminutive polyp, appearing as a small, rounded sessile elevation.

Endoscopic Findings

At endoscopy, polyps are characterized by location and size, as well as whether they are sessile or pedunculated. No endoscopic features, however, can be relied on, especially in small polyps, to distinguish adenomas from nonneoplastic polyps.[1]

Diminutive Polyps

Diminutive polyps are the earliest stage of evolution of all polyps; they are less than 5 mm in size and sessile (Fig. 12–1). Their small size permits the endoscopist to remove them completely with biopsy forceps, despite their being sessile. The pathologic specimen that results from a diminutive polyp contains multiple tissue fragments with the central lesion and surrounding normal colorectal mucosa. Endoscopic removal of diminutive polyps is safe; the only complication is significant hemorrhage, which occurs in less than 1% of cases and only when hot biopsy is used.[2]

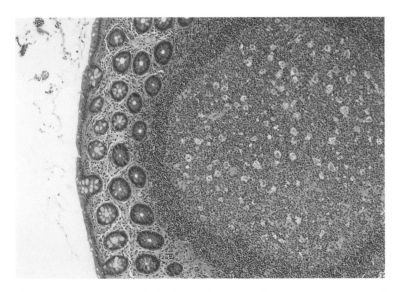

Figure 12–2. Hyperplastic lymphoid nodule in colonic mucosa. This is a common cause of a small sessile diminutive polyp.

Thirty percent to 60% of diminutive polyps are tubular or tubulovillous adenomas,[2–4] another 30–40% are hyperplastic polyps. The remainder are mucosal tags and lymphoid aggregates (Fig. 12–2), with other polyp types such as malakoplakia[5] (Fig. 12–3), heterotopic gastric mucosa[6] (Fig. 12–4), colitis cystica profunda (Chapter 10), and pneumatosis intestinalis (Fig. 12–5; also see Chapter 8) being rare.[2] The chance that a diminutive polyp is a villous adenoma is less than 1%. The chance of finding severe dysplasia or cancer in a diminutive polyp is generally considered to be under 1%, although a recent study reported a 2.4% occurrence of invasive carcinoma in flat adenomas smaller than 6 mm in diameter.[7]

The rate of growth of diminutive polyps is variable. A study that followed diminutive polyps over a 2-year period showed that

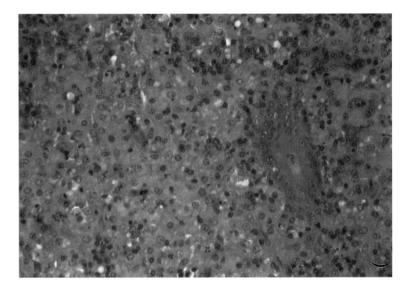

A

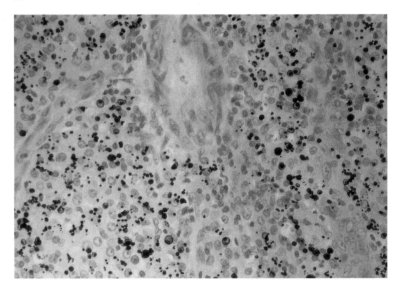

B

Figure 12–3. A: Malakoplakia of the colonic mucosa, showing a crypt surrounded by a diffuse collection of histiocytic cells with abundant cytoplasm that contains numerous, rounded, pale blue cytoplasmic Michaelis-Gutmann bodies. Some of these are as large as a nucleus and some have a typical targetoid appearance, resembling a nucleus with a nucleolus. B: Malakoplakia, von Kossa's stain, showing the typical appearance of Michaelis-Gutmann bodies, some of which have a targetoid appearance.

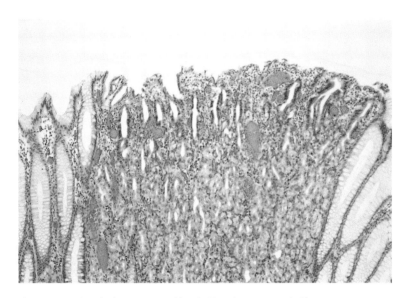

Figure 12–4. Rectal polyp in a 4-year-old male. The polyp is composed of heterotopic gastric mucosa, consisting of gastric glands with parietal cells in rectal mucosa.

over 90% remained the same size.[8] On the other hand, another study showed growth rates of 2–4 mm/y in some tubular adenomas, with no evidence of regression in any diminutive polyp.[9]

Their high frequency and very low risk of malignancy has led to debate over: (1) whether it is necessary to remove all diminutive polyps that are found at endoscopy,[8] and (2) whether it is adequate to simply fulgurate diminutive polyps without submitting them for pathologic examination.[4] Neither of these choices is recommended. If fulguration is entertained, it should be limited to patients in whom a plan of surveillance has already been established by finding prior histologically documented adenomas.[4]

Pedunculated Polyps

Pedunculated polyps are suspended from the mucosal surface by a stalk whose circumference is small enough to permit polypectomy by snaring the stalk at endoscopy. The length of the stalk varies; pedunculated polyps are sometimes classified

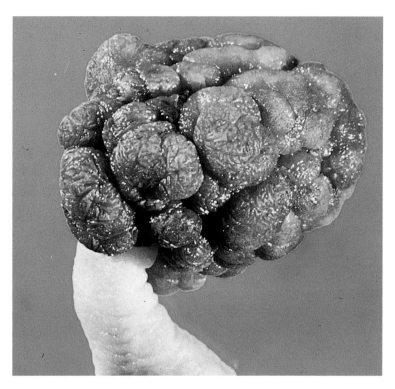

Figure 12–6. Pedunculated colonic polyp with a long stalk. Note the relatively normal colonic mucosa lining the stalk, with gross abnormality beginning at the point at which the head of the stalk begins.

into long- and short-stalked polyps based on whether the length of the stalk is more or less than 2 cm (Figs. 12–6 and 12–7). Pedunculated polyps are received complete by the pathologist with the rounded head of the polyp at one end and the cauterized stalk base at the other end.

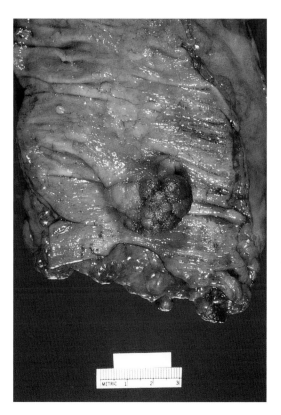

Figure 12–7. Pedunculated polyp with a short stalk in colon resected for adenocarcinoma elsewhere in the colon.

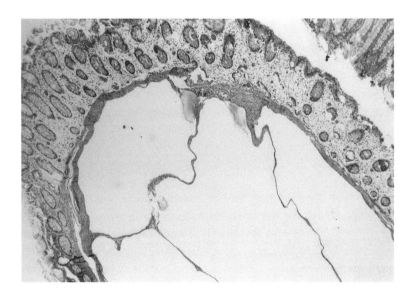

Figure 12–5. Polypoid mucosa in pneumatosis intestinalis, showing gas spaces in the submucosa.

As polyps increase in size, the probability that they are adenomas increases, as well as the probability that they have a villous component. Adenomas and serrated adenomas account for more than 95% of polyps larger than 1 cm. Rarely, larger polyps are hyperplastic polyps, mesenchymal neoplasms (lipomas, stromal tumors), or carcinoid tumors.

Large Sessile Polyps

Large sessile polyps have mucosal attachment or a base that is too wide for polypectomy by snaring (Figs. 12–8 and 12–9). Unlike a diminutive polyp, large sessile polyps are too large for

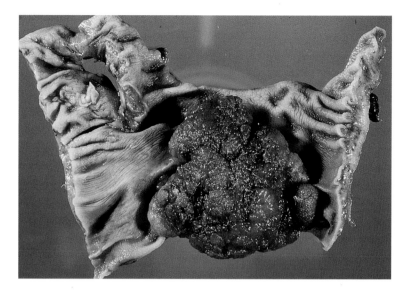

Figure 12–9. Large sessile polyp of the colon with a more papilliform surface. This was a benign villous adenoma.

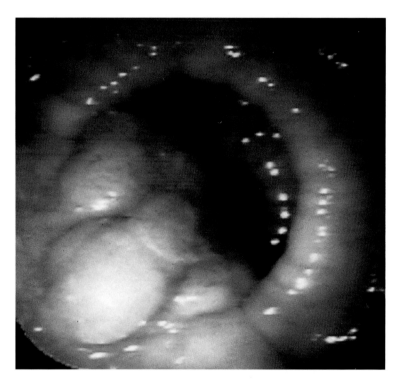

A

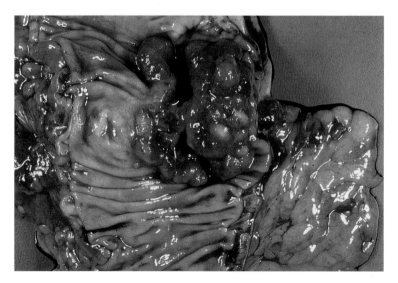

B

Figure 12–8. A: Large, sessile colonic polyp at endoscopy. B: Large, sessile polyp of the colon with a smooth surface. On microscopy, this was a benign tubulovillous adenoma. (Part A: Courtesy of Aslam Godil, MD, Dept. of Gastroenterology, Loma Linda University, CA).

complete removal at endoscopy. The pathologic specimen from large sessile polyps encountered at endoscopy consists of multiple tissue fragments from the lesion, usually with no surrounding normal mucosa. Unlike in diminutive polyps and pedunculated polyps, the objective of the endoscopist in examining large sessile lesions is to establish an accurate pathologic diagnosis by adequate biopsy rather than complete excision. Over 95% of clinically encountered large sessile polyps are adenomas or serrated adenomas. Giant inflammatory polyps in idiopathic inflammatory bowel disease (see Chapter 11), infectious processes such as tuberculosis (see Chapter 8), and the polypoid phase of solitary rectal ulcer syndrome (see Chapter 10) can produce large sessile polyps that are nonneoplastic.

Colorectal Polyps of Epithelial Origin

Hyperplastic Polyp

Hyperplastic polyps commonly present as sessile polyps that are less than 1 cm in size (Fig. 12–10A). More rarely, they may be pedunculated or large sessile polyps. An increased incidence of hyperplastic polyps is associated with intake of more than 30 g alcohol per day, cigarette smoking, and increased intake of animal fat.[10] Hyperplastic polyps are not associated with any risk of malignant transformation. In any given patient, however, hyperplastic polyps frequently coexist with adenomas and, rarely, adenocarcinoma. This association with neoplastic polyps may be increased when multiple, large (over 1 cm), hyperplastic polyps are present.[11]

Hyperplastic polyps are the result of increased cell proliferation in the cells at the crypt base, which often show nuclear enlargement. The crypts increase in length, and the lining cells toward the surface become enlarged due to cytoplasmic distension with mucin. The nuclei in the superficial cells remain basal without enlargement or hyperchromasia. The crypt lumen typically becomes dilated and serrated toward the surface (Fig. 12–10B).

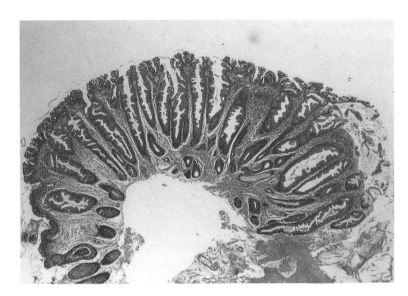

A

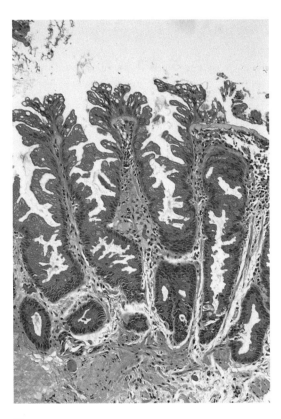

B

Figure 12–10. A: Sessile hyperplastic polyp of the colon. B: Hyperplastic polyp of the colon, showing the serrated lumina of the superficial part of the crypt lined by mucin-distended cells with normal nuclei. The cells at the crypt bases show proliferative features with larger nuclei and dense cytoplasm without vacuolated mucin.

In properly oriented sections, the diagnosis is easy. In tangentially cut sections, hyperplastic polyps can mimic adenomas, particularly if the section is horizontal across the active crypt base region (Fig. 12–11). Doubt can be resolved by examining the surface cells, which show hyperplastic change. This is the reverse of adenomas, in which adenomatous change tends to occur first in the cells near the surface.

Large hyperplastic polyps should be thoroughly sampled

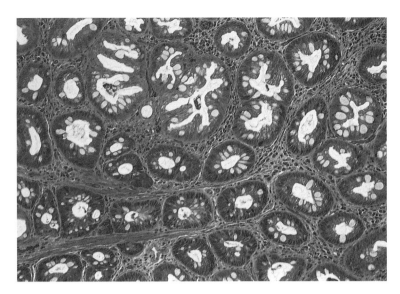

Figure 12–11. Hyperplastic polyp of the colon, horizontally cut. Part of the polyp shows the typical serrated lumina and mucin-distended lining cells from the superficial crypt. Part shows the more proliferative crypt base in cross section, which resembles adenomatous change.

and carefully examined for evidence of focal adenomatous change (serrated adenoma). Hyperplastic polyps sometimes show evidence of acute and chronic inflammation and, rarely, surface erosion. In the latter event, they may resemble inflammatory pseudo-polyps associated with idiopathic inflammatory bowel disease, and in order to make the correct diagnosis it is important to know that the lesion was an isolated finding in otherwise normal colorectal mucosa. Also, ulcerated hyperplastic polyps show reactive epithelial changes (Fig. 12–12); these must not be mistaken for adenomatous change, which may result in a misdiagnosis as mixed hyperplastic adenomatous polyp.

Juvenile Polyp

Colorectal juvenile polyps (or juvenile retention polyps; hamartomatous polyps) occur predominantly in children and adoles-

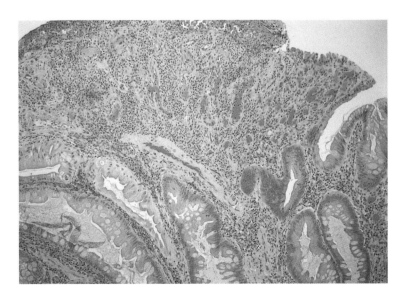

Figure 12–12. Hyperplastic polyps with surface erosion, granulation tissue, and reactive change in crypts at ulcer base.

cents. Rare cases occur in older persons. Juvenile polyps account for 85% of colorectal polyps in children and are the most common cause of rectal bleeding in children.[12] They are common lesions, found in approximately 1% of children. Most patients have a solitary polyp and over 80% of polyps are located in the rectosigmoid colon. Rarely, juvenile retention polyps occurring more proximally form the apex of an intussusception. Multiple juvenile polyps exceeding 10 in number indicate juvenile polyposis.

Juvenile polyps are small, sessile or larger, pedunculated polyps that can be removed at colonoscopy. They are characterized histologically by disorganized crypts that are distended by retained intraluminal mucin to form microcystic structures (Fig. 12–13A and B). Surface erosion and acute inflammation are common and responsible for hemorrhage (Fig. 12–13C). The interior of the polyp contains chronic inflammatory cells, fibrosis, and irregular smooth muscle, which separate the dilated crypts. The crypts are lined by cytologically normal, somewhat flattened epithelial cells.

Solitary juvenile polyps occurring in children do not predispose to future development of new juvenile polyps and have no association with adenomas or colorectal cancer in either the patient or first-degree relatives.[13]

Inflammatory Myoglandular Polyp

Inflammatory myoglandular polyp is an uncommon polyp in the colon,[14] usually discovered during a screening examination. Less than half the patients present with rectal bleeding or occult blood positivity. At endoscopy, these are solitary polyps that occur usually in the left colon, most commonly in the sigmoid. A case has been reported in the terminal ileum, resulting in intussusception.[15] They are pedunculated, red in color, and have a smooth surface, but are generally indistinguishable from pedunculated tubular adenomas. They vary in size, and can exceed 2 cm; they frequently have a long stalk. Inflammatory myoglandular polyps are defined by their histology: they are characterized by hyperplastic distorted crypts with a tendency to

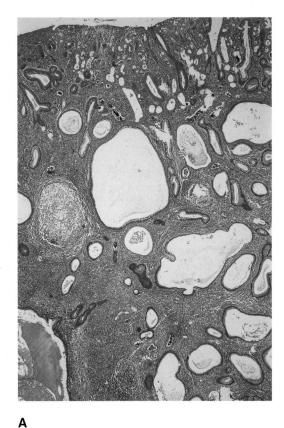

A

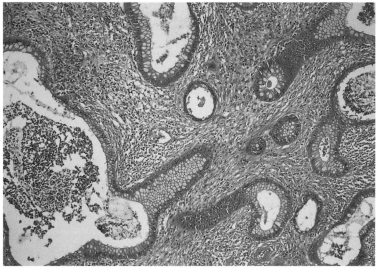

B

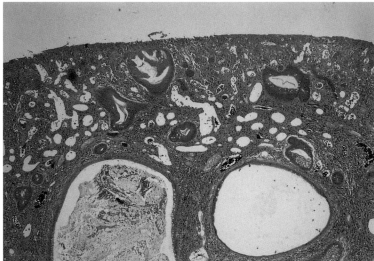

C

Figure 12–13. A: Juvenile polyp, showing the cystically dilated and distorted crypts filled with mucin, surrounded by fibrosis and inflammatory cells. B: Juvenile polyp, showing cystically dilated crypt lined by flattened epithelium without dysplasia. There is stromal fibrosis and acute inflammation. C: Surface erosion and inflammation in a juvenile polyp.

cystic dilatation, inflammatory granulation tissue in the lamina propria, and proliferation of smooth muscle. They are distinguished from juvenile polyps, inflammatory fibroid polyps, and hamartomas of Peutz-Jeghers syndrome by the presence of abundant smooth muscle cells. They are distinguished from polypoid variants of solitary rectal ulcer syndrome by their location. They have no malignant potential.

Colorectal Adenoma

Adenomas are the commonest pathologic type of colorectal polyp and are most important because they are the precursor lesion for colorectal adenocarcinoma. They occur with increasing frequency with increasing age, and in high-risk countries such as United States, 50–65% of people over age 65 have colorectal adenomas detected at autopsy.[16] Colorectal adenomas occur rarely in children without familial adenomatous polyposis.[17] Adenoma risk is associated with a diet rich in animal fat and low in fiber, high alcohol intake, and cigarette smoking.[4] The genetic changes associated with adenomas are considered in the adenoma–carcinoma sequence in Chapter 13.

When detected endoscopically, 26–29% of adenomas are smaller than 1 cm.[4] Large adenomas tend to occur in older patients and in the distal colon. Adenomas tend to be multiple (Fig. 12–14), particularly in older patients, 30–50% of whom have more than one adenoma.[4] Because multiple sporadic adenomas rarely exceed 20 in number and almost never exceed 50, they can be reliably differentiated from familial adenomatous polyposes, in which the number of adenomas almost always exceeds 100. Most adenomas are discovered during screenings using flexible sigmoidoscopy or colonoscopy. Some are associated with surface erosion and bleeding, either clinical or occult.

Adenomas are defined by the presence of adenomatous change, which is a cytologic change in the crypt epithelial cells that is equivalent to low-grade epithelial dysplasia (Fig. 12–15). The earliest adenoma is recognized as an aberrant crypt that has an elliptical opening and is lined by cells showing adenomatous change. Adenomatous change usually occurs first in the most superficial region of the crypt nearest to the surface (Fig. 12–16). The affected cells have an increased rate of proliferation and are characterized by stratification within the affected crypt, increased nuclear size, and depletion of cytoplasmic mucin. The enlarged nuclei are ovoid and show hyperchromasia and increased mitotic activity. The affected crypts are initially simple with round lumina, and the nuclei of the lining cells show normal polarity where the long axis of the ovoid nucleus is perpendicular to the basement membrane of the crypt (see Fig. 12–15).

Adenomas have two architectural patterns: tubular and villous. In the tubular architecture, the adenomatous crypts resemble normal crypts, extending downward from the surface epithelium, forming tubular structures that appear rounded when sectioned horizontally (Fig. 12–17). In the villous architecture, the adenomatous epithelium lines finger-like villi that appear to project up from the surface epithelium and have a fibrovascular core (Fig. 12–18). Based on the amount of the two patterns, colonic adenomas are classified as tubular (<25% vil-

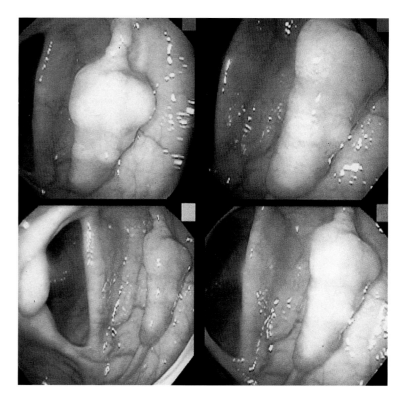

A

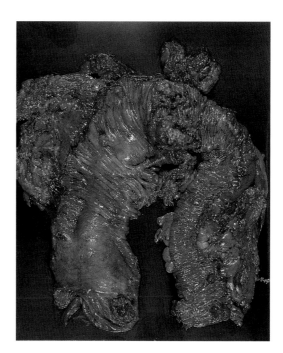

B

Figure 12–14. A: Multiple polyps at colonoscopy. B: Specimen of a colectomy for a large, fungating adenocarcinoma of the transverse colon, showing six other polyps (all adenomas by microscopy) distributed throughout the colon.

lous pattern), tubulovillous (Fig. 12–19) (25–75% villous pattern), and villous (>75% villous pattern). By these criteria, 80–87% of colonic adenomas are tubular, 8–16% are tubulovillous, and 3–6% are villous.[18] A villous architecture tends to be found more frequently in larger adenomas and is associated with a higher risk of malignancy.

The growth rate of colorectal adenomas and the risk and

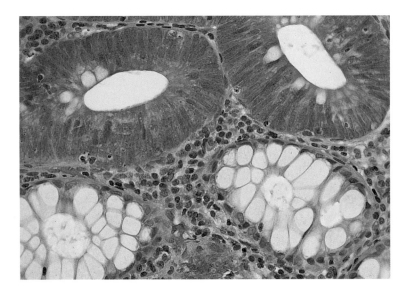

Figure 12–15. Adenomatous change in colonic crypts showing the cytologic change that defines adenoma (ie, low-grade dysplasia) compared with normal colonic mucosa. The adenomatous crypt shows cell stratification, mucin depletion in cytoplasm, and enlarged hyperchromatic nuclei. The nuclear polarity is normal, with the longitudinal axes of the cigar-shaped nuclei being arranged perpendicular to the basement membrane.

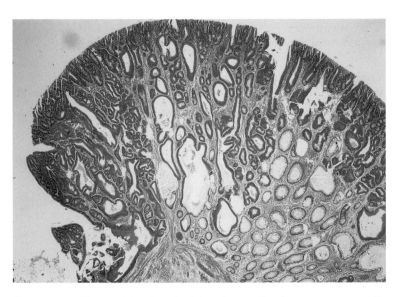

Figure 12–17. Adenoma of the colon with tubular architecture. The adenomatous crypts resemble normal colonic crypts, except for their larger size, distortion, and adenomatous change.

interval of malignant transformation vary widely. Over 90% of diminutive adenomas show no significant change over several years[8]; the minority grow 2–4 mm/y.[9] The cumulative risk for cancer in an adenoma smaller than 1 cm has been calculated as 2.5% at 5 years, 8% at 10 years, and 24% at 20 years.[19]

The likelihood of invasive carcinoma in an adenoma is greatest with larger (more than 2 cm) polyps, when a villous component or high-grade dysplasia is present on histologic examination.[4,18] Invasive carcinoma is preceded by high-grade dysplasia (ie, severe dysplasia and carcinoma in situ). High-

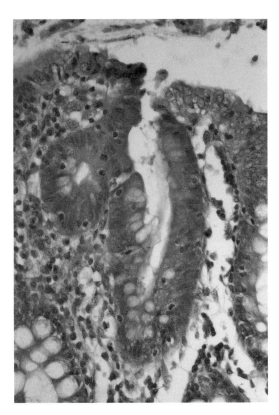

Figure 12–16. Dysplastic crypt focus. This is characterized by adenomatous change in a single crypt at the point of its opening. This is the earliest change in the adenoma–carcinoma sequence. This section is from a colon removed for familial adenomatous polyposis which is the type of specimen that commonly shows this change.

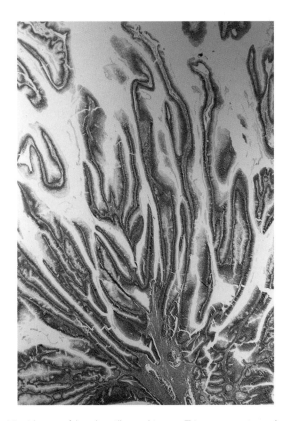

Figure 12–18. Adenoma of the colon, villous architecture. This was an area in a pedunculated adenoma that had admixed tubular elements exceeding 25% of the polyp (tubulovillous adenoma).

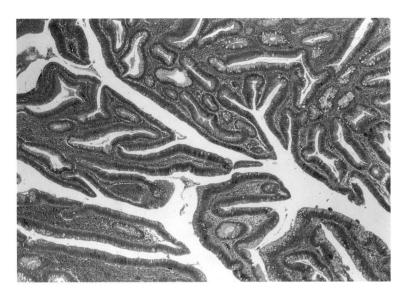

Figure 12–19. Adenoma of the colon, mixed tubular and villous pattern. The diagnosis of tubulovillous adenoma can be made when the villous component in the entire polyp is 25–75% of the volume of the lesion. Tubulovillous adenomas can occur as diminutive, pedunculated, and large sessile polyps.

grade dysplasia is characterized by the presence of severe cytologic abnormality of the adenomatous cells with nuclear irregularity, size variation, increased hyperchromasia with abnormal chromatin distribution, and atypical mitotic figures (Fig. 12–20A). Severe cytologic abnormality must be associated with either loss of nuclear polarity (Fig. 12–20B) or gland complexity to establish a diagnosis of high-grade dysplasia. Gland complexity is characterized by luminal bridging and cribriform change in the affected crypts (Fig. 12–20C). The next stage of malignancy in a polyp is invasion of the lamina propria by the carcinoma (Fig. 12–21). When invasion is restricted to the lamina propria without extension through the muscularis mucosae into the submucosa, a diagnosis of intramucosal carcinoma is made. In the colon and rectum, intramucosal carcinoma is not associated with any risk of metastasis; this is due to the absence of significant lymphatic channels in the colonic mucosa.

Metastatic risk, and therefore definitive carcinoma, occurs only when the carcinoma infiltrates into the submucosa through the muscularis mucosae. When this happens, the carci-

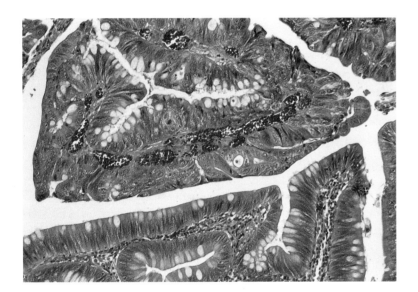

A

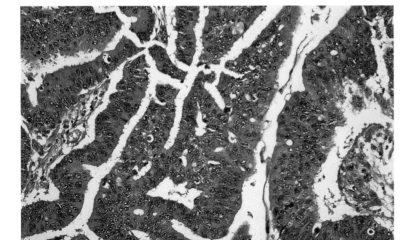

B

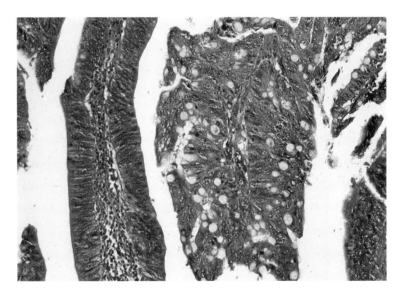

C

Figure 12–20. A: High-grade dysplasia in a villous adenoma, showing severe cytologic atypia of the lining cells associated with loss of nuclear polarity. The nuclei lining the crypt are rounded, and their long axes are no longer perpendicular to the basement membrane. Adenomatous villi without high-grade dysplasia are present at the bottom for comparison. B: High-grade dysplasia in a colonic adenoma, showing severe cytologic abnormality associated with early gland complexity, which is seen as the development of secondary lumina caused by epithelium bridging the lumen of the crypts. C: High-grade dysplasia in colonic adenoma, showing severe cytologic abnormality, loss of nuclear polarity, and complex glands with cribriform change.

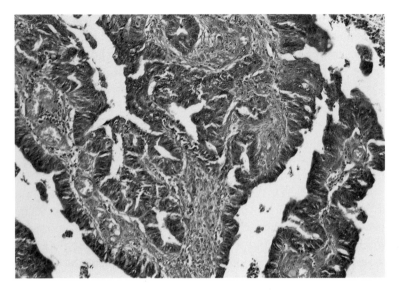

Figure 12–21. Intramucosal carcinoma in a colonic adenoma, showing infiltration of the lamina propria by glands showing features of high-grade dysplasia. The glands have an irregular outline. Intramucosal carcinoma has no metastatic potential, and its separation from high-grade dysplasia has no practical value.

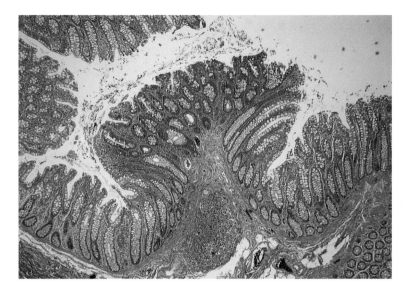

Figure 12–23. Diminutive tubular adenoma showing a raised lesion with surface adenomatous change and the beginning of stalk formation. This would appear endoscopically as a sessile lesion and be removed piecemeal.

noma has access to submucosal lymphatics, which represent the first route of metastasis in colorectal carcinoma.

Morphologic Types of Colorectal Adenoma

DIMINUTIVE ADENOMA. Colorectal adenomas may present as diminutive adenomas that are smaller than 5 mm (Figs. 12–22 and 12–23). The pathologic specimen from a diminutive adenoma consists of several pieces of tissue containing adenomatous epithelium and surrounding uninvolved colonic mucosa. Because the lesion is removed piecemeal, the pathologic examination cannot provide assessment of completeness of removal of the adenoma; this must be ensured by gross examination at the time of endoscopy.

Diminutive adenomas are almost always tubular; villous architecture is seen in less than 0.5% cases. Severe dysplasia or cancer is present less than 1% of the time.[7]

FLAT ADENOMA. Flat adenoma consists of a mucosal plaque smaller than 1 cm that frequently shows a central depression. The adenomatous epithelium is present on the surface over normal crypt bases, and the lesion thickness is less than twice the normal mucosal thickness[20] (Fig. 12–24). When first reported in

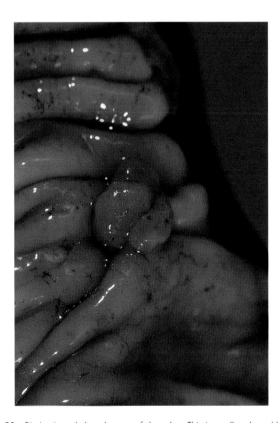

Figure 12–22. Diminutive tubular adenoma of the colon. This is small and would be removed piecemeal with the biopsy forceps.

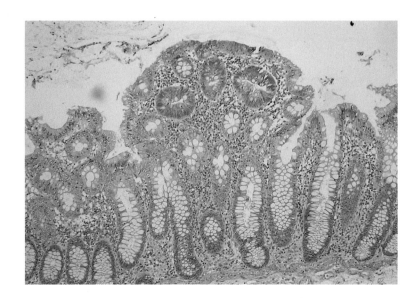

Figure 12–24. Flat adenoma of the colon. The mucosa is essentially flat, and the adenomatous change is restricted to the superficial part of the mucosa and is less than twice the mucosal thickness.

Europe, they were said to have a high-grade dysplasia rate of 42%; a higher 2.4% rate of invasive cancer has also been reported.[7] Questions have been raised regarding these rates of high-grade dysplasia and invasive cancer.[21] Flat adenomas are rarely reported as such in the United States; it is likely that they are included within the diagnosis of diminutive adenoma.

PEDUNCULATED ADENOMA. Most colorectal adenomas present as pedunculated polyps with a well-defined stalk of varying length at the top of which is the expanded rounded head of the polyp (Fig. 12–25). Eighty percent of pedunculated adenomas are tubular adenomas. Tubulovillous adenomas tend to be common among the larger polyps. A purely villous architecture is uncommon in pedunculated adenomas. The stalk of a pedunculated adenoma is usually lined at least partly by normal colorectal mucosa. Adenomatous change usually begins close to the place where the stalk joins the head (called the neck region of the polyp) and covers the entire head of the polyp (Figs. 12–25 and 12–26). Snaring, which removes the polyp close to its mucosal attachment, therefore commonly removes all the adenomatous epithelium.

Pathologic assessment of a pedunculated polyp requires that it be sectioned in such a way as to produce a section through the center of the polyp including the entire stalk and head of the polyp. It is not necessary to ink the base of the stalk because the polypectomy margin can be recognized by cautery artefact (Fig. 12–27). The practice of cutting the base of the stalk horizontally for margin evaluation is also discouraged; this provides an inferior assessment of the polyp margin and leads to problems if the polyp is not oriented correctly.

The pathologic diagnosis of a pedunculated adenoma should provide information regarding: (1) polyp size, (2) type (ie, tubular, tubulovillous, or villous), (3) the presence or absence of high-grade dysplasia and malignancy, and (4) where possible, whether the adenoma has been completely excised. Excision of the adenoma is complete if the base of the stalk is completely surrounded by nonadenomatous normal colorectal mucosa.

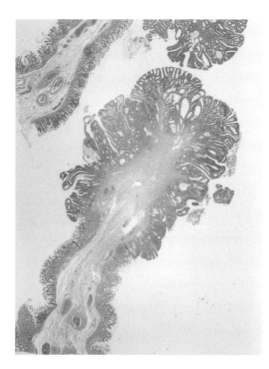

Figure 12–26. Pedunculated adenoma of the colon, showing stalk lined by normal epithelium with adenomatous change in the head region. The base is surrounded by normal mucosa, indicating complete removal. The stalk is clear of tumor.

Varying degrees of inflammation, both acute and chronic, may be seen in a pedunculated adenoma. This must be distinguished from dysplastic polypoid lesions occurring in idiopathic inflammatory bowel disease, which is best done by the endoscopic information that the polyp occurred in otherwise normal colonic mucosa.

LARGE SESSILE ADENOMA. Large sessile adenomas have the highest incidence of malignancy among all colorectal adenomas. Because their relative frequency is low, however, these large, sessile adenomas account for a small number of colorectal cancers overall. Sessile adenomas occur most commonly in the rectum and can

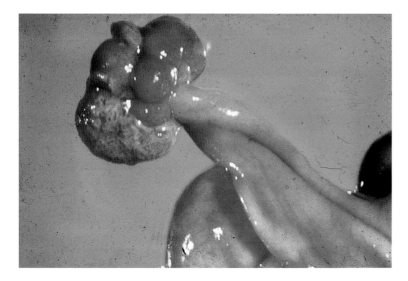

Figure 12–25. Pedunculated, long-stalked adenoma. Note the gross surface ulceration in the head of the polyp; this is common and usually the result of inflammation and does not signify malignancy.

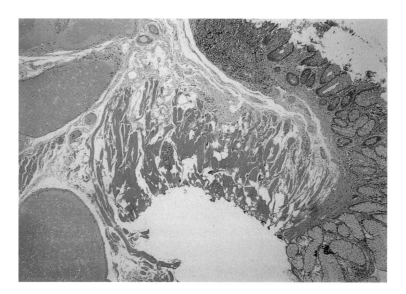

Figure 12–27. Cautery artefact at base of stalk, which identifies the resection margin.

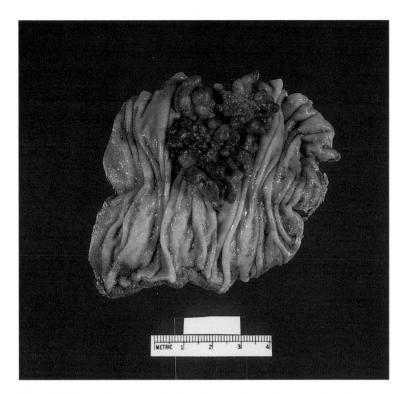

Figure 12–28. Locally resected rectal villous adenoma with the typical velvety finger-like appearance of the surface.

reach a large (10 cm) size (Fig. 12–28; see Figs. 12–8 and 12–9). They have a soft velvety appearance; they can be so soft that low rectal sessile adenomas are sometimes missed on digital rectal examination. The incidence of malignancy in large, sessile adenomas increases with size, and lesions larger than 3 cm have a reported prevalence of invasive cancer involving the submucosa of 60%.[22]

Most sessile adenomas are villous or tubulovillous (Figs. 12–29 and 12–30). Because these lesions are too large to remove completely at endoscopy, they should be extensively sampled. The resulting pathologic specimen consists of multiple pieces from the adenoma. The pathologic report of a large, sessile adenoma should include (1) pathologic type, and (2) the presence or absence of high-grade dysplasia or malignancy. Size assessment is not possible in such piecemeal samples, and these lesions are incompletely removed at endoscopy.

Large, sessile adenomas need to be surgically removed. Colonic and high to midrectal tumors can be resected by segmental colon resection and anterior resection, respectively. When they occur in the low rectum and do not show invasive carcinoma in biopsy samples and there is no clinical, endoscopic, or endoscopic ultrasound evidence to suggest malignancy, local complete excision by a technique such as transanal endoscopic microsurgery (TEM) is indicated[23] (see Fig. 12–28; also see Chapter 13). For circumferential tumors in the low rectum, circumferential mucosectomy may be used.[24] Invasive carcinoma is sometimes first found in the resected specimen; pathologic examination of the entire specimen is the only way in which adenocarcinoma can be definitely excluded in a large, sessile adenoma.

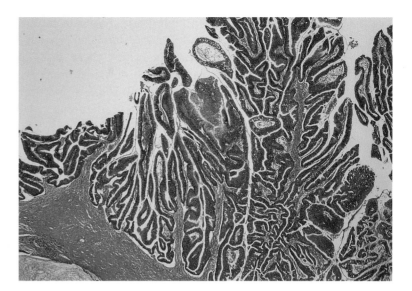

A

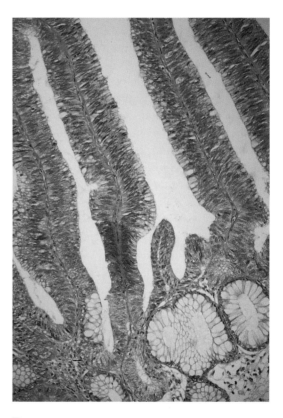

B

Figure 12–29. A: Adenoma of the colon, villous architecture, sessile. The long, finger-like villi lie on the muscularis mucosae. B: Villous adenoma, showing long finger-like villi lined by adenomatous epithelium.

Carcinomatous Adenomas. Carcinomatous adenomatous polyps contain invasive adenocarcinoma that has invaded through the muscularis mucosae to involve the submucosa. High-grade dysplasia and intramucosal carcinoma (see Figs. 12–20 and 12–21) have no metastatic capability and are therefore cured by polypectomy.

CARCINOMATOUS DIMINUTIVE ADENOMAS. Invasive carcinoma occurs in less than 1% of diminutive adenomas; a higher percentage of

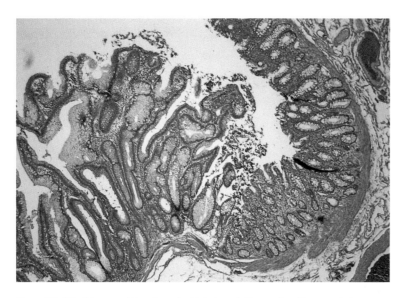

Figure 12–30. Adenoma of the colon, mixed tubular and villous pattern. The muscularis mucosae under the adenoma is continuous with the muscularis mucosae of the normal colonic mucosa at the edge of the lesion.

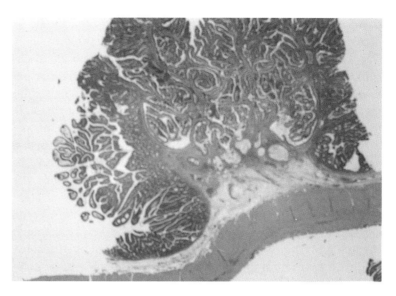

Figure 12–32. Stalk invasion in a pedunculated adenoma, showing extension of irregular nests of the invasive tumor into the head of the polyp.

flat adenomas are reported to have high-grade dysplasia and invasive carcinoma. When present in the usual piecemeal mucosal biopsy specimen from such a lesion, it is difficult to assess whether the invasion is restricted to the mucosa or submucosal invasion has occurred. Endoscopic ultrasound findings and whether carcinoma can be detected in an immediate rebiopsy of the site of initial polypectomy determine whether colonic resection is necessary.

CARCINOMATOUS PEDUNCULATED ADENOMAS. Pedunculated adenomas carry within their stalks an attenuated muscularis mucosae. The muscularis mucosae is well defined in the stalk of the polyp. Its appearance in the head of the stalk varies; it may become attenuated, split into layers, or be hyperplastic (Fig. 12–31). The

interior of the stalk is composed of an upward extension of submucosa and contains blood vessels and lymphatics. The submucosa is sometimes not clearly demarcated from the muscularis mucosae in the head of the polyp when the muscularis mucosae has become a poorly defined, nonlinear structure.

A carcinomatous pedunculated adenoma is characterized by invasive carcinoma extending through the muscularis mucosae into the substance of the stalk (Figs. 12–32 and 12–33). Definite involvement of the connective tissue of the stalk head must be present for invasion to be diagnosed. In tangentially sectioned polyps with an irregular muscularis mucosae, it is not uncommon to see adenomatous glands at the base of the mucosa being surrounded by muscle; this does not represent invasion unless clear extension is present below the muscle into the soft

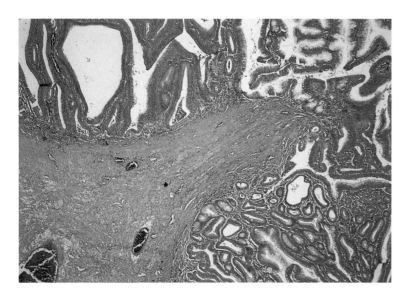

Figure 12–31. Head of a pedunculated adenoma, showing hyperplastic smooth muscle of the muscularis muscosae under the adenomatous mucosa.

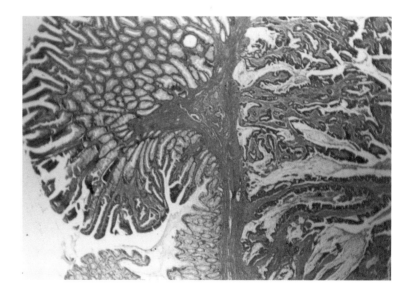

Figure 12–33. Stalk invasion in a pedunculated adenoma. This shows one side of the neck of the polyp where normal mucosa changes to adenomatous epithelium in the expanded polyp head with the underlying muscularis mucosae. In the interior of the stalk below the muscularis mucosae, an invasive carcinoma is evident.

tissue of the stalk head. The diagnosis of stalk invasion should be highly specific and made only when it is definitely present.

True stalk invasion must be distinguished from gland entrapment in the stalk ("pseudo-stalk invasion"), which is believed to result from torsion of the polyp (Fig. 12–34A). Pseudoinvasion is typically characterized by the presence in the stalk head of distorted adenomatous glands without malignant features; the glands are usually surrounded by lamina propria and associated with mucin extravasation, hemorrhage, and the presence of hemosiderin pigment (Fig. 12–34B, C). When the adenomatous glands that are displaced show features of high-grade dysplasia, the differentiation can be difficult (Figs. 12–35 and 12–36). Recently, expression of stromelysin-3 (ST3), one of the metalloproteinase family of enzymes detected by in situ hybridization or immunohistochemistry,[25] was shown to be helpful in differentiating true invasion (ST3-positive) from pseudoinvasion (ST3-negative).

The degree of stalk invasion is defined by Haggitt levels (Fig. 12–37)[26]:

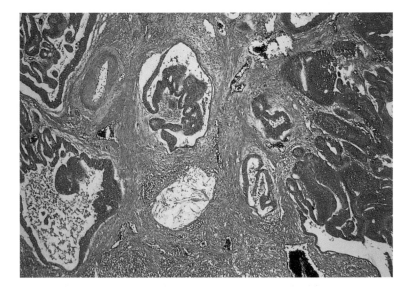

Figure 12–35. Pseudo-stalk invasion, showing mucin lakes and irregular glands with features of high-grade dysplasia surrounded by muscle and fibrosis in the stalk head. This is difficult to distinguish from true stalk invasion.

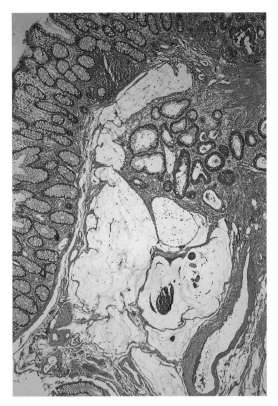

A

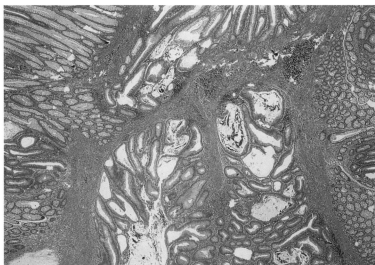

B

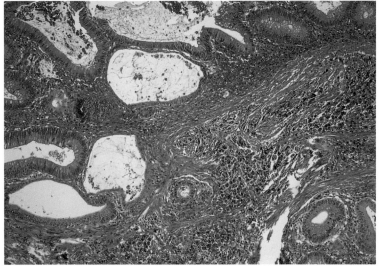

C

Figure 12–34. A: Pseudo-stalk invasion in a pedunculated adenoma, showing entrapment of adenomatous glands in the stalk. Note the normal mucosa and muscularis mucosae lining the stalk. B: Pseudo-stalk invasion, showing adenomatous glands in the stalk associated with hemorrhage and large mucin lakes. C: Pseudo-stalk invasion, showing adenomatous glands surrounded by lamina propria that contains hemosiderin; the glands lack features of high-grade dysplasia and malignancy.

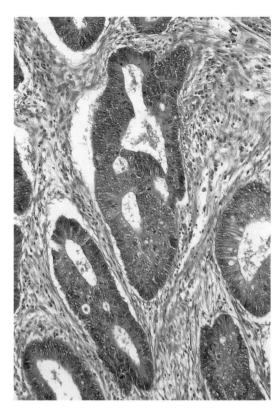

Figure 12–36. True stalk invasion, showing irregular malignant glands infiltrating the stalk surrounded by a desmoplastic stroma.

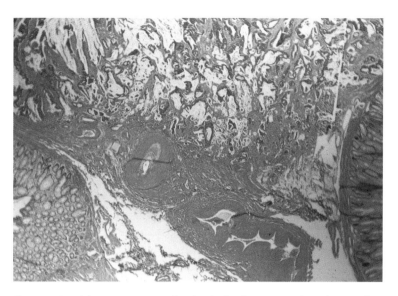

Figure 12–38. Adenocarcinoma in a pedunculated polyp. Section across the neck region of the polyp, showing extension of the invasive carcinoma to the level of the neck region (level 1) with the stalk being clear.

Level 1: invasion restricted to the head of the polyp.

Level 2: invasion of the stalk below the level of the neck (point where the stalk expands into the head), but with the basal part of the stalk uninvolved (Fig. 12–38).

Level 3: invasion of the stalk base without invasion of the colorectal submucosa below the level of the polyp base.

Level 4: tumor involving the colorectal submucosa.

It is important to recognize that these levels were defined in colectomy specimens in which the polyps were still attached to the colon. It is not possible in practice to differentiate between levels 3 and 4 on a polypectomy specimen; this must be done on the colonic resection specimen that should result when a colonic adenoma has stalk invasion extending to involve the base.

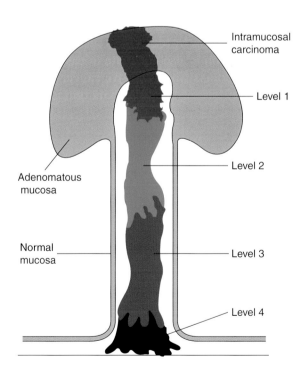

Figure 12–37. Diagram of pedunculated adenoma of the colon, showing levels of invasion. Level 1: carcinoma in mucosa, infiltrating the stalk with invasion limited to the stalk head (red). Level 2: carcinoma in stalk below neck region, but sparing the basal region (blue). Level 3: carcinoma involving stalk base but above level of colonic submucosa (purple). Level 4: carcinoma involving the colonic submucosa (black). Note that in a polypectomy specimen, level 3 (basal margin of polypectomy positive for carcinoma) cannot be distinguished from level 4.

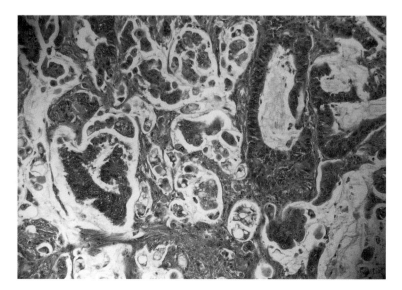

Figure 12–39. Carcinomatous polyp in which the malignant element is poorly differentiated, composed of small cell clusters with high nuclear grade and extracellular mucin.

The management of a carcinomatous polyp depends on the risk that residual carcinoma is present in either the polypectomy site or regional lymph nodes. The following factors have been identified as indicative of a high risk of residual tumor and are therefore used as indications for colectomy: (1) poorly differentiated adenocarcinoma (Fig. 12–39), (2) invasion by tumor of lymphovascular structures in the stalk (Fig. 12–40), and (3) the presence of tumor at, or within, 2 mm of the cauterized base of the stalk, which is the polypectomy margin (Fig. 12–41). When none of these risk factors are present, the likelihood of finding residual carcinoma in a colectomy specimen is 1–2%, and the risk of disease recurrence with simple follow-up is very small.[27] For this reason, it is generally recommended that colectomy is not required for carcinomatous adenomatous polyps without these risk indicators.[28]

Evaluation of involvement of the base can sometimes be difficult, most often because of imperfect sectioning of the polyp associated with malorientation, which precludes determination of the exact relationship of the invasive tumor to the margin. Even with well-oriented sections, it must be recognized that a considerable amount of heat is applied by the cautery at the margin. Small foci of cauterized tumor at or close to the margin may appear as unrecognizable basophilic structures, leading to interpretive difficulty (see Fig. 12–41).

CARCINOMATOUS LARGE, SESSILE ADENOMAS. At endoscopy, carcinomatous sessile adenomas are commonly indistinguishable from their benign counterparts; the diagnosis of malignancy is made by microscopic examination of random biopsy samples or in a resected specimen. Less commonly, a sessile adenoma may show a gross abnormality in part of its surface that indicates a likelihood of malignant transformation, permitting directed sampling from this region (Fig. 12–42). When invasive carcinoma extends through the muscularis mucosae in large, sessile adenomas, they are in the colonic submucosa (Fig. 12–43). When

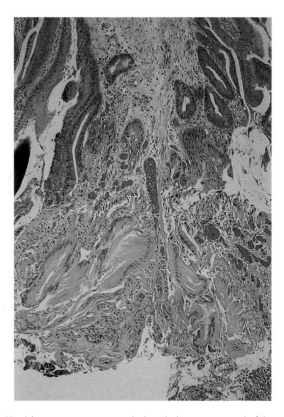

Figure 12–41. Adenocarcinoma present at the base (polypectomy margin) of the stalk. Note the cautery artefact in the malignant glands at the base. This is evidence of incomplete resection of the malignant tumor and is an indication for colonic resection.

invasive carcinoma is present in a biopsy from a sessile adenoma and when clinical or endoscopic ultrasound features indicate that invasion is limited to the rectal wall, the tumor can usually be resected locally by techniques such as TEM[23] (see Fig. 12–28). Local resection is also adequate in cases thought to be benign villous adenomas when invasive cancer is found in the resection specimen, as long as the deep margin is free of tumor.

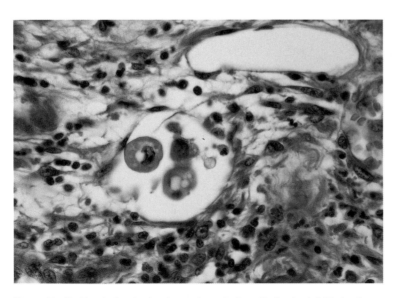

Figure 12–40. Vascular invasion by adenocarcinoma in the stalk, showing individual malignant cells in a small vessel in the stalk.

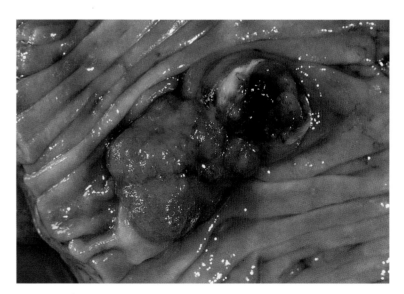

Figure 12–42. Adenocarcinoma developing in a sessile adenoma. Note the ulcerated appearance of the part of the tumor that has undergone malignant transformation compared with the smooth surface of the benign component.

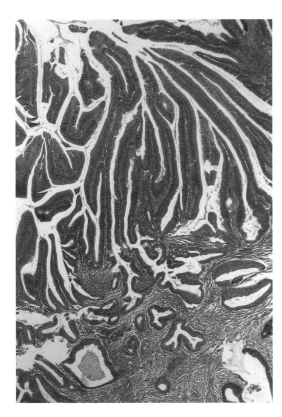

Figure 12–43. Adenocarcinoma developing in a villous adenoma, showing irregular malignant glands at the base of the villous component. The malignant glands are in the colonic submucosa (level 4) as soon as they invade the muscularis mucosae in sessile adenomas.

The pathologic handling of these local resection specimens is described in Chapter 13. With more deeply invasive low rectal tumors, abdominoperineal resection is indicated, as for any other deeply invasive adenocarcinoma of the rectum.

Principles for Surveillance in Patients with Colorectal Adenomas. When the first colorectal adenoma detected during a screening flexible sigmoidoscopy is larger than 1 cm, or there is more than one adenoma, an immediate follow-up colonoscopy is indicated because 30–50% of these patients have other adenomas in the more proximal colon.[4] When the adenoma detected by flexible sigmoidoscopy is single, smaller than 1 cm, tubular, and has no high-grade dysplasia, the justification for a follow-up colonoscopy is lessened.

After the first positive colonoscopy has cleared the colon of all adenomas, a decision must be made regarding long-term surveillance. Risk factors for the development of metachronous adenomas and therefore for placing the patient under surveillance are (1) a positive family history of colon cancer, (2) greater than 1 cm size of adenomas; (3) the presence of multiple adenomas, irrespective of size, (4) the presence of a villous or tubulovillous architecture, and (5) the presence of high-grade dysplasia.[7] At present, surveillance is not recommended if the finding at the first colonoscopy is a single tubular adenoma smaller than 1 cm.

Clearing the colon of adenomas and postpolypectomy surveillance has been shown to effectively decrease the incidence of colorectal carcinoma.[29]

Serrated Adenoma

Serrated adenomas (mixed hyperplastic adenomatous polyps) are a specific histologic form of colorectal polyp. They vary in size from 2 mm to over 2 cm. They occur as diminutive, sessile polyps; pedunculated polyps; and large, sessile polyps. The small lesions are indistinguishable from hyperplastic polyps endoscopically. Serrated adenomas occur predominantly (75%) in the rectosigmoid region. Serrated adenomas have a frequency of high-grade dysplasia and carcinoma that is similar to that for adenomas.[30]

Histologically, serrated adenomas have the architecture of a hyperplastic polyp, being characterized by elongated and dilated crypts lined by enlarged cells that line serrated lumina (Fig. 12–44A). The lining cells show nuclear enlargement and adenomatous change associated with the mucin hypersection[31] (Fig. 12–44B). This change occurs throughout the crypt. The extent of adenomatous change in a serrated adenoma is variable, and large areas of the polyp may show features of hyperplasia only. Complete histologic examination of hyperplastic polyps is essential to exclude serrated adenoma to avoid misdiagnosis of the premalignant serrated adenoma as a hyperplastic polyp.

COLORECTAL POLYPOSIS SYNDROMES

A large number of syndromes are characterized by the presence of multiple colorectal polyps (Table 12–2). These are classified by the pathologic types of polyps into hamartomatous polyposis syndromes and adenomatous polyposis syndromes. Apart from the difference in the pathology of the polyps, the major difference between these two types is that the incidence of adenocarcinoma is low in the hamartomatous polyposes compared with the adenomatous polyposes.

Hamartomatous Polyposis Syndromes

Hamartomas are mass lesions resulting from a disorderly proliferation of tissue elements normally present at that site. Intestinal hamartomas are usually composed of disordered crypts that show varying degrees of hyperplasia and cystic change and smooth muscle. Inflammation and fibrosis are commonly present.

Peutz-Jeghers Syndrome

Peutz-Jeghers syndrome[32] is characterized by gastrointestinal hamartomatous polyps associated with pigmented macules on the skin around the mouth and eyes and in the buccal mucosa (Fig. 12–45). More rarely, macules are present in the extremities and perianal area. The brown macules appear in early childhood and are 1–2 mm in size. Histologically, the macules show increased melanin pigment in the basal layer of the epidermis and increased dermal melanophages. Peutz-Jeghers syndrome is inherited as an autosomal-dominant trait; neither the genetic

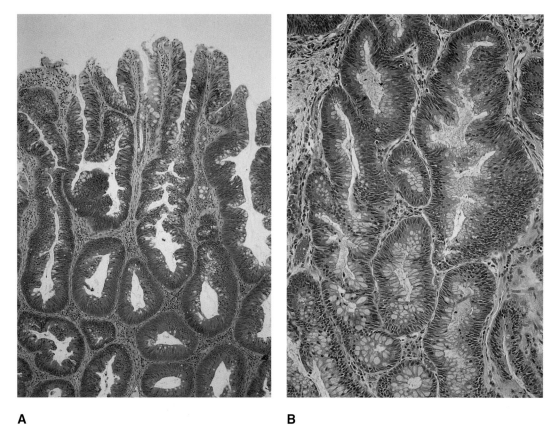

A   **B**

Figure 12–44. A: Serrated adenoma, showing the serrated crypt architecture of a hyperplastic polyp with the lining cells showing evidence of adenomatous change. B: Serrated adenoma, showing adenomatous change of the lining cells.

defect nor the chromosomal location of the abnormal gene have been determined. The condition is uncommon; approximately 600 cases have been reported.

Multiple polyps are found throughout the gastrointestinal tract, with maximal frequency of occurrence being in the jejunum (Fig. 12–46), followed by the colon and then the stomach (Fig. 12–47). Rare cases with a solitary polyp have occurred in families with the syndrome. The polyps appear in the first decade of life and range in size from 1–3 cm. The smaller polyps are sessile, whereas the large ones are peduculated and have a

TABLE 12–2. COLONIC POLYPOSES AND RELATED SYNDROMES

	Inheritance Pattern	Mutated Gene	Intestinal Lesions	Extraintestinal Lesions
Hamartomatous Polyposes				
Peutz-Jeghers syndrome	AD	?	Intestinal hamartomas	Pigmented macules in skin and mouth
Familial juvenile polyposis	AD	?	Juvenile polyps	None
Cronkhite-Canada syndrome	None	0	Juvenile polyps	Severe disease, often fatal
Cowden's disease	AD	?	Hamartomas	Skin tumors, breast and thyroid cancers
Adenomatous Polyposes				
Familial adenomatous polyposis	AD	*APC*	Colorectal adenomas	Gastric fundic polyps; and duodenal adenomas and CA
Gardner's syndrome	AD	*APC*	Same as FAP	Same as FAP +; skull osteomas; skin tumors; desmoid tumors; CHRPE
Turcot's syndrome, 66%	AD	*APC*	Same as FAP	PNET of CNS
33%	AR	MMR genes	Same as FAP	Glioblastoma multiforme
Attenuated adenomatous polyposis coli	AD	*APC*	Fewer polyps	None
Hereditary nonpolyposis colorectal carcinoma,				
type I	AD	MMR genes	Familial CRC	None
type II (cancer family syndrome)	AD	MMR genes	Familial CRC	Multiorgan cancers

Abbreviations: AD = autosomal-dominant; APC = adenomatous polyposis coli; CA = cancer; FAP = familial adenomatous polyposis; CHRPE = congenital hypertrophy of the retinal pigmented epithelium; PNET = primitive neuroectodermal tumor; CNS = central nervous system; AR = autosomal-recessive; MMR = mismatch repair; CRC = colorectal cancer.

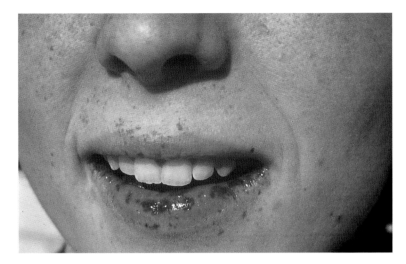

Figure 12–45. Peutz-Jeghers syndrome showing melanin pigmentation of circumoral skin.

typical frond-like appearance, with a long slender stalk. On microscopy, the polyps are a complex mass of disorganized and hyperplastic mucosal glands containing secretory and absorptive enterocytes and Paneth cells. Bundles of smooth muscle arborize through the polyp, dividing the glandular element into lobules (Fig. 12–48). Dysplasia is rare (Fig. 12–49). Extension into the submucosa and superficial muscularis externa ("pseudo-invasion") may occur. Gastric polyps are frequently multiple, large, and have the appearance of hyperplastic gastric polyps.

Patients commonly present in the second and third decades of life with recurrent bouts of intussusception associated with abdominal pain (see Fig. 12–46). Bleeding with anemia also occurs. Rarely, hamartomatous polyps occur in the nasal cavity, bronchus, and urinary bladder.

Reported extraintestinal manifestations, apart from pigmented macules around the mouth and eyes and in the buccal mucosa, are

1. Benign ovarian sex cord tumor with annular tubules is present bilaterally in most affected patients, usually as incidental microscopic findings.
2. In females, well-differentiated adenocarcinoma (adenoma malignum variant) of the endocervix occurs.
3. In males, bilateral Sertoli cell tumor of the testis occurs.
4. A general increased incidence of malignant neoplasms, including breast, ovarian, pancreatic and gallbladder carcinomas, has been observed in patients with Peutz-Jeghers syndrome.

Peutz-Jeghers syndrome is associated with a 2–3% risk of developing gastrointestinal malignancies.[33] These are most common in the colon, followed by the duodenum, jejunum, and stomach. Colorectal carcinomas occur at a younger age (median age around 40 years) than in the general population, suggesting that malignancy is in some way related to a preexisting polyp rather than to the coincidental development of an unre-

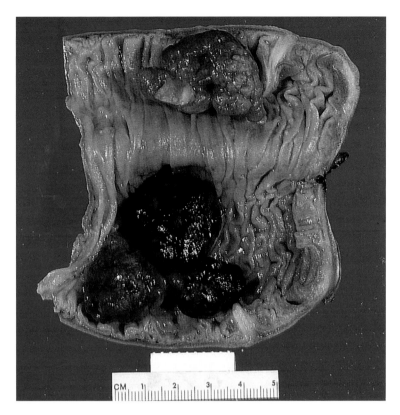

Figure 12–46. Resected jejunum in Peutz-Jeghers syndrome showing two large polyps (hamartomatous by microscopy). One of the polyps shows discoloration due to hemorrhagic necrosis resulting from intussusception, which was the indication for surgery.

lated colonic adenoma. Carcinomas of the small intestine rarely develop in hamartomatous polyps.

Familial Juvenile Polyposis

Sporadic juvenile polyps are common colorectal polyps in children. Patients with sporadic polyps usually have a single polyp, with a maximum of five polyps, which are restricted to the

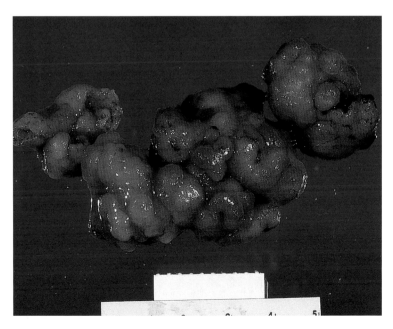

Figure 12–47. Gastric polyp in Peutz-Jeghers syndrome. This is unusually large.

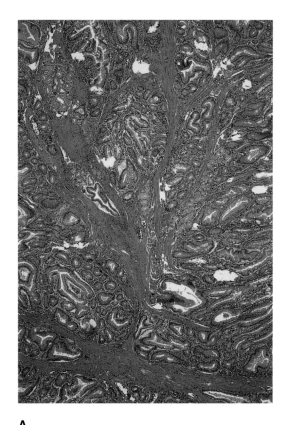

A

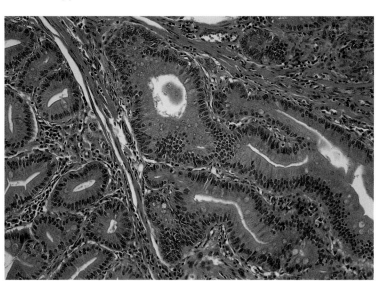

B

Figure 12–48. A: Jejunal hamartoma in Peutz-Jeghers syndrome, showing typical arborizing pattern of smooth muscle within the polyp. B: Jejunal hamartoma in Peutz-Jeghers syndrome, showing cytologically normal, disorganized glandular proliferation.

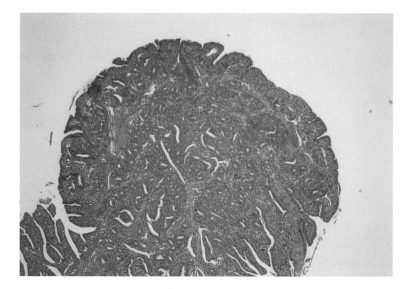

A

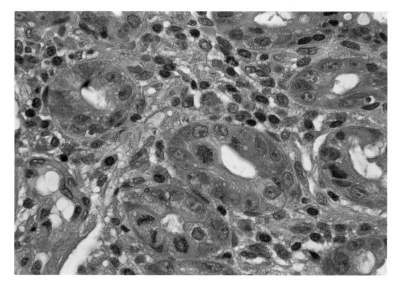

B

Figure 12–49. A: Small polyp in Peutz-Jeghers syndrome, showing gland crowding and epithelial dysplasia. B: Severe epithelial dysplasia in a Peutz-Jeghers polyp. The lining cells show severe cytologic abnormality, loss of polarity, and increased mitotic activity. Peutz-Jeghers polyps in the small intestine rarely become malignant.

colon and rectum. Juvenile polyposis is diagnosed when a patient has more than six polyps or polyps in the stomach and small bowel in addition to the colorectum, and when a patient in a family with familial juvenile polyposis develops any juvenile polyp.[34] In the fully developed disease, hundreds of juvenile polyps are found throughout the gastrointestinal tract with a maximal incidence in the colon. Juvenile polyps in the stomach are identical to gastric hyperplastic polyps.

The polyps, which are identical histologically to sporadic juvenile polyps, range from diminutive sessile polyps to pedunculated polyps that can reach a size of 3 cm. Symptoms usually appear in the third decade and include bleeding, intussusception, and protein-losing enteropathy.

Familial juvenile polyposis is rare and accounts for a third of all cases of juvenile polyposis. It is inherited as an autosomal-dominant trait. The affected gene is unknown.

Patients with familial juvenile polyposis have an increased incidence of colorectal adenocarcinoma; the risk has been estimated to be as high as 23%. The larger polyps in familial juvenile polyposis harbor foci of dysplasia and villous change, which probably represent the source of malignant transformation. According to some authorities, the risk of malignancy is high enough to justify prophylactic colectomy.[35]

Cronkhite-Canada Syndrome

Cronkhite-Canada syndrome is a nonfamilial condition characterized by the presence of juvenile polyps of the gastrointestinal tract, brown skin macules, generalized alopecia, and atrophy of the nails.[36] The median age of disease onset is approximately 60 years. The disease commonly presents acutely with diarrhea, often with severe bleeding, abdominal pain, and protein-losing enteropathy. The disease is commonly severe, progressing to malnutrition and immunodeficiency, and death can occur within months of disease onset. There is no effective treatment. Survival is uncommon, but spontaneous remissions have been reported.

Hundreds of polyps are present throughout the entire gastrointestinal tract from stomach to rectum. The polyps range from diminutive polyps to 3 cm in diameter and tend to be sessile even when large. Histologically, the polyps resemble juvenile polyps. Cronkhite-Canada syndrome is different from all other polyposis syndromes in that the mucosa between the polyps is abnormal, showing edema, inflammation, gland distortion, and vascular ectasia. Adenomatous change and adenocarcinoma occur, with an incidence of 15%.

Cowden's Disease

Cowden's disease (multiple hamartoma and neoplasia syndrome) is a rare disease inherited as an autosomal-dominant trait.[37] It is characterized by (1) Multiple hamartomas of the skin; multiple facial tricholemmomas appearing in the second decade of life is typical. Café-au-lait spots, epidermoid cysts, and basal cell carcinomas also occur. (2) Multiple verrucoid squamous papillomas in the oral cavity. (3) Hamartomatous polyps in the gastrointestinal tract occur in 30–60%. These occur through the GI tract, including esophagus, and include juvenile polyps and various types of nonepithelial polyps, such as lymphoid polyps, lipomas, and ganglioneuromas.

There is no increased risk of gastrointestinal tract cancer in Cowden's disease; however, 50% of patients develop breast cancer, and 10% develop thyroid cancer. Over 50% of patients have goiters. Also reported are numerous extraintestinal mesenchymal neoplasms, such as lipomas, benign vascular tumors, neurofibromas, and meningiomas.

Other Hamartomatous Polyposis Syndromes

Multiple mucosal neurofibromas involving small intestine, stomach, and colon occur in 25% of patients with generalized neurofibromatosis.[38] Neurofibrosarcomas of the intestine have been reported.

Intestinal ganglioneuromatosis consists of multiple hamartomas involving the submucosal and myenteric nerve plexuses, causing thickening of the affected bowel wall and motility disorders.[39] This is most commonly associated with multiple endocrine neoplasia, type IIb (medullary carcinoma of the thyroid and pheochromocytoma), in which small ganglioneuromas occur from lips to rectum (see Chapter 14). It can also occur as an autosomal-dominant isolated entity or be associated with familial juvenile polyposis and Cowden's disease.

Ruvalcaba-Myhre-Smith syndrome is a variant of familial juvenile polyposis in which the intestinal juvenile polyps are associated with macrocephaly, developmental delay, and pigmented macules on the penis.[40]

A rare form of nonfamilial polyposis characterized by multiple gastrointestinal hyperplastic polyps[41] has been reported. This resembles familial adenomatous polyposis and must be separated from that entity by histologic examination.

A rare familial disease characterized by multiple inflammatory fibroid polyps of the small intestine and stomach (Devon polyposis syndrome)[42] has been reported.

Adenomatous Polyposis Syndromes

All adenomatous polyposis syndromes are characterized by inheritance of a single abnormal gene that results in the presence of multiple colorectal adenomatous polyps,[34,43] Three variant syndromes (familial adenomatous polyposis, Gardner's syndrome, and Turcot's syndrome) are defined by the presence of different extracolonic manifestations. Inherited adenomatous polyposis syndromes are important not only from a practical standpoint, but also because they have been largely responsible for the understanding of the genetic basis of colorectal carcinoma. These adenomatous polyposis syndromes are rare; they affect 1 in approximately 10,000 persons worldwide.

Familial Adenomatous Polyposis

Familial adenomatous polyposis (FAP), also known as adenomatous polyposis coli (APC) and familial polyposis coli (FPC) is characterized by the presence of multiple adenomatous polyps in the colon and rectum. The number of polyps is usually innumerable (in the thousands, Figs. 12–50 and 12–51), but cases with fewer polyps are reported. All cases have more than 100 colorectal polyps, a fact that permits clear separation from patients who have multiple sporadic colorectal adenomas. Microscopically, all types of adenomas are present, including single dysplastic crypts; flat adenomas; and sessile and pedunculated adenomas with tubular, tubulovillous, and villous architecture. Polyps also occur in the stomach and duodenum in virtually all patients. Over 90% of gastric polyps are fundic gland polyps. Duodenal polyps, distal gastric antral polyps, and small-intestinal polyps are usually adenomas. Although the mutation is in the germline, colorectal adenomas are not present at birth; they develop in the second decade of life, with rectal bleeding being the most common presenting symptom.

Untreated, FAP invariably leads to increasing dysplasia and colorectal cancer (Fig. 12–52). Seven percent of patients have developed cancer by age 21 years, 50% at 39 years, and 90% by 45 years.[44] There is a 10–12% risk of developing periampullary duodenal carcinoma (Fig. 12–53). The incidence of gastric and small-intestinal cancers apart from the periampullary region is low.

FAP results from the autosomal-dominant inheritance of a single mutated gene in the long arm of chromosome 5 between Giemsa-stained bands 21 and 22 that is called the *APC* gene.[45]

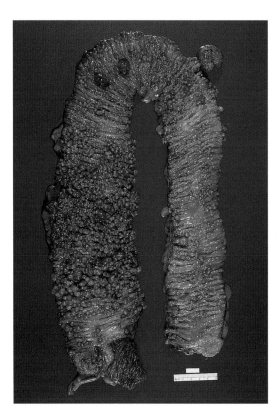

Figure 12–50. Colon in familial adenomatous polyposis, showing innumerable polyps in the colonic mucosa. Some polyps are larger and stand out.

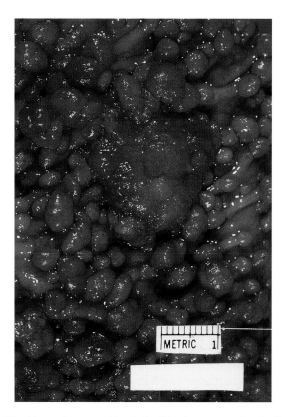

Figure 12–52. Adenocarcinoma occurring in familial adenomatous polyposis. The carcinoma appears as an ulcer in the midst of numerous polyps.

This mutated gene is in the germline and can be distinguished from all other genetic defects found in the adenoma–carcinoma sequence. APC codes for a 2843 amino acid protein, which has a tumor suppressor function but whose exact function is unclear. APC protein interacts with microtubules and β-catenin, a protein involved in cell adhesion. The exact location of the *APC* gene mutation influences the disease phenotype; an *APC* mutation in the midportion of exon 15 is associated with greater numbers of adenomas, and one at codon 1309 is associated with earlier onset of adenomas and cancer. Differences in the locus

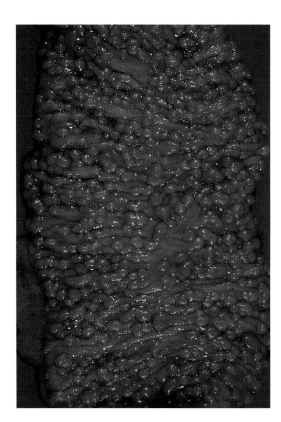

Figure 12–51. Colon in familial adenomatous polyposis, showing multiple small polyps with only small amounts of normal mucosal surface visible between the polyps.

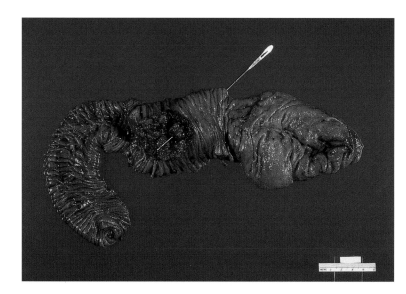

Figure 12–53. Periampullary carcinoma of the duodenum occurring in a patient with familial adenomatous polyposis 12 years after colectomy.

of the mutation may also be partly responsible for the variant syndromes of FAP. Genetic testing is now commercially available to detect the germline defect in FAP.

Gardner's Syndrome

Gardner's syndrome is a variant of FAP associated with a germline mutation of the *APC* gene and shows intestinal manifestations identical to those in FAP. The frequency of extraintestinal lesions differentiate Gardner's syndrome from FAP; this distinction becoming less important as the genetic similarity between the two conditions is being recognized. FAP and Gardner's syndrome have the identical mutation in the *APC* gene in terms of nature and location. The increased expression of extraintestinal lesions in Gardner's syndrome, however, breeds true in families, and it is postulated that some additional modifying gene is present in these families.

The extraintestinal lesions in Gardner's syndrome are:

1. Osteomas, most commonly seen in the mandible and other skull bones.
2. Skin tumors, including epidermoid cysts and fibromas.
3. Desmoid-type fibromatosis (Fig. 12–54), most commonly of the retroperitoneum and mesentery, which occur in 10% of patients.
4. Supernumerary teeth.
5. Congenital hypertrophy of the retinal pigmented epithelium (CHRPE).

Turcot's Syndrome

In Turcot's syndrome, the intestinal polyposis is associated with central nervous system neoplasms. The intestinal lesions are identical to adenomatosis polyposis coli. One case encountered at our institution was characterized by colorectal carcinomas in two sisters aged 8 and 14 years, one of whom had developed a cervical cord glioblastoma multiforme 6 months previously (Fig. 12–55).

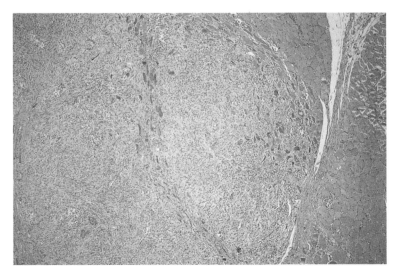

Figure 12–54. Abdominal fibromatosis (desmoid tumor) in patient with Gardner's syndrome. This is composed of a fibroblastic proliferation of low cellularity that extensively infiltrates the muscle.

Turcot's syndrome is not a homogeneous entity; two thirds of cases are caused by *APC* gene mutations, and one third by mutation of mismatch repair genes that characterize hereditary nonpolyposis colorectal cancer (HNPCC). Patients with *APC* gene mutations develop primitive neuroectodermal tumors, such as medulloblastomas, malignant astrocytomas, and ependymomas, whereas those with mismatch repair gene mutations develop glioblastoma multiforme.[46]

Attenuated Adenomatous Polyposis Coli

Attenuated adenomatous polyposis coli (AAPC) is a variant of FAP that arises from an *APC* mutation located distal to 5,′ in contrast to FAP in which the mutation is located proximal to 5.′[47] These patients have fewer colorectal adenomas (mean: 30) and develop adenomas and carcinoma approximately 10 years later than patients with typical FAP (Fig. 12–56). Seventy percent of the colorectal adenomas occur proximal to the splenic flexure. The risk of colon cancer is very high, but may be less than 100%.

Screening and Management of Adenomatous Polyposis Syndromes

Families with known FAP should be offered genetic testing.[48] A negative test has a high enough predictive value of disease absence that further screening is not necessary. Patients who are

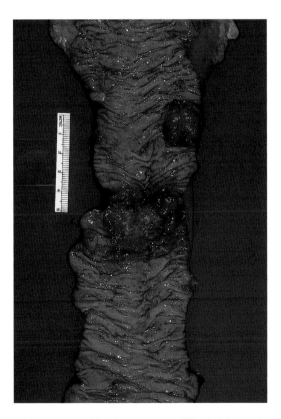

Figure 12–55. Adenocarcinoma of the colon in an 8-year-old female. Only one other polyp is visible grossly, but numerous microscopic adenomatous crypts were present in grossly normal colonic mucosa. This patient had a cervical cord glioblastoma multiforme 6 months previously, and a sister, 12 years old, had multiple colonic polyps with an adenocarcinoma. The parents were normal, indicating the autosomal-recessive type of Turcot's syndrome.

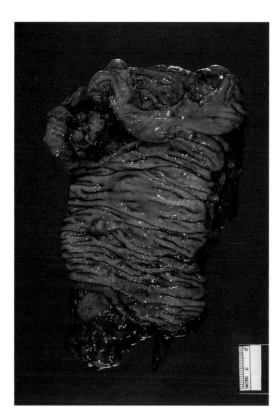

Figure 12–56. Colon carcinoma in 38-year-old male with a positive family history of colon cancer, showing pattern of involvement in attenuated adenomatous polyposis of the colon. The right-sided adenocarcinoma is associated with a few large adenomas.

positive for the mutated *APC* gene should be screened by flexible sigmoidoscopy every 1–2 years until age 35 years, starting at age 10. Prophylactic colectomy should be planned as soon as the diagnosis of adenomatous polyposis is made. No clear guidelines exist for the age at which colectomy should be performed; early teenage years are the safest. The procedure of choice is colectomy with mucosal proctectomy and ileoanal pouch construction. If colectomy with ileorectal anastomosis is performed, adenomas recur in the rectum and need to be excised regularly by surveillance proctoscopy. Sulindac, an antiinflammatory drug, has been shown to control rectal polyps in some patients.[49] Upper gastrointestinal screening for duodenal adenocarcinoma is also necessary in patients with a diagnosis of FAP and Gardner's syndrome.

In AAPC, screening can be started at age 20 years because of the later onset of disease. Screening must be by colonoscopy, however, because of the high incidence of proximal lesions in AAPC.

HEREDITARY NONPOLYPOSIS COLORECTAL CANCER

Hereditary nonpolyposis colorectal cancer (HNPCC or Lynch syndrome) is the most common form of hereditary colon cancer, responsible for 1–5% of all colorectal carcinomas.[50] It is an autosomal-dominant disease characterized by a high familial

incidence of colorectal cancer. Cancer tends to occur at a younger age (median 45 years), and 70% of the tumors occur proximal to the splenic flexure. HNPCC is diagnosed according to the following strict criteria (Amsterdam criteria): (1) at least three family members with colorectal carcinoma, at least two being first-degree relatives; (2) at least two generations with colorectal carcinoma; and (3) at least one colorectal carcinoma patient younger than 50 years old at diagnosis. Over 70% of families that meet these criteria have a genetic mutation associated with HNPCC.[43]

Patients with HNPCC do not have colonic polyposis. They may have one or a few colorectal adenomas. Adenomas in HNPCC are larger, occur at an earlier age, occur more often in the right colon, are more often multiple, and more often have a villous histology than sporadic colorectal adenomas. The lifetime risk of developing colorectal carcinoma is 80% and 45% of patients have synchronous or metachronous second primary colorectal carcinomas. Pathologically, colorectal carcinomas in HNPCC have a higher frequency of mucinous and poorly differentiated types and are associated with a marked lymphocytic response.[51]

HNPCC is subclassified into (1) Lynch syndrome I, in which cancers occur only in the colorectum; and (2) Lynch syndrome II, in which cancers of the endometrium, stomach, pancreas, ovary, small intestine, and kidney occur in addition to colorectal carcinomas ("cancer family syndrome").

Colorectal carcinomas occurring in HNPCC show microsatellite instability. Microsatellites are repeating DNA sequences distributed throughout the genome. Microsatellite instability is a difference in the length of microsatellites between tumor DNA and nontumor DNA from the same patient. Microsatellite instability is also present in 12–15% of sporadic colorectal carcinomas.[52] The finding of microsatellite instability in HNPCC tumors led to the discovery that HNPCC was the result of the presence in the germline of mutant genes involved in DNA mismatch repair (MMR). Errors of 1–5 base pair lengths commonly occur during DNA replication; MMR is the mechanism for repairing these errors by removing the errant DNA length and replacing it with the appropriately structured DNA. Four genes have so far been identified that play a role in the DNA mismatch repair process: *hMLH1* (chromosome 3p), *hMSH2* (chromosome 2p), *hPMS1* (chromosome 2q), and *hPMS2* (chromosome 7p). The presence of mutations in any of these four genes result in HNPCC; *hMLH1* and *hMSH2* mutations are responsible for the majority of cases. As expected, tumors in HNPCC show numerous DNA errors, also called a positive replication error phenotype (RER+). The increased rate of development of DNA errors is believed to translate into an acceleration of the adenoma–carcinoma sequence in patients with HNPCC.

Genetic screening is now available for HNPCC,[48] but is recommended only in families that meet the strict Amsterdam diagnostic criteria for the disease. Prophylactic colectomy should be offered to HNPCC gene carriers, because their lifetime risk of developing colorectal carcinoma is 80%. The alternative is lifetime colonoscopic screening beginning at age 25 years or

5 years less than the youngest family member with colon cancer. Colonoscopy should be repeated every 2 years. Females with Lynch syndrome II should be encouraged to have their children early and consider total hysterectomy and bilateral salpingo-oophorectomy because of the risk of endometrial and ovarian cancer.[53]

References

1. Granqvist S, Gabrielsson N, Sunderlin P. Diminutive colonic polyps: Clinical significance and management. *Endoscopy.* 1979;1: 36–42.

2. Weston AP, Campbell DR. Diminutive colonic polyps: Histopathology, spatial distribution, concomitant significant lesions, and treatment complications. *Am J Gastroenterol.* 1995; 90:1–2.

3. Tsai CJ, Lu DK. Small colorectal polyps: Histopathology and clinical significance. *Am J Gastroenterol.* 1995;90:988–994.

4. Itzkowitz SH. Gastrointestinal adenomatous polyps. *Semin Gastrointest Dis.* 1996;7:105–116.

5. Radin DR, Chandrasoma P, Halls JM. Colonic malakoplakia. *Gastrointest Radiol.* 1984;9:359–361.

6. Wolff M. Heterotopic gastric epithelium in the rectum. A report of three cases with a review of 87 cases of gastric heterotopia in the alimentary canal. *Am J Clin Pathol.* 1971;55:604–616.

7. Rossini FP, Arrigoni A, Pennanzio M. Treatment and follow-up of large bowel adenoma. *Tumori.* 1995;81:38–44.

8. Ueyama T, Kawamoto K, Iwashita I, et al. Natural history of minute sessile colonic adenomas based on radiographic findings. Is endoscopic removal of every colonic adenoma necessary? *Dis Colon Rectum.* 1995;38:268–272.

9. Bersentes K, Fennerty MB, Sampliner RE, et al. Lack of spontaneous regression of tubular adenomas in two years of follow-up. *Am J Gastroenterol.* 1997;92:1117–1120.

10. Kearney J, Giovannucci E, Rimm EB, et al. Diet, alcohol, and smoking and the occurrence of hyperplastic polyps of the colon and rectum (United States). *Cancer Causes Control.* 1995;6:45–56.

11. Warner AS, Glick ME, Fogt F. Multiple large hyperplastic polyps of the colon coincident with adenocarcinoma. *Am J Gastroenterol.* 1994;89:123–125.

12. Ko FY, Wu TC, Hwang B. Intestinal polyps in children and adolescents: A review of 103 cases. *Acta Paediatr Sinica.* 1995;36: 197–202.

13. Kapetanakis AM, Vini D, Plitsis G. Solitary juvenile polyps in children and colon cancer. *Hepatogastroenterology.* 1996;43:1530–1531.

14. Nakamura S, Kino I, Akagi T. Inflammatory myoglandular polyps of the colon and rectum. A clinicopathological study of 32 pedunculated polyps, distinct from other types of polyps. *Am J Surg Pathol.* 1992;16:772–779.

15. Griffiths AP, Hopkinson JM, Dixon MF. Inflammatory myoglandular polyp causing ileo-ileal intussusception. *Histopathology.* 1993;23:596–598.

16. Rickert RR, Auerbach O, Garfinkel L, et al. Adenomatous lesions of the large bowel. An autopsy survey. *Cancer.* 1979;43:1847–1857.

17. Yamamoto K, Tanaka T, Kuno K, et al. Carcinoma of the colon in children: Case report and review of the Japanese literature. *J Gastroenterol.* 1994;29:647–652.

18. O'Brien MJ, Winawer SJ, Zauber AG, et al. The National Polyp Study: Patient and polyp characteristics associated with high grade dysplasia in colorectal adenomas. *Gastroenterology.* 1990;98:371–379.

19. Stryker SJ, Wolff BG, Culp CE, et al. Natural history of untreated colonic polyps. *Gastroenterology.* 1987;98:1009–1013.

20. Muto T, Bussey HJR, Morson BC. The evolution of cancer of the colon and rectum. *Cancer.* 1975;36:2251–2270.

21. O'Brien MJ, Gibbons D. The adenoma–carcinoma sequence in colorectal carcinoma. *Surg Clin North Am.* 1996;5:513–530.

22. Ishikawa M, Mibu R, Nakamura K, et al. Correlation between macroscopic morphologic features and malignant potential of colorectal sessile adenomas. *Dis Colon Rectum.* 1996;39: 1275–1281.

23. Stipa S, Chiavellati L, Nicolanti V, et al. Microscopic endoluminal tumorectomy. *Dis Colon Rectum.* 1994;37:S81–85.

24. Whitlow CB, Beck DE, Gathright JB. Surgical excision of large rectal villous adenomas. *Surg Oncol Clin North Am* 1996;5:723–734.

25. Mueller J, Mueller E, Arras E, et al. Stromelysin-3 expression in early (pT1) carcinomas and pseudoinvasive lesions of the colorectum. *Virchows Arch.* 1997;430:213–219.

26. Haggitt RC, Glotzbach RE, Soffer EE, et al. Prognostic factors in colorectal carcinomas arising in adenomas. Implications for lesions removed by endoscopic polypectomy. *Gastroenterology.* 1985;89:328–336.

27. Frei JV. Endoscopic large bowel polypectomy. Adequate treatment for some completely removed, minimally invasive lesions. *Am J Surg Pathol.* 1985;9:355–359.

28. Whitlow C, Gathright JB Jr, Herbert SJ, et al. Long term survival after treatment of malignant colonic polyps. *Dis Colon Rectum.* 1997;40:929–934.

29. Winawer SJ, Zauber AG, Ho MN, et al. Prevention of colorectal cancer by colonoscopic polypectomy. *N Engl J Med.* 1993;329: 1977–1981.

30. Jaramillo E, Watanabe M, Rubio C, et al. Small colorectal serrated adenomas: Endoscopic findings. *Endoscopy.* 1997;29:1–3.

31. Urbanski SJ, Kossakowska AE, Marcon N, et al. Mixed hyperplastic adenomatous polyps—An underdiagnosed entity. *Am J Surg Pathol.* 1984;8:551–556.

32. Kitagawa S, Townsend BL, Hebert AA. Peutz-Jeghers syndrome. *Dermatol Clin.* 1995;13:127–133.

33. Flageole H, Raptis S, Trudel JL, et al. Progression toward malignancy of hamartomas in a patient with Peutz-Jeghers syndrome: Case report and literature review. *Can J Surg.* 1994;37:231–236.

34. Kuwada SK, Burt RW. The clinical features of the hereditary and nonhereditary polyposis syndromes. *Surg Oncol Clin North Am.* 1996;5:553–567.

35. Jarvinen H, Franssila KO. Familial juvenile polyposis coli: Increased risk of colorectal cancer. *Gut.* 1984;24:333–339.

36. Daniel ES, Ludwig SL, Lewin KJ, et al. The Cronkhite-Canada syndrome: An analysis of clinical and pathologic features and therapy in 55 patients. *Medicine.* 1982;61:293–309.

37. Salem OS, Steck WD. Cowden's disease (multiple hamartoma and neoplasia syndrome): A case report and review of the English literature. *J Am Acad Dermatol.* 1983;8:686–696.

38. Hochberg FH, Dasilva AB, Galdobini J, et al. Gastrointestinal involvement in von Recklinghausen's neurofibromatosis. *Neurology.* 1974;24:1144–1151.

39. d'Amore ESG, Manivel JC, Pettinato G, et al. Intestinal ganglioneuromatosis: Mucosal and transmural types. *Hum Pathol.* 1991;22:276–286.

40. DiLiberti JH, Weleber RG, Budden S. Ruvalcaba-Myhre-Smith

syndrome: A case with probable autosomal dominant inheritance and additional manifestations. *Am J Med Genet.* 1983;15:491–495.

41. Williams GT, Arthur JF, Bussey HJR, et al. Metaplastic polyps and polyposis of the colorectum. *Histopathology.* 1980;4:155–170.

42. Allibone RO, Nanson JK, Anthony PP. Multiple and recurrent inflammatory fibroid polyps in a Devon family ("Devon polyposis syndrome"): An update. *Gut.* 1992;33:1004–1005.

43. Burt RW. Familial risk and colorectal cancer. *Gastroenterol Clin North Am.* 1996;25:793–803.

44. Burt RW, DeSario JA, Cannon-Albright L. Genetics of colon cancer: Impact of inheritance on colon cancer risk. *Annu Rev Med.* 1995;46:371–379.

45. Powell SM. Familial polyposis syndromes. Advances in molecular genetic characterization. *Surg Oncol Clin North Am* 1996;5:569–587.

46. Hamilton SR, Liu B, Parsons RE, et al. The molecular basis of "Turcot's Syndrome." *N Engl J Med.* 1995;332:839–847.

47. Spirio L, Olschwang S, Groden J, et al. Alleles of the APC gene: An attenuated form of familial polyposis. *Cell.* 1993;75:951–957.

48. Burt RW. Screening of patients with a positive family history of colorectal cancer. *Gastrointest Endosc Clin North Am.* 1997;7:65–79.

49. Winde G, Schmid KW, Schlegel W, et al. Complete reversion and prevention of rectal adenomas in colectomized patients with familial adenomatous polyposis by rectal low dosage sulindac maintenance treatment. *Dis Colon Rectum.* 1995;38:813–830.

50. Lynch HT, Smyrk T, Lynch J. An update of HNPCC (Lynch syndrome). *Cancer Genet Cytogenet.* 1997;93:84–99.

51. Messerini L, Mori S, Zampi G. Pathologic features of hereditary nonpolyposis colorectal cancer. *Tumori.* 1996;82:114–116.

52. Marra G, Boland CR. Hereditary nonpolyposis colorectal cancer: The syndrome, the genes, and historical perspectives. *J Natl Cancer Inst.* 1995;87:1114–1125.

53. Lynch HT, Smyrk T, Lynch J. Overview of natural history, pathology, molecular genetics and management of HNPCC (Lynch syndrome). *Int J Cancer.* 1996;69:38–43.

13

COLORECTAL MALIGNANT NEOPLASMS

Patricia Dalton and Parakrama Chandrasoma

Adenocarcinoma constitutes over 90% of malignant neoplasms of the colon and rectum. The remainder are neoplasms of the neuroendocrine cells, mainly carcinoid tumors; direct invasion of the colon and rectum by other visceral malignancies, such as carcinomas of the prostate, urinary bladder, and uterus; and metastatic tumors, such as malignant melanoma.

COLORECTAL ADENOCARCINOMA

Incidence

Colorectal carcinoma (CRC) is second only to lung cancer as a cause of cancer death in the United States. In 1994, there were an estimated 149,000 new cases and 56,000 deaths from CRC.

The incidence for carcinomas in the colon increased during the 1973–1987 period, whereas the incidence of rectal carcinoma remained constant.[1] Colorectal carcinoma is slightly more common in males. Sporadic CRC occurs over the age of 50 years. When CRC occurs at a younger age, the likelihood of a germline genetic abnormality is significant.

The cause of CRC is unknown and most likely multifactorial. Dietary factors associated with both benign adenoma frequency and CRC include high intake of animal fat and low intake of fiber. These account for the geographic variation in adenoma incidence and CRC, which are neoplasms that are much more prevalent in affluent societies such as those in the United States and Western Europe than in the developing countries of Asia and Africa.[2] Geographic variation is not due to genetic factors because migrants from one area to another assume the risk of their new domicile.

Precursor Lesions

The Adenoma–Carcinoma Sequence

It is accepted that the vast majority of CRC passes through a recognizable premalignant adenoma phase (Fig. 13–1).[2] The adenoma begins as a diminutive polyp; as it increases in size it takes on either a pedunculated or sessile macroscopic appearance and a tubular or villous microscopic architecture. Adenomatous change, which defines an adenoma, is equivalent to low-grade epithelial dysplasia.

Adenomas that progress toward CRC develop high-grade

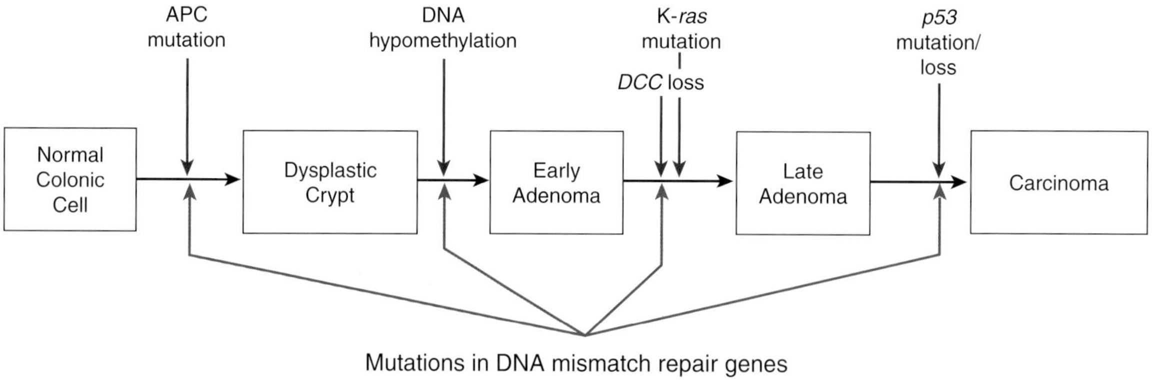

Figure 13–1. The adenoma–carcinoma sequence of colorectal carcinoma. The changes in the upper part are those associated with the LOH pathway for colorectal carcinoma, which is responsible for 85 to 95% of these cancers. The other 10–15% (the RER pathway) are associated with microsatellite instability.

dysplasia, which is histologically defined (see Chapter 12). The occurrence of high-grade dysplasia in clinically encountered adenomas is approximately 5%. The risk of high-grade dysplasia increases as the polyp size increases and the histologic villous element increases (Table 13–1). The number of adenomas with high-grade dysplasia that progress to invasive carcinoma is unknown because adenomas with high-grade dysplasia are removed at the time of detection. It is known, however, that the presence of high-grade dysplasia in a removed adenoma increases the patient's risk for future CRC, suggesting that high-grade dysplasia is an intermediate stage between adenoma and invasive carcinoma. The fact that residual adenoma is found in more than two thirds of small carcinomas that have not invaded beyond the submucosa[3] also suggests that the adenoma–carcinoma sequence is the common pathway of developing CRC.

Flat Colorectal Adenoma

The concept that CRC invariably arises as an orderly progression from small adenoma to large adenoma to high-grade dysplasia to invasive cancer has been questioned by the recognition of flat adenomas of the colon. Flat adenomas are smaller than 1 cm in size, frequently have a depressed center, and have a 10–15% rate of high-grade dysplasia and 2–3% incidence of invasive carcinoma.[4] Flat adenomas are translucent, making their detection at colonoscopy difficult. The use of high-resolution video endoscopy and chromoscopy facilitates their detection.[5]

These flat adenomas, although they go through the adenoma–carcinoma sequence, appear to do so unusually rapidly without a large-size intermediate adenoma. Coupled with the fact that the smaller lesions can be missed at conventional screening colonoscopy, they can represent lesions that first present as flat invasive adenocarcinomas ("de novo CRC"). Some suggest that the flat adenoma–carcinoma sequence has been underestimated in the etiology of CRC.[5,6] Other authorities question the concept of an accelerated adenoma–carcinoma sequence in flat adenomas.[2,7] Flat adenomas are not commonly recognized in the United States. When detected, they are very likely called diminutive adenomas.

Chronic Ulcerative Colitis

Patients with chronic ulcerative colitis have an increased risk of CRC. The development of carcinoma in ulcerative colitis is more akin to the sequence in flat adenomas than the usual adenoma–carcinoma sequence. Dysplasia commonly develops in a flat mucosa and progresses to high-grade dysplasia without being endoscopically detectable. Adenocarcinoma that occurs in ulcerative colitis tends to be flat and invasive more frequently and is much more difficult to detect endoscopically at an early stage.

Genetic Basis

Germline Defects

Understanding the genetic (inherited) basis of CRC has been facilitated by the study of familial adenomatous polyposis (FAP) and hereditary nonpolyposis colorectal cancer (HNPCC) (see Chapter 12). FAP is a disease caused by the inheritance of a mutant adenomatous polyposis coli gene, *APC*, on chromosome 5q21–22 resulting in the genesis of innumerable colorectal adenomas at an early age with a 100% likelihood of developing CRC.

HNPCC results from germline mutations in one of several DNA mismatch repair genes, *hMLH1, hMSH2, hPMS1,* and *hPMS2,* located on chromosomes 2, 3, and 7. The abnormality in the DNA mismatch repair genes permits tumor cells to accumulate multiple DNA errors. This is known as the positive replication error phenotype of CRC (RER+). The genomic instability is most easily recognized by the occurrence of DNA sequence errors in microsatellites (microsatellite instability). HNPCC is clinically associated with a high familial likelihood of CRC occurring in younger (<50 years) patients; the cancers tend to be

TABLE 13–1. ODDS RATIO FOR HIGH-GRADE DYSPLASIA IN ADENOMAS: EFFECTS OF SIZE AND VILLOUS COMPONENT

	<0.5 cm	0.5–1 cm	>1 cm
Tubular (0% villous)	1	3.1	7.3
Tubular (<25% villous)	2.9	8.8	21.2
Tubulovillous (25–75% villous)	3.6	11	26.4
Villous (>75% villous)	8.2	25.1	60

The reference category is a diminutive tubular adenoma without any villous architecture, which is given a risk of 1.

TABLE 13–2. ACQUIRED GENETIC CHANGES IN THE ADENOMA–CARCINOMA SEQUENCE

Gene Involved	Normal Mucosa	Small (<1 cm) Adenoma	Large (>1cm)/Villous	Adenoma with HGD	Invasive Carcinoma
LOH Pathway					
APC Allele 1	Normal	Mutant	Mutant	Mutant	Mutant
Allele 2	Normal	Normal	Normal	Loss	Loss
K-ras Allele 1	Normal	Normal	Mutant	Mutant	Mutant
Allele 2	Normal	Normal	Normal	Normal	Normal
DCC Allele 1	Normal	Normal	Normal	Loss	Loss
Allele 2	Normal	Normal	Normal	Normal	Loss
p53 Allele 1	Normal	Normal	Normal	Mutant	Mutant
Allele 2	Normal	Normal	Normal	Normal	Loss
RER Pathway					
DNA mismatch repair genes	Normal	Mutated	Mutated	Mutated	Mutated

Abbreviations: HGD = high-grade dysplasia; LOH = loss of heterozygosity; *APC* = adenomatous polyposis coli (gene); *DCC* = deleted in colon cancer (gene).

multiple and involve the proximal colon. HNPCC has been estimated to be responsible for as many as 5% of all CRC.

There is a definite familial clustering of CRC in patients with sporadic CRC.[8] The likelihood of a positive family history increases with the following factors: (1) younger age of occurrence of CRC (<45 years), (2) proximal location of CRC, (3) presence of multiple adenomas and villous histology of adenomas associated with CRC. Patients with this familial tendency to develop CRC are believed to account for up to 50% of sporadic CRC. Although there are epidemiologic suggestions of an inherited basis for these cases and mild mutations of the *APC* gene and mismatch repair genes have been suggested as possible causes, no germline genetic defects have yet been identified in these patients.[8]

Acquired Genetic Changes

Over 95% of CRC occur in patients who do not have an inherited (germline) genetic abnormality. These cases result from unidentified environmental factors that produce a series of genetic alterations in a colorectal epithelial cell destined to become neoplastic.

The Loss of Heterozygosity Pathway. The first alteration in the adenoma–carcinoma sequence is a mutation of one allele of the *APC* gene on chromosome 5q21–22 (Table 13–2, Fig. 13–1) in a crypt stem cell. This results in adenomatous change (low-grade dysplasia) and disordered proliferation of the altered clone of cells, first recognized as a microscopic dysplastic aberrant crypt focus (see Chapter 12).[9] Aberrant crypt foci are not visible macroscopically; they are identified by microscopic examination of whole mounts of colonic mucosa as elongated crypts whose upper part is lined by epithelial cells showing adenomatous change. Continued growth results in a diminutive adenoma. DNA hypomethylation, an epigenetic event that may facilitate the expression of these genetic changes, is also a feature of early adenomas.[10]

Numerous other genetic abnormalities occur in the intermediate stages of the adenoma–carcinoma sequence (see Fig. 13–1). K-*ras* mutations, which may occur in hyperplastic polyps and the smallest adenomas, increase in frequency to more than 50% in larger adenomas, in adenomas with villous architecture, and adenomas with high-grade dysplasia. The *DCC* (deleted in colon cancer) gene on chromosome 18q is also commonly lost in larger adenomas.[11] K-*ras* and *DCC* gene abnormalities are not associated with malignant transformation of an adenoma.

Genetic alteration of the *p53* gene on chromosome 17 is presently thought to be responsible for malignant transformation in an adenoma. Mutations in *p53* first involve one allele, an event that appears to be followed by deletion of the *p53* locus on the other allele, resulting in *p53* inactivation. Inactivation of *p53*, which is seen in only 3% of large adenomas, is present in 75% of invasive carcinomas.[12]

The Replication Error Pathway. A second pathway leading to sporadic CRC involves acquired mutations in DNA mismatch repair genes, the same genes that are responsible for HNPCC. These tumor cells show microsatellite instability and multiple DNA replication errors (RER+). RER+ tumors comprise all CRC in HNPCC and 10–15% of sporadic CRC in patients who do not have the germline genetic abnormality of HNPCC. RER+ colorectal carcinoma has distinct pathologic characteristics[2,13]:

1. They are more frequently large exophytic growths.
2. They are preponderantly in the right colon.
3. Histologically, they are solid, poorly differentiated carcinomas with no gland formation, and have an often marked lymphocytic host response.
4. They have less frequent expression of carcinoembryonic antigen.
5. They have a lower incidence of *p53* mutations.
6. Stage for stage, they have a better prognosis than RER– tumors.

RER+ adenomas have been demonstrated in patients with RER+ carcinomas, suggesting that the RER pathway is a second molecular pathway for the adenoma–carcinoma sequence.

Diagnosis

Clinical Features

Early clinical features of CRC include alteration in bowel habits and anemia resulting from chronic blood loss. Late clinical features of CRC, such as overt rectal bleeding, colonic obstruction, the presence of a mass, and weight loss, usually signify late-stage disease.

Screening

Because early detection greatly influences survival in CRC, mass population screening has been recommended in many high-risk populations. Screening is aimed at identifying a group of patients at high enough risk for CRC to justify regular colonoscopy during which all adenomas are removed (Fig. 13–2). The extensive National Polyp Study established that regular colonoscopic polypectomy in a selected high-risk group results in a dramatic reduction in the incidence of CRC in this group.[14]

Patients with familial adenomatous polyposis (FAP) and HNPCC, and patients with chronic ulcerative colitis are known to be at high risk by virtue of their diseases. Family members of patients with FAP and HNPCC can be tested genetically to establish inheritance of the genetic abnormality. Ideally, prophylactic total colectomy, mucosal proctectomy, and ileoanal anastomosis should be performed on these patients before they develop CRC. Particularly in ulcerative colitis, however, colorectal carcinoma still occurs in some patients before colectomy is performed; not infrequently the cancers are not early-stage cancers.[15]

Screening for sporadic CRC is unsatisfactory. Several different screening methods have been advocated.

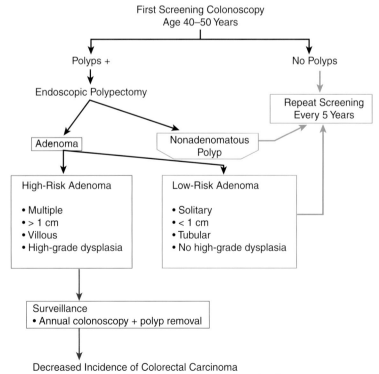

Figure 13–2. Screening algorithm for colorectal carcinoma.

Fecal Occult Blood Testing. Digital rectal examination is an excellent screening test for low rectal carcinomas and should be part of any physical examination in patients older than 40 years. Fecal hemoccult testing is done at the time of the rectal examination. It is a very unsatisfactory screening test. Thirty to 50% of patients with a documented CRC have a negative test. Three to 5% of all patients have a positive hemoccult test; of these, only 5–10% will have CRC, and a further 25% will have a benign adenoma. The great majority of patients who are hemoccult-positive are therefore subjected to considerable anxiety and an uncomfortable and expensive endoscopic procedure that is not without complications.

Flexible Sigmoidoscopy or Colonoscopy. Flexible sigmoidoscopy or colonoscopy is an alternative screening method and is recommended by the American Cancer Society for all persons at age 50 years (see Fig. 13–2). If flexible sigmoidoscopy is used, it must be followed immediately by a colonoscopy if a high-risk lesion is found in the distal colon. Endoscopy permits accurate identification of colorectal polyps, which can be removed for histologic examination. Polyps that signify a high risk for CRC are adenomas larger than 1 cm, multiple adenomas, adenomas with villous histology, and adenomas with high-grade dysplasia. Patients with any of these high-risk adenomas should have annual colonoscopy with clearance of all polyps. Individuals without high-risk adenomas are advised to have a repeat screening every 3–5 years.

Although this screening protocol decreases CRC in the screened population, the total number of people entering such screening programs will ultimately determine the success screening will have in decreasing the overall incidence of CRC in the population. Acceptance of colonoscopy and cost constraints will have to change significantly in most populations to affect CRC incidence.

Genetic Testing. Genetic testing is recommended only for: (1) kindred of those with familial polyposis syndrome and HNPCC to see whether they have the inherited genetic defect; (2) patients with sporadic CRC who satisfy the Amsterdam criteria for HNPCC (see Chapter 12). Seventy percent of such patients will have DNA mismatch repair gene defects that characterize HNPCC. No genetic testing exists for the 95% of patients with sporadic CRC who have no detectable germline defect. Testing the tumor cells from resected CRC for microsatellite instability or DNA mismatch gene mutations has been suggested as a method of diagnosis of HNPCC; this is not feasible, however, because the majority of cancers with the RER+ phenotype are sporadic CRC with acquired mutations of DNA mismatch repair genes.

Pathologic Diagnosis

The diagnosis of colorectal carcinoma is established by histologic examination of a biopsy specimen (Fig. 13–3). Rarely, in cases with tight strictures, endoscopic biopsy is not possible, and the diagnosis must be made intraoperatively. Carcinomatous polyps are considered in Chapter 12.

This section is confined to the diagnosis of lesions that

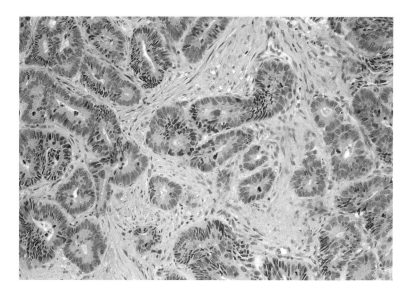

Figure 13–3. Colon biopsy specimen from a mass lesion, showing replacement of normal mucosa by a poorly differentiated adenocarcinoma, consisting of irregular nests of malignant cells surrounded by desmoplasia. Focal mucin production indicates that this is an adenocarcinoma.

present as tumor masses, ulcers, or strictures that are endoscopically suspected of being carcinomas (Fig. 13–4). Not all endoscopic tumors and ulcerative lesions suggestive of carcinoma are malignant; we have encountered amebomas, hyperplastic cecal tuberculosis, and giant inflammatory polyps that were thought to be carcinoma at endoscopy. Strictures that are suspected of being malignant not infrequently have a nonneoplastic basis, such as diverticulitis and Crohn's disease.

In nonobstructed cases, the tumor surface can be visualized and biopsy specimens taken from the surface and edge of the lesion. Pathologic diagnosis of the vast majority of well-differenti-

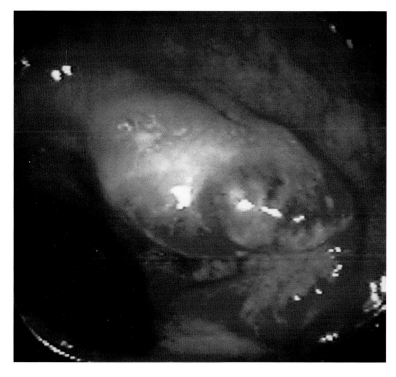

Figure 13–4. Colon carcinoma at colonoscopy, showing a large mass lesion with focal ulceration. (Courtesy of Aslam Godil, MD, Dept. of Gastroenterology, Loma Linda University, CA.)

ated colorectal carcinomas presents few problems to the pathologist. Rarely, infiltration of the rectum by an adenocarcinoma of the prostate or endometrioid carcinoma of the uterus or ovary may result in diagnostic confusion. In these cases, recognition that the tumor is not associated with dysplastic changes in the colorectal mucosa, the histologic features, and immunoperoxidase staining (eg, for prostate-specific antigen) may be helpful.

Carcinomatous strictures present diagnostic difficulty when the narrowing is so tight that it is difficult to pass the endoscope sufficiently to visualize the tumor and obtain adequate specimens. In these cases, samples are frequently taken from the lower limit of the tumor and may be more difficult to interpret than usual (Fig. 13–5). False-negative biopsy specimens may also result, necessitating intraoperative diagnosis in resec-

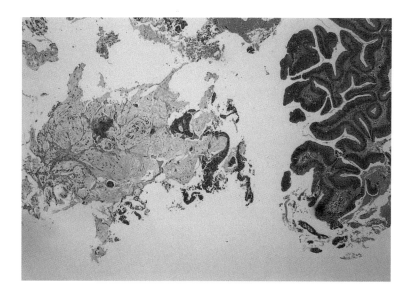

A

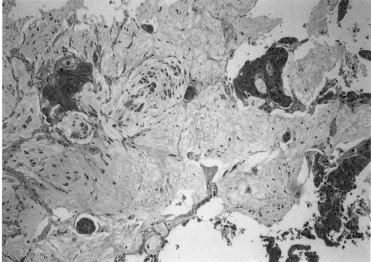

B

Figure 13–5. A: Biopsy specimen from a malignant stricture of the sigmoid colon showing one piece from a villoglandular adenoma and a second piece of tissue in which malignant epithelial cells are suspended in abundant extracellular mucin. B: Higher power micrograph of part A, showing malignant cytologic features in the cells suspended in the mucin. Biopsy samples such as this, without surrounding tissue, are difficult to evaluate in many cases.

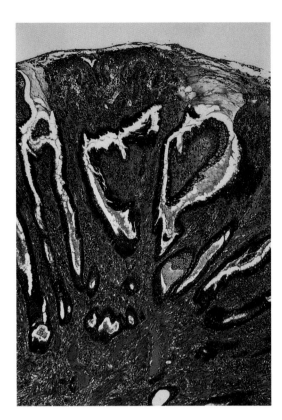

Figure 13–6. Solitary rectal ulcer syndrome, showing villous features with cytologic features of reactive atypia. When associated with colitis cystica profunda, this can mimic adenocarcinoma.

tions that have been performed without a preoperative diagnosis of cancer.

The most significant cause of a false-positive diagnosis of well-differentiated adenocarcinoma is solitary rectal ulcer syndrome. In the hyperplastic phase of this disease, the epithelium can show villous features with significant atypia that can be mistaken for a villous adenoma (Fig. 13–6). When colitis cystica profunda coexists and atypical glands are entrapped in the submucosa, there is a real danger of misdiagnosis as adenocarcinoma.

Poorly differentiated adenocarcinoma of the colon (Fig. 13–7) must be distinguished from other poorly differentiated malignant neoplasms, such as malignant lymphoma (CD45+, keratin−), metastatic malignant melanoma (keratin±, S100 protein+, HMB45+), epithelioid gastrointestinal stromal neoplasms (keratin±, vimentin+, CD34+), and poorly differentiated neuroendocrine neoplasms (keratin±, chromogranin+, neuron-specific enolase+). Immunoperoxidase staining is very helpful (Fig. 13–7C).

Brush cytology has been described as a useful adjunct to diagnosis of rectal cancer (see Chapter 18).[16] The increased cost and the presence of rare false-positive diagnoses probably does not justify recommending this technique for routine use.

Preoperative Staging

Availability of endoscopic ultrasonography permits preoperative staging of CRC. It is also feasible to perform ultrasound-guided core needle biopsies on suspicious-looking pararectal lymph nodes in patients with rectal cancer.[17] Ultrasound-guided needle biopsies of lymph nodes provides material adequate for diagnosis in most cases with reasonable diagnostic accuracy. In patients with low rectal carcinomas in whom a localized excision is being considered, intraoperative staging information is invaluable.

Treatment

Surgery is the primary treatment modality for colorectal carcinoma. For tumors of the colon, this entails a segmental resection. Anterior resection is used for high rectal tumors; with newer methods of anastomosis using stapling devices, anterior resection can be performed for midrectal tumors as well. The principles of resection include en bloc removal of the segment of colon containing tumor with adequate margins along with the lymphatic drainage and any invaded adjacent structures. In rectal tumors, a 2-cm distal mucosal margin is considered adequate because lymphatic drainage from the rectum is upward, limiting the likelihood of submucosal tumor distal to the tumor's edge. Although these surgical principles are firmly established, variation in patient outcomes in the hands of different surgeons suggests that differences of technique are common and may play an important role in patient survival.[18]

Laparoscopic colon resection for benign disease has been feasible since 1990. It has been shown that laparoscopic colectomy for treatment of colon carcinoma permits an adequate oncologic resection with surgical margins and number of retrieved draining lymph nodes being equivalent to conventional colectomy.[19] Reports of a high incidence of abdominal wall recurrences at the trochar site and peritoneal carcinomatosis, however,[20] have raised serious concerns about laparoscopic resection for colon cancer.

Rectal carcinomas that are too low for anterior resection have traditionally been treated by abdominoperineal resection. Laparoscopic abdominoperineal resections have also been reported with satisfactory outcomes.[21] Although abdominoperineal resections are still necessary for larger and more invasive rectal carcinomas, there is a tendency to use transanal sphincter-sparing local resections of earlier stage rectal carcinomas. In general, tumors smaller than 4 cm with invasion restricted to the rectal wall are amenable to local resection. The most elegant technique for local resection is transanal endoscopic microsurgery, (TEM)[21] which provides full access to the rectum under gas insufflation via a stereoscopic telescope. This technique permits full-thickness local rectal wall excision with repair of the mural defect. TEM is now the preferred form of local treatment for large sessile polyps of the rectum and early rectal carcinomas.

Pathologic Features

Intraoperative Consultation

Intraoperative pathologic consultation is rarely necessary in colon resections for carcinoma. In rectal tumors, it is often necessary to examine the resection specimen to ensure that clear

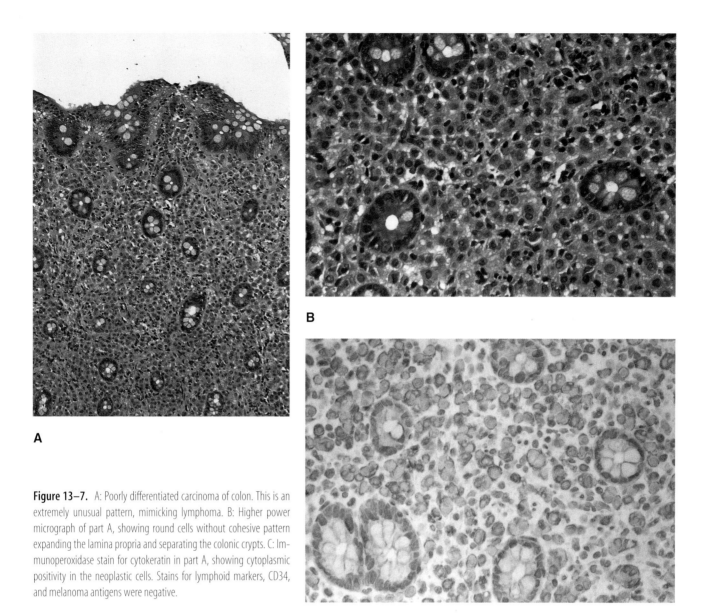

Figure 13–7. A: Poorly differentiated carcinoma of colon. This is an extremely unusual pattern, mimicking lymphoma. B: Higher power micrograph of part A, showing round cells without cohesive pattern expanding the lamina propria and separating the colonic crypts. C: Immunoperoxidase stain for cytokeratin in part A, showing cytoplasmic positivity in the neoplastic cells. Stains for lymphoid markers, CD34, and melanoma antigens were negative.

mucosal tissue extends for at least 2 cm between the distal tumor edge and the distal surgical margin. Frozen sections are rarely needed.

In local transanal resections, the pathologist should receive the specimen immediately after resection so that it can be pinned out prior to fixation; otherwise tissue contraction makes margin evaluation difficult.

Pathologic Examination of the Resected Specimen

The aims of pathologic examination of the resected specimen are

1. To provide an accurate gross description.
2. To confirm the diagnosis and histologically type and grade the neoplasm.
3. To determine the extent of local invasion and express this according to some form of pathologic staging system.
4. To assess the lymph nodes.

5. To determine the presence or absence of lymphovascular invasion.
6. To assess the adequacy of the resection by evaluating surgical margins.
7. To provide the best estimate of prognosis.

The results of this assessment are incorporated into the surgical pathology report, which must be concise, accurate, and comprehensive (Table 13–3).

Gross Description. A careful gross description is a crucial part of the pathology report. It represents the only permanent record of the resected specimen, which is generally discarded after it has been sampled for microscopy and the pathology report has been issued. The gross description should have

1. The dimensions of the specimen, which must include the length of colon or surface dimensions of a localized rectal resection, and the surrounding soft tissues.

TABLE 13–3. THE PATHOLOGY REPORT FOR COLORECTAL CARCINOMA

Pathology Laboratory Information

Patient Demographic Information   Dates
Pathology Number
Clinical Data (including physicians involved)
Specimens Submitted

Intraoperative Consultation Results (including frozen sections)
Gross Description
Tumor
    Obligatory: Location: Cecum/ ascending colon/ hepatic flexure/ transverse colon/ splenic flexure/
             descending colon/ sigmoid colon/ rectum
    Desirable: (a) Tumor size; gross type
              (b) Circumferential/ anterior/ posterior
              (c) Relationship to serosal surface
              (d) Relationship to surgical margin
Extent of Surgery
    Obligatory: (a) Segmental colectomy/ Total colectomy/ Abdominoperineal resection/
                Transanal local resection
             (b) Removal of other organs
             (c) Length of removed colon
             (d) Distance of tumor edges from ends of resection
    Desirable: Extent of lymphadenectomy

Microscopic Description and Diagnosis

Histomorphology
    Obligatory: (a) Histologic type and degree of differentiation
               (b) Lymphovascular invasion
Staging/primary tumor
    Obligatory: Depth of infiltration (Tis–T4)
    Desirable: Microscopic serosal involvement
Staging/lymph nodes
    Obligatory: TNM lymph node status (N0–N3)
    Desirable: Number of nodes examined and number involved.
Surgical margin
    Obligatory: Microscopic surgical margin status.

Other lesions in the specimen, if any: idiopathic inflammatory disease, polyps, etc.

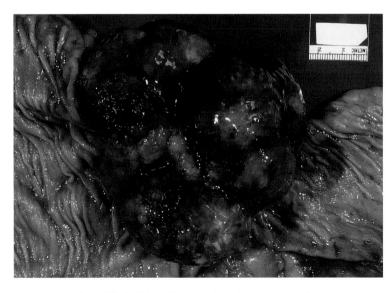

Figure 13–8. Polypoid intraluminal mass in the ascending colon.

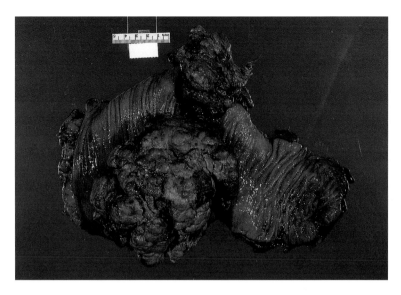

Figure 13–9. Large polypoid mass in the transverse colon.

2. The macroscopic characteristics of the tumor, including size, surface area of involvement, and location within the circumference (eg, anterior or posterior or circumferential).
3. The relationship of the tumor to the mucosal margins; for this purpose, routinely marking the distal margin at surgery with a suture is recommended.
4. A record of any incidental lesions, particularly polyps; if none is found, a statement to this effect should be included.
5. The gross impression of a section through the tumor in terms of macroscopic features, estimated invasiveness, and relationship to serosal surfaces and inked soft tissue margins.

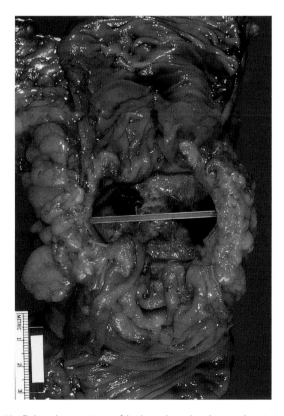

Figure 13–10. Tight malignant stricture of the descending colon, showing ulcerative mucosal lesion with circumferential infiltration of the colonic wall.

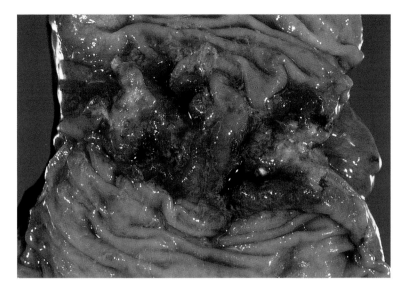

Figure 13–11. Circumferential ulcerative mass in the sigmoid colon associated with narrowing.

6. A description of the nodal dissection and a statement of how many nodes were found and where they were located.
7. A description of the sections taken from the specimen for microscopy; a letter or number key that identifies the location of each section is essential.

Colorectal carcinoma has three main macroscopic patterns of tumor growth. Right-sided colon cancers tend to be large exophytic tumors that involve part of the circumference of the wall and project into the lumen (Figs. 13–8 and 13–9). Left-sided colon cancers tend to be circumferential lesions with mucosal ulceration and thickening of the wall, causing luminal

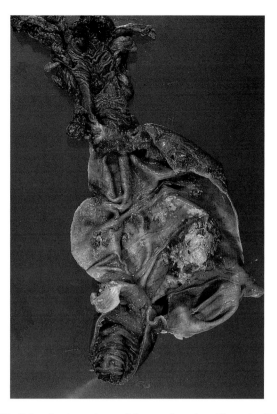

Figure 13–13. Tight-stricturing carcinoma of the ascending colon with massive dilatation of the cecum, indicative of obstruction. Note that the terminal ileum is of normal caliber.

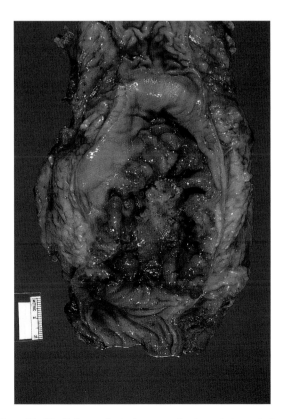

Figure 13–12. Malignant ulcer in the rectum, showing typical everted edges.

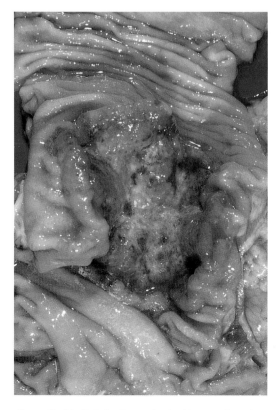

Figure 13–14. Typical malignant ulcer involving ascending colon.

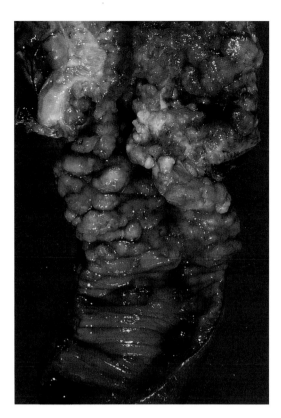

Figure 13–15. Unusual gross appearance of colon carcinoma, showing multinodular involvement of the mucosa with ulceration and stricture formation due to infiltration of the wall.

narrowing ("applecore," or "napkin ring" tumors) (Figs. 13–10 and 13–11). Rectal cancers tend to be either exophytic tumors or malignant ulcers that are characterized by a central crater surrounded by raised indurated edges (Fig. 13–12). There are many exceptions to these generalizations (Figs. 13–13 and 13–14). Some colon cancers do not fit any of these stereotypic morphologic types (Fig. 13–15). Early colorectal carcinomas resemble polypoid adenomas or sessile adenomas with evidence of infiltration at the base of the polyp on microscopic examination (Figs. 13–16 and 13–17).

Colorectal carcinomas can be multifocal; in approximately 10% of cases, a second primary occurs in some other part of the colon (Fig. 13–18). Synchronous primaries must be excluded by colonoscopy in all cases of colorectal cancer. Care must be taken to ascribe separate primaries to two positive biopsy specimens from different sites in the colon; the possibility of a single large tumor infiltrating two places in the colon, with or without a colocolic fistula must be considered (Fig. 13–19). Invasion into adjacent organs such as small intestine, stomach, and urinary bladder may be present; in these cases, the resection specimen may include parts of these organs in continuity with the colorectal tumor (Fig. 13–20).

Histologic Types of Colorectal Carcinoma. Approximately 85% of colorectal carcinomas are well and moderately differentiated adenocarcinomas (Table 13–4) (Fig. 13–21). These are composed of irregularly infiltrating malignant glands. The cells are columnar and have elongated ("cigar-shaped") nuclei. The invasive tumor is usually surrounded by a desmoplastic response (Fig. 13–21A). Focal necrosis is common, and mitotic activity is variable.

The customary grading of colorectal adenocarcinoma recognizes well, moderately, and poorly differentiated adenocarcinoma, corresponding to grades 1, 2, and 3. Well-differentiated (grade 1) adenocarcinoma consists of simple glands with orderly and uniform nuclei (see Fig. 13–21A). Moderately differentiated adenocarcinoma consists of more complex glands with cribriform structure and nuclei that are more disorderly and pleomorphic (Fig. 13–21B). Poorly differentiated carcinoma has either a diffuse or solid growth pattern without gland formation (Fig. 13–22).

The vast majority of tumors have varying mixtures of these grade patterns, and no quantitative definitions are available that indicate how tumors with a mixed pattern should be graded. If grading is done according to the worst grade seen in a tumor, irrespective of quantity, the bias will be toward high-grade tumors, and well-differentiated carcinoma will be very

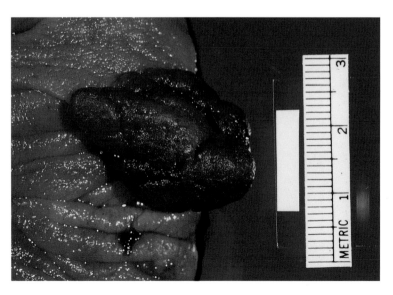

Figure 13–16. Polypoid adenocarcinoma. This is indistinguishable from a large adenoma. Differentiation is by the presence of invasive carcinoma involving the stalk or submucosa.

TABLE 13–4. FREQUENCIES OF COLORECTAL CARCINOMA BY HISTOLOGIC TYPE

Type of Carcinoma	Frequency (%)
Adenocarcinoma, well and moderately differentiated	76
Mucinous adenocarcinoma	10
Adenocarcinoma in villous adenoma	5.1
Adenocarcinoma in adenomatous polyp	4.2
Papillary adenocarcinoma	1.1
Signet ring cell adenocarcinoma	0.3
Undifferentiated carcinoma	0.2
Adenocarcinoma in familial adenomatous polyposis	0.1
Unspecified and other types	3

Adenocarcinoma occurring in hereditary nonpolyposis colorectal cancer and chronic ulcerative colitis are included within the various histologic types in this table.

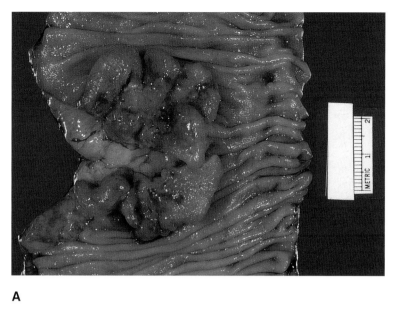

A

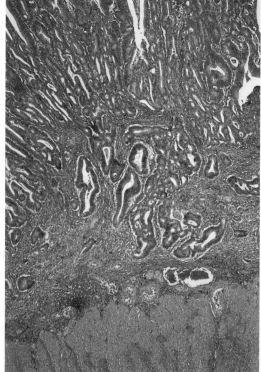

C

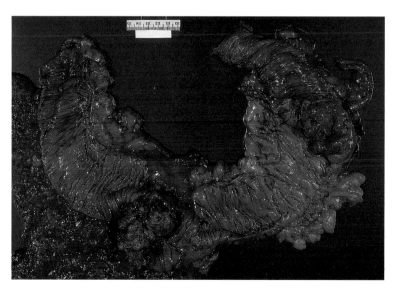

B

Figure 13–17. A: Adenocarcinoma of the colon. This is indistinguishable at endoscopy from a villous adenoma. B: Cut section of tumor in part A, showing minimal invasion at one point. C: Villous adenoma of the colon with invasive carcinoma at the base, extending to the interphase between submucosa and muscularis externa.

Figure 13–18. Synchronous carcinomas in transverse and ascending colon.

rare. For these reasons, histologic grading of colorectal carcinoma is inconsistent among pathologists. In particular, the distinction between well- and moderately differentiated adenocarcinoma is very arbitrary. It has been suggested recently that it would be more meaningful to divide the moderately differentiated carcinomas into moderately/well (Mw) and moderately/poorly (Mp) subtypes and recognize two grades (well + Mw and poorly + Mp).[22] Removal of the intermediate grade in any three-grade histologic system usually improves consistency (eg, low- and high-grade dysplasia is more consistent than mild, moderate, and severe dysplasia).

The only other type of colorectal adenocarcinoma commonly encountered is mucinous adenocarcinoma, which accounts for about 10% of colorectal carcinomas (Fig. 13–23). This is defined by the presence of large lakes of extracellular mucin in which are suspended groups and strips of well-differentiated adenocarcinomatous cells. At least 50% of the volume

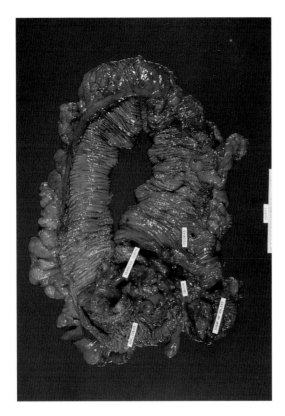

Figure 13–19. Large carcinoma involving the sigmoid colon, cecum, and terminal ileum. At colonoscopy, a biopsy was performed at its sigmoid location and cecal location, suggesting two separate primary tumors.

of the tumor must be composed of this mucinous tumor type for the designation mucinous carcinoma to be applied. Mucinous carcinoma must be distinguished from signet ring cell carcinoma, which can also have mucin lakes, but the cells associated are poorly differentiated signet ring cells (Fig. 13–24). Mucinous carcinoma has been reported to have a worse biologic behavior than usual colorectal adenocarcinoma, but a bet-

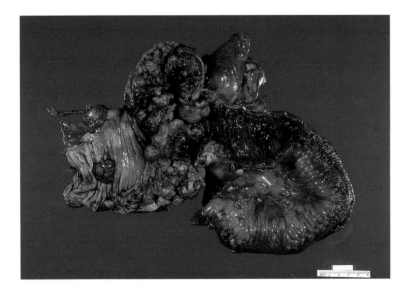

Figure 13–20. Adenocarcinoma of the high rectum, showing an obstructing carcinoma with marked dilatation of the proximal colon. The tumor has infiltrated through the wall to involve the urinary bladder, which is seen as a nodular mass of tumor.

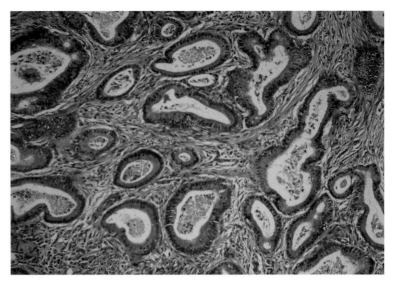

A

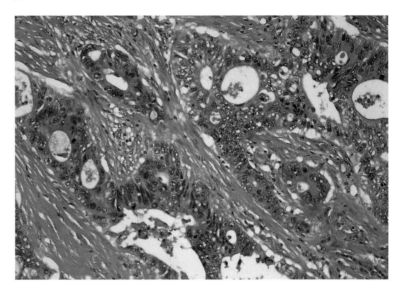

B

Figure 13–21. A: Well-differentiated adenocarcinoma of the colon, characterized by invasive simple malignant glands surrounded by desmoplasia. B: Moderately differentiated adenocarcinoma of colon, showing complex infiltrating malignant glands.

ter prognosis than signet ring cell carcinoma.[23,24] Rare signet ring cell carcinomas have a linitis plastica growth pattern, in which the muscle wall is diffusely infiltrated by a desmoplastic process with signet ring cells that can be difficult to recognize (Fig. 13–25).[25]

Other histologic types of colorectal carcinoma include adenosquamous carcinoma[26] (Fig. 13–26A), squamous carcinoma[27] (Fig. 13–26B and C), spindle cell (sarcomatoid or metaplastic) carcinoma[28] (Fig. 13–27), and clear cell adenocarcinomas[29] (Fig. 13–28). A β-human chorionic gonadotropin-producing glassy cell variant of adenosquamous carcinoma[30] and an α-fetoprotein-producing hepatoid-type of carcinoma[31] have been described as primary colonic tumors. Neuroendocrine carcinoma, including small cell undifferentiated carcinoma and composite adenocarcinoma-carcinoid are considered

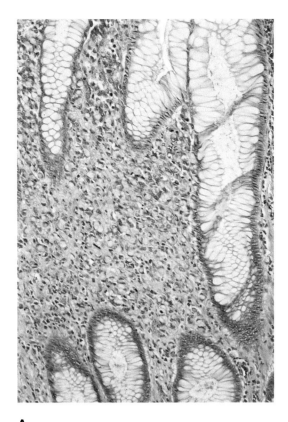

A

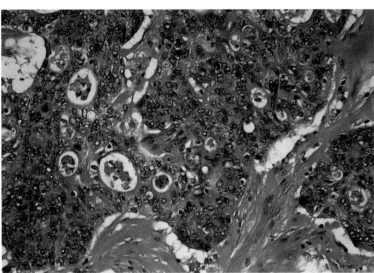

B

Figure 13–22. A: Poorly differentiated adenocarcinoma, consisting of malignant cells diffusely expanding the lamina propria. B: Poorly differentiated adenocarcinoma, solid pattern without significant gland formation.

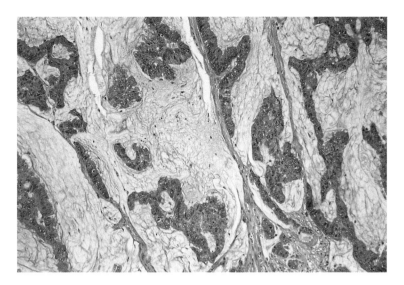

Figure 13–23. Mucinous carcinoma, consisting of well-differentiated malignant glandular elements in the extracellular mucinous lakes.

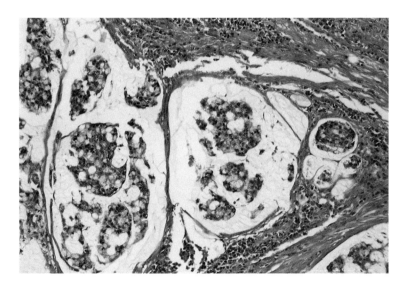

A

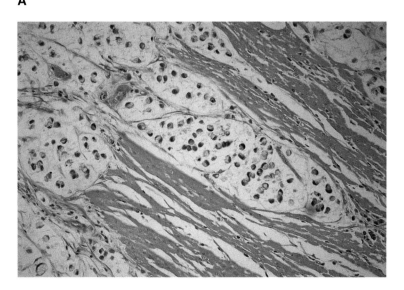

B

Figure 13–24. A: Poorly differentiated adenocarcinoma with clusters of signet ring cells in lakes of extracellular mucin. B: Signet ring cell carcinoma invading the colonic muscle. The tumor cells are single signet ring cells surrounded by extracellular mucin.

separately later in this chapter. Because of their rarity, when these histologic types of CRC are encountered, the question of whether these neoplasms represent metastases to the colon should be asked. This is best answered by looking for a primary tumor elsewhere (Fig. 13–26C) (eg, lung and uterine cervix in squamous carcinoma, lung in small cell undifferentiated carcinoma, and kidney in clear cell adenocarcinoma).

Colorectal carcinomas occurring in patients younger than 45 years old tend to be more infiltrative than usual, have a dis-

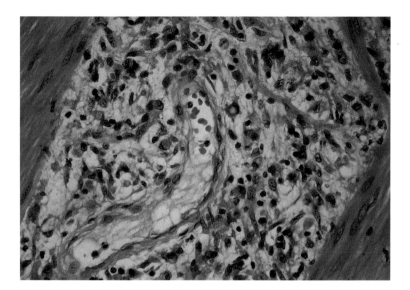

Figure 13–25. Poorly differentiated adenocarcinoma with inflammation and desmoplasia infiltrating muscle wall. Malignant cells are difficult to identify in this field.

proportionate number of signet ring cell and poorly differentiated adenocarcinomas, and have a higher occurrence of nodal metastases at presentation.[32] The higher occurrence of these negative factors makes prognosis worse in young patients.

Pathologic Staging. Pathologic staging is an expression of the degree of invasion and metastatic spread of the tumor. Accurate staging depends on the presence of a vertical section of the tumor to demonstrate the depth of invasion of the colorectal wall and on a thorough dissection of the lymph nodes in the specimen.

Evaluation of depth of invasion is not difficult in a well-oriented section. Invasion through the muscularis mucosae into the submucosa and extension into the muscle wall are easily recognized (Fig. 13–29A and B). When tumor extends into pericolic fat, full-thickness muscle invasion is easy to identify (Fig. 13–29C). When the tumor evokes a desmoplastic response, it is important to identify the external plane of the muscle wall and evaluate the limit of tumor invasion in relation to this plane (Fig. 13–29D). In some cases, the desmoplastic reaction may destroy the muscle over a large area, making it difficult to identify the plane of the outer surface of the muscle wall. Careful examination and good judgment are needed in such cases to differentiate between partial-thickness and full-thickness invasion of the muscle wall, which is a crucial staging criterion. In difficult cases, trichrome stain is helpful to distinguish muscle from collagen.

Three different systems are used for staging colorectal carcinoma, each having their advocates in different parts of the world (Table 13–5). In Europe, Dukes' system[33] is widely used. In the United States, the Astler-Coller system[34] is used in addition to Dukes' system, although a recommendation has been made that both systems be supplanted with the more detailed tumor, node, metastasis (TNM) system.[35] Because the various designations of tumor stage have different meanings within these systems, it is crucial to state which system is being used.

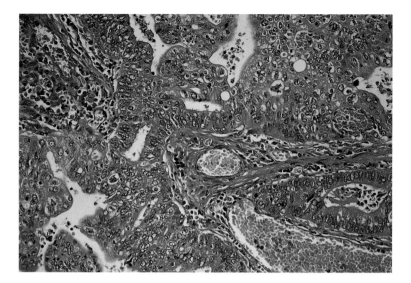

A

B

C

Figure 13–26. A: Adenosquamous carcinoma. B: Colonic biopsy specimen, showing squamous carcinoma. C: Colonic biopsy specimen, showing extensive involvement of the mucosa by squamous carcinoma. Note that the mucosal crypts are normal. This patient had a history of uterine squamous carcinoma; this most likely represents a metastatic tumor.

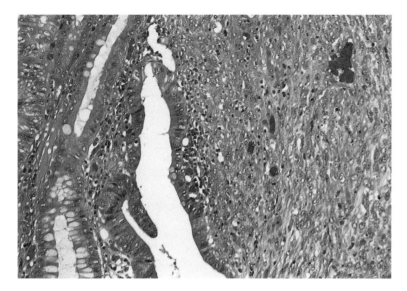

A

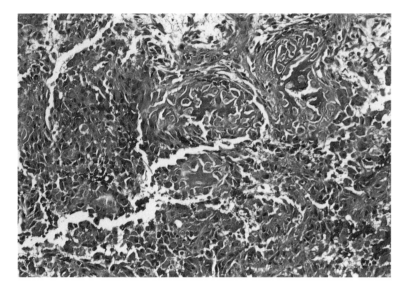

B

Figure 13–27. A: Carcinosarcoma of the colon, showing a malignant spindle cell tumor adjacent to adenocarcinoma. B: Carcinosarcoma of colon, showing osteosarcomatous differentiation with malignant cells surrounded by calcified osteoid.

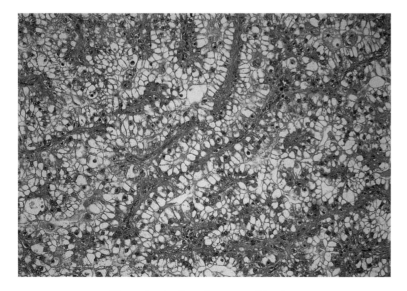

Figure 13–28. Clear cell carcinoma of the colon.

TABLE 13–5. STAGING CRITERIA OF COLORECTAL CANCER AS APPLIED BY THE DIFFERENT STAGING SYSTEMS

	Dukes'	Astler-Coller	TNM
Tumor invasion restricted to mucosa	A	A	Tis,N0
Tumor restricted to submucosa, node negative	A	B1*	T1,N0
Tumor restricted to submucosa, node positive	C	C1*	T1,N1–3†
Tumor restricted to muscle wall, node negative	A	B1	T2,N0
Tumor restricted to muscle wall, node positive	C	C1	T2,N1–3†
Tumor completely through muscle wall, node negative	B	B2	T3,N0
Tumor completely through muscle wall, node positive	C	C2	T3,N1–3†
Tumor involving adjacent organs, node negative	B	B2	T4,N0
Tumor involving adjacent organs, node positive	C	C2	T4,N1–3†
Distant metastases present irrespective of any other factors	D	D	T1–4,N0–3,M-1

Abbreviation: TNM = tumor, node, metastasis.
*Astler-Coller's original system did not include a category of invasion restricted to the submucosa; this was inserted into the system later and has a significance within this system that is equivalent to partial muscle wall invasion.
†N1 = 1–3 positive pericolic lymph nodes; N2 = 4 or more positive pericolic lymph nodes; N3 = positive node along any major named vascular trunk or a positive apical node (when marked at surgery).

The Dukes' system of staging is the simplest. Cancers restricted to the colorectal wall are stage A, those that invade outside the muscularis externa are stage B, those with positive nodes are stage C, and those that have distant metastases are stage D. The Astler-Coller system is similar, except that it provides a better distinction between minimally invasive tumors in terms of their nodal status. This is advantageous because the extent of wall invasion and nodal status are independent prognostic factors.

Although the TNM system is much more accurate in terms of its definition, it suffers the major disadvantage of being too cumbersome for general use. There is also argument about whether subdivision of tumors into so many different staging categories has practical value. To answer the second criticism, the TNM system has a stage grouping that brings it into line with the Dukes' system (Table 13–6). The TNM system is rec-

TABLE 13–6. STAGE GROUPING IN THE TNM STAGING SYSTEM AND ITS CORRELATION WITH THE OTHER SYSTEMS AND SURVIVAL

TNM Stage Grouping	TNM Criteria	Dukes'	Astler-Coller	5-year Survival Rate (%)
Stage 0	Tis N0 M0	A	A	100
Stage I	T1 N0 M0	A	B1	90
	T2 N0 M0	A	B1	80
Stage II	T3 N0 M0	B	B2	55
	T4 N0 M0	B	B2	45
Stage III	AnyT N1–3 M0	C	C1/C2	40
Stage IV	AnyT AnyN M1	D	D	<5

Abbreviation: TNM = tumor, node, metastasis.

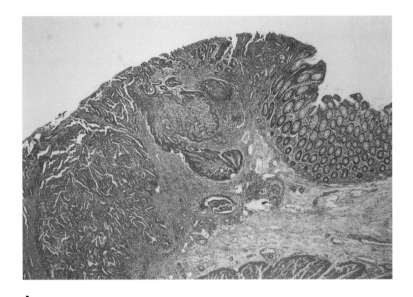

A

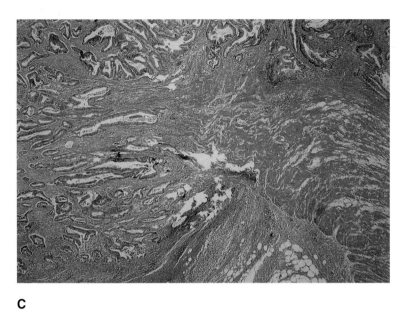

C

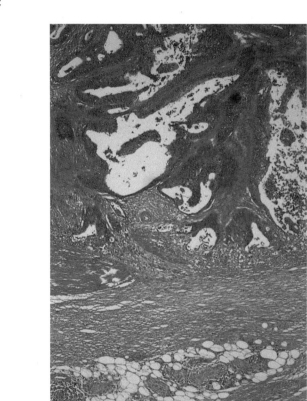

D

B

Figure 13–29. A: Adenocarcinoma of colon, showing invasion of submucosa. The muscularis mucosae, penetration of which defines submucosal involvement, is seen under the normal colonic mucosa. B: Adenocarcinoma of the colon, infiltrating the muscle wall. C: Adenocarcinoma of the colon, extending through full thickness of colonic wall to involve pericolic fat. D: Adenocarcinoma of the colon with full-thickness muscle wall invasion. The tumor is separated only by desmoplastic collagen from the pericolic fat. There is no muscle between tumor and pericolic connective tissue.

ommended in the United States and is the system used in most specialized cancer centers in this country.

From the pathologist's standpoint, it is advisable to have all the characteristics used for staging in the pathology report, so that if the patient is later evaluated in another medical center where a different system is used, the appropriate stage in that system can be determined by simply reading the report.

A frequent staging problem relates to satellite tumor nodules that are encountered in pericolic fat, which are indistinguishable on gross examination from a small lymph node (Fig.

13–30). These are nodules of tumor separate from the primary tumor that on microscopy do not have any lymphoid tissue associated with the tumor. By convention, satellites are recorded as positive lymph nodes if they are identified at gross examination. Satellites detected during microscopic examination that are smaller than 3 mm are equated to pericolic invasion.

Lymph Node Assessment. Assessment of lymph nodes is crucial to staging, decisions regarding adjuvant therapy, and evaluation of prognosis. Although the majority of metastases are found in en-

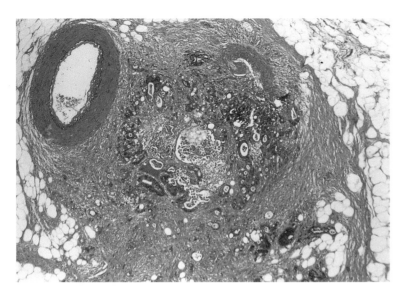

Figure 13–30. Satellite nodule in pericolic fat, consisting of a nodular mass of adenocarcinoma without association with lymph node tissue.

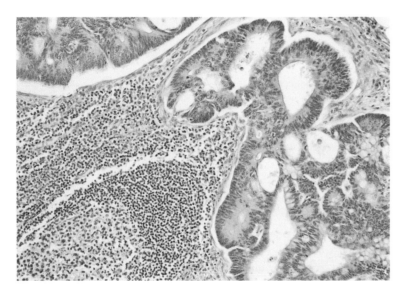

Figure 13–31. Metastatic adenocarcinoma in grossly enlarged pericolic lymph node.

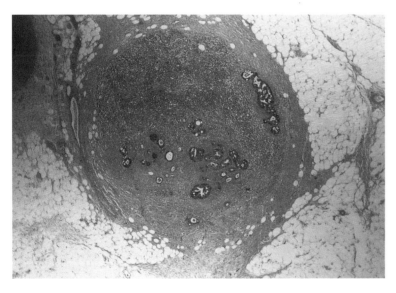

Figure 13–32. Metastatic adenocarcinoma in a small lymph node found in pericolic fat.

larged lymph nodes (Fig. 13–31), some are found in minute nodes in the pericolic fat (Fig. 13–32). Lymph nodes are found in the pericolorectal adipose tissue, mesocolon, and mesorectum and can be present at any point between the bowel wall and the margin of resection. There is no substitute for careful dissection of this predominantly adipose tissue to find lymph nodes. Fat-clearing techniques, when used, increase the harvest of nodes,[36] but are not routinely employed.

The number of lymph nodes present in a colectomy specimen varies with location, patient, and the extent of surgery. The number of nodes found in a specimen is probably determined most by the amount of effort put in by the pathologist to this task. Goldstein and colleagues[37] reported that the number of lymph nodes recovered from specimens increased in 1992 compared with the earlier 40-year period; this is about the time when the number of positive nodes became widely recognized as being an important prognostic indicator in colorectal carcinoma.

Lymph nodes are easy to find in patients with positive nodes because they are enlarged and firmer than normal. They are more difficult to find when not grossly involved by tumor. These nodes can harbor microscopic metastases, however, and are crucial to recover from a specimen. Recommendations for the minimum number of lymph nodes that must be recovered from a resection specimen to ensure node negativity varies between 12 and 17.[37,38]

Each lymph node found should be documented in terms of size and location; this is best done with a diagram of the specimen. Each node is sectioned, and half of it is submitted in a labeled cassette; multiple nodes from a localized region can be included in one cassette. One histologic section from each node is examined microscopically for evidence of metastases. This routine has been established for reasons of practicability and cost. Some evidence suggests that a more thorough examination of the nodes by submitting all the tissue and taking sections at multiple levels of the block increases the rate of positivity in lymph nodes.[39] The use of immunoperoxidase stains in negative lymph nodes permits identification of micrometastases that are not identifiable by routine light microscopy (Fig. 13–33).[40]

A potential cause of false-positive diagnosis of lymph node positivity is the presence of endosalpingiosis in lymph nodes in female patients. These are usually found in the periphery of the node as small glandular spaces lined by flattened epithelial cells without cytologic features of malignancy.

Assessment of Lymphovascular Invasion.
Lymphovascular invasion is not of prognostic value, and its presence does not direct any change in treatment in the usual colorectal adenocarcinoma (Fig. 13–34). Lymphovascular invasion by carcinoma is of practical value in two situations: (1) In patients with carcinomatous polyps, the presence of lymphovascular invasion in the stalk is an indication for surgical resection irrespective of any other factor. (2) In localized resections of low rectal carcinomas, the presence of lymphovascular invasion has been suggested as an

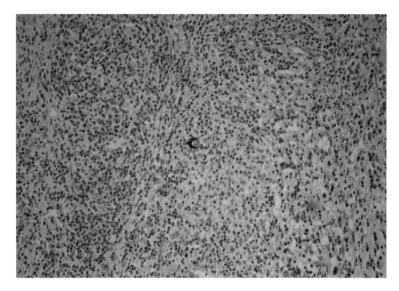

A

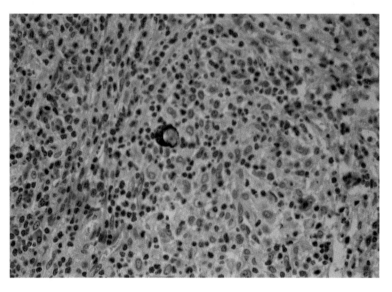

B

Figure 13–33. A: Histologically negative lymph node, stained by immunoperoxidase for cytokeratin, showing a single positive cell indicative of micrometastasis. B: High power showing malignant cytologic features of the keratin positive cell.

indication that the patient needs further therapy. The presence of perineural invasion is not uncommonly seen in colorectal carcinoma (Fig. 13–35); this is not of established prognostic significance.

Assessment of Surgical Margins. All segments of resected colon and rectum have a proximal and distal margin composed of colorectum, or perianal skin in the case of an abdominoperineal resection of the rectum.

For purposes of evaluation of the other surgical margins, colorectal resections can be divided into three specimen types (Fig. 13–36):

1. The transverse and sigmoid colon are suspended in the peritoneal cavity by a mesocolon. Except for the mesocolonic at-

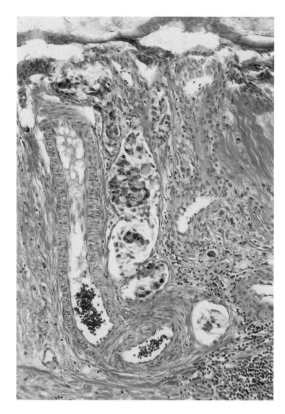

Figure 13–34. Lymphovascular invasion in colon carcinoma.

tachment, these segments of colon are covered entirely by peritoneum, with only a small amount of pericolic fat between the muscle wall and peritoneal mesothelium. The only surgical margin in these colonic segments is the point of separation of the base of the mesocolon from the posterior abdominal wall. Penetration through the colonic wall may involve the peritoneal surface, and this should be documented, but this is a surface involvement, not a margin involvement. The surgical margin at the base of the mesocolon is rarely involved by tumor unless positive lymph nodes are present there.

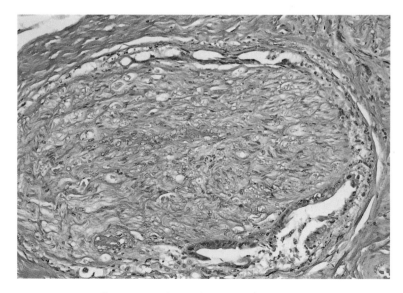

Figure 13–35. Perineural invasion in colon carcinoma.

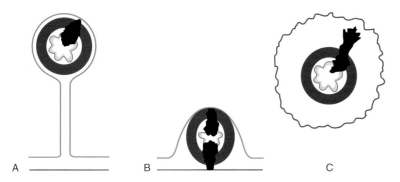

Figure 13–36. Diagram of different types of colorectal specimens, classified according to factors affecting evaluation of surgical margins. A: Colon suspended in the peritoneal cavity by a mesocolon (eg, sigmoid and transverse colon). A transmural tumor at any point in the circumference can involve the serosa (*green*), causing peritoneal seeding. The surgical margin (*red*) is separated from the tumor by the mesocolon. B: Colon in the retroperitoneum, covered by the peritoneum of the paracolic gutters in its anterior half (eg, ascending and descending colon). Anterior tumors involve serosa, whereas posterior tumors involve the retroperitoneum with risk of surgical margin involvement. C: Rectum below the peritoneal relationship. The external surface of this specimen consists of a surgical margin where the rectum is separated from the rest of the pelvic structures.

2. The cecum, ascending colon, and descending colon are located in the paracolic gutters. The anterior half of the colonic wall is covered by peritoneum; the posterior half is separated from the abdominal wall by pericolic connective tissue. The entire posterior surface represents a surgical margin. This must be carefully inked and the relationship of tumor to this margin documented grossly and microscopically. Involvement of the peritoneal surface by a carcinoma involving the anterior wall should also be documented, but this does not represent a positive surgical margin. It is a matter of concern that posterior margin assessment in this type of specimen is not widely addressed in the literature.

3. The rectum is located below the pelvic peritoneal reflection and therefore does not have a peritoneal surface. The rectum is removed from the side and posterior wall of the pelvis and separated anteriorly from the uterus and vagina (in females) or bladder and prostate (in males). The rectum therefore has a radial surgical margin that covers the entire circumference. This entire margin should be inked and its relationship to the tumor must be established by careful gross and microscopic examination. In some centers, the rectal resection specimen is fixed in situ for 3 days after inking the margin and then cut in as whole-mount sections, which permit elegant evaluation of the relationship of the tumor to all its margins. This technique requires outsize cassettes, microtomes adapted to cut large blocks, and 4″ × 3″ glass slides, and is rarely used in the United States.

Assessment of Local Resections of Low Rectal Carcinomas. Transanal resections are being increasingly performed for large low rectal adenomas and low rectal carcinomas with invasion that is clinically restricted to the submucosa.[21] These specimens present a special problem to the pathologist. The ideal specimen, commonly produced when the surgery is done by the TEM technique, consists of a rectangular piece of mucosa-covered rectal tissue that is submitted in one piece (see Fig. 12–38). The tumor is in the center, and there is a rim of uninvolved mucosa on all sides. The depth of rectal wall submitted varies, but the specimen commonly contains the full thickness of the wall with pericolic connective tissue. The specimen must be submitted to the pathologist immediately after removal with sutures that provide orientation of the specimen. Transanal resection specimens that are suboptimal in being fragmented or submitted in formalin are very difficult to evaluate appropriately.

The pathologist inks the deep surgical margin (multicolor inks can be used to identify deep, anterior, posterior, and left and right lateral margins), and then pins out the specimen on a cork board using multiple pins to pull out the mucosal edges and compensate for the tissue contraction that might give the impression of a false-positive margin. The specimen is fixed overnight and cut in completely. This technique is necessary to provide accurate information regarding depth of invasion and document that the mucosal margins are clear in these limited resections.

TEM specimens have been evaluated by criteria that are more detailed that those used for standard colorectal cancers[41]:

1. The gross pattern of growth is reported as polypoid or nonpolypoid.
2. The grade of the tumor is determined by the deepest invasive tumor as well, moderately well (Mw), moderately poorly (Mp) and poorly differentiated.
3. The presence or absence of lymphatic invasion is recorded.
4. When invasion is limited to the submucosa, the level of invasion within the submucosa is classified into superficial submucosal (sm-s) and deep submucosal (sm-d) based on whether invasion was confined to the superficial 50% of the submucosa or not.

In early rectal carcinomas, the risk of lymph node positivity increases with a nonpolypoid growth pattern, poorly or moderately poorly differentiated tumor, the presence of lymphatic invasion, and deep submucosal or muscle wall invasion.[22] The recognition of any of these adverse indicators may result in an extended surgical resection or adjuvant therapy.[41,42]

Assessment of Prognosis

Prognosis of colorectal carcinoma is most significantly predicted by the pathologic stage (see Table 13–6). Within each individual stage, however, patients can be further stratified by the presence or absence of a large number of other factors, which act as independent prognostic indicators (Table 13–7).[43–51]

Patients who have adverse risk indicators are considered for adjuvant chemotherapy. In 1990, the National Institutes of Health Consensus Conference made the following recommendations regarding adjuvant chemotherapy[52]: Patients with TNM stage III colon cancer and stage II/III rectal cancer are at high enough risk to warrant adjuvant therapy. A combination of flu-orouracil and levamisole was advocated for colon cancer; combined postoperative chemotherapy and radiation was advocated for rectal cancer. The statement also suggested that many of the factors listed in Table 13–6 as "factors not routinely used" may define subsets of patients with stage II colon cancer whose risk may be high enough to merit testing adjuvant chemotherapy. Oncologists sometimes use lymph node micrometastases, cytoplasmic *p53* accumulation, 18q deletion, and aneuploidy in their clinical decision-making process in patients with stage II colon cancer.

Treatment Failure

Types of Treatment Failure

Three types of treatment failure occur after surgery for CRC, with or without adjuvant chemotherapy.

Locoregional Failure. Locoregional failure is a recurrence of tumor in or around the anastomotic site (Fig. 13–37). Locoregional failure results from positive surgical margins whether or not margin positivity was detected at the initial pathologic examination. Locoregional recurrence correlates best with the degree of invasion of the colorectal wall by the tumor; the more extensively tumors infiltrate pericolic or perirectal connective tissue, the greater the likelihood of undetected soft tissue margin positivity. After anastomosis, the viable tumor cells that remain multiply in the pericolic and perirectal connective tissue, producing tumor masses that remain silent for a long

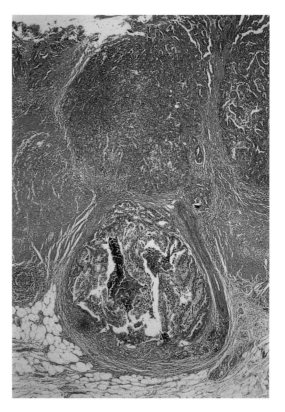

Figure 13–37. Recurrent adenocarcinoma at an anastomotic region, showing a large mass involving the pericolic fat extending through the colonic wall to cause mucosal ulceration.

time. Involvement of the colorectal wall at the site of anastomosis and the ability to detect tumor at colonoscopy are late features.

In low rectal tumors that have a relatively small distal surgical margin and in carcinomas treated by local resections of the rectum, which frequently have small surgical margins, locoregional recurrence may be due to undetected intestinal margin involvement. In such cases, recurrence results in changes visible at endoscopy at a much earlier stage.

Peritoneal Metastasis. Peritoneal metastasis is the result of seeding of the peritoneal cavity by the tumor prior to surgery. Involvement of the peritoneal cavity occurs with colonic tumors that are related to a peritoneal surface (eg, transverse and sigmoid colon tumors, anterior wall ascending and descending colon tumors), and which invade through the full thickness of the wall to involve the serosal lining. Involvement of the peritoneal cavity can be assessed at the time of surgery by cytologic examination of peritoneal lavage and serosal scrapings[53] (Fig. 13–38). This is rarely done.

Distant Metastasis. Distant metastases may manifest in lymph nodes more proximal to those in the field of initial surgery and elsewhere in the body (most commonly liver, lungs, brain, and bone) due to hematogenous spread (Fig. 13–39). Occurrence of

TABLE 13–7. FACTORS USED AS INDEPENDENT PROGNOSTIC INDICATORS IN COLORECTAL CARCINOMA

Routinely Used Factors
Pathologic stage: The strongest criterion
Histologic grade: Poorly differentiated carcinoma (including signet ring cell carcinoma) is worst; well-differentiated carcinoma is best; mucinous carcinoma is intermediate.

Experimental Factors Not in Routine Use
Micrometastases in histologically negative nodes demonstrated by cytokeratin immunostaining is an adverse marker[39]
Micrometastases in bone marrow and peritoneal cavity detected by multiple antibody immuno-staining is an adverse factor[40]
HER-2/neu (*p185*) overexpression is an adverse factor[41]
Cytoplasmic *p53* accumulation demonstrated by immunohistochemical staining is an adverse factor[42]
Aneuploidy is an adverse factor in Dukes' stage B tumors[43]
Allelic loss of chromosome 18q is a strong adverse factor in TNM stage II and III cancers[44]
Higher levels of tumor angiogenesis is an adverse factor[45]
Low levels of intratumoral CD57-positive natural killer cells is an adverse factor[46]
A preoperative serum carcinoembryonic antigen value > 5 ng/mL is an adverse factor[47]

Abbreviation: TNM = tumor, node, metastasis.

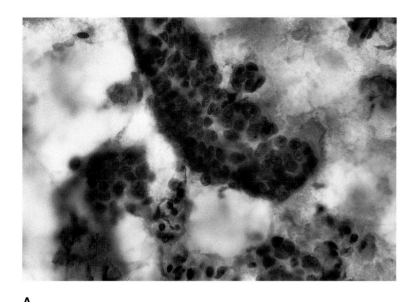

A

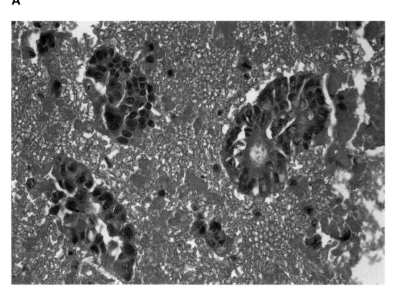

B

Figure 13–38. Metastatic colon carcinoma in the peritoneal cavity. A: Smear of ascitic fluid, showing a cluster of malignant glandular cells. The cells are well differentiated and do not have features that permit definitive diagnosis of primary site as colon. B: Cell block preparation, showing well-differentiated adenocarcinoma. The cytologic features are suggestive of a gastrointestinal primary.

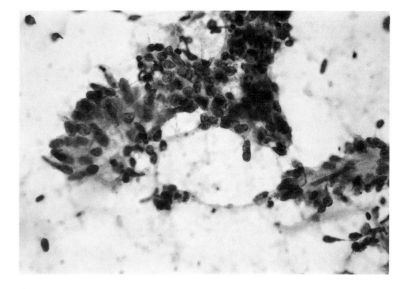

A

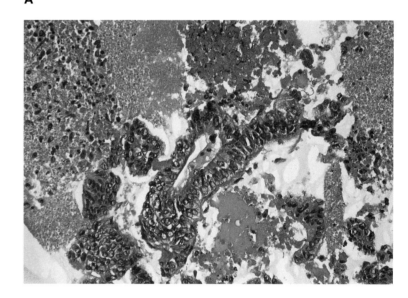

B

Figure 13–39. A: Fine-needle aspiration of a liver nodule, showing the typical columnar cells with cigar-shaped nuclei that is predictive for a colon primary. B: Cell block preparation of metastatic colon adenocarcinoma in liver.

distant metastases correlate best with stage of disease, particularly lymph node status.

Detection of Treatment Failures

The occurrence of symptoms is the most common method whereby treatment failures manifest.[54] There is no satisfactory method for detecting treatment failures at a time when treatment can significantly affect the further course of the disease. Serial serum assays for carcinoembryonic antigen (CEA), CT scans, radionuclide liver scans, and colonoscopy have all been recommended and are done, usually with unsatisfactory results in prolonging survival in those patients that fail treatment.

Serum CEA is the most widely used test for detection of recurrence. Elevated serum CEA levels occur in approximately 60% of patients who develop recurrences, often before the recurrence becomes manifest clinically. The maximum sensitivity of serum CEA elevation is in the detection of hepatic metastases.[55] In addition to the significant false-negative rate, false-positive elevation of serum CEA also occurs.[56] In about 1% of patients followed for colorectal carcinoma, resection of a recurrence detected by an elevated CEA is associated with long-term survival.[56]

The most important test in the follow-up of patients treated for CRC is routine colonoscopic surveillance for the occurrence of a metachronous second primary colorectal carcinoma, an event which occurs in 5–10% of patients.

COLORECTAL NEUROENDOCRINE TUMORS

Neuroendocrine tumors of the colorectum constitute a spectrum of malignant neoplasm from the most differentiated (carcinoid tumor) through atypical carcinoid tumors, goblet cell carcinoid tumors (adenocarcinoid), to poorly differentiated neuroendocrine carcinoma. Many adenocarcinomas also contain small numbers of neuroendocrine cells, but these are of no practical importance because biologically they behave the same as adenocarcinoma. Composite adenocarcinoma-carcinoid tumors composed of approximately equal amounts of adenocarcinoma and well-differentiated carcinoid tumor are very rare in the colorectum.

Carcinoid Tumors

Carcinoid tumors occur throughout the colon and rectum. Although the appendix is widely held to be the commonest gas-

trointestinal location for carcinoid tumors, rectal carcinoids account for more than 50% of gastrointestinal carcinoids in some series.[57] Colorectal carcinoid tumors are malignant neoplasms whose risk of metastasis vary greatly with the location and size of the tumor.

Rectal Carcinoid Tumors

Rectal carcinoid tumors usually occur in patients older than age 40 years and commonly present as a solitary, small nodule covered with intact mucosa. They are discovered during rectal examination of asymptomatic patients or during examination for other benign anorectal disease. Rectal carcinoids are not hormonally active. They do not produce carcinoid syndrome even when liver metastases are present.

Ninety percent of rectal carcinoid tumors are smaller than 2 cm. Rectal carcinoids that are smaller than 2 cm have a very low risk of metastasis. There is no guarantee that any rectal carcinoid will not metastasize; however, because lymph node

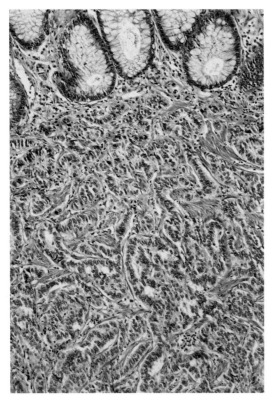

A

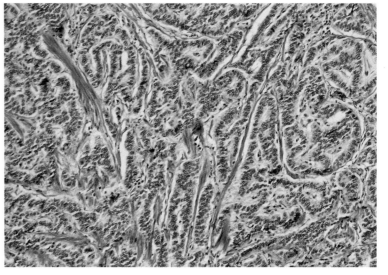

B

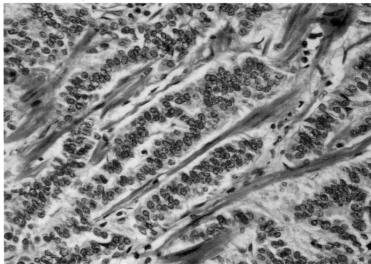

C

Figure 13–40. A: Rectal carcinoid tumor, showing involvement of deep mucosa and submucosa with overlying intact mucosa. B: Rectal carcinoid tumor, showing a trabecular pattern. C: Higher power micrograph of part B, showing small cells with uniform round nuclei arranged in a trabecular pattern.

metastasis has been reported with a 1-mm rectal carcinoid located entirely in the submucosa.[58]

Tumors smaller than 1 cm can be treated with endoscopic polypectomy and fulguration; this can be done in the first examination if the nature of the tumor is recognized clinically. When a polypectomy reveals a rectal carcinoid and the pathologic examination reveals margin involvement, a second procedure with repeat biopsy of the base and fulguration is necessary. Rectal carcinoids that are 1–2 cm in size may require local transanal surgical excision after biopsy.

Rectal carcinoid tumors that are ulcerated, associated with rectal bleeding, or larger than 2 cm in size, or that show increased mitotic activity or microscopic evidence of muscle invasion have a high risk of metastasis and should be treated with a standard cancer resection after biopsy. Such tumors constitute approximately 10% of rectal carcinoid tumors.

Microscopically, rectal carcinoid tumors are circumscribed but unencapsulated nodules that involve the deep mucosa and submucosa (Fig. 13–40A). Extension into the muscle is limited to the large tumors. The tumor commonly has a nested or trabecular pattern (Fig. 13–40B and C). Microacinar structures are common (Fig. 13–41). The cells are small and uniform with typical round nuclei with granular chromatin. Cytologic atypia and significant mitotic activity (atypical carcinoid tumor) are rare. Rectal carcinoids show positivity with chromogranin A, neuron-specific enolase, and synaptophysin.

The main differential diagnostic problem is the possibility of rectal involvement by an adenocarcinoma of the prostate. The differentiation between these is complicated by the fact that 80% of rectal carcinoid tumors show positive staining with prostatic acid phosphatase. Stain for prostate-specific antigen is negative, and neuroendocrine markers are positive in rectal carcinoid; this immunophenotype and the histologic appearance should be used to make the distinction.[59]

Carcinoid Tumors of the Colon

Colonic carcinoids occur in a wide age range, with a mean age at diagnosis of 60 years. They are rare, with the cecum accounting for about 50% of colonic carcinoid tumors and the remainder distributed throughout the rest of the colon.[60] Multiple carcinoid tumors occur in 10% of patients. Grossly, the smaller tumors present incidentally at endoscopy as smooth-surfaced

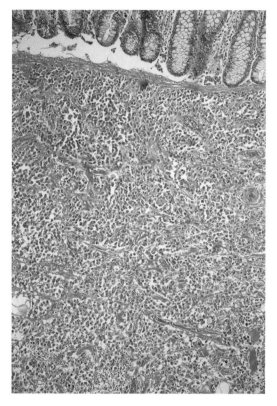

A

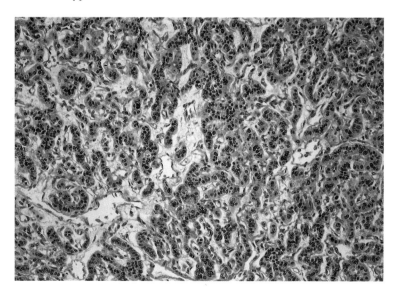

B

Figure 13–42. Colonic carcinoid tumor. A: Submucosal mass of small cells with round nuclei. The tumor has a more diffuse architecture than the usual nested pattern. This tumor diffusely infiltrated the wall and metastasized to the liver. B: Trabecular architecture and significant cytologic atypia. This tumor also metastasized.

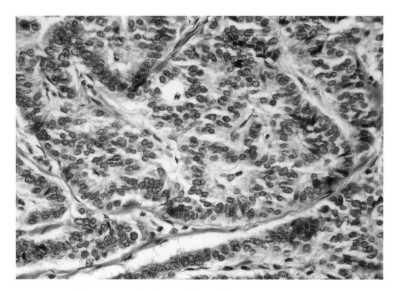

Figure 13–41. Rectal carcinoid tumor, showing microacinar pattern.

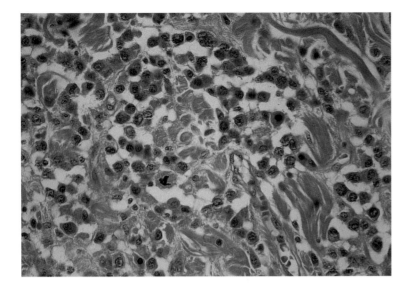

A

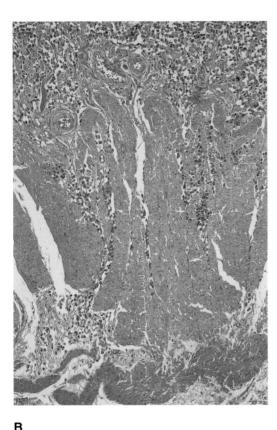

B

Figure 13–43. A: Malignant carcinoid tumor of the colon, showing small round cells arranged in an infiltrative pattern. The cells show nuclear atypia and mitotic activity. B: Irregular invasion of the muscle wall by malignant carcinoid tumor of the colon.

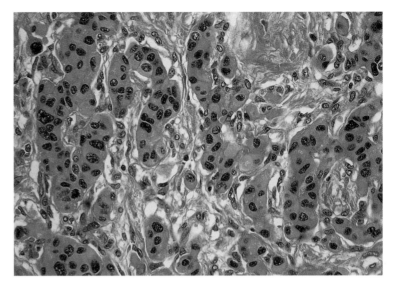

A

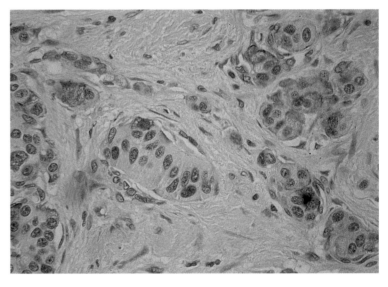

B

Figure 13–44. A: Poorly differentiated large-cell neuroendocrine carcinoma of the colon. The tumor shows malignant cytology with a suggestion of a nested architecture. B: Neuroendocrine carcinoma of the colon shown in part A.

polyps. The larger tumors show ulceration and resemble other malignant neoplasms. Microscopically, they have a typical nested, trabecular, or microacinar appearance (Fig. 13–42). Cytologic atypia, increased mitotic activity, ulceration, and muscle invasion occur in larger tumors (Fig. 13–43). Vascular invasion is frequently present, even in smaller tumors.

Colonic carcinoid tumors have a greater malignant potential than rectal carcinoids. Even tumors less than 2 cm in size have a significant metastasis rate. The vast majority of colonic carcinoids are found when their size is greater than 2 cm, when the risk of metastasis is high. The usual treatment for almost all colonic carcinoid tumors is a standard colon resection, including the lymphatic drainage. Local resection may be considered for a colonic carcinoid smaller than 2 cm but appears to be an inferior treatment when surgical risk is compared with benefit.[59] The overall prognosis of colonic carcinoids is poor, with a 5-year survival rate of less than 40%.

Patients with colorectal carcinoids have an increased risk of developing colorectal adenocarcinoma. For this reason, surveillance is indicated.

Goblet Cell Carcinoid

Goblet cell carcinoid commonly occurs only in the appendix (see Chapter 9). It is a rare tumor in the colorectum. Tumors composed of signet ring cells that occur in the colon are overwhelmingly poorly differentiated adenocarcinomas; some of these have interspersed endocrine cells, but this does not alter their behavior, which is that of a poorly differentiated adenocarcinoma.

Poorly Differentiated Neuroendocrine Carcinoma

Poorly differentiated neuroendocrine carcinoma includes large-cell neuroendocrine carcinoma and small-cell neuroendocrine carcinoma. Large-cell neuroendocrine carcinomas resemble poorly differentiated colorectal adenocarcinomas in all respects and can be differentiated from them only by ultrastructural demonstration of dense core granules or immunohistochemical demonstration of chromogranin A, neuron-specific enolase, and synaptophysin (Fig. 13–44). The recognition of large-cell neuroendocrine carcinomas from adenocarcinomas is not of great practical importance because the treatment and prognosis of the two are similar.

Small-cell neuroendocrine carcinomas are rare. When encountered, the question usually arises that they may represent a metastasis from a primary lung tumor because this histologic pattern is common in the lung. There is no way to pathologically differentiate between a primary and metastatic small-cell neuroendocrine carcinoma of the colorectum; differentiation is best done by excluding a lung primary by clinical testing. Small-cell neuroendocrine carcinomas are highly aggressive neoplasms with early hematogenous spread. Many patients first present with liver metastases. Few patients survive 1 year, even with aggressive chemotherapy.

References

1. Thomas RM, Sobin LH. Gastrointestinal cancer. *Cancer* (Supp). 1995;75:154–170.
2. O'Brien MJ, Gibbons D. The adenoma-carcinoma sequence in colorectal neoplasia. *Surg Oncol Clin North Am.* 1996;5:513–530.
3. Eide TJ. Remnants of adenomas in colorectal carcinomas. *Cancer.* 1983;51:1866–1872.
4. Muto T, Kamiya J, Sawada T, et al. Small "flat adenoma" of the large bowel with special reference to its clinicopathologic features. *Dis Colon Rectum.* 1985;28:847–851.
5. Jaramillo E, Watanabe M, Slezak P, et al. Flat neoplastic lesions of the colon and rectum detected by high resolution video endoscopy and chromoscopy. *Gastrointest Endosc.* 1995;42:114–122.
6. Riddell RH. Flat adenomas and carcinoma: Seeking the invisible? (Editorial) *Gastrointest Endosc.* 1992;38:721–723.
7. Lanspa SJ, Rouse J, Smyrk T, et al. Epidemiologic characteristics of the flat adenoma of Muto: A prospective study. *Dis Colon Rectum.* 1992;35:543–546.
8. Burt RW. Screening of patients with a positive family history of colorectal cancer. *Gastrointest Endosc Clin North Am* 1997;7: 65–79.
9. Pretlow TP, Barrow BJ, Ashton WS, et al. Aberrant crypts: Putative preneoplastic foci in human colonic mucosa. *Cancer Res.* 1991;51:1564–1567.
10. Goelz SE, Vogelstein B, Hamilton SR, et al. Hypomethylation of DNA from benign and malignant human colon neoplasms. *Science.* 1985;228:187–190.
11. Vogelstein B, Fearon ER, Hamilton SR, et al. Genetic alterations during colorectal tumor development. *N Engl J Med.* 1988;319: 525–532.
12. Yanoshita RK, Konishi M, Ito S, et al. Genetic changes of both p53 alleles associated with the conversion from colorectal adenoma to early carcinoma in familial adenomatous polyposis and non-familial adenomatous polyposis patients. *Cancer Res.* 1992;52: 3965–3971.
13. Kim H, Jung JK, Park JH, et al. Immunohistochemical characteristics of colorectal carcinoma with DNA replication errors. *J Korean Med Sci.* 1996;11:137–143.
14. Winawer SJ, Zauber AG, Ho MN, et al. Prevention of colorectal cancer by colonoscopic polypectomy. *N Engl J Med.* 1993;329: 1977–1981.
15. Pitsch RJ, Becker JM, Dayton MT. The occurrence of colon cancer in patients with known premalignant colonic mucosal diseases. *J Surg Res.* 1994;57:293–298.
16. Farouk R, Dodds J, MacDonald AW, et al. Feasibility study for use of brush cytology as a complementary method for diagnosis of rectal cancer. *Dis Colon Rectum.* 1997;40:609–613.
17. Milsom JW, Czyrko C, Hull TL, et al. Preoperative biopsy of pararectal lymph nodes in rectal cancer using endoluminal ultrasonography. *Dis Colon Rectum.* 1994;37:364–368.
18. Fengler SA, Pearl RK. Technical considerations in the surgical treatment of colon and rectal cancer. *Semin Surg Oncol.* 1994;10: 200–207.
19. Franklin ME Jr, Rosenthal D, Norem RF. Prospective evaluation of laparoscopic colon resection versus open colon resection for adenocarcinoma. A multicenter study. *Surg Endosc.* 1995;9:811–816.
20. Jacquet P, Averbach AM, Jacquet N. Abdominal wall metastasis and peritoneal carcinomatosis after laparoscopic-assisted colectomy for colon cancer. *Eur J Surg Oncol.* 1995;21:568–570.
21. Stipa S, Chiavellati L, Nicolanti V, et al. Microscopic endoluminal tumorectomy. *Dis Colon Rectum.* 1994;37:S81–85.
22. Tanaka S, Haruma K, Teixeira CR, et al. Endoscopic treatment of submucosal invasive colorectal carcinoma with special reference to risk factors for lymph node metastasis. *J Gastroenterol.* 1995;30:710–717.
23. Sacco GB, Fardelli R, Campora E, et al. Primary mucinous adenocarcinoma and signet ring cell carcinomas of colon and rectum. *Oncology.* 1994;51:30–34.
24. Anthony T, George R, Rodriguez-Bigas M, et al. Primary signet ring cell carcinoma of the colon and rectum. *Ann Surg Oncol.* 1996;3:344–348.
25. Shirouzu K, Isomoto H, Morodomi T, et al. Primary linitis plastica carcinoma of the colon and rectum. *Cancer.* 1994;74:1863–1868.
26. Novello P, Duvillard P, Grandjouan S, et al. Carcinomas of the colon with multidirectional differentiation. *Dig Dis Sci.* 1995;40: 100–106.
27. Vraux H, Kartheuser A, Haot J, et al. Primary squamous-cell carcinoma of the colon: A case report. *Acta Chir Belg.* 1994;94:318–320.
28. Isimbaldi G, Sironi M, Assi A. Sarcomatoid carcinoma of the colon. Report of the second case with immunohistochemical study. *Pathol Rest Pract.* 1996;192:483–487.
29. Rubio CA. Clear cell adenocarcinoma of the colon. *J Clin Pathol.* 1995;48:1142–1144.
30. Aru A, Rasmussen LA, Federspiel B, et al. Glassy cell carcinoma of

the colon with human chorionic gonadotropin production. A case report with immunohistochemical and ultrastructural analysis. *Am J Surg Pathol.* 1996;20:187–192.

31. Hocking GR, Shembrey M, Hay D, et al. Alpha-fetoprotein producing adenocarcinoma of the sigmoid colon with possible hepatoid differentiation. *Pathology.* 1995;27:277–279.

32. Cusack JC, Giacco GC, Clearly K, et al. Survival factors in 186 patients younger than 40 years old with colorectal adenocarcinoma. *J Am Coll Surg.* 1996;183:105–112.

33. Dukes CE. The classification of cancer of the rectum. *J Pathol Bacteriol.* 1932;35:322–332.

34. Astler VA, Coller FA. The prognostic significance of direct extension of carcinoma of the colon and rectum. *Ann Surg.* 1954;139:846–852.

35. Beahrs OH, Henson DE, Hulter RV. *Colon and Rectum: AJCC Manual for Staging of Cancer,* 4th ed. Philadelphia, JB Lippincott, 1992. pp. 75–82.

36. Scott KW, Grace RH. Detection of lymph node metastases in colorectal carcinoma before and after fat clearance. *Br J Surg.* 1989;76:1165–1167.

37. Goldstein NS, Sanford W, Coffey M, et al. Lymph node recovery from colorectal resection specimens removed for adenocarcinoma. Trends over time and a recommendation for a minimum number of lymph nodes to be recovered. *Am J Clin Pathol.* 1996;106:209–216.

38. Fielding LP, Arsenault PA, Chapuis PH, et al. Working party report to the World Congress of Gastroenterology, Sydney, 1990. *J Gastroenterol Hepatol.* 1991;6:325–344.

39. Wilkinson EJ, Hause L. Probability in lymph node sectioning. *Cancer.* 1974;33:1269–1274.

40. Cutait R, Alves VA, Lopes LC, et al. Restaging of colorectal cancer based on the identification of lymph node micrometastases through immunoperoxidase staining of CEA and cytokeratins. *Dis Colon Rectum.* 1991;34:917–920.

41. Tanaka S, Yokota T, Saito D, et al. Clinicopathologic features of early rectal carcinoma and indications for endoscopic treatment. *Dis Colon Rectum.* 1995;38:959–963.

42. Bleday R, Breen E, Jessup JM, et al. Prospective evaluation of local excision for small rectal cancers. *Dis Colon Rectum.* 1997;40:388–392.

43. Bertoglio S, Percivale P, Gambini C, et al. Cytokeratin immunostaining reveals micrometastasis in negative hematoxylin-eosin lymph nodes of resected stage I-II (pT2–pT3) colorectal cancer. *J Chemother.* 1997;9:119–120.

44. Juhl H, Kalthoff H, Kruger U, et al. Immunocytologic detection of micrometastatic cells in patients with gastrointestinal tumors. *Zentralbl Chir.* 1995;120:116–122 (German).

45. Kapitanovic S, Radosevic S, Kapitanovic M, et al. The expression of p185(HER-2/*neu*) correlates with the stage of disease and survival in colorectal cancer. *Gastroenterology.* 1997;112:1103–1113.

46. Bosari S, Viale G, Bossi P, et al. Cytoplasmic accumulation of p53 protein: An independent prognostic indicator in colorectal adenocarcinomas. *J Natl Cancer Inst.* 1994;86:681–687.

47. Takanishi DM, Hart J, Covarelli P, et al. Ploidy as a prognostic factor in colonic adenocarcinoma. *Arch Surg.* 1996;131:587–592.

48. Jen J, Kim H, Piantadosi S, et al. Allelic loss of chromosome 18q and prognosis in colorectal cancer. *N Engl J Med.* 1994;331:213–221.

49. Saclarides TJ, Speziale NJ, Drab E, et al. Tumor angiogenesis and rectal carcinoma. *Dis Colon Rectum.* 1994;37:921–926.

50. Coca S, Perez-Piqueras J, Martinez D, et al. The prognostic significance of intramural natural killer cells in patients with colorectal carcinoma. *Cancer.* 1997;79:2320–2328.

51. Slentz K, Senagore A, Hibbert J, et al. Can preoperative and postoperative CEA predict survival after colon cancer resection? *Am Surg.* 1994;60:528–532.

52. NIH Consensus Conference. Adjuvant therapy for patients with colon and rectal cancer. *JAMA.* 1990;264:1444–1450.

53. Uras C, Altinkaya E, Yardimci H, et al. Peritoneal cytology in the determination of free tumour cells within the abdomen in colon cancer. *Surg Oncol.* 1996;5:259–263.

54. Peethambaram P, Weiss M, Loprinzi CL, et al. An evaluation of postoperative follow-up tests in colon cancer patients treated for cure. *Oncology.* 1997;54:287–292.

55. McCall JL, Black RB, Rich CA, et al. The value of serum carcinoembryonic antigen in predicting recurrent disease following curative resection of colorectal cancer. *Dis Colon Rectum.* 1994;37:875–881.

56. Lucha PA Jr, Rosen L, Olenwine JA, et al. Value of carcinoembryonic antigen monitoring in curative surgery for recurrent colorectal carcinoma. *Dis Colon Rectum.* 1997;40:145–149.

57. Jetmore AB, Ray JE, Gathright JB Jr, et al. Rectal carcinoids: The most frequent carcinoid tumor. *Dis Colon Rectum.* 1992;35:717–725.

58. Seow CF, Ho J. Tiny carcinoids may be malignant. *Dis Colon Rectum.* 1993;36:309–310.

59. Stinner B, Kisker O, Zielke A, et al. Surgical management for carcinoid tumors of small bowel, appendix, colon, and rectum. *World J Surg.* 1996;20:183–188.

60. Ballantyne GH, Savoca PE, Flannery JT, et al. Incidence and mortality of carcinoids of the colon. Data from the Connecticut Tumor Registry. *Cancer.* 1992;69:2400–2405.

14

MESENCHYMAL TUMORS OF THE GASTROINTESTINAL TRACT

Milton Kiyabu

▶ CHAPTER OUTLINE

GASTROINTESTINAL STROMAL NEOPLASMS

Gastrointestinal stromal (GIST) tumors are the most common mesenchymal neoplasms of the gastrointestinal tract. They are found throughout the GI tract from the esophagus to the rectum. Although generally solitary, multiple tumors have been reported, particularly in human immunodeficiency virus (HIV)-infected individuals.[1–3] GIST can present as submucosal, intramural, or subserosal tumors (Figs. 14–1, 14–2, and 14–3). In some cases, they have an "hourglass" configuration, with submucosal and serosal masses connected by a narrow area across the muscle wall of the intestine (see Figs. 14–2 and 14–3).

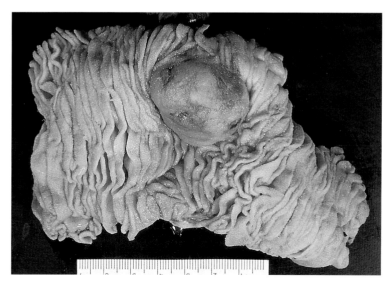

Figure 14–1. GI stromal tumor of the small intestine, showing a submucosal mass protruding into the lumen.

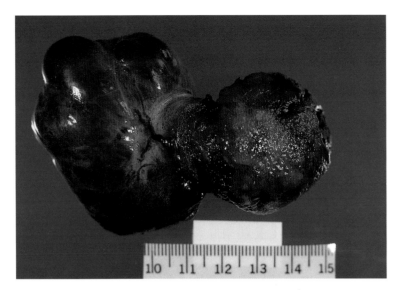

Figure 14–2. Gastric GI stromal tumor showing a large dumbbell-shaped tumor mass. The constriction corresponds to the gastric wall, with the ulcerated mucosal component to the right and the serosal component to the left.

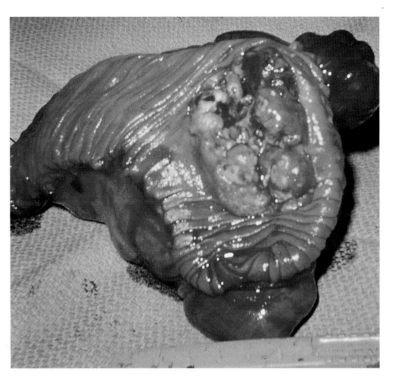

Figure 14–4. GI stromal tumor of the small intestine, showing ulcerated mucosal mass.

Larger submucosal tumors frequently show an area of ulceration of the overlying mucosa (Fig. 14–4). On cut section, GIST are usually well circumscribed, gray-white fleshy tumors that commonly have a vague lobulated appearance due to the presence of thickened septa of muscle derived from the muscularis externa (Figs. 14–5 and 14–6).

Microscopically, GIST are generally composed of spindle-shaped cells arranged in a variety of architectural patterns, including herringbone, storiform, and hemangiopericytoma-like patterns (Fig. 14–7). More rounded epithelioid cells are commonly present (Fig. 14–8), either admixed with spindle cells or forming the dominant cellular element in the tumor. Cellularity varies from low with abundant intercellular collagen to highly cellular. The degree of pleomorphism and mitotic activity also varies considerably from tumor to tumor (Fig. 14–9). Secondary degenerative changes are common, including stromal myxomatous change, hyalinization (Fig. 14–10A), calcification (Fig. 14–10B and C) and microcystic change (Fig. 14–11).

Stout originally classified GIST as smooth muscle tumors because of their resemblance to smooth muscle and because of their origin in the muscle wall of the GI tract.[4,5] He extended the term even to those epithelioid tumors whose cells did not bear a close resemblance to smooth muscle cells, calling these leiomyoblastomas.[6] It is apparent, however, that the majority of GIST

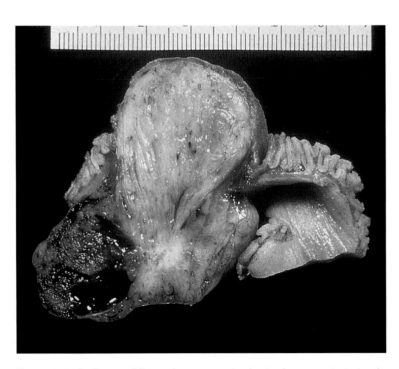

Figure 14–3. Small-intestinal GI stromal tumor, cut section showing the tumor projecting into the lumen and extending across the wall to form a large serosal mass. The tumor has a "dumbbell" appearance, the narrow part of which is the intramural part.

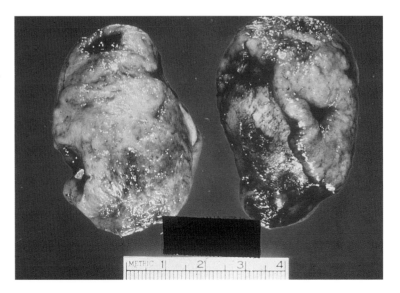

Figure 14–5. Gastric GI stromal tumor, cut surface showing typical lobulated appearance.

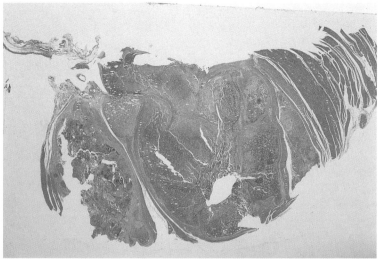

A

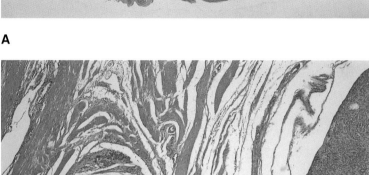

B

Figure 14–6. A: GI stromal tumor, intramural component, showing lobulation resulting from separation of tumor nodules by bands of muscle. B: Lobulated pattern of GI stromal tumor with nodules of tumor separated by muscle bands.

do not have evidence of an origin from smooth muscle cells. Myofibrils are rarely seen on special histochemical stains, and the cytoplasm of the cells in many cases is clear or amphophilic rather than eosinophilic.

Recent ultrastructural and immunohistochemical studies have not resolved the issue of histogenesis of these tumors[7-13] (Table 14–1). In the majority of cases, no specific differentiation can be seen either on electron microscopy or immunohistochemistry. In some cases, myogenic differentiation is seen, as indicated by actin or desmin immunoreactivity.[10,12] In other cases, neurogenic differentiation is seen, based primarily on S100 protein immunoreactivity.[7,11] Some studies have concluded that these tumors are immunohistochemically diverse, depending on their location in the GI tract.[11] Because of the present uncertainty regarding the histogenesis of this group of neoplasms, it has become customary to use the noncommittal designation of gastrointestinal stromal tumors.[14] The term

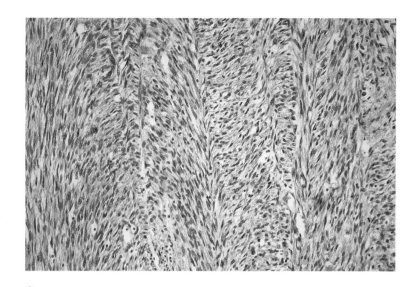

A

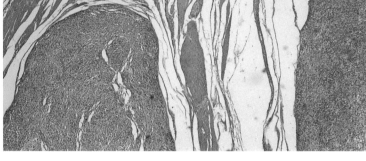

B

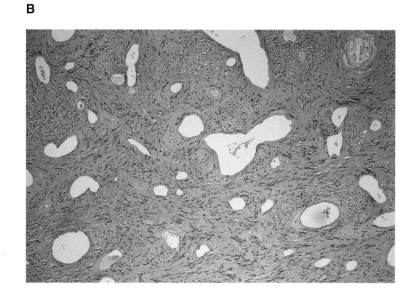

C

Figure 14–7. A: GI stromal tumor, showing the typical "herringbone" arrangement of the neoplastic spindle cells. The tumor is cellular, cytologically uniform, and has no necrosis or mitotic activity. B: Cellular GI stromal tumor, showing a more disorganized, somewhat storiform arrangement of the neoplastic spindle cells. C: GI stromal tumor, showing a tumor of low cellularity with a hemangiopericytoma-like architecture.

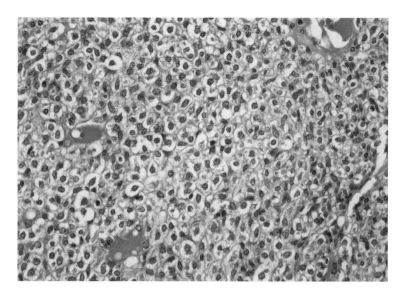

Figure 14–8. Cellular GI stromal tumor composed of epithelioid cells. The cells have uniform round nuclei with a clear cytoplasm.

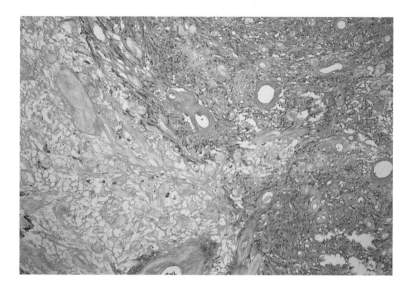

A

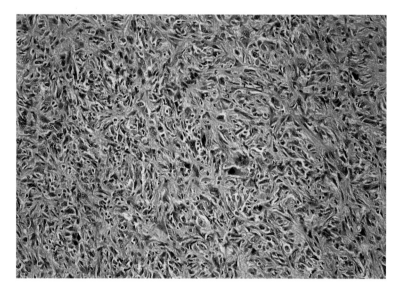

Figure 14–9. Highly cellular GI stromal tumor with marked cytologic atypia and pleomorphism.

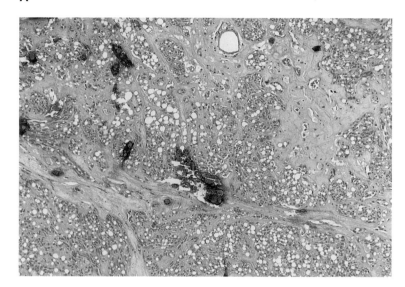

B

TABLE 14–1. IMMUNOHISTOCHEMICAL PROFILES OF COMMON GI TRACT NEOPLASMS

Neoplasm	Keratin	CLA	Vimentin	CD34	Desmin	S100 Protein
Carcinoma	+	−	−*	−	−	−
Lymphoma	−	+	+	−	−	−
GIST	−†	−	+	+	−‡	−‡
Nerve sheath	−	−	+	−	−	+
Granular cell	−	−	+	−	−	+

Abbreviations: GI = gastrointestinal; CLA = common leukocyte antigen (CD45); GIST = gastrointestinal stromal tumor.
*Spindle cell carcinomas may be immunoreactive for keratin and vimentin.
†Epithelioid variants of GIST may be immunoreactive for keratin.
‡Occasional GIST may be immunoreactive for desmin or muscle-specific actin; some may be S100 protein-positive, often focally.

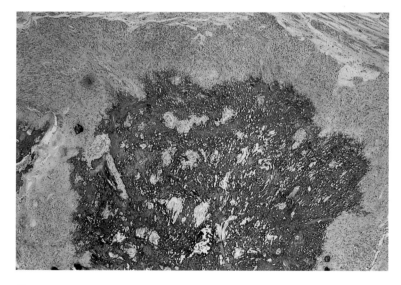

C

Figure 14–10. A: Hyaline degeneration in a GI stromal tumor. Thick-walled vessels are evident. The appearance bears a superficial resemblance to an ancient schwannoma. This was S100 protein-negative. B: Hyaline degeneration and calcification in a GI stromal tumor. C: Extensive calcification in GI stromal tumor.

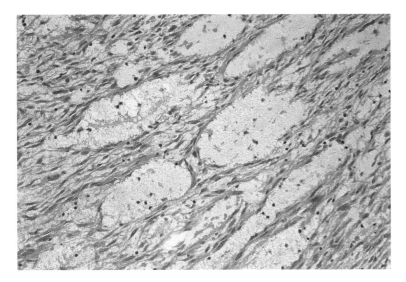

Figure 14–11. Microcystic degeneration in GI stromal tumor.

"leiomyoblastoma" is no longer used; these tumors are designated epithelioid GIST.

In addition to their marked heterogeneity, GIST have site-specific characteristics that determine prognosis and are therefore best considered according to their location.

Esophageal GIST

Esophageal GIST are the most common mesenchymal neoplasms of the esophagus. The vast majority of esophageal GIST are located in the muscularis externa, with rare tumors situated in the submucosa, and are less than 2 cm in size; most tumors are smaller than 1 cm (Fig. 14–12).[15] These may present incidentally as a polypoid lesion and may be found in biopsy sam-

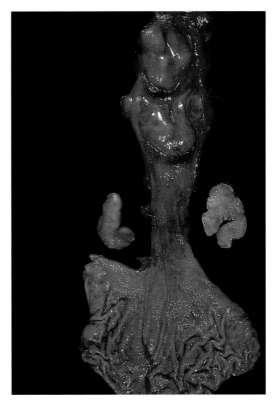

A

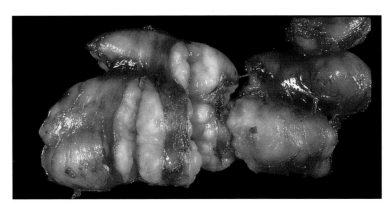

B

Figure 14–12. A: Large esophageal GI stromal tumor involving the middle third of the esophagus. B: Cut surface of the dissected tumor in part A, showing fleshy, lobulated surface. The tumor histologically was of low cellularity and had well-differentiated smooth muscle, raising the question of whether this was a large leiomyoma or a GI stromal tumor.

ples, esophagectomy specimens, or at autopsy (Figs. 14–13 and 14–14). The tumors are well circumscribed. The cells are arranged in fascicles and show almost complete smooth muscle differentiation of the neoplastic cells (Fig. 14–15). The cytoplasm has an eosinophilic fibrillary appearance that stains positively with trichrome stain and has strong immunoreactivity for desmin and muscle-specific actin. There is no cytologic atypia or mitotic activity. These tumors are therefore true leiomyomas. They are benign (Table 14–2).

The occurrence of malignant GIST is rare in the esophagus. Malignant GIST tend to be large (>2 cm), bulky tumors with marked cellularity, necrosis, mitotic activity, and pleomorphism; they usually cause dysphagia and not infrequently have

TABLE 14–2. CRITERIA FOR CLASSIFICATION OF GI STROMAL TUMORS

Esophagus

Benign: <2 cm in size; with smooth muscle differentiation; no mitotic figures.

Malignant (very rare): >2 cm in size; no smooth muscle differentiation; cytologic atypia, increased mitotic activity (number of cases in literature too small for reliable criteria).

Stomach

Benign: Incidental, asymptomatic; <2 cm; paucicellular; no mitotic activity.

GIST of uncertain malignant potential: Clinically symptomatic; cellular; <5 mitotic figures/10 hpf; necrosis absent.

Low-grade malignant gastric GIST: Clinically symptomatic; cellular; 5–9 mitotic figures/10 hpf *or* tumor necrosis.

High-grade malignant gastric GIST: Clinically symptomatic; cellular; 10 or more mitotic figures/10 hpf.

Small and Large Intestine

Benign: Rectal leiomyomatous polyp.

Intestinal GIST of uncertain malignant potential: Cellular; <5 cm in size; <5 mitotic figures/10 hpf.

Low-grade malignant intestinal GIST: Cellular; larger than 5 cm in size *or* 5–9 mitotic figures/10 hpf *or* tumor necrosis.

High-grade malignant intestinal GIST: Cellular; 10 or more mitotic figures/10 hpf.

Abbreviations: GI = gastrointestinal; GIST = gastrointestinal stromal tumor.

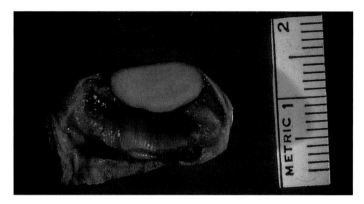

Figure 14–13. Cross section of esophagus at autopsy, showing an incidentally found leiomyoma.

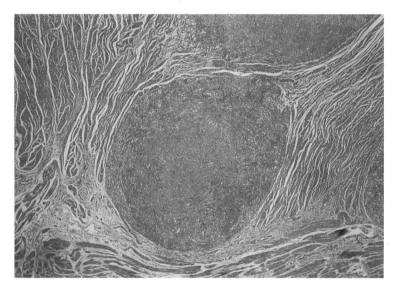

Figure 14–14. Intramural leiomyoma of the distal esophagus, incidentally found in an esophagectomy specimen from a patient with an esophageal adenocarcinoma.

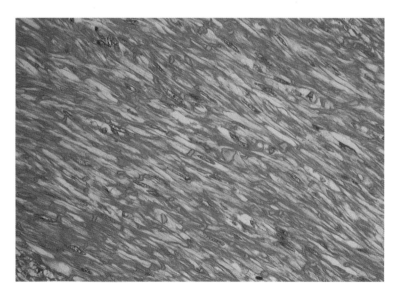

Figure 14–15. Esophageal leiomyoma, showing well-differentiated smooth muscle cells with abundant fibrillary eosinophilic cytoplasm.

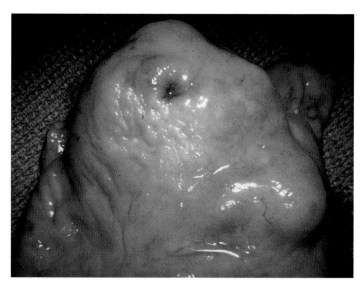

Figure 14–16. GI stromal tumor of the stomach, mucosal surface, showing a large mass covered by mucosa protruding into the lumen with ulceration at the dome.

evidence of metastasis at the time of presentation. They usually do not show evidence of smooth muscle differentiation on immunohistochemistry and are therefore malignant GIST.

GIST of the Stomach

The stomach is the most common site of occurrence of GIST. Gastric GIST may be found incidentally during upper GI radiography, endoscopy, or abdominal computed tomography (CT) scan. When these tumors are smaller than 2 cm, have no mitotic activity, and show no evidence of necrosis, they are classified as benign gastric GIST.

Gastric GIST neoplasms may present with evidence of upper GI bleeding, manifesting as hematemesis or melena. Slow bleeding from the ulcerated surface of a GIST may produce anemia, which is a common presentation. Larger tumors may be felt as an epigastric mass. Endoscopically and grossly, the tumors are submucosal nodular masses with an area of mucosal ulceration at the dome (Fig. 14–16). They have the typical lobulated appearance on their cut surface (Fig. 14–17). The mucosal

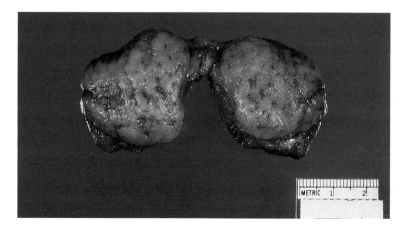

Figure 14–17. Gastric GI stromal tumor, bisected cut surface, showing typical fleshy appearance with lobulation.

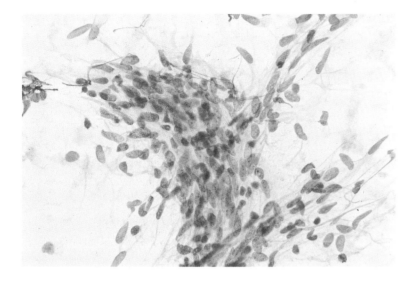

A

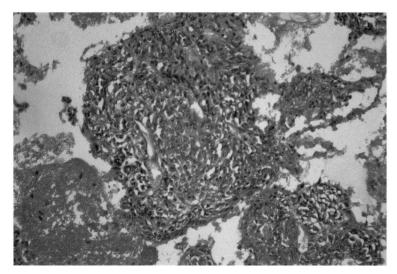

B

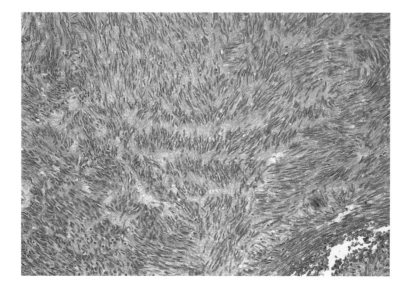

C

Figure 14–18. A: Smear of fine-needle aspiration of a liver mass, showing a metastatic gastric stromal neoplasm composed of spindle cells. B: Smear of liver fine-needle aspiration, showing metastatic epithelioid GI stromal tumor. Note the rounded cells. C: Cell block preparation from specimen whose smear is illustrated in part B, showing epithelioid GI stromal tumor. This patient had a gastric primary tumor.

ulceration at the dome of the tumor may be large as well as deep, extending into the body of the tumor; this process is probably accentuated in the stomach because of the acidity of the gastric contents. Biopsies frequently produce only necrotic tissue from the ulcer base and uninvolved mucosa. With deep ulceration of the tumor, the endoscopic appearances may be confusing; we have experienced one deeply ulcerated gastric GIST in which the endoscope was passed through the mouth of the ulcer into the tumor cavity; biopsy specimens from the depths of the ulcer in this case included tumor and normal splenic tissue, which formed the base of the ulcerated tumor.

Gastric GIST may be submucosal, intramural, or subserosal; subserosal masses may be largely exophytic, and their origin from the gastric wall may not be apparent on CT scan examination. We have encountered gastric GIST misinterpreted preoperatively as retroperitoneal tumors and hepatic tumors. These large tumors not uncommonly undergo fine-needle aspiration biopsy under radiologic guidance. The first diagnosis may sometimes be made by fine-needle aspiration of a liver metastasis (Fig. 14–18).

Microscopically, gastric GIST are generally composed of a uniform population of spindle cells with a fascicular growth pattern. Minimal cytologic atypia is the rule. Nuclear palisading is a common finding (Fig. 14–19), similar to that seen in soft tissue schwannomas; tumors with nuclear palisading are almost invariably S100 protein-negative. Perinuclear cytoplasmic vacuoles are often present both in formalin-fixed sections and smears of fine-needle aspiration biopsies; these are areas devoid of glycogen and mucin on electron microscopy. A subset of gastric GIST are composed entirely of epithelioid cells with variable amounts of clear to eosinophilic cytoplasm (Fig. 14–20). These cells have uniform, centrally located nuclei and usually have a compact, nested, or trabecular arrangement. When cellular discohesion is present, GIST may mimic malignant lymphomas. Some epithelioid tumors have myxomatous stroma and a single cell pattern (Fig. 14–21), mimicking myxoid sarco-

Figure 14–19. GI stromal neoplasm of the stomach composed of a cellular proliferation of spindle cells showing nuclear palisading. This was S100 protein-negative and CD34-positive.

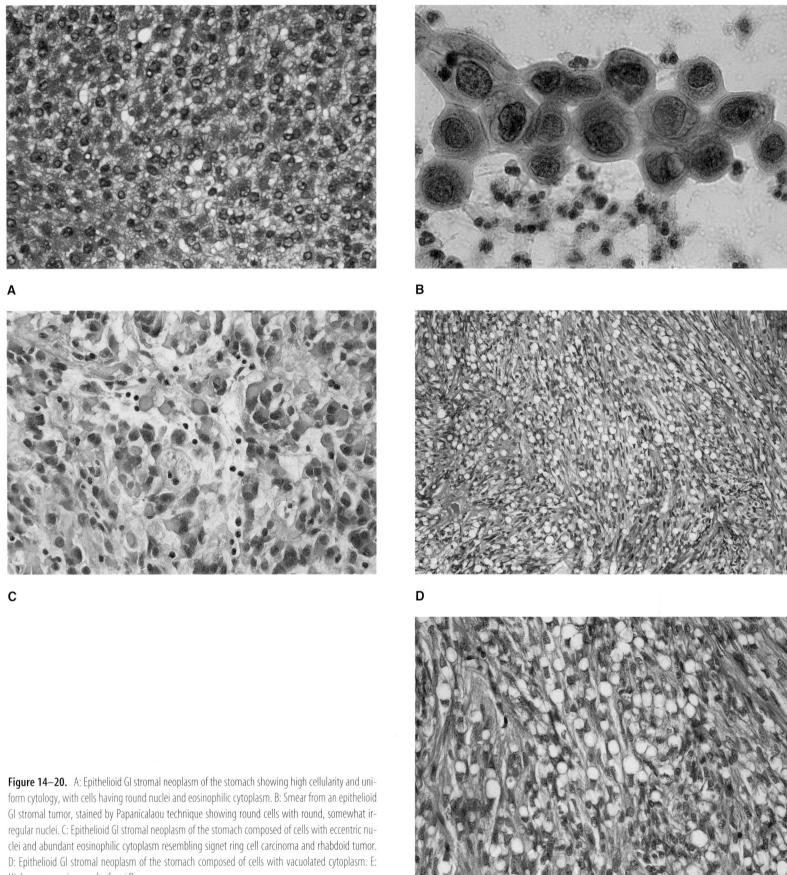

Figure 14–20. A: Epithelioid GI stromal neoplasm of the stomach showing high cellularity and uniform cytology, with cells having round nuclei and eosinophilic cytoplasm. B: Smear from an epithelioid GI stromal tumor, stained by Papanicalaou technique showing round cells with round, somewhat irregular nuclei. C: Epithelioid GI stromal neoplasm of the stomach composed of cells with eccentric nuclei and abundant eosinophilic cytoplasm resembling signet ring cell carcinoma and rhabdoid tumor. D: Epithelioid GI stromal neoplasm of the stomach composed of cells with vacuolated cytoplasm. E: Higher power micrograph of part D.

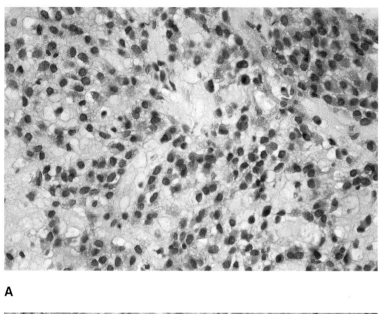

A

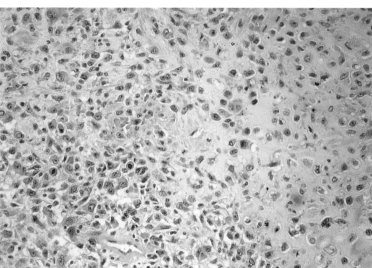

B

Figure 14–21. A: Epithelioid GI stromal neoplasm of the stomach with abundant myxoid stroma separating the neoplastic cells. This appearance mimics myxoid sarcomas of soft tissue. B: Epithelioid GI stroma with myxomatous stroma, resembling a chondroid neoplasm.

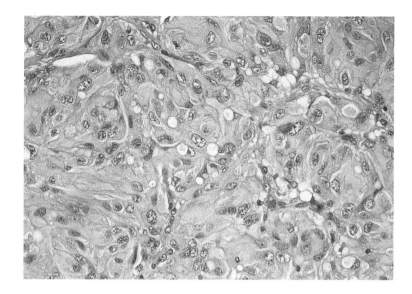

A

B

Figure 14–22. A: Epithelioid GI stromal neoplasm of the stomach composed of large, cohesive, epithelioid cells with focally vacuolated cytoplasm arranged in nests. This appearance can mimic poorly differentiated carcinoma and metastatic malignant melanoma. B: Epithelioid GI stromal neoplasm, Papanicalaou stained smear, showing rounded cells with signet ring features.

mas.[16] Rarely, the cells have eccentric nuclei, resulting in a resemblance to signet ring cells (Fig. 14–22). The microscopic differentiation can usually be made accurately on morphologic criteria; in difficult cases, staining for epithelial mucin (absent in GIST; present in signet ring cell carcinoma), and immunoperoxidase staining for keratin, CD34, and CD45 is confirmatory. Epithelioid GIST can show keratin positivity (Fig. 14–23), but this is usually focal and weak. Positivity with vimentin and CD34 is a constant finding in gastric GIST and diagnostically useful.[17] Stains for desmin, muscle-specific actin, and actin may show variable focal positivity.

Carney described a group of patients who had gastric epithelioid leiomyosarcoma (malignant gastric GIST), functioning extraadrenal paraganglioma, and pulmonary chondroid hamar-

toma.[18,19] This is known as Carney's triad. These tumors are either synchronous or metachronous. Most of the patients were younger than age 20.

Gastric GIST show marked variation in histologic features; histologic parameters, particularly necrosis and mitotic rate, can be used to predict biologic behavior.[20–23] When appropriately treated by complete surgical removal with wide margins, gastric GIST have an overall 5-year survival rate of approximately 70%. Most patients who develop recurrences or metastases have large, high-grade malignant tumors and present with recurrences within 2 years of initial treatment; late recurrence after initial successful treatment may rarely occur with low-grade tumors.[24]

All symptomatic GIST are potentially malignant (see Table 14–2). They can be classified into the following:

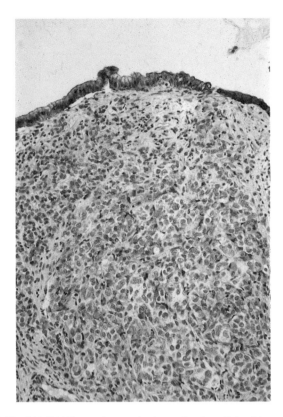

Figure 14–23. Epithelioid GI stromal tumor, showing cytokeratin positivity of the neoplastic cells. Note the much more intense positivity in the overlying flattened epithelium.

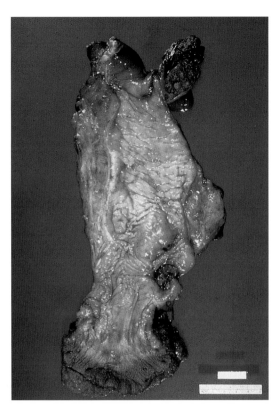

Figure 14–25. GI stromal tumor of the low rectum, presenting as an ulcerated mass without much intraluminal mass effect. This is an unusual gross appearance for a GI stromal tumor.

1. Gastric GIST of uncertain malignant potential: this is a cellular neoplasm with a mitotic rate less than 5/10 hpf and absent necrosis. These tumors have a nearly 100% survival if adequately treated; however, with inadequate surgery, recurrence and metastasis may occur.
2. Low-grade malignant gastric GIST: this is a cellular neoplasm of any size that contains 5–9 mitotic figures/10 hpf or shows coagulative tumor cell necrosis. Many large gastric GIST have necrotic tissue in the area of ulceration; this does not fall within the definition of coagulative tumor cell necro-

sis. Low-grade gastric GIST have a low risk of recurrence and metastatic disease after adequate surgery.
3. High-grade gastric GIST: this is a cellular neoplasm with 10 or more mitotic figures/10 hpf, irrespective of any other factor. High-grade gastric GIST has a high risk of recurrence and metastasis, even after adequate surgery.

The mitotic rate is the best predictor of malignancy in gastric GIST. Because the mitotic activity differs so greatly in different areas of the tumor, extensive microscopic sampling is

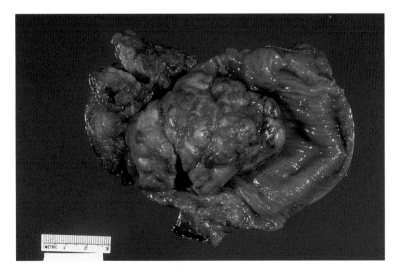

Figure 14–24. Large GI stromal tumor of the small intestine projecting into the lumen. The tumor was transmural with a serosal component.

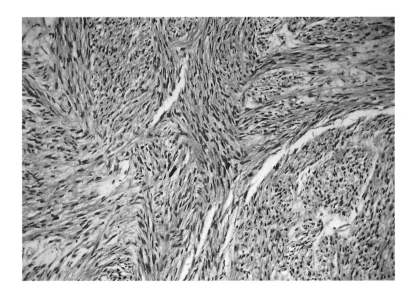

Figure 14–26. GI stromal tumor of the intestine, showing a cellular spindle cell proliferation.

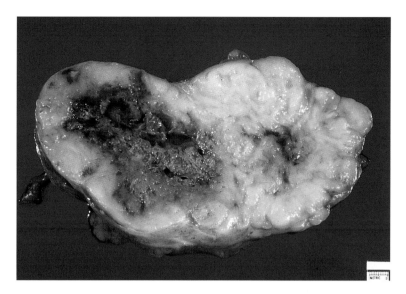

Figure 14–27. Intestinal GI stromal tumor, showing a large area of necrosis.

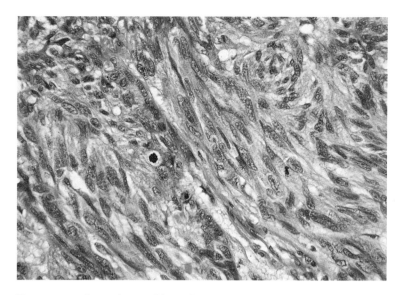

Figure 14–29. GI stromal tumor of the small intestine, showing high cellularity, cytologic atypia, and mitotic figures.

necessary in all gastric GIST. Mitotic counting must be done systematically and in many areas of the tumor; the final count is the highest count obtained in the most active area. Flow cytometric assessment of DNA content and ploidy are useful in predicting biologic behavior in gastric GIST.[25–27]

Gastric GIST must be treated with complete excision with a margin of at least 2 cm around the gross extent of the tumor. This must include a 2-cm margin at all levels of the stomach wall, including the intramural component. With large tumors, adequate resection usually entails a partial gastrectomy. Wedge resection is possible for smaller tumors, but these should be carefully controlled with intraoperative examination, including frozen section, to ensure that the intramural tumor extent is not underestimated. There is no effective chemotherapy or radiation.

Small- and Large-Intestinal GIST

Intestinal GIST are almost always detected because they are symptomatic, either due to bleeding or intestinal obstruction. Obstruction may be the result of encroachment on the lumen by the tumor or due to torsion, angulation, or intussusception. In contrast to gastric GIST, intestinal GIST are generally smaller at time of diagnosis, but are at significantly higher risk for a more malignant biologic course.[22] For this reason, any intestinal GIST larger than 5 cm should be regarded as malignant, irrespective of any histologic criterion (see Table 14–2).

Intestinal GIST have gross and microscopic features similar to those described for gastric GIST (Figs. 14–24 and 14–25). Intestinal GIST, however, generally have a greater degree of cytologic atypia and pleomorphism, higher mitotic rate, and

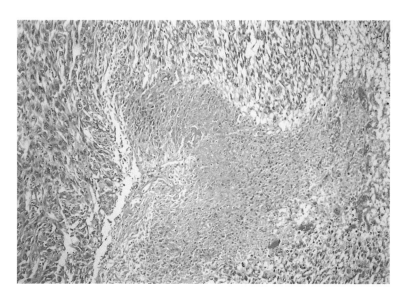

Figure 14–28. GI stromal tumor of small intestine, showing coagulative tumor cell necrosis. The tumor adjacent to the necrosis is highly cellular with pleomorphism and mitotic activity.

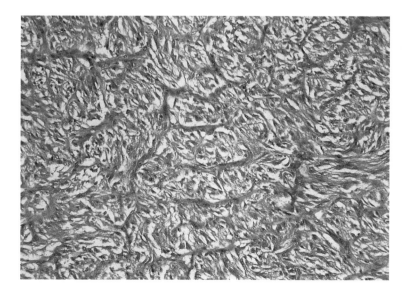

Figure 14–30. GI stromal tumor of small intestine, showing organoid pattern, consisting of nests of epithelioid cells separated by fibrovascular stroma. This condition mimics paraganglioma. The tumor was CD34-positive and chromogranin-negative.

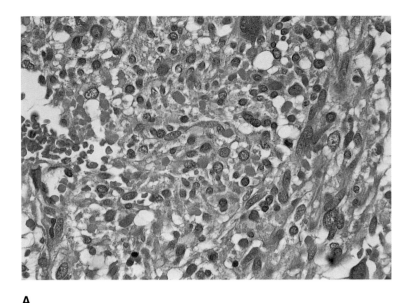

A

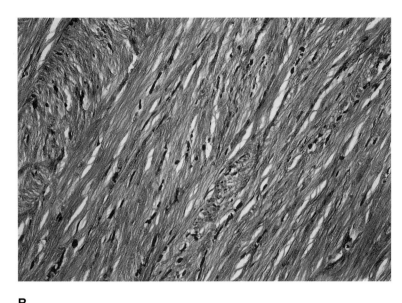

B

Figure 14–31. A: Epithelioid GI stromal tumor of the small intestine, showing high cellularity and cytologic atypia. Large, rounded cytoplasmic inclusions are evident in many cells, representing skeinoid fibers. B: GI stromal tumor of the small intestine, stained with digested PAS, showing skeinoid fibers in the neoplastic cells appearing as irregular round-to-oval inclusions.

necrosis than gastric GIST (Figs. 14–26 through 14–29). Two histologic features are unique to intestinal GIST. First, some small-intestinal GIST have an organoid growth pattern (Fig. 14–30) similar to that seen in gangliocytic paraganglioma of the duodenum.[28] This is characterized by compact clusters of neoplastic cells separated by thin fibrous septa. This pattern may be present focally or may constitute the major histologic pattern of the tumor. Second, many small-intestinal GIST contain intracytoplasmic inclusions called skeinoid bodies (Fig. 14–31A).[29] Skeinoid bodies are periodic acid–Schiff (PAS)-positive and resistant to diastase digestion (Fig. 14–31B). Ultrastructurally, they are composed of tangled fibers of uncertain origin, resembling skeins of yarn. Skeinoid bodies are believed to be an ultrastructural marker of neural differentiation.

Intestinal GIST are much more unpredictable than gastric GIST, and no intestinal GIST can be guaranteed to have a benign biologic behavior.[30–32] Intestinal GIST fall into the following classifications: (1) Intestinal GIST of uncertain malignant potential: this tumor is smaller than 5 cm with a mitotic rate of less than 5/10 hpf. (2) Low-grade malignant intestinal GIST: this is larger than 5 cm *or* contains 5–9 mitotic figures/10 hpf *or* demonstrates tumoral necrosis. (3) High-grade malignant intestinal GIST: this tumor has 10 or more mitotic figures/10 hpf, irrespective of any other criterion.

Intestinal GIST are treated with segmental resection of the

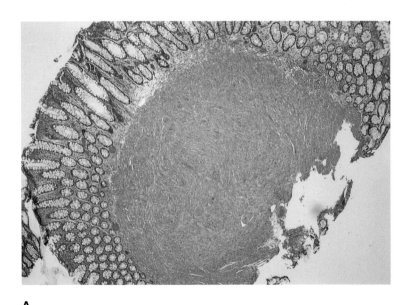

A

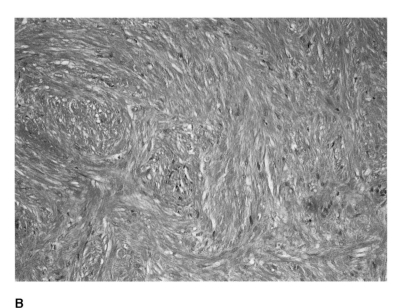

B

Figure 14–32. A: Leiomyomatous polyp of the rectum. B: Higher power micrograph of part A, showing a leiomyoma, consisting of well-differentiated, cytologically benign, smooth muscle cells with abundant eosinophilic cytoplasm.

tumor containing part of the small or large intestine. The overall 5-year survival rate is approximately 40%. The presence of aneuploidy by flow cytometric DNA analysis correlates with poor survival. Flow cytometry is most useful in distinguishing tumors in the low-grade malignant and uncertain malignant potential categories; although aneuploidy is less common in these tumors than in high-grade tumors, they provide more valuable prognostic information.[25–27]

A clinically and pathologically distinct rectal neoplasm that is a well-differentiated leiomyoma arises in the muscularis mucosae (Fig. 14–32). These leiomyomatous rectal polyps are usually submucosal, covered by normal mucosa, and smaller than 2 cm.[30] They are detected as incidental findings during rectal or endoscopic examination, are invariably benign, and are treated by endoscopic polypectomy. Histologically, they are uniform, of low cellularity, and lack mitotic activity and necrosis.

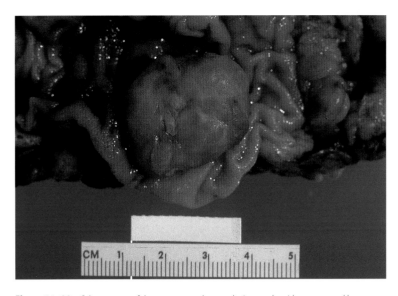

Figure 14–33. Schawnnoma of the transverse colon, producing a polypoid mass covered by mucosa projecting into the lumen.

GASTROINTESTINAL AUTONOMIC NERVE TUMOR

Gastrointestinal autonomic nerve tumors (GANT) are a neurogenic subset of GIST.[33–35] They have been reported primarily in the stomach and small intestine, and most cases have been malignant. Morphologically and immunohistochemically, GANT are identical to the more common GIST. They can be recognized only with electron microscopy. GANT cells display neuronal-type differentiation with the formation of synaptic-like terminals; schwannian differentiation is not seen. Based on these features, GANT is believed to arise from the myenteric plexus.

PERIPHERAL NERVE SHEATH TUMORS

Schwannoma and Neurofibroma

Peripheral nerve sheath tumors of the GI tract are uncommon, even in patients with von Recklinghausen's disease (Figs. 14–33 and 14–34). In patients with von Recklinghausen's disease, a variety of tumors occurs, including neurofibroma, schwannoma, GIST, ganglioneuroma, and ganglioneurofibroma.[36–38]

The majority of GI tract schwannomas occur in the stomach.[39] Unlike their soft tissue counterparts, gastric schwannomas have a more compact fascicular cell arrangement, including a storiform pattern (Fig. 14–35A). Nuclear palisading is uncommon in gastric schwannoma, and its presence strongly indicates a GIST. Aggregates of small lymphocytes are often a prominent feature in gastric schwannoma, usually along and within the perimeter; this feature is a strong predictor that a gastric spindle cell tumor is a schwannoma and should lead to confirmatory testing for S100 protein by immunoperoxidase (Fig. 14–35B). Similar lymphocytic aggregates have been reported in GANT.[34]

In sites other than the stomach, schwannomas frequently show nuclear palisading (Fig. 14–36A). Because peripheral nerve sheath tumors cannot be reliably differentiated from GIST on morphologic grounds, it is probably advisable to perform immunoperoxidase staining for CD34 and S100 protein in all GI tract spindle cell neoplasms.[17] This separates out the rare peripheral nerve sheath tumors (Fig. 14–36B) (S100 protein-positive CD34-negative) from the more common GIST (CD34-positive S100 protein +/−). This has practical value because histologically benign peripheral nerve sheath tumors of the GI tract have a benign biologic behavior in contrast to GIST, which may be potentially malignant despite a benign histology. In patients with von Recklinghausen's disease, a diffuse neural proliferation may occur, either involving a localized region such as the appendix (Fig. 14–37) or involving the intestine more dif-

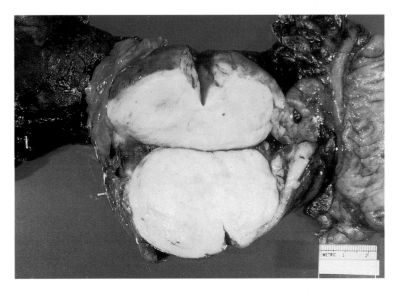

Figure 14–34. Schwannoma in the serosal aspect of the colon, cut surface, showing encapsulated mass with a yellow color on the cut surface.

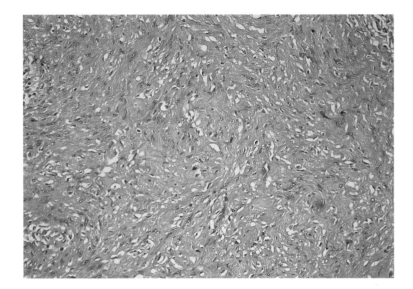

A

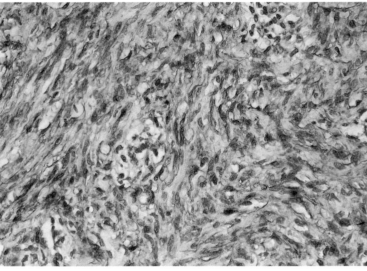

B

Figure 14–35. A: Schwannoma of the stomach, showing spindle cell proliferation without nuclear palisading. Immunoperoxidase staining is required to differentiate this tumor from GIST. B: S100 protein positivity by immunoperoxidase staining in a gastric schwannoma.

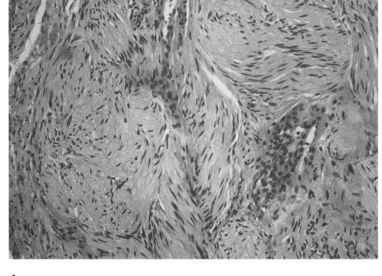

A

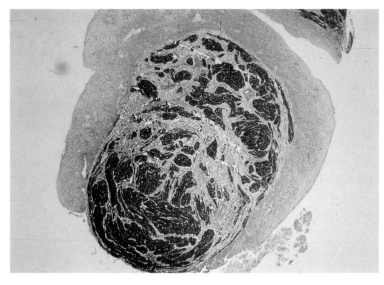

B

Figure 14–36. A: Neurofibroma of the esophagus, presenting as a polypoid mass, which was removed by endoscopy. The spindle cells are uniform with the wavy nuclei typical of neurofibroma and nuclear palisading. B: Esophageal neurofibroma, stained by immunoperoxidase for S100 protein, showing strong positivity. This is a low-power photograph, showing the polypoid nature of this mass, which is covered by squamous epithelium.

fusely. Rarely, sarcomatous transformation may occur in a GI tract neurofibroma; this occurs mainly in patients with von Recklinghausen's neurofibromatosis.

Granular Cell Tumor

Granular cell tumors (previously called granular cell myoblastomas) are uncommon GI tract neoplasms that are probably derived from peripheral nerve; they are also called granular cell schwannomas. They have a distinctive patient profile; most patients are African-American, female, and between ages 40 and 60. These neoplasms occur throughout the GI tract; the favored sites are esophagus, colon (Fig. 14–38), and stomach (see Chapter 5).[40] They may occur as solitary or multiple tumors; when

multiple, they can occur in many different parts of the GI tract.[41–43] Smaller granular cell tumors are asymptomatic and found incidentally at endoscopy; larger tumors may cause dysphagia (esophagus), upper GI bleeding (stomach), or lower GI bleeding (colon). Granular cell tumors also occur in the terminal bile duct and are a cause of obstructive jaundice associated with a periampullary mass.

Granular cell tumors commonly occur as submucosal tumors with an intact overlying mucosa (Fig. 14–39). Rarely, ulceration occurs at the dome of the tumor. Cut section reveals a well-circumscribed, gray-white, fleshy tumor (see Fig. 14–38B). When the tumor is large and when mucosal ulceration is present at the dome, granular cell tumors are grossly indistinguishable from GIST.

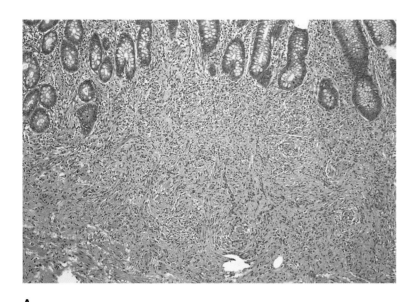

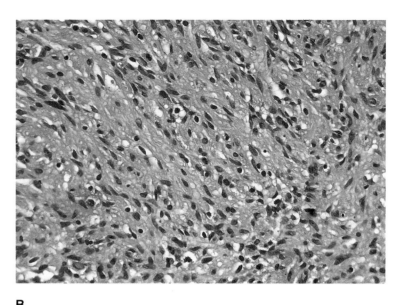

Figure 14–37. A: Diffuse neurofibroma of the appendix, showing a diffuse proliferation of neural spindle cells in the deep mucosa. This patient had von Recklinghausen's neurofibromatosis. B: Higher power micrograph of part A.

Microscopically, granular cell tumors have an expansile growth pattern with an infiltrative edge. Although mainly submucosal, extension of the tumor as single cells into the overlying mucosa is common (Fig. 14–40). The tumor mass is composed of large polygonal cells with small vesicular nuclei and abundant, coarsely granular, eosinophilic cytoplasm (Fig. 14–41A). The cells are arranged in nests and singly, and a vari-able amount of intercellular collagen is present (Fig. 14–41B). Mitotic activity is not present. Cytoplasmic granularity can be accentuated by PAS stain. The cells show strong immunoreactivity for S100 protein (Fig. 14–41C); they are negative for keratin, desmin, and muscle specific-actin; stain for carcinoembryonic antigen may be positive.[44,45]

Mucosal biopsy samples taken over the nodular mass at

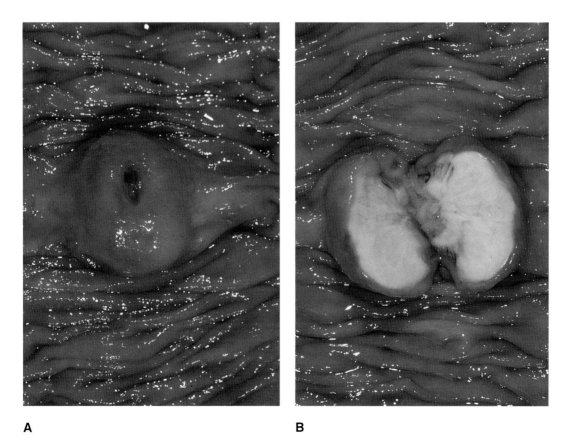

Figure 14–38. A: Polypoid granular cell tumor in the transverse colon. This is covered by mucosa and shows a small ulcer at the dome of the lesion. B: Cut section of the tumor in part A, showing the dense, white, cut surface typical of a granular cell tumor.

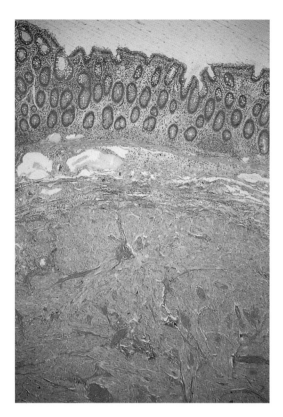

Figure 14–39. Granular cell tumor of the colon, showing the tumor in the submucosa without any extension into the mucosa, which is normal.

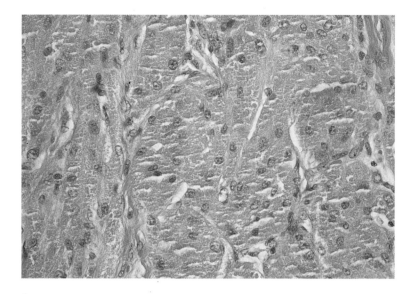

A

endoscopy not uncommonly show infiltration of the lamina propria by single granular cells, producing an easily missed but diagnostic appearance in endoscopic biopsies (see Fig. 14–40). When the cells are recognized, they can easily be characterized by staining for S100 protein.

Granular cell tumors are almost invariably benign; malignancy has been reported rarely.[46] It is difficult to predict malignant behavior in a granular cell tumor; the presence of any mitotic activity represents the only predictor of aggressive

B

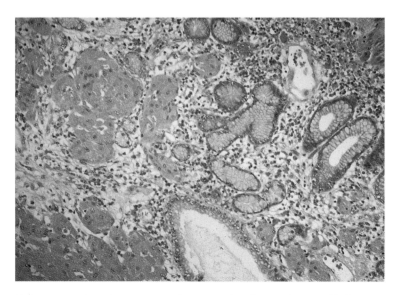

Figure 14–40. Gastric biopsy specimen, showing granular cell tumor, characterized by large neoplastic cells with abundant granular eosinophilic cytoplasm in the lamina propria.

C

Figure 14–41. A: Granular cell tumor, showing large cells with granular cytoplasm and small nuclei. B: Granular cell tumor with hyalinization. C: Granular cell tumor, immunoperoxidase stain shows strongly positive for S100 protein.

behavior. There are rare reported instances of benign granular cell tumors coexisting with other malignant neoplasms in the GI tract, including gastric adenocarcinoma[47] and esophageal squamous carcinoma.[48]

When a granular cell tumor is encountered, it is advisable to document immunoreactivity for S100 protein. Very rarely, adult rhabdomyoma,[49] rhabdomyosarcoma,[50] and alveolar soft part sarcoma[51] occur in the GI tract. Although these superficially resemble granular cell tumors, they can be distinguished both by typical morphology (eg, alveolar pattern and PAS-positive cytoplasmic crystals in alveolar soft part sarcoma), immunohistochemical staining (muscle tumors are S100 protein-negative, desmin-positive, actin-positive; alveolar soft part sarcoma is S100 protein-negative, desmin-negative, actin-negative), and electron microscopy (myofilaments in muscle tumors; typical crystals in alveolar soft part sarcoma). Primary gastric rhabdomyosarcomas are commonly associated with adenocarcinoma, suggesting that they may represent metaplastic gastric adenocarcinoma.[50]

Ganglioneuroma

Ganglioneuromas are rare GI tumors. Composed of varying proportions of ganglion cells and spindle cells of neural derivation, they can be found throughout the GI tract, but are most common in the colon and rectum. Two principal forms of presentation, focal ("solitary") and diffuse, are reported.[52–54]

Focal ganglioneuroma presents as solitary or multiple discrete polyps. Ganglioneuromatous polyps may occur as a sole abnormality or be associated with other types of multiple colonic polyposis.[55,56] Ganglioneuromatous polyps are usually smaller than 2 cm. Focal ganglioneuromas occur in the mucosa as a benign spindle cell proliferation (which shows S100 protein immunoreactivity) in which are found scattered mature ganglion cells, which are large cells with granular cytoplasm and a large round excentric nucleus with a prominent nucleolus (Fig. 14–42). The presence of ganglion cells can be accentuated with

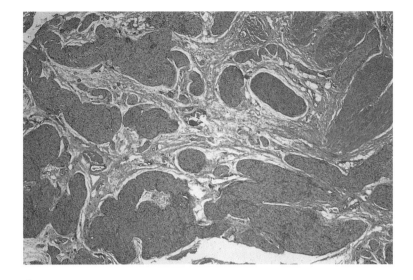

A

B

C

Figure 14–43. A: Plexiform ganglioneurofibroma of the colon. This was a diffuse thickening of the colonic wall in a 4-year-old girl with severe constipation (chronic intestinal pseudo-obstruction). B: Higher power micrograph of part A, showing neural elements containing ganglion cells. C: Patient with multiple endocrine adenomatosis type IIb, showing mucosal neuromas in the tongue. This patient had bilateral pheochromocytomas of the adrenal gland and medullary carcinoma of the thyroid.

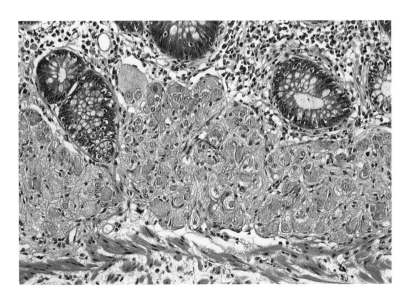

Figure 14–42. Mucosal ganglioneuroma in the colon. This was an incidental finding in a colon removed for adenocarcinoma.

immunoperoxidase staining for neuron-specific enolase. The crypts adjacent to the ganglioneuromatous proliferation commonly show proliferative changes resembling hyperplastic and retention polyps.

The diffuse form of intestinal ganglioneuromatosis (also called intestinal neuronal dysplasia) presents as ill-defined nodules resembling plexiform neurofibromas; these may be either intramural or transmural (Fig. 14–43A and B). The majority of these patients have stigmata of multiple endocrine neoplasia (type IIb) or von Recklinghausen's neurofibromatosis (Fig. 14–43C).[57-60] They commonly present with chronic intestinal pseudo-obstruction caused by intestinal dysmotility, manifested by constipation and megacolon. Microscopically, proliferation of the enteric nerve plexuses is seen, mainly in the myenteric plexus. The neural spindle cell and ganglion cell proliferation expands the myenteric plexus, diffusely producing a multinodular or confluent mass; when severe, this proliferation may produce diffuse thickening of the intestinal wall.

GANGLIOCYTIC PARAGANGLIOMA

Gangliocytic paragangliomas occur almost exclusively in the second portion of the duodenum.[61-63] They are invariably benign, although some of these tumors have been associated with other neoplasms, including adenocarcinoma, neurofibromatosis, and carcinoid tumors.[64,65]

Gangliocytic paraganglioma usually presents as a duodenal polyp; although commonly small, these can become large and be associated with upper gastrointestinal hemorrhage secondary to ulceration of the overlying mucosa.

Microscopically, they are characterized by three distinctive patterns:

1. An organoid pattern, resembling the "zellballen" (nest-like clusters) appearance of a paraganglioma (Fig. 14–44A). This consists of plexiform nests of small neuroendocrine cells separated by thin fibrovascular septa. The cells have round-to-oval nuclei, delicately stippled chromatin, and inconspicuous nucleoli. The amount of cytoplasm varies. These cells show immunoreactivity for neuron-specific enolase and are variably somatostatin-positive. Stain for S100 protein shows scattered sustentacular cells in the periphery of the cell nests in the manner typical of paragangliomas.
2. An epithelioid ribbon, or festoon, pattern resembling carcinoid tumors, in which similar neuroendocrine cells are arranged in cords, ribbons, and trabeculae (Fib. 14–44B). The cells are often aligned perpendicular to the long axis of the groupings. Presence of this festooning pattern is very useful in separating gangliocytic paraganglioma from GIST, which can also have a trabecular or organoid histologic pattern.
3. A histologically benign spindle cell proliferation with neural differentiation (immunoreactive for S100 protein) with scattered ganglion cells resembling ganglioneuroma (Fig.

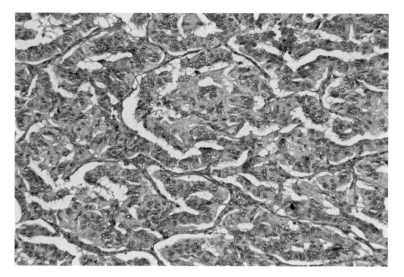

A

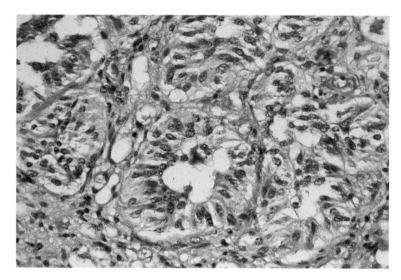

B

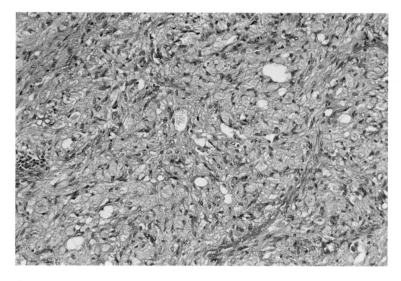

C

Figure 14–44. A: Gangliocytic paraganglioma of the duodenum, showing an organoid pattern resembling the typical "zellballen" appearance of paraganglioma. The cells are fairly uniform. B: Gangliocytic paraganglioma, showing ribbon-like arrangement of cells resembling a carcinoid tumor. C: Diffuse ganglioneuromatous pattern in a gangliocytic paraganglioma of the duodenum. Ganglion cells are not prominent.

14–44C). The ganglion cells are large with abundant, finely granular cytoplasm and large, round, excentric nuclei with prominent nucleoli. These ganglion cells are seen singly and in small clusters within the spindle cell element, but can also be seen as scattered cells in the other two histologic elements. The ganglion cells are immunoreactive for neuron-specific enolase.

Although the individual patterns of gangliocytic paraganglioma may occur in duodenal GIST, duodenal carcinoid tumors, and ganglioneuroma, the combination of these three histologic patterns defines gangliocytic paraganglioma.

TUMORS OF ADIPOCYTES

Lipomas can occur anywhere in the GI tract (Fig. 14–45); the majority are found in the cecum and ascending colon.[66,67] The majority of lipomas are smaller than 2 cm and found incidentally during endoscopy; they are yellow, have a submucosal location, and are covered by normal mucosa. Small GI tract lipomas are usually removed endoscopically. Larger lipomas of the GI tract can be recognized specifically by CT scan because of their fat density.

Large lipomas may become pedunculated polyps and be the apex of an intussusception (Fig. 14–46). Intestinal obstruction and rectal bleeding secondary to intussusception is the most common clinical presentation for a colonic lipoma. When intussusception occurs, secondary changes occur within the lipoma, including infarction, myxomatous change, ulceration, and inflammation; these result in loss of attenuation on CT scan and may result in a failure to recognize the mass at the apex of the intussusception as a lipoma preoperatively.[68]

Grossly and microscopically, lipomas are composed of mature adipose tissue within the submucosa (Fig. 14–47). The mere presence of adipocytes in the submucosa is not diagnostic of lipoma; scattered fat cells can be present normally in the submucosa of the GI tract. Prominent accumulation of fat cells in the ileocecal valve can produce a mass-like enlargement of the valve, known as lipohyperplasia. Lipomas associated with mucosal ulceration or those found at the apex of an intussusception frequently show marked degenerative histologic changes, including infarction, inflammation, myxomatous stromal change, and nuclear atypia in the stromal cells (Fig. 14–48). These changes must not be interpreted as representing malignancy.

Gastric xanthelasma is a common endoscopic finding; it appears as a small yellow focus in the mucosa that may mimic a small lipoma (see Chapter 4). Microscopically, xanthelasma consists of a collection of foamy macrophages in the mucosa, usually immediately beneath the surface. A change that can mimic colonic lipoma microscopically is mucosal pneumatosis intestinalis ("pseudo-lipomatosis").[69] Endoscopically, this appears as small white-to-yellow plaques 0.2–4 cm in size; microscopically, biopsy specimens of these plaques reveal multiple unlined spaces within the lamina propria. These spaces do not

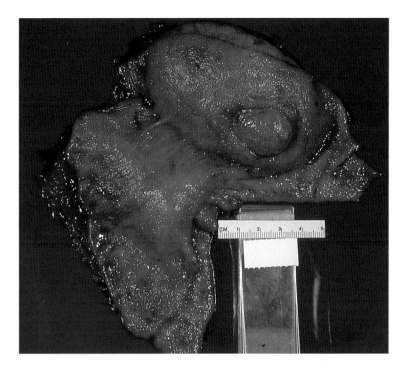

A

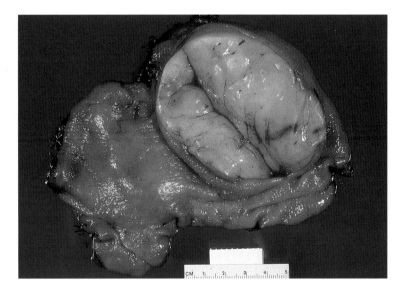

B

Figure 14–45. A: Gastric lipoma, showing a large submucosal mass covered by mucosa that shows focal ulceration. B: Gastric lipoma, cut section, showing the large tumor composed of fat.

contain lipid on histochemical and electron microscopic examination; they are believed to be mucosal gas spaces created during endoscopy, probably secondary to insufflation of the colon (see Chapter 8).

Primary liposarcomas of the GI tract are extremely rare[70]; it is possible that many of the cases reported are really GIST. On small endoscopic biopsy samples, variants of epithelioid GIST with abundant myxoid stroma can resemble myxoid liposarcoma. The cells of these epithelioid GIST, however, have abundant eosinophilic or clear cytoplasm rather than the vacuolated cytoplasm of lipoblasts. Immunoreactivity for CD34 in epithelioid GIST permits reliable separation from liposarcoma, which is CD34-negative.

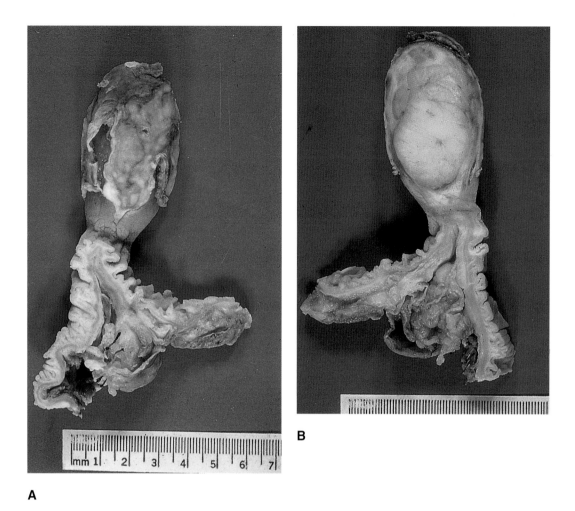

Figure 14–46. A: Colonic lipoma producing a polypoid mass that acted as the apex of an intussusception. The apex of the polyp is discolored and shows an exudate associated with ulceration. B: Tumor in part A after bisection, showing changes associated with intussusception at the apical part of the tumor.

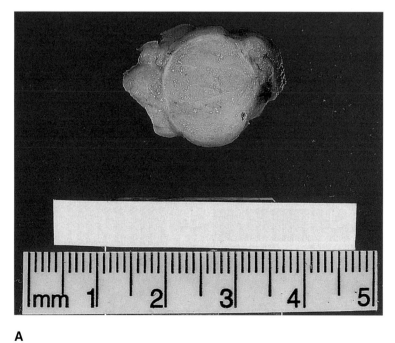

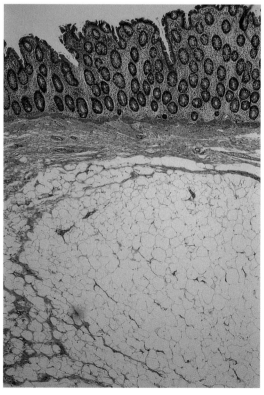

Figure 14–47. A: Submucosal lipoma removed at colonoscopy. B: Lipoma, showing tumor in the submucosa with overlying normal colonic mucosa.

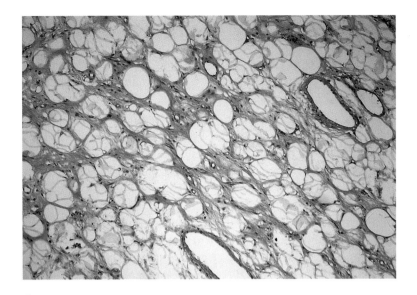

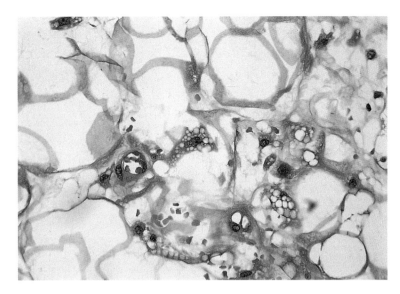

A   **B**

Figure 14–48. A: Lipoma with degenerative changes, characterized by focal myxomatous change. B: Lipoma with degenerative changes and scattered atypical cells with vacuolated cytoplasm resembling lipoblasts.

VASCULAR TUMORS

Neuromuscular and Vascular Hamartoma

Hamartomas composed of a haphazard admixture of bundles of smooth muscle, neural elements including ganglion cells, and ectatic blood vessels, have been reported in the small intestine. They are submucosal polypoid tumors and may cause obstruction and bleeding.[71,72] They should be differentiated from extensively degenerated GIST by an absence of CD34 positive cells by immunoperoxidase staining.

Hemangioma

Hemangiomas are rare GI tract tumors (Fig. 14–49); they may be solitary or multiple, and occur throughout the GI tract.[73] They may be associated with hemangiomas elsewhere in the body, most commonly in the skin; however, less than 2% of patients with cutaneous hemangiomas have GI tract hemangiomas. Arteriovenous malformations are larger lesions that may occur in any layer of the intestinal wall (Fig. 14–50).

In addition to sporadic tumors, hemangiomas of the GI tract may be seen in several rare syndromes[74]:

1. Klippel-Trenaunay syndrome: hemangiomas of the lower extremity and GI tract.
2. Osler-Weber-Rendu disease (hereditary hemorrhagic telangiectasia): familial disease characterized by telangiectasias of the mucous membranes associated with repeated gastrointestinal hemorrhage.
3. Blue rubber bleb nevus syndrome: cavernous hemangiomas of the skin and GI tract. The cutaneous hemangiomas are bluish and feel like "rubber nipples."

4. Maffucci syndrome: hemangiomas associated with multiple enchondromas.
5. Kasabach-Merritt syndrome: triad of hemangioma, thrombocytopenia, and bleeding diathesis.

GI tract hemangiomas are of three types:

1. Capillary hemangiomas are small, appearing as a cherry red spot on the mucosa at endoscopy. They occur most commonly in the stomach and small intestine, and are usually asymptomatic. Rarely they produce occult GI bleeding.
2. Cavernous hemangioma, which is usually large and symptomatic, presenting with GI hemorrhage or intestinal obstruction. They most commonly occur in the sigmoid colon and

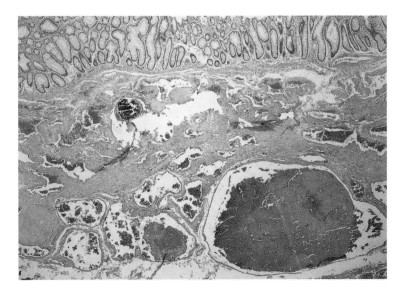

Figure 14–49. Hemangioma of the rectum, showing submucosal cavernous vascular spaces with focal thrombosis.

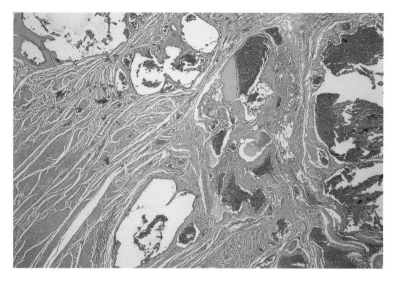

A

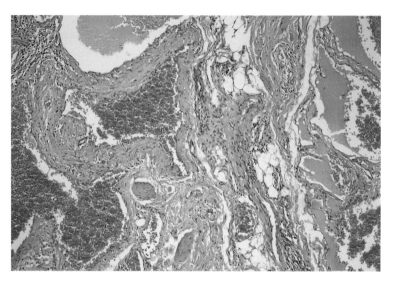

B

Figure 14–50. A: Arteriovenous malformation of the colonic wall, showing vascular spaces of varying size and wall thickness. Colonic muscle wall elements are present around and between the vascular spaces. B: Higher power micrograph of part A, showing an arteriolar vessel and larger thin-walled vessels in the arteriovenous malformation.

rectum and appear as submucosal tumors with petechial hemorrhages in the overlying mucosa. Mucosal ulceration is rare. Cavernous angiomas may undergo thrombosis; when large and thrombosis is extensive, a bleeding diathesis may result from consumption thrombocytopenia and hypofibrinogenemia.[73]

3. Mixed capillary–cavernous hemangiomas.

Cavernous hemangioma must be distinguished from the much commoner colonic angiodysplasia, a very common lesion occurring mainly in the right side of the colon that is responsible for many cases of lower GI bleeding in the elderly. The distinction is made by radiologic findings; angiodysplasia rarely forms a recognizable mass lesion when the affected colonic segment is resected, unlike cavernous hemangioma, which is a grossly defined tumor mass.

Glomus Tumor

Glomus tumors are extremely rare in the GI tract; most reported cases have been in the stomach (Fig. 14–51).[75] Glomus tumors are 1–4 cm in size and located predominantly in the muscular wall, mimicking GIST grossly. Microscopically, they are composed of a uniform population of small, polygonal cells in nests separated by vascular channels. The neoplastic cells have sharp, well-defined cell borders; central nuclei; and clear-to-amphophilic cytoplasm. The vascular network is best seen at the periphery of the tumor and can be accentuated by reticulin stain. The main tumor to be differentiated from the glomus tumor is an epithelioid GIST; this differential diagnosis is best resolved by immunohistochemical staining (GIST is CD34-positive, actin-negative, whereas the glomus tumor is CD34-negative, actin-positive). Glomus tumors are benign.

Kaposi's Sarcoma

Kaposi's sarcoma almost always occurs in immunocompromised patients, most commonly those with HIV-related immunodeficiency and after organ transplantation. Kaposi's sarcoma of the GI tract is common in patients with cutaneous Kaposi's sarcoma, but may occur without cutaneous involvement; in the latter case, GI tract Kaposi's sarcoma may represent the first AIDS-defining condition in an HIV-positive patient.

GI tract Kaposi's sarcoma presents as red nodular lesions that are usually 0.5–1.5 cm in size (Fig. 14–52); lesions occur throughout the GI tract and may be solitary, but are frequently multiple.[76] More rarely, large nodules with mucosal ulceration may occur. They are commonly submucosal with an overlying normal mucosa; in these cases, mucosal biopsy samples taken from an endoscopically obvious lesion may be negative. Mucosal infiltration by Kaposi's sarcoma is not uncommon, however, and in these cases, mucosal biopsy is positive. In rare cases, Kaposi's sarcoma may present as diffuse ulceration of the mucosa, mimicking ulcerative colitis.[77]

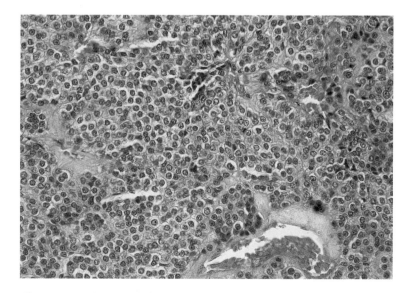

Figure 14–51. Glomus tumor of the stomach, showing typical uniform round cells around vessels.

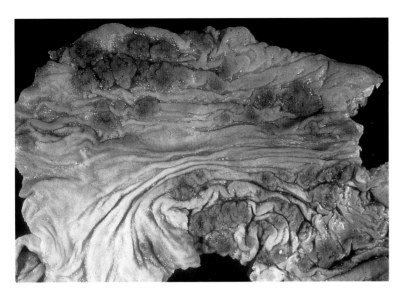

Figure 14–52. Stomach at autopsy in a patient with AIDS, showing multiple brownish plaque/nodular lesions of Kaposi's sarcoma.

Microscopically, Kaposi's sarcoma is characterized by a spindle cell proliferation with slit-like vascular spaces associated with extravasated erythrocytes and hemosiderin pigment (Fig. 14–53A). Eosinophilic, PAS-positive cytoplasmic globules of varying size may be seen in the proliferating endothelial cells (Fig. 14–53B).[78] These changes are diagnostic when they occur in a submucosal nodule. In a mucosal biopsy specimen, these changes are difficult to distinguish from granulation tissue associated with a healing ulcer; Kaposi's sarcoma is usually not associated with surface ulceration and the neoplastic proliferation is seen to splay out the normal mucosal glands. Sometimes, patients with mucosal infection with cytomegalovirus show an associated proliferation of the affected vessels that may mimic Kaposi's sarcoma; the presence of cytomegalovirus inclusions permits this diagnosis. The differentiation of proliferative cy-

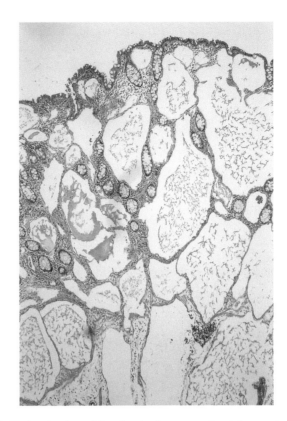

Figure 14–54. Lymphangioma of the colon, showing cavernous lymphatic spaces in the mucosa. Note the residual colonic crypts between the cavernous spaces.

tomegalovirus vasculitis from Kaposi's sarcoma, however, may not be completely clear because Kaposi's sarcoma is sometimes associated with cytomegalovirus infection.

Hemangiopericytoma

Primary hemangiopericytomas are extremely rare in the GI tract. Most of the reported cases have been in the small intes-

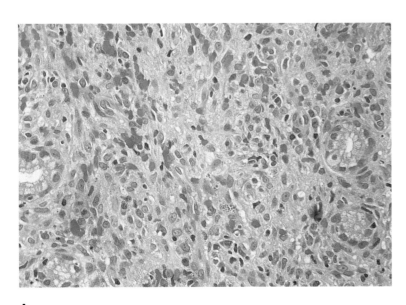

A

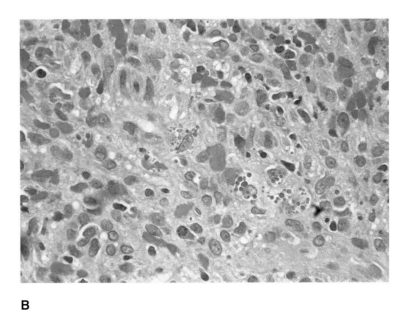

B

Figure 14–53. A: Kaposi's sarcoma of the stomach, showing spindle cell proliferation in the lamina propria associated with erythrocyte extravasation. B: Higher power micrograph of part A, showing hyaline globules in the cytoplasm of the endothelial cells.

tine.[79–81] Most GI tumors with the histologic appearance of a hemangiopericytoma are really GISTs. A diagnosis of hemangiopericytoma should be considered only when a GI tumor is composed entirely of hemangiopericytomatous histology and are CD34-negative. Even in these cases, a controversy arises about whether these represent CD34-negative GISTs rather than hemangiopericytoma. A few CD34-positive hemangiopericytomas have been reported, but how these differ from GISTs with a hemangiopericytomatous architecture is unclear.

Angiosarcoma

Angiosarcomas are extremely rare in the GI tract.[82–84] A spectrum of histologic pattern occurs, ranging from the typical anastomosing vascular channels lined by malignant endothelial cells that frequently show papillary change, to more solid, less obviously vascular lesions with malignant spindle-shaped and epithelioid cells. The predominantly solid angiosarcomas are frequently mistaken on morphologic examination for poorly differentiated carcinomas, metastatic malignant melanomas, and malignant GISTs. Immunoperoxidase staining is useful in establishing the diagnosis of angiosarcoma (vimentin-positive, factor VIII-positive, CD31-positive, CD34-positive, S100 protein-negative, HMB45-negative).[85,86] Epithelioid angiosarcomas may express keratin immunoreactivity[87] leading to potential confusion with poorly differentiated carcinoma; however, carcinomas do not coexpress CD34 and factor VIII. The positivity of angiosarcoma with CD34 may cause diagnostic confusion with malignant GIST unless the entire panel of stains is performed.

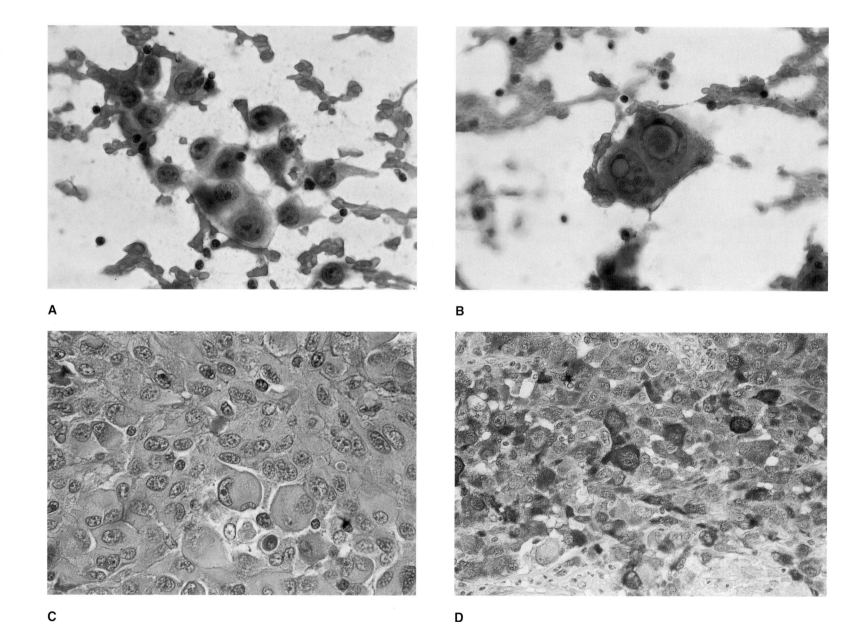

A

B

C

D

Figure 14–55. A: Metastatic melanoma, smear, showing pigmented malignant cells. B: Metastatic melanoma, smear, showing large malignant cell with cytoplasmic pigment and an intranuclear pseudo-inclusion that also contains melanin pigment. C: Metastatic melanoma in the small intestine, achromatic, showing poorly differentiated malignant cells without pigment. The cells have large nuclei with prominent nucleoli and abundant glassy eosinophilic cytoplasm. D: Metastatic malignant melanoma, showing strong S100 protein positivity in immunoperoxidase stain.

Lymphangioma

Lymphangiomas are rare tumors of the GI tract (Fig. 14–54). They are usually asymptomatic, forming small submucosal nodules that are found incidentally. Microscopically, they are composed of dilated, thin-walled channels, often accompanied by small lymphocytic aggregates. On small endoscopic biopsy specimens, lymphangiomas can be mistaken for intestinal lymphangiectasia, both primary and secondary. Intestinal lymphangiectasia involves the small intestine and is recognizable as a dilatation of the preexisting mucosal lymphatic channels; the normal architecture of the mucosa is maintained. Primary intestinal lymphangiectasia does not form a mass; it is a histologic mucosal change that is sometimes associated with malabsorption syndrome (see Chapter 7).

METASTATIC NEOPLASMS

Metastatic neoplasms involving the wall of the intestine may clinically and grossly resemble GIST. The most common of these is metastatic malignant melanoma, which is not an uncommon tumor in the intestine. Most patients have a known history of melanoma, but in some patients, this history is not known at the time of examination, only being elicited by direct questioning after the pathologic diagnosis of metastatic melanoma has been made. Malignant melanoma commonly involves the submucosa and muscle wall of the intestine, producing a mass that not uncommonly causes intestinal obstruction or bleeding. Microscopically, the diagnosis is obvious when melanin pigment is present (Fig. 14–55). In achromatic tumors, the malignant proliferation of spindle-shaped and epithelioid cells can resemble GIST. The typical nuclear features of melanoma, which include round nuclei with prominent nucleoli and the presence of intranuclear pseudoinclusions, are diagnostically helpful, but may be absent (Fig. 14–55C). Differentiation from GIST and other malignant neoplasms depends on positive staining of melanoma with vimentin, S100 protein, and HMB45 (Fig. 14–55D). Rare melanomas are negative for both S100 protein and HMB45 by immunoperoxidase; also rarely, melanomas express immunoreactivity for keratin. In these cases, the differentiation of metastatic melanoma from poorly differentiated carcinoma can be very difficult.

Another specific metastatic sarcoma that can create confusion is a low-grade endometrial stromal sarcoma. We have experienced two such cases in which patients presented with large tumors in the sigmoid colon that were thought clinically to be colonic GIST. Mucosal biopsies showed nests of spindle cells within vascular channels, and the resection specimen showed this intravascular pattern of spindle cell sarcoma throughout the full thickness of the colonic wall. This appearance was so distinctive for low-grade endometrial stromal sarcoma ("endolymphatic stromal myosis") that a review of the past pathology of these patients was made. Both had prior hysterectomies diagnosed as "cellular leiomyoma," which on review were reclassified as low-grade endometrial stromal sarcoma.

References

1. Chadwick EQ, Connor EJ, Hanson CS, et al. Tumors of smooth-muscle origin in HIV-infected children. *JAMA*. 1990;263:3182–3184.
2. McLoughlin LC, Nord KS, Joshi VV, et al. Disseminated leiomyosarcoma in a child with acquired immune deficiency syndrome. *Cancer*. 1991;6:2618–2621.
3. Radin DR, Kiyabu M. Multiple smooth-muscle tumors of the colon and adrenal gland in an adult with AIDS. *AJR*. 1992;159:545–546.
4. Stout AP. Tumors of the stomach. In *Atlas of Tumor Pathology*, section 6, fasc 21. Washington DC, Armed Forces Institute of Pathology, 1953.
5. Golden T, Stout AP. Smooth muscle tumors of the gastrointestinal tract and retroperitoneal tissues. *Surg Gynecol Obstet*. 1941;73:784–810.
6. Stout AP. Bizarre smooth muscle tumors of the stomach. *Cancer*. 1962;15:400–409.
7. Mazur MT, Clark HB. Gastric stromal tumors. Reappraisal of histogenesis. *Am J Surg Pathol*. 1983;7:507–519.
8. Evans DJ, Lampert IA, Jacobs M. Intermediate filaments in smooth muscle tumors. *J Clin Pathol*. 1983;36:57–61.
9. Hjermstad EM, Sobin LH, Helwig EB. Stromal tumors of the gastrointestinal tract: Myogenic or neurogenic? *Am J Surg Pathol*. 1987;11:383–386.
10. Saul SH, Rast ML, Brooks JJ. The immunohistochemistry of gastrointestinal stromal tumors. Evidence supporting an origin from smooth muscle. *Am J Surg Pathol*. 1987;11:464–473.
11. Pike AM, Lloyd RV, Appelman MD. Cell markers in gastrointestinal stromal tumors. *Hum Pathol*. 1988;19:830–834.
12. Ueyama T, Quo K-J, Hashimoto H, et al. A clinicopathologic and immunohistochemical study of gastrointestinal stromal tumors. *Cancer*. 1992;69:947–955.
13. Ma CK, De Peralta MN, Amin MB, et al. Small intestinal stromal tumors. A clinicopathologic study of 20 cases with immunohistochemical assessment of cell differentiation and the prognostic role of proliferation antigens. *Am J Clin Pathol*. 1997;108:641–651.
14. Appleman HD. Smooth muscle tumors of the gastrointestinal tract. What we know now that Stout didn't know. *Am J Surg Pathol*. 1986; 10(Suppl 1)83–99.
15. Takubo K, Nakagawa H, Tsuchiya S, et al. Seedling leiomyoma of the esophagus and esophagogastric junction zone. *Hum Pathol*. 1981;12:1006–1010.
16. Suster S, Sorace D, Moran CA. Gastrointestinal stromal tumors with prominent myxoid matrix. Clinicopathologic, immunohistochemical, and ultrastructural study of nine cases of a distinctive morphologic variant of myogenic stromal tumor. *Am J Surg Pathol*. 1995;19:59–70.
17. Miettinen N, Virolainen M, Maarit-Sarloma-Rikala. Gastrointestinal stromal tumors—value of CD34 antigen in their identification and separation from true leiomyomas and schwannomas. *Am J Surg Pathol*. 1995;19:207–216.
18. Carney JA. The triad of gastric epithelioid leiomyosarcoma, functioning extra-adrenal paraganglioma, and pulmonary chondroma. *Cancer*. 1979;43:374–382.
19. Carney JA. The triad of gastric epithelioid leiomyosarcoma, pul-

monary chondroma, and functioning extra-adrenal paraganglioma: A five-year review. *Medicine.* 1983;62:159–169.

20. Appleman MD, Meiwig EB. Gastric epithelioid leiomyoma and leioymosarcoma (leiomyoblastoma). *Cancer.* 1976;38:708–728.

21. Appleman MD, Helwig EB. Sarcomas of the stomach. *Am J Clin Pathol.* 1977;67:2–10.

22. Ranchod N, Kempson RL. Smooth muscle tumors of the gastrointestinal tract and retroperitoneum. *Cancer.* 1977;39:255–262.

23. Shiu NH, Earr GM, Papachtistou DN, et al. Myosarcomas of the stomach: Natural history, prognostic factors and management. *Cancer.* 1982;49:177–187.

24. Miller KA, Ribnitz ME, Roth SI. Late recurrence (33 years) of a gastric epithelioid stromal tumor (leiomyoblastoma) with low malignant potential. *Arch Pathol Lab Med.* 1988;112:86–90.

25. Tsushima K, Rainwater LM, Goellner JR. Leiomyosarcomas and benign smooth muscle tumors of the stomach: Nuclear DNA patterns studied by flow cytometry. *Mayo Clin Proc.* 1987;62:275–280.

26. Kiyabu MT, Bishop PC, Parker JW, et al. Smooth muscle tumors of the gastrointestinal tract. Flow cytometric quantitation of DNA and nuclear antigen content and correlation with histologic grade. *Am J Surg Pathol.* 1988;12:954–960.

27. Cunningham RE, Federspiel EM, McCarthy WE, et al. Predicting prognosis of gastrointestinal smooth muscle tumors. Role of clinical and histologic evaluation, flow cytometry, and image cytometry. *Am J Surg Pathol.* 1993;17:588–594.

28. Goldblum JR, Appelman MD. Stromal tumors of the duodenum. A histologic and immunohistochemical study of 20 cases. *Am J Surg Pathol.* 1995;19:71–80.

29. Min K-W. Small intestinal stromal tumors with skeinoid fibers. Clinicopathological, immunohistochemical, and ultrastructural investigations. *Am J Surg Pathol.* 1992;16:145–155.

30. Walsh TM, Mann CV. Smooth muscle neoplasms of the rectum and anal canal. *Br J Surg.* 1984;71:597–599.

31. Evans HL. Smooth muscle tumors of the gastrointestinal tract. A study of 56 cases followed for a minimum of 10 years. *Cancer.* 1985;56:2242–2250.

32. McGrath PC, Neifeld JP, Lawrence W, et al. Gastrointestinal sarcomas. Analysis of prognostic factors. *Ann Surg.* 1987;206:706–710.

33. Herrera GA, Cerezo L, Jones JE, et al. Gastrointestinal autonomic nerve tumors. 'Plexosarcomas.' *Arch Pathol Lab Med.* 1989;113:846–853.

34. Lauwers GY, Erlandson RA, Casper ES, et al. Gastrointestinal autonomic nerve tumors. A clinicopathological, immunohistochemical, and ultrastructural study of 12 cases. *Am J Surg Pathol.* 1993;17:887–897.

35. Shek TWM, Luk ISC, Loong F, et al. Inflammatory cell-rich gastrointestinal autonomic nerve tumor. An expansion of its histologic spectrum. *Am J Surg Pathol.* 1996;20:225–331.

36. Raszkowski HJ, Hufner RF. Neurofibromatosis of the colon: A unique manifestation of von Recklinghausen's disease. *Cancer.* 1971;27:134–142.

37. Mochberg FM, Dasilva AB, Qaldabini J, et al. Gastrointestinal involvement in von Recklinghausen's neurofibromatosis. *Neurology.* 1974;24:1144–1151.

38. Schaldenbrand JD, Appelman HD. Solitary solid stromal gastrointestinal tumors in von Recklinghausen's disease with minimal smooth muscle differentiation. *Hum Pathol.* 1984;15:229–232.

39. Daimaru Y, Kido H, Hashimoto H, et al. Benign schwannoma of the gastrointestinal tract: A clinicopathologic and immunohistochemical study. *Hum Pathol.* 1988;19:257–264.

40. Johnston J, Helwig SB. Granular cell tumors of the gastrointestinal tract and perianal region. A study of 74 cases. *Dig Dis Sci.* 1981;26:807–816.

41. Schwartz DT, Gaetz HP. Multiple granular cell myoblastomas of the stomach. *Am J Clin Pathol.* 1965;44:453–457.

42. Kanabe S, Watanabe I, Lotuaco L. Multiple granular-cell tumors of the ascending colon: Microscopic study. *Dis Colon Rectum.* 1978;21:322–328.

43. Fried KS, Arden JL, Gouge TM, et al. Multifocal granular cell tumors of the gastrointestinal tract. *Am J Gastroenterol.* 1984;79:751–755.

44. Buley ID, Gatter KC, Kelley PMA, et al. Granular cell tumors revisited. An immunological and ultrastructural study. *Histopathology.* 1988;12:263–274.

45. Nazur MT, Shultz JJ, Myers JL. Granular cell tumor. Immunohistochemical analysis of 21 benign tumors and one malignant tumor. *Arch Pathol Lab Med.* 1990;114:692–696.

46. Matsumoto H, Kojima Y, Inoue T, et al. A malignant granular cell tumor of the stomach: Report of a case. *Surg Today.* 1996;26:119–122.

47. Yamaguchi K, Maeda S, Kitamura K. Granular cell tumor of the stomach coincident with two early gastric carcinomas. *Am J Gastroenterol.* 1989;84:656–659.

48. Joshi A, Chandrasoma P, Kiyabu M. Multiple granular cell tumors of the gastrointestinal tract with subsequent development of esophageal squamous carcinoma. *Dig Dis Sci.* 1992;37:1612–1618.

49. Box JC, Newman CL, Anastasiades KD, et al. Adult rhabdomyoma: Presentation as a cervicomediastinal mass (case report and review of the literature). *Am. Surg.* 1995;61:271–276.

50. Fox KR, Moussa SM, Mitre RJ, et al. Clinical and pathologic features of primary gastric rhabdomyosarcoma. *Cancer.* 1990;66:772–778.

51. Yagihashi S, Yagihashi N, Hase Y, et al. Primary alveolar soft part sarcoma of the stomach. *Am J Surg Pathol.* 1991;15:399–406.

52. Shekitka KM, Sobin LH. Ganglioneuromas of the gastrointestinal tract. Relation to von Recklinghausen's disease and other multiple tumor syndromes. *Am J Surg Pathol.* 1994;18:250–257.

53. Gleason IOW, Beauchemin J, Bursk A. Polypoid ganglioneuromatosis of the large bowel. *Arch Neurol.* 1962;6:242–247.

54. Donnelly WH, Sieber WK, Yunis EJ. Polypoid ganglioneurofibromatosis of the large bowel. *Arch Pathol.* 1969;87:537–541.

55. Mendelsohn S, Diamond MP. Familial ganglioneuromatous polyposis of the large bowel. Report of a family with associated juvenile polyposis. *Am J Surg Pathol.* 1984;8:515–520.

56. Weidner N, Flanders DJ, Mitros FA. Mucosal ganglioneuromatosis associated with multiple colonic polyps. *Am J Surg Pathol.* 1984;8:779–786.

57. Carney JA, Go VLW, Sizemore GW, et al. Alimentary-tract ganglioneuromatosis. A major component of the syndrome of multiple endocrine neoplasia, Type 2b. *N Engl J Med.* 1976;295:1287–1291.

58. Carney JA, Mayles AB. Alimentary tract manifestations of multiple endocrine neoplasia, type 2b. *Mayo Clin Proc.* 1977;52:543–548.

59. Deschryver-Kecskemeti K, Clouse RE, Goldstein MN, et al. Intestinal ganglioneuromatosis. A manifestation of overproduction of nerve growth factor? *N Engl J Med.* 1983;308:635–639.

60. Feinstat T, Tesluk H, Schuffler MD, et al. Megacolon and neurofibromatosis: A neuronal intestinal dysplasia. Case report and review of the literature. *Gastroenterology.* 1984;86:1573–1579.

61. Reed RJ, Daroca PJ, Harkin JC. Gangliocytic paraganglioma. *Am J Surg Pathol.* 1977;1:207–216.

62. Perrone T, Sibley RK, Rosai J. Duodenal gangliocytic paraganglioma. An immunohistochemical and ultrastructural study and a hypothesis concerning its origin. *Am J Surg Pathol.* 1985;9:31–41.

63. Scheithauer BW, Nora FE, LeChago J, et al. Duodenal gangliocytic paraganglioma. Clinicopathologic and immunohistochemical study of 11 cases. *Am J Clin Pathol.* 1986;86:559–565.

64. Anders KH, Glasgow BJ, Lewin KJ. Gangliocytic paraganglioma associated with duodenal adenocarcinoma. Case report with immunohistochemical evaluation. *Arch Pathol Lab Med.* 1987;111:49–52.

65. Stephens M, Williams GT, Jasani B, et al. Synchronous duodenal neuroendocrine tumours in von Recklinghausen's disease—a case report of co-existing gangliocytic paraganglioma and somatostatin-rich glandular carcinoid. *Histopathology.* 1987;11:1331–1340.

66. Castro EB, Stearns MW. Lipoma of the large intestine: A review of 45 cases. *Dis Colon Rectum.* 1972;15:441–444.

67. Fernandez MJ, Davis RP, Nora PF. Gastrointestinal lipomas. *Arch Surg.* 1993;118:1081–1084.

68. Buetow PC, Buck SL, Carr NJ, et al. Intussuscepted colonic lipomas: Loss of fat attenuation on CT with pathologic correlation in 10 cases. *Abdom Imag.* 1996;21:153–156.

69. Snover DC, Sandstad J, Hutton S. Mucosal pseudolipomatosis of the colon. *Am J Clin Pathol.* 1985;84:575–580.

70. Atik N, Whittlesey RH. Liposarcoma of jejunum. *Ann Surg.* 1957;146:837–842.

71. Smith CET, Filipe MI, Owen WJ. Neuromuscular and vascular hamartoma of small bowel presenting as inflammatory bowel disease. *Gut.* 1986;27:964–969.

72. Kwasnik EM, Tahan SR, Lowell JA, et al. Neuromuscular and vascular hamartoma of the small bowel. *Dig Dis Sci.* 1989;34:108–110.

73. Lyon DT, Mantia AG. Large-bowel hemangioma. *Dis Colon Rectum.* 1987;27:404–414.

74. Fenoglio-Preiser CM, Lantz PE, Listrom MB. *Gastrointestinal Pathology. An Atlas and Text.* New York, Raven Press, 1989.

75. Appelman HD, Heiwig EB. Glomus tumors of the stomach. *Cancer.* 1969;23:203–213.

76. Friedman SL, Wright TL, Altman DF. Gastrointestinal Kaposi's sarcoma in patients with acquired immunodeficiency syndrome. *Gastroenterology.* 1985;89:102–108.

77. Biggs BA, Crowe SM, Lucas CR, et al. AIDS related Kaposi's sarcoma presenting as ulcerative colitis and complicated by toxic megacolon. *Gut.* 1987;28:1302–1306.

78. Senba M, Itakura H, Yamashita H, et al. Eosinophilic globules in Kaposi's sarcoma. A histochemical, immunohistochemical, and ultrastructural study. *Acta Pathol Jpn.* 1986;36:1327–1333.

79. Burke JS, Ranchod N. Hemangiopericytoma of the esophagus. *Hum Pathol.* 1981;12:96–100.

80. Genter B, Mir R, Strauss R. Hemangiopericytoma of the colon: report of a case and review of the literature. *Dis Colon Rectum.* 1982;25:149–156.

81. Ball ABS, Strong L, Hastings A. Malignant haemangiopericytoma of the terminal ileum presenting with peritonitis and transcoelomic metastases. *Br J Surg.* 1984;71:161–162.

82. Ordonez NG, del Junco GW, Ayala AG, et al. Angiosarcoma of the small intestine: An immunoperoxidase study. *Am J Gastroenterol.* 1983;78:218–221.

83. Taxy JB, Battifora H. Angiosarcoma of the gastrointestinal tract. A report of three cases. *Cancer.* 1988;62:210–216.

84. Smith JA, Bhathai PS, Cuthbertson AM. Angiosarcoma of the colon. Report of a case with long-term survival. *Dis Colon Rectum.* 1990;33:330–333.

85. De Young BR, Wick MR, Fitzgibbon JF, et al. CD31. An immunospecific marker for endothelial differentiation in human neoplasms. *Appl Immunohistochem.* 1993;1:97–100.

86. Sirgi KE, Wick MR, Swanson PE. B72.3 and CD34 immunoreactivity in malignant epithelioid soft tissue tumors. Adjuncts in the recognition of endothelial neoplasms. *Am J Surg Pathol.* 1993;17:179–185.

87. Gray MH, Rosenberg AF, Dickerson GR. Cytokeratin expression in epithelioid vascular neoplasms. *Hum Pathol.* 1990;21:212–217.

15

MALIGNANT LYMPHOMAS OF THE GASTROINTESTINAL TRACT

Joel Chan

NORMAL LYMPHOID TISSUE

Stomach

Well-developed lymphoid follicles with germinal centers are not found in normal gastric mucosa (Fig. 15–1).[1] Occasional small aggregates of lymphocytes can occur without germinal centers; these are usually found in the deep mucosa adjacent to the muscularis mucosae.[2] Lymphoid aggregates are found throughout the stomach but most commonly in the distal antrum. The presence of well-formed reactive follicles in the superficial gastric mucosa is a direct consequence of infection with *Helicobacter pylori* (Fig. 15–2).[2,3] Thus, "normal" gastric mucosa-associated lymphoid tissue (MALT) represents an abnormal histologic finding.

Intestine

The lamina propria of the small and large intestine is populated by plasma cells, histiocytes, and scattered B and T lymphocytes. Unlike the stomach, the intestine normally has well-developed lymphoid follicles. In the large intestine, the follicles are scattered (Fig. 15–3); in the small intestine, they are aggregated to form large Peyer's patches (Fig. 15–4).

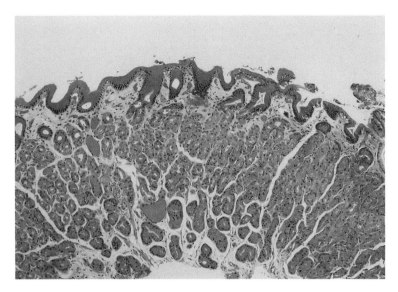

Figure 15–1. Relatively normal-appearing gastric mucosa showing a very sparse mononuclear inflammatory infiltrate.

The lymphoid follicles occur in the mucosa and submucosa. Just as in the normal lymph node, these follicles are surrounded by a mantle zone of small B lymphocytes (Fig. 15–5). Unlike the lymph node, there is often an identifiable zone of small to medium-sized B lymphocytes, centrocyte-like cells, or monocytoid B cells with moderate amounts of cytoplasm surrounding the mantle zones and forming marginal zones.[4] This marginal zone of lymphocytes can sometimes focally extend

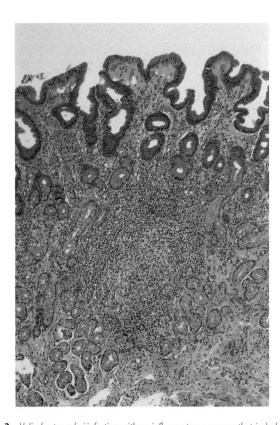

Figure 15–2. *Helicobacter pylori* infection with an inflammatory response that includes the formation of follicles and an increase in the number of lymphocytes within the lamina propria. Compared with lymphomas of MALT, the lymphocytic infiltrate here is not dense.

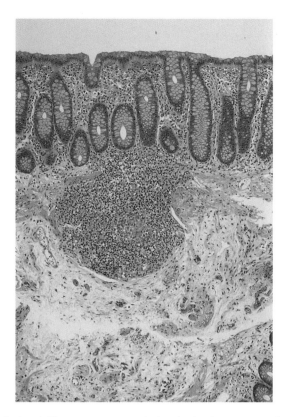

Figure 15–3. Lymphoid aggregates are present in the colon, but they are not as well developed as those seen in the small intestine.

upward to infiltrate the overlying epithelium and to form small collections of intraepithelial B cells (Fig. 15–6).[5]

Intraepithelial T lymphocytes are normally present, especially in the small intestine. The number of these intraepithelial lymphocytes decreases distally. It is appropriate to find approximately 20 lymphocytes per 100 epithelial cells in the jejunum, whereas in the ileum approximately 13 lymphocytes occur per 100 epithelial cells.[6]

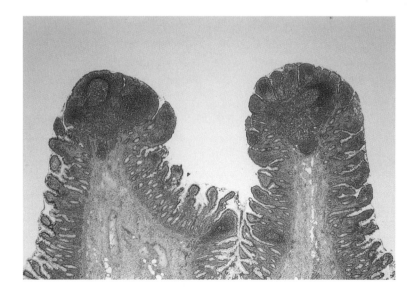

Figure 15–4. Large lymphoid aggregates are normal findings in the small intestine, where they coalesce to form Peyer's patches.

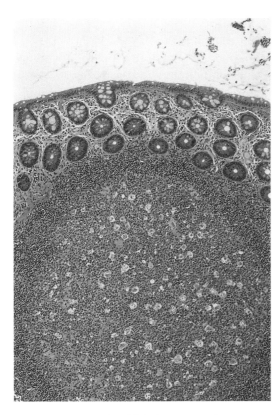

Figure 15–5. This benign colonic lymphoid follicle shows a germinal center composed of a mixture of small and large lymphocytes and tingible body macrophages. The mantle zone composed of small lymphocytes rims the germinal center.

CLASSIFICATION OF GI TRACT LYMPHOMAS

There is no universally agreed upon histological scheme for classifying gastrointestinal lymphomas. The original approach assigned a diagnosis based on their closest histological nodal-based counterpart. In Europe, gastrointestinal lymphomas are often classified in accordance with the updated Kiel classification[7] (Table 15–1). Isaacson and colleagues, who first proposed the concept of the mucosal-associated lymphoid tissue (MALT) lymphoma, proposed a separate scheme (Table 15–2).[8] In the United States, the Working formulation is the most widely used histological classification (Table 15–3).

These classification schema are not satisfactory when considering gastrointestinal lymphomas, however, because primary GI lymphomas have unique clinicopathologic characteristics. In the stomach, the low-grade B-cell lymphoma of MALT, depending on its constituent lymphocytes, can be classified as small lymphocytic, diffuse small cleaved cell, or diffuse mixed small- and large-cell lymphoma. These are unsatisfactory diagnoses considering that the latter two classes represent intermediate-grade lymphomas by the Working formulation. Furthermore, the nodal-based monocytoid B-cell lymphoma, which is currently thought to be the nodal counterpart of MALT lymphomas, is not recognized under the Working formulation.

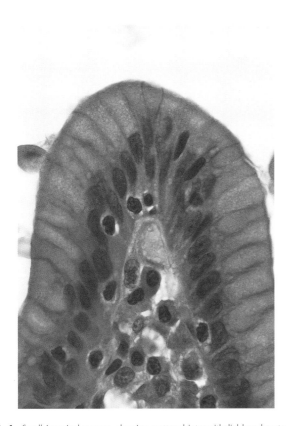

Figure 15–6. Small-intestinal mucosa, showing scattered intraepithelial lymphocytes among the villous epithelial cells. Normal intraepithelial lymphocytes are seen as single cells without nuclear atypia.

TABLE 15–1. UPDATED KIEL CLASSIFICATION

B Cell

Low Grade
   Lymphocytic
   Hairy-cell leukemia
   Lymphoplasmacytic/cytoid (LP immunocytoma)
   Plasmacytic
   Centroblastic/centrocytic—follicular, diffuse

High Grade
   Centroblastic
   Immunoblastic
   Large-cell anaplastic (Ki-1+)
   Burkitt's lymphoma
   Lymphoblastic

T Cell

Low Grade
   Lymphocytic—chronic lymphocytic and prolymphocytic leukemia
   Small, cerebriform cell—mycosis fungoides, Sezary's syndrome
   Lymphoepithelioid (Lennert's lymphoma)
   Angioimmunoblastic (AILD)
   T zone
   Pleomorphic, small cell

High Grade
   Pleomorphic, medium and large cell
   Immunoblastic
   Large-cell anaplastic (Ki-1+)
   Lymphoblastic

TABLE 15–2. PROPOSED ISAACSON CLASSIFICATION

B Cell
    Low-grade B-cell lymphoma of MALT
    High-grade B-cell lymphoma of MALT, with or without evidence of a low-grade component
    Mediterranean lymphoma (immunoproliferative small-intestinal disease), low grade, mixed, or
        high grade
    Malignant lymphoma centrocytic (lymphomatous polyposis)
    Burkitt-like lymphoma
    Other types of low- or high-grade lymphoma corresponding to peripheral lymph node equivalents
T Cell
    Enteropathy-associated T-cell lymphoma (EATL)
    Other types unassociated with enteropathy

In lieu of the Working formulation, we use a three-tiered grading system (see Table 15–3). Because the purpose of any classification system is to provide clinicians with prognostically useful information, we choose an appellation that conveys the aggressiveness of the lesion. When appropriate, we use the diagnosis of "low-grade B-cell lymphoma of MALT" to convey the low-grade behavior of this lesion to clinicians. When focal areas of transformation occur, this finding is addended to the preceding diagnosis. When the higher grade lymphomatous areas comprise the majority of the lesion, then the lymphoma is classified as a high-grade lymphoma of MALT.

With a high-grade lymphoma, an attempt is made to identify a low-grade component with the assumption that the high-grade lymphoma evolved from a low-grade lesion. A residual low-grade lymphoma is not always identifiable, however, so it is uncertain whether these lesions represent a de novo high-grade lymphoma. Tumors composed entirely of high-grade lymphoma are classified according to their nodal-based counterparts per the Working formulation, for example, as an immunoblastic lymphoma.

We believe that this system is in keeping with studies showing that stratification of gastric MALT lymphomas into low grade, low grade with focal areas of transformation, and high-grade lymphomas has prognostic significance.

Other primary gastrointestinal lymphomas show unique clinicopathologic features. Multiple lymphomatous polyposis is a primary intestinal mantle cell lymphoma. Although it has the same histologic and immunophenotypic expression as nodal-based mantle cell lymphoma, it has a distinct clinical progression.[9] Immunoproliferative small-intestinal disease (IPSID) can be considered a special form of MALT lymphoma that is intimately associated with α-heavy-chain disease.[10,11] Enteropathy-associated T-cell lymphoma (EATL) arises in the setting of celiac disease.[12] Neither IPSID nor EATL can be adequately de-

TABLE 15–3. SUGGESTED CLASSIFICATION SCHEME AND A COMPARISON WITH VARIOUS CLASSIFICATION SCHEMES

Working Formulation	Updated Kiel Classification	REAL Classification	Suggested Classification
B-Cell lymphomas:			
Low-grade lymphomas			
Small lymphocytic;	Lymphocytic	Extranodal marginal zone	Low-grade lymphoma of MALT
Diffuse, small cleaved;		B-cell lymphoma	
Diffuse, mixed small and large			
	Lymphoplasmacytic/cytoid		IPSID
	(LP immunocytoma)		
Small lymphocytic;	Centrocytic	Mantle cell lymphoma	Multiple lymphomatous polyposis (MLP)
Follicular, small cleaved cell;			
Diffuse, small cleaved;			
Diffuse, mixed, small and large;			
Diffuse, large cleaved			
High-grade lymphomas			
Diffuse large cell, immunoblastic	Centroblastic; immunoblastic	Diffuse large B-cell lymphoma	High-grade lymphoma of MALT
Small noncleaved, Burkitt's;	Burkitt's	Burkitt's lymphoma;	Burkitt; Burkitt-like
Small noncleaved non-Burkitt's		High-grade B-cell lymphoma, Burkitt-like	
T-Cell lymphomas			
Diffuse, small cleaved;		Intestinal T-cell lymphoma	Enteropathy-associated T-cell lymphoma
Diffuse, mixed small and large;			(EATL)
Diffuse, large			
Large-cell immunoblastic			

Abbreviations: MALT = mucosa-associated lymphoid tissue. IPSID = immunoproliferative small intestinal disease.

scribed or classified in accordance with any of the current schema.

The revised European-American lymphoma (REAL) classification is a newly proposed scheme (see Table 15–3).[13] Using morphologic, immunologic, and genetic techniques currently available, REAL tries to reclassify lymphomas in accordance with their normal counterpart. This scheme recognizes some of the primary gut lymphomas as specific entities having a unique biology and natural course.

MALT LYMPHOMAS

Primary extranodal lymphomas account for up to 40% of all non-Hodgkin's lymphomas.[14] Lymphomas of the gastrointestinal tract constitute the majority of primary extranodal lymphomas, and most of these arise in the stomach.[15] Considering gastric neoplasms as a whole, however, lymphoma is a relatively rare tumor, accounting for only 7% of all primary gastric malignant neoplasms.[16]

The concept of MALT lymphoma was proposed by Isaacson and Wright in 1983 to describe a distinct group of extranodal lymphomas arising in MALT sharing similar clinicopathologic characteristics.[17] The gastrointestinal tract accounts for the vast majority of MALT lymphomas, but these have been reported to occur in a variety of other tissues, such as the lung, thyroid, salivary, and lacrimal glands.

MALT lymphomas, as a group, because of their tendency to remain localized for long periods, respond well to local therapy, such as surgery, and have excellent long-term disease-free survival rates.[18] Because of their indolent nature, they have a much better prognosis than similar histologic grade nodal-based lymphomas.[19] Their propensity to remain localized for long periods is thought to be secondary to the inherently epitheliotropic nature of lymphoid cells to specifically target their respective organs.[20] A unique occurrence to MALT lymphoma as a group, which is distinctly different from nodal-based lymphomas, is its ability to present metachronously or synchronously with MALT lymphomas at other sites.[21]

Gastric Malt Lymphomas

The stomach is thought to have some lymphoid inflammatory cells but no lymphoid follicles or well-developed MALT.[1,2] In the stomach, the development of MALT is usually associated with *Helicobacter pylori* infection (Figs. 15–7 and 15–8). In the evolution of MALT lymphoma, it is thought that *H. pylori* infection leads to the development of MALT.[22] Arising from this MALT is a neoplastic clone that, with the help of *H. pylori* antigen-driven T cells, proliferates and becomes the early MALT lymphoma.[22,23] A considerable body of evidence supports this concept:

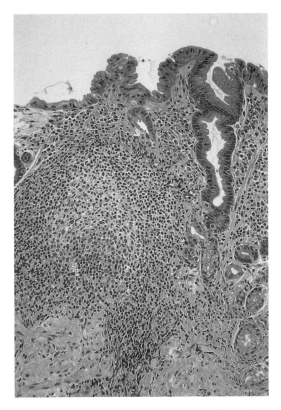

Figure 15–7. Chronic antral gastritis secondary to *Helicobacter pylori* infection, showing lymphocytic infiltration of the mucosa with a reactive follicle.

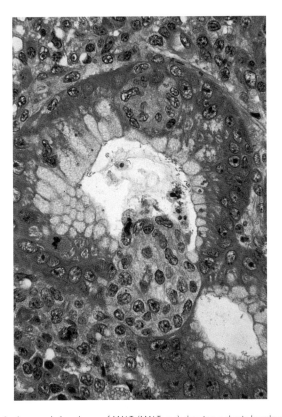

Figure 15–8. Low-grade lymphoma of MALT (MALToma) showing a classic lymphoepithelial lesion. The gland lumen shows numerous eosinophilic, rod-shaped *H. pylori*. At the 12 o'clock and 6 o'clock positions of the gland, groups of atypical-appearing lymphocytes are evident invading the gland.

1. Nearly 90% of gastric MALT lymphomas have evidence of *H. pylori* infection.[22,24]
2. A significant proportion of gastric MALT lymphomas regress following eradication of *H. pylori* by antibiotic treatment.[25–27]
3. Reported cases of lymphoma have relapsed following reinfection with *H. pylori.*[28]
4. Evidence of active chronic gastritis, a finding almost always associated with *H. pylori* infection, can almost always be identified in the uninvolved gastric mucosa adjacent to MALT lymphomas.[24]

B-cell primary gastric lymphomas of MALT differ from lymphomas that arise from lymph nodes and secondarily involve the stomach. Whereas nodal lymphomas secondarily involving the stomach are disseminated diseases, primary lymphomas of MALT remain localized to the stomach for a long time. Nodal metastasis occurs in up to one third of patients,[29] but usually after a long period of localized disease.[30]

One recent study using a population-based registry to compare nodal-based non-Hodgkin's lymphoma (NHL) with gastric MALT lymphoma found that gastric MALT lymphoma was more likely to be localized at presentation, had a significantly lower recurrence rate, and a significantly better disease-free survival rate than nodal NHL. Overall survival did not differ significantly between these two groups, however.[31]

In other series, nodal-based monocytoid B-cell lymphomas have been reported to have very similar morphologic and immunophenotypic characteristics to primary gastric MALT lymphomas (Fig. 15–9). Unlike primary gastric MALT lymphomas, however, which are usually localized diseases, nodal monocytoid B-cell lymphomas usually present with widespread disease, including bone marrow involvement, and have lower disease-free survival rates.[32,33]

Clinical Presentation

Low-grade MALT lymphomas tend to occur in patients older than 50, with a peak occurrence in the seventh decade of life. Symptoms are nonspecific and include epigastric pain, dyspepsia, and nausea and vomiting.[34]

On endoscopic examination, the appearance of low-grade MALT lymphoma can mimic that of benign conditions such as chronic gastritis and peptic ulcer disease.[34,35] Thickening of mucosal folds, irregular nodularity producing a cobblestone effect, and ulceration are common features (Figs. 15–10 and 15–11). Gastric masses are rarely found in low-grade lymphomas, but are common in high-grade lymphomas (Fig. 15–12), in which the endoscopic features may resemble gastric carcinoma.[35,36] The pyloric antrum and the prepylorus is the most common site for MALT lymphoma, followed by the gastric body and the fundus. Multiple foci of lymphoma are a frequent occurrence.[37] Due to this multifocality, local excision can leave behind small foci of neoplastic lymphocytes, which can be the source of later relapse.[38]

Pathologic Features in Endoscopic Biopsies

Low-Grade MALT Lymphoma. Histologically, on lower power view, most cases show a dense lymphocytic infiltrate in the mucosa that involves the submucosa (Fig. 15–13). Mucosal ulceration is common. Reactive lymphoid follicles are usually present (Fig. 15–14) and can be so florid that the appearance mimics a follicular lymphoma.[19,39] Low-grade MALT lymphomas usually do not invade below the submucosa.

The neoplastic lymphoid infiltrate is classically referred to as "centrocyte-like" in appearance.[19] Centrocyte-like lymphocytes resemble follicular center centrocytes or small cleaved cells that have small, irregularly shaped nuclei with scant to

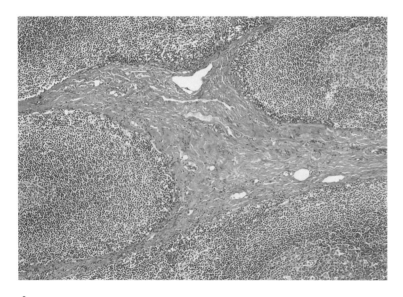

A

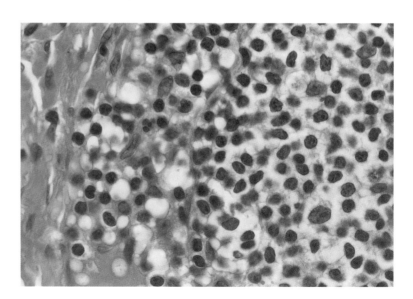

B

Figure 15–9. A: Nodal-based monocytoid B-cell lymphoma, showing hyalinized sinuses surrounded by islands of pale monocytoid B cells. B: Higher power micrograph of part A, showing typical monocytoid B-cell morphology.

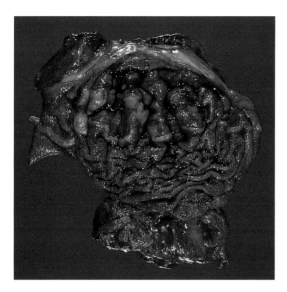

Figure 15–10. This gastric low-grade MALToma presents as enlarged rugal folds. Low-grade lymphomas usually present as thickenings of the folds or as erosions.

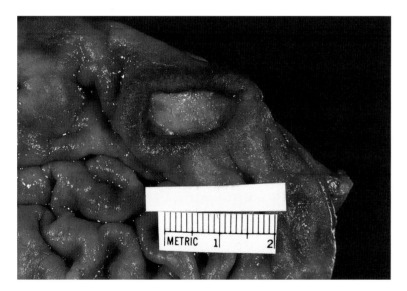

Figure 15–11. Another gastric low-grade MALToma presents as enlarged rugal folds, with a focal, large area of ulceration.

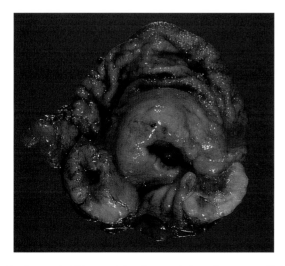

Figure 15–12. Compared with low-grade lymphomas, which usually present as thickenings or ulcers, high-grade lymphomas often present as mass lesions. This gastric high-grade MALToma presented as a tumor with an overlying central ulceration.

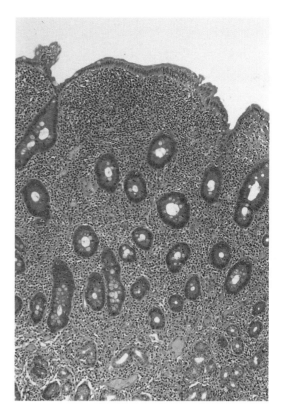

Figure 15–13. The superficial and deep glands show intestinal metaplasia secondary to chronic *H. pylori* gastritis. A diffuse lymphoplasmacytic infiltrate infuses the entire lamina propria. No identifiable lymphoepithelial lesions or benign reactive follicles are evident, however. These features are not always present in MALT.

moderate amounts of cytoplasm (Fig. 15–15).[40] The neoplastic lymphoid cells, however, can show a spectrum from these centrocyte-like cells to monocytoid B cells, which have abundant clear to amphophilic cytoplasm and well-defined cytoplasmic borders (Fig. 15–16).[33,34]

Lymphoepithelial cells are a typical feature of MALT lym-

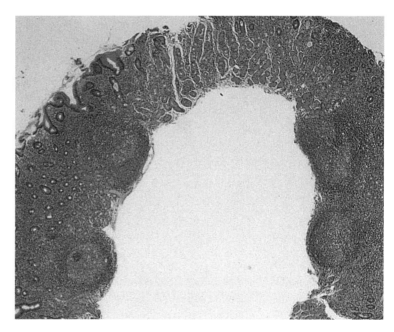

Figure 15–14. Stomach, MALT-lymphoma. Compared with Figure 15–13, the dense lymphoplasmacytic infiltrate here is accompanied by several benign, reactive lymphoid follicles.

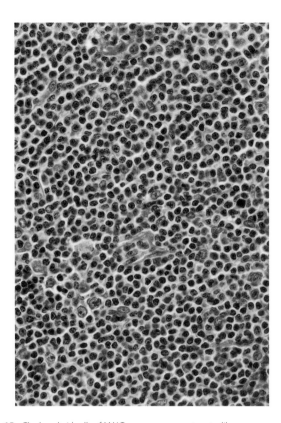

Figure 15–15. The lymphoid cells of MALT can appear as centrocyte-like or as monocytoid B cells. In this example of low-grade lymphoma of MALT, the lymphoid cells are small, with slightly irregular nuclear contours and scant cytoplasm.

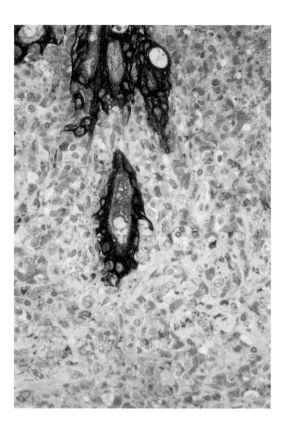

Figure 15–17. Immunoperoxidase staining for keratin often highlights lymphoepithelial lesions. Here the lymphoid cells appear as pale cells infiltrating the positively stained (brown) epithelium.

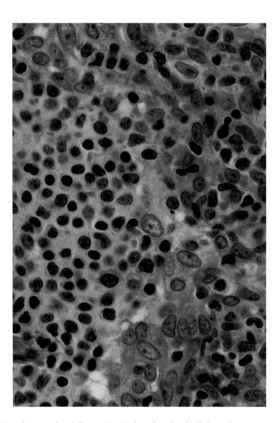

Figure 15–16. Compared with Figure 15–15, these lymphoid cells have the appearance of the classic monocytoid B cells. The lymphoid cells have round to slightly irregular nuclear contours and moderate amounts of pale cytoplasm.

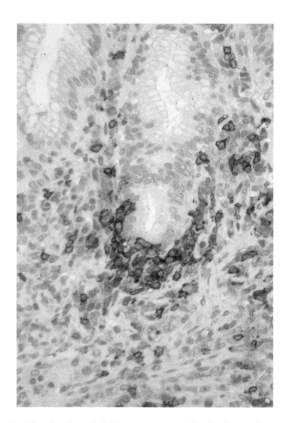

Figure 15–18. Often, lymphoepithelial lesions are not readily identified. In these situations, immunoperoxidase staining can be helpful. In this example, staining for CD20 antigen highlights the infiltrating lymphoid cells.

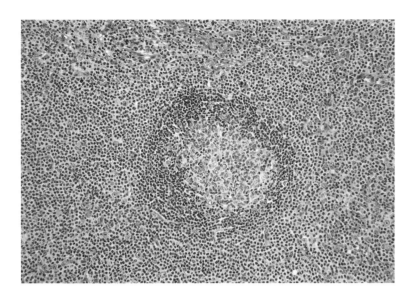

Figure 15–19. Benign reactive follicles can be seen in both chronic *H. pylori* gastritis and in MALT-omas. Here the benign reactive follicle is rimmed by a mantle zone and surrounded by a broad zone of monocytoid B cells.

phomas.[17,19,41] These are formed by the invasion of glands by the neoplastic centrocyte-like cells and lead to distortion and eventual destruction of the gland (Figs. 15–17 and 15–18).

The lamina propria is usually markedly expanded as the lymphomatous infiltrate grows around reactive follicles (Fig.

15–19), which are more frequently seen in lower grade lymphomas. The malignant lymphocytes tend to partially or completely colonize these reactive follicles (Fig. 15–20); when complete colonization occurs, the histological appearance mimics a follicular lymphoma.[19,42]

Approximately 30% of low-grade MALT lymphomas show plasmacytic differentiation (Fig. 15–21). The plasma cell component is usually subepithelially located and intermixed with the centrocyte-like lymphocytes or monocytoid B cells. These plasma cells do not contribute to the formation of lymphoepithelial lesions.[19] Occasionally, the plasmacytoid lymphocytes can display nuclear atypia with Dutcher and Russell bodies. In extreme cases, the plasma cells can constitute the predominant population, and the lesion can be misdiagnosed as a plasmacytoma.

High-Grade Primary Gastric Lymphoma. High-grade lymphomas are characterized by a diffuse proliferation of large transformed cells with a high mitotic rate (Figs. 15–22 and 15–23). These cells diffusely infiltrate the lamina propria, separating and destroying the gastric glands. When the biopsy specimen shows a malignant neoplasm composed of diffuse sheets of malignant cells, immunoperoxidase staining for CD45 and cytokeratin may be needed to distinguish high-grade lymphoma from poorly differentiated carcinoma.

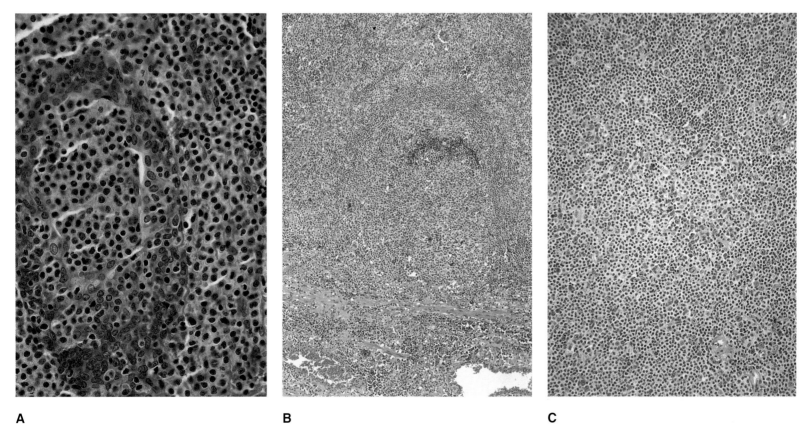

A　　　　　　　　　　**B**　　　　　　　　　　**C**

Figure 15–20. A: This follicle shows partial colonization by monocytoid B cells. The surrounding monocytoid B cells have small, round, dark nuclei with moderate amounts of pale cytoplasm. The residual follicular cells have been pushed to the side and appear as a dark rim. B: This follicle also shows partial colonization by monocytoid B cells. The residual follicular cells remain as a thin rim of small, dark cells. C: Complete colonization of the follicle has occurred. Here a vague nodularity is evident. The residual follicular lymphocytes appear as a focus of small lymphocytes at the top of the nodule. In addition, this colonized follicle also shows numerous large lymphoid cells and could possibly represent a focus of transformation to a high-grade lymphoma.

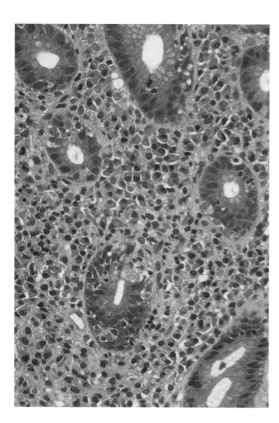

Figure 15–21. Stomach MALT lymphoma, showing lymphoepithelial lesions surrounded by lymphocytes and numerous plasma cells. Such plasmacytic differentiation is common in MALT lymphomas.

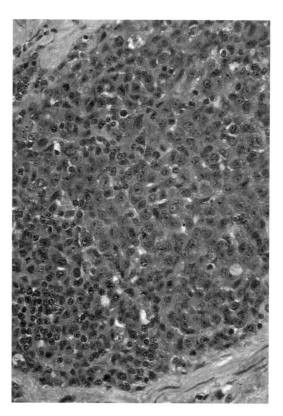

Figure 15–23. This high-grade immunoblastic lymphoma is composed of large lymphoid cells with large nuclei, prominent central nucleoli, and moderate amounts of cytoplasm.

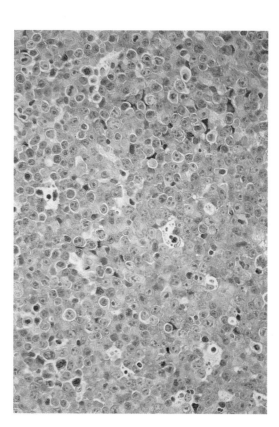

Figure 15–22. This is an example of a small noncleaved, non-Burkitt's lymphoma (Burkitt's-like lymphoma, or sporadic lymphoma). The lesion shows a diffuse proliferation of medium-size lymphocytes with scant cytoplasm, round nuclear contours, and one to three prominent nucleoli. In the background, numerous macrophages are filled with cellular debris ("tingible body marcophages"), which at scanning power would impart a "starry sky" appearance to the lesion.

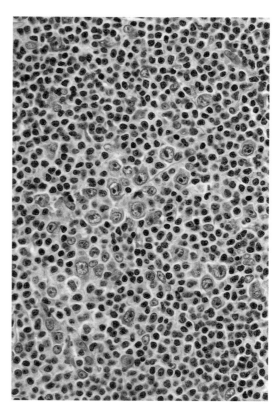

Figure 15–24. A cluster of immunoblasts is evident amidst smaller lymphoid cells. Such foci of high-grade lymphoma can arise from a background of a low-grade lymphoma of MALT. Given their prognostic significance, such foci should be reported.

High-grade gastric lymphomas may or may not have evidence of a preexisting low-grade MALT lymphoma (Figs. 15–24 and 15–25).

Genetic Features

Low-grade B-cell lymphomas arising from MALT show clonal immunoglobulin heavy-chain and light-chain rearrangements.[43] This feature has important diagnostic significance, because Southern blot analysis of endoscopic specimens for immunoglobulin (Ig) gene rearrangement has proven monoclonality in cases that showed no histologic criteria for a diagnosis of malignant lymphoma.[44] Gene rearrangement studies can be performed on endoscopic biopsy samples with as little as 20 mg of tissue, but the results are more consistent with larger samples weighing 40–60 mg.[45]

MALT lymphomas do not show rearrangement of the *bcl*-1 gene or expression of the cyclin D1 protein,[43] which is a characteristic finding of mantle cell lymphomas. Rearrangement of the *bcl*-2 gene has been documented, however, and its frequency of expression shown to be inversely proportional to the grade of the tumor.[46,47] Low-grade tumors almost always express *bcl*-2, but only less than 50% of the high-grade tumors express *bcl*-2. In addition, those high-grade lymphomas with identifiable low-grade components usually stain positively for *bcl*-2 within the low-grade component.[47]

Expression of p53 protein is sometimes demonstrable, especially in the higher grade lymphomas. Only 6% of low-grade

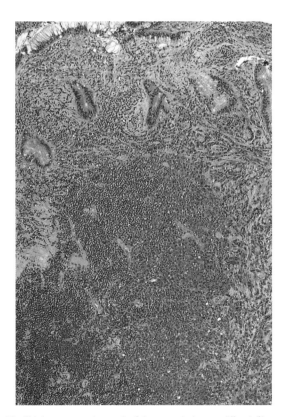

Figure 15–25. This low power micrograph of the stomach shows a diffuse infiltrate of neoplastic lymphoid cells. The paler cells on the right represent a high-grade lymphoma, which arose from the lower grade lymphoma evident on the left side. Given that this lesion shows a majority of the high-grade component, it is most appropriate to diagnose it as a high-grade lymphoma of MALT.

lymphomas express p53 protein, but this increases to 12% for low-grade tumors showing focal high-grade transformation, and to 31% for high-grade lymphomas. Patients with lymphomas positive for p53 protein have a worse prognosis than those who have p53-negative lymphomas.[46] Expression of p53 protein has been found in extremely inflamed benign gastric mucosa, however. Thus, positive staining for p53 should not be used indiscriminately as a marker for dysplasia or malignancy.[48]

Neoplastic lymphoid cells are negative for the c-*myc* gene rearrangement.[49] Trisomy 13 is the most commonly demonstrable cytogenetic abnormality, occurring in up to 60% of cases.[50] Other, less commonly seen genetic abnormalities include t(11;18) and t(1;14).[51]

Immunophenotypic Expression

The neoplastic cells of MALT lymphomas usually have the following antigen profile: CD5-negative,[52] *bcl*-1- or cyclin D1-negative, CD10-negative, CD20-positive (Table 15–4) (Fig. 15–26A). MALT lymphomas can sometimes show aberrant expression of the T-lymphocyte antigen CD43 (Fig. 15–26B).[53]

Pathologic (Biopsy) Differential Diagnosis

Atypical Lymphoid Infiltrate Secondary to H. pylori Gastritis.
When an atypical lymphoid infiltrate is present without definitive morphologic criteria of MALT lymphoma (lymphoepithelial lesions and a dense lymphocytic infiltrate with centrocyte-like cells or monocytoid B cells), the differential diagnosis between *H. pylori* gastritis and an early MALT lymphoma can be difficult (Fig. 15–27). Reactive follicles are not helpful because they can be seen in both conditions.

Two optional courses of action are available: (1) The patient is treated with antibiotics to eradicate *H. pylori*, and the biopsy is repeated. In most cases, the lymphoid infiltrate regresses rapidly, and these lesions most likely represent *H. pylori* gastritis. When the atypical lymphoid infiltrate persists, immunologic and molecular testing for MALT lymphoma is undertaken. (2) Immunoperoxidase testing for CD20, CD43, and immunoglobulin light chains is performed. The presence of cells coexpressing CD20 and CD43, and the presence of plasma cell monoclonality permits a diagnosis of MALT lymphoma. In cases of persisting doubt, a repeat biopsy with a large sample should be obtained for immunoglobulin gene rearrangement; this has been shown to demonstrate monoclonality in early MALT lymphomas not meeting definitive morphologic criteria for biopsy diagnosis.[44]

Pseudo-Lymphoma.
The term "pseudo-lymphoma" was used in the past to describe gastric lesions showing histologic features between lymphoid hyperplasia and malignant lymphoma. The presence of reactive follicles, plasma cells, and a mixed population of lymphocytes were considered suggestive of this reactive process. We no longer use the term "pseudo-lymphoma." Using current morphologic and immunohistochemical methods, these lesions can be classified as either reactive or neoplastic.

TABLE 15–4. IMMUNOPHENOTYPIC FEATURES OF COMMON B-CELL LYMPHOMAS

Lymphoma Type:	CD5	CD10	CD20	CD23	CD43	*bcl-1/PRAD1/Cyclin D1*	*bcl-2*
MALT	−	−	+	−	+/−	−	+/−
Follicular	−	+	+	−	−	−	+
Mantle cell/MLP	+	−	+	−	+/−	+	−
Small lymphocytic	+	−	+	+	+	−	−
Burkitt's/Burkitt's-like	−	−	+	−	−	−	+/−

Abbreviations: MALT = mucosa-associated lymphoid tissue; MLP = multiple lymphomatous polyposis.

Most archival cases coded as pseudo-lymphoma in the past are reclassifiable as MALT lymphomas.[54]

Non-MALT Lymphomas. Nodal follicular center cell lymphomas can secondarily involve the stomach as part of their dissemination. Unlike MALT lymphomas, in which the neoplastic follicles result from secondary colonization of reactive follicles by the neoplastic cells, follicular center cell lymphomas consists of neoplastic follicles that are closely packed, or back to back, and lack a surrounding mantle zone (Fig. 15–28A). In many cases of MALT lymphoma, colonization of the follicle is incomplete, and there is evidence of at least some elements of the original reactive follicle. Because both MALT and follicular lymphomas can express *bcl*-2, care must be taken when interpreting *bcl*-2 posi-

tivity in the follicles (Fig. 15–28B). Positivity for CD10 supports a diagnosis of follicular center cell lymphoma over low-grade MALT lymphoma (see Table 15–4).[55] Secondary involvement of the stomach by disseminated nodal lymphoma becomes evident during clinical staging of gastric lymphoma (see the following section).

Mantle cell lymphomas or multiple lymphomatous polyposis can involve the stomach (Fig. 15–29). The infiltrate in these lymphomas consists of small lymphocytes with nuclei reminiscent of centrocyte-like cells. Like MALT lymphomas, the neoplastic lymphoid cells coexpress CD20 and CD43. Unlike low-grade MALT lymphomas, however, the infiltrate is monomorphous in appearance and also shows expression of CD5 and *bcl*-1 or PRAD1/cyclin D1.

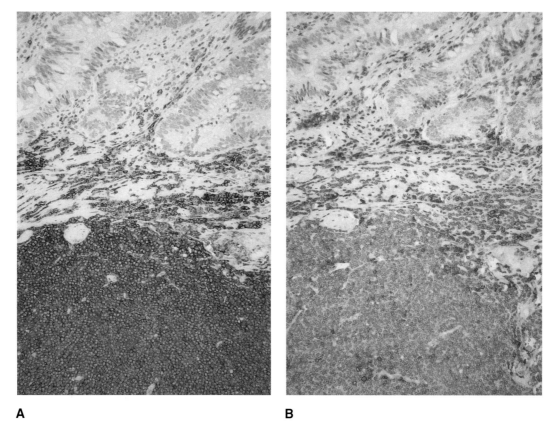

A   **B**

Figure 15–26. A: The neoplastic lymphoid cells of this gastric MALToma stain strongly for CD20 (a B-lymphocyte marker) by immunoperoxidase technique. B: The same lymphoma depicted in part A stains positively for CD43, a T-lymphocyte marker. Compared with the staining for CD20, the intensity of staining and the number of positive cells is less. Such aberrant expression of antigens is supportive of the diagnosis of lymphoma.

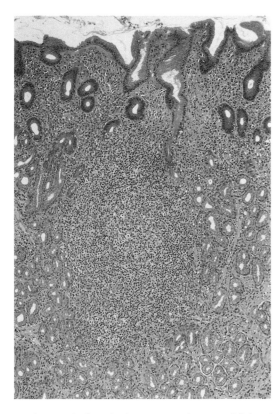

Figure 15–27. In this example of *H. pylori* chronic gastritis, the reactive follicle in the center is surrounded by monocytoid B cells, some of which are infiltrating overlying and adjacent glands to form lymphoepithelial lesions. The lamina propria contains a dense infiltrate of plasma cells and monocytoid B cells. These features are very suggestive of a MALToma. Immunoperoxidase staining of gene rearrangement studies would be helpful in proving monoclonality of the infiltrate.

Signet Ring Cell Carcinoma. Foveolar epithelial cells that have disaggregated secondary to infiltration by neoplastic lymphocytes in MALT lymphomas may appear as single mucin-positive, keratin-positive epithelial cells that resemble signet ring cells, leading to a misdiagnosis as carcinoma.[56]

Treatment

It is difficult to draw conclusions about the effectiveness of surgery, chemotherapy, and radiation, either alone or in combination, in treating MALT lymphomas because there are no multicenter studies comparing these various modalities. The histologic classifications of these tumors, the staging systems that have been used, and the treatment protocols vary from study to study, making comparisons impossible. For example, few series analyze treatment outcomes based on the concept of the MALT lymphoma. Most series use either the Working formulation or the updated Kiel classification (see Table 15–3) in assigning histologic grades. Various staging systems, including the tumor, node, metastasis (TNM) system, Ann Arbor system,[57] and the Musshoff modified Ann Arbor system,[58] have been used. Because of the lack of consensus regarding treatment, the frequency with which the pathologist receives a gastrectomy specimen after an endoscopic diagnosis of gastric MALT lymphoma varies among institutions.

Clinical staging should be carefully performed after a diag-

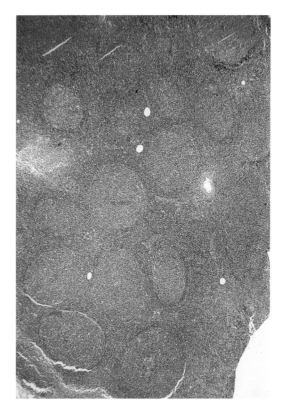

A

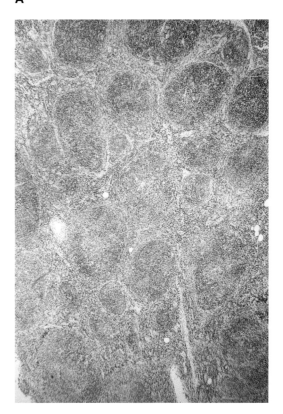

B

Figure 15–28. A: In this gastric follicular lymphoma, numerous follicles are evident without readily identifiable mantle zones. Without the mantle zones the follicles appear to fuse. B: Staining the same lymphoma for *bcl*-2 by immunoperoxidase highlights the neoplastic follicles. Benign, reactive follicles do not stain for *bcl*-2.

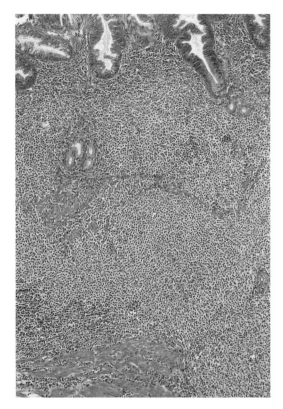

A

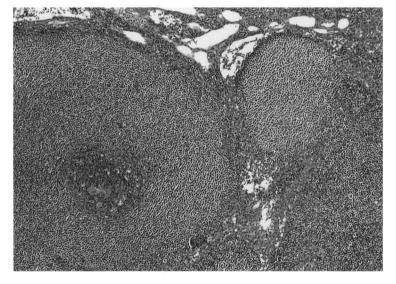

B

Figure 15–29. A: Gastric mantle cell lymphoma presenting as a diffuse lymphoid infiltrate. The low power and microscopic appearance of the neoplastic lymphoid infiltrate could lead to an erroneous diagnosis of MALT lymphoma. Note the absence of mantle cell nodules, which are classically found in mantle cell lymphomas (see part B and Fig. 15–43). B: The involved gastric lymph node showed numerous mantle cell nodules. Some nodules, such as the one depicted here, had residual germinal centers that were rimmed by an expanded mantle zone.

nosis of gastric MALT lymphoma. The Musshoff modification of the Ann Arbor staging system is presently recommended[58] (Table 15–5). Clinical staging should include a careful history and physical examination, including endoscopy, routine biochemical and hematologic studies, chest radiograph, computed tomography (CT) scan of the abdomen, bone marrow biopsy,

TABLE 15–5. MUSSHOFF MODIFIED ANN ARBOR STAGING SYSTEM

Stage	Criteria
E-I	Localized involvement of one or more GI site(s) on one side of the diaphragm without lymph node involvement
E-I$_1$	Lymphoma confined to the mucosa and submucosa
E-I$_2$	Lymphoma extending beyond the submucosa
E-II	Localized involvement of one or more GI site(s) with any depth of infiltration into the gut wall accompanied by nodal involvement on one side of the diaphragm
E-II$_1$	Involvement of contiguous regional lymph nodes
E-II$_2$	Involvement of noncontiguous, but regional, lymph nodes
E-III	Localized involvement of the GI tract with lymph node involvement on both sides of the diaphragm; splenic involvement
E-IV	Disseminated involvement of non-GI tract organs

Note: The prefix "E" denotes extranodal involvement by lymphoma.

and indirect laryngoscopy of Waldeyer's ring. Endoscopic ultrasonography should be done in centers where this technique is available. Endoscopic ultrasonography provides information relating to the depth of tumor invasion into the gastric wall and the presence of perigastric nodal enlargement.[59] The distinction between enlarged reactive lymph nodes and nodal involvement by lymphoma cannot be made by ultrasonography.

Disease in states E-III (positive nodes above the diaphragm) or stage E-IV (involvement of non-GI tract organs) is treated with primary chemotherapy in all centers. It is difficult to determine whether these patients have systemic nodal-based lymphomas involving the stomach or disseminated primary gastric lymphomas; this distinction is not critical in practice.

Antibiotic treatment to eradicate *H. pylori* has been shown to cause regression of MALT lymphomas and is considered the first line of treatment for stage E-I$_1$ lesions (restricted to mucosa and submucosa). Tumors that show complete regression can be followed; many of these cases relapse.[60] It was shown in a prospective study that less than 10% of patients with primary gastric lymphoma can be treated with antibiotic therapy alone.[61]

Patients with locoregional disease (stages E-I and E-II) are subjected to laparotomy in many, but not all centers.[62] Some centers use primary chemotherapy or radiation therapy (or both) even for these early-stage tumors. The surgical procedure of choice in these cases is subtotal gastrectomy with regional node removal and sampling of nodes outside the resection limits. In patients who have a final pathologic staging of E-I$_1$ and have clear surgical resection margins, some data suggest that surgery alone is curative.[63] The need for chemotherapy or radiation in these cases is controversial. When surgical margins are positive or when tumor invasion is more advanced than stage E-I$_1$, chemotherapy and radiation are indicated.

Prognostic Factors

Histologic grade is an important prognostic factor.[36] Low-grade B-cell MALT lymphomas are associated with a better prognosis and likelihood of survival than low-grade MALT lymphomas showing foci of higher grade lymphoma. High-grade lymphomas in which the low-grade lymphoma constitutes a minority of the lesion, or in which no low-grade component is identifiable, have a poor prognosis. For gastric low-grade B-cell lymphomas of MALT treated with various therapies, the survival rate at 5 years is 91–96% and at 10 years is 75–89%.

According to some authorities, pathologic stage is a better prognostic indicator than histologic grade of tumor.[64,65] Overall, patients with lymphomas localized to the stomach (stage E-I) had a better 5-year survival rate of 95% compared with a rate of 79–82% for patients with lymph node involvement (stage E-II).[66-70]

Depth of gastric wall infiltration is an adverse prognostic factor, significantly correlating with lymph node involvement.[70] The prognosis for stage E-I$_1$, with a 90% 5-year survival, was superior to stage E-I$_2$, which had only a 54% 5-year survival rate.[64] Cogliatti's group[67] showed that infiltration of the tumor into the serosa decreased the 5-year survival rate from 80% to 54%. Within stage E-II, a distinct worsening of prognosis took place in stage E-II$_2$ patients compared with stage E-II$_1$ patients.[64] Disease in patients with stage E-II$_2$ (positive regional but noncontiguous lymph nodes) behaves more like disseminated disease rather than locoregional disease.

In general, irrespective of the therapeutic modality, patients who have an initial complete remission are most likely to have long-term survival.

Intestinal Malt Lymphomas

The lymphomas of the small intestine and colon can be considered as MALT lymphomas in that they probably arise from the native lymphoid tissue of their respective organs. They display the same histologic, immunophenotypic, molecular, and genetic features of gastric MALT lymphomas.[71] Unlike the MALT lymphomas of the stomach, few studies have characterized intestinal lymphomas in light of the MALT lymphoma concept, so information on these lesions is limited. This dearth of information is related to the fact that the small intestine is not accessible to endoscopy.

In discussing intestinal lymphomas, distinction is made between lymphomas of MALT and multiple lymphomatous polyposis (MLP), immunoproliferative small-intestinal disease (IPSID), and enteropathy-associated T lymphoma (EATL), which have distinct clinicopathologic features. Although all these entities very likely arise from intestinal MALT, MLP, IPSID, and EATL are considered separately because they have distinctive clinical features.

As a group, most intestinal lymphomas of MALT arise in the small intestine. Unlike their gastric counterpart, they tend to present with local lymph node involvement and are more frequently high-grade malignancies[62,64] with a lower overall 5-year survival rate.[62,64,72] Important prognostic indicators for both small- and large-intestine lymphomas are clinicopathologic stage, histologic grade, and tumor resectability.[62,64,72,73]

Small-intestinal lymphomas occur in patients in the sixth and seventh decades who present with abdominal pain, weight

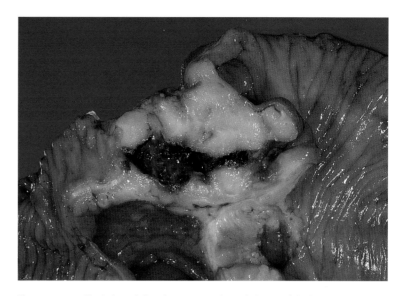

Figure 15–30. This high-grade lymphoma presented as a thickening of the ileocecal valve, which led to symptomatology secondary to obstruction.

loss, and bowel obstruction. Grossly, most small-intestinal B-cell lymphomas are high grade and appear as exophytic or annular, constricting tumors of large size (Figs. 15–30 and 15–31). Up to 30% of small-intestinal lymphomas are T-cell lymphomas; these tend to appear as thickened plaques, strictures, or ulcers.[72]

Colorectal lymphomas of MALT are almost always B-cell lymphomas and commonly occur in patients older than 50.[73] These tumors may complicate long-standing chronic ulcerative colitis.[74] Grossly, colorectal lymphomas of low grade appear as a

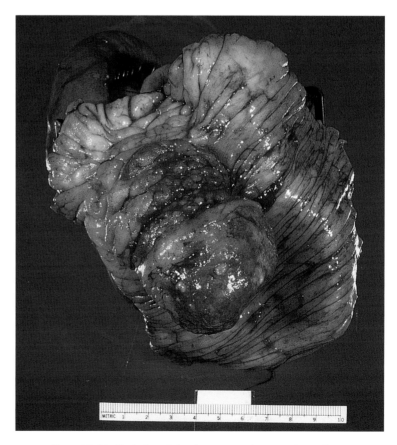

Figure 15–31. This high-grade lymphoma presented as a mass-forming lesion.

solitary mass involving the mucosa with variable muscle invasion. Higher grade tumors are usually large masses with ulceration.

Small-intestinal lymphomas are encountered by the pathologist as a resected segment of tumor containing bowel. Preoperatively, many of these cases do not have a specific diagnosis. Pathologic diagnosis by morphologic and immunophenotypic criteria should establish the appropriate designation (Fig. 15–32), histologic grade, and pathologic stage according to the TNM classification for small-bowel cancer (see Chapter 8).

In contrast, colorectal lymphomas first come to the attention of the pathologist as an endoscopic biopsy specimen (Fig. 15–33). The criteria for diagnosis of low-grade MALT lymphoma are similar to those for gastric lesions, that is, the presence of a dense atypical lymphoid infiltrate in the mucosa and submucosa with a mixed population of lymphocytes with centrocyte-like or monocytoid B-cell features, colonization of normal reactive follicles in the mucosa by neoplastic lymphocytes, the presence of plasmacytoid cells, and the presence of lymphoepithelial lesions (Fig. 15–34).

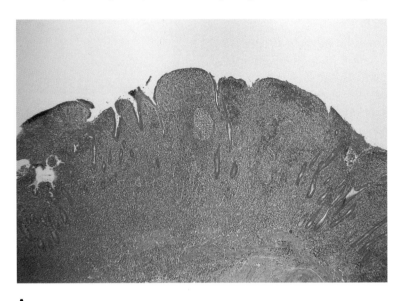

A

B

C

Figure 15–32. A: The intense lymphoid infiltrate infuses the lamina propria, leading to widening and partial obliteration of the villi. B: Small-intestinal MALT lymphoma, showing diffuse mucosal lymphocytic infiltrate involving the villi and extending into the submucosa. C: Small-intestinal MALT lymphoma, showing diffuse mucosal lymphocytic infiltrate involving the villi and extending into the submucosa.

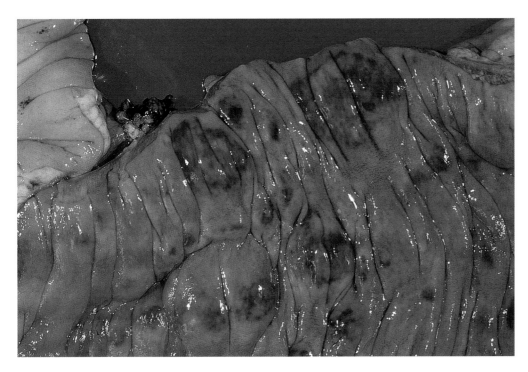

Figure 15–33. Lymphoma presented as multiple surface erosions. No mass lesions were identified.

The colonic mucosa and submucosa normally contain lymphoglandular structures that have crypts in close association with lymphoid tissue, often extending into the submucosa. These should not be mistaken for lymphoepithelial lesions or submucosal extension of the tumor. Immunoperoxidase staining to document coexpression of CD20 and CD43 by the neoplastic cells or light-chain staining to establish monoclonality in plasma cells are valuable diagnostic techniques. In cases of difficulty, the biopsy can be repeated to obtain specimens for immunoglobulin gene rearrangement studies.

High-grade colorectal lymphoma is easier to diagnose at endoscopy; these malignant neoplasms may need immunoperoxidase staining (CD45, keratin) to distinguish them from poorly differentiated adenocarcinoma (Figs. 15–35 and 15–36). High-grade colorectal lymphomas are usually diffuse large-cell lymphomas, Burkitt-like lymphomas, or immunoblastic lymphomas.[72,73,75] Some of these high-grade tumors may show residual areas of low-grade MALT lymphoma.

Colorectal lymphomas are treated by primary chemotherapy or radiation (or both) or segmental resection. Resected specimens are staged according to the TNM system used for colorectal adenocarcinoma (see Chapter 13).

GI INVOLVEMENT BY NODAL-BASED LYMPHOMAS

Secondary gastrointestinal involvement by nodal-based lymphoma is common. Compiled from autopsy reviews, nodal-based lymphomas or lymphocytic leukemia involve the GI tract in up to 60% of cases.[76] Most of these patients, however, have subclinical or terminal involvement of the gastrointestinal tract and do not present clinically with a GI tract lymphoma. Rates of gastrointestinal tract involvement are lower when clinical detection methods are used. Endoscopic evidence of gastroduodenal involvement is reported in 16–27% of patients with disseminated nodal-based non-Hodgkin's lymphomas and in less than 5% of Hodgkin's lymphoma.[77,78]

By site, the stomach is the most common site for dissemination of nodal-based lymphoma, followed by the small intestine.[77] Of the low-grade non-Hodgkin's lymphomas, the most common histologic types are small-lymphocytic (Fig. 15–37) and plasmacytoid lymphomas; most of the secondary higher grade lymphomas are diffuse large-cell (Fig. 15–38) and small, noncleaved cell lymphomas (Fig. 15–39).[77]

IMMUNOPROLIFERATIVE SMALL-INTESTINAL DISEASE

Immunoproliferative small-intestinal disease (IPSID) is an entity of the non-Western world seen primarily in the Middle East, Mediterranean countries, and Asia.[79–81] The disease has also been reported from Mexico.[82] In some Middle Eastern countries, IPSID is the most common form of primary small-intestinal lymphoma.[83] Classically, it is associated with α-heavy-chain disease, with high levels of α-heavy chain in the serum.[84,85] IPSID tends to have a long clinical course with extraabdominal extension and high-grade lymphomatous transformation occurring in the late stages of the disease.[86]

Clinical Presentation

IPSID predominantly affects young adults, primarily in the 20–40-year age group. Patients often present with malabsorption syndrome; common symptoms are abdominal pain,

Figure 15–34. A: Compared with gastric MALTomas, intestinal lymphomas have fewer identifiable lymphoepithelial lesions. In this colonic MALToma, a dense lymphoid infiltrate is present that pushes up into the overlying epithelium. No lymphoepithelial lesions are identifiable. B: Rectal MALT lymphoma, showing lymphoid cells infiltrating the lamina propria and separating rectal crypts. No lymphoepithelial lesions are evident. C: Colonic MALT lymphoma, showing a high-grade component (*right side*) arising from a low-grade lymphoma (*left side,* periglandular). D: Recognizable lymphoepithelial lesions, such as seen here, are often difficult to identify in intestinal MALT lymphomas. E: Colonic MALT lymphoma, showing numerous residual follicles, which are distorted but still recognizable amid the lymphomatous infiltrate. F: Colon MALT lymphoma, showing a diffuse lymphoid infiltrate extending through the full thickness of the colonic wall into the serosal fat.

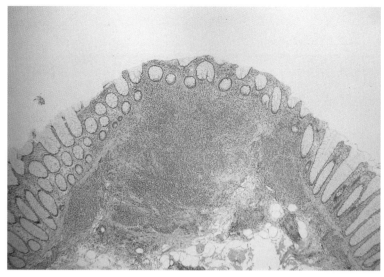

A

B

C

D

E

F

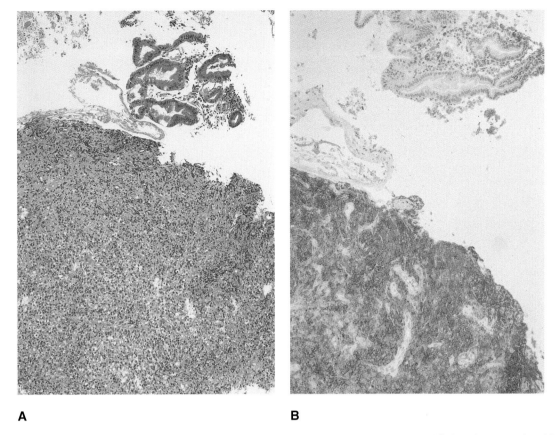

Figure 15–35. A: On small biopsy samples differentiation between high-grade carcinomas and lymphomas can be difficult. In this specimen loss of the overlying epithelium is evident. The underlying neoplastic infiltrate appears as large cells with large nuclei and moderate amounts of cytoplasm. The lack of identifiable gland formation favors a diagnosis of lymphoma. B: Immunoperoxidase staining for CD20 (B-cell marker) of the same biopsy specimen seen in part A reveals that the infiltrating cells are B lymphocytes. Staining for CD45 (common leukocyte antigen) achieves similar results.

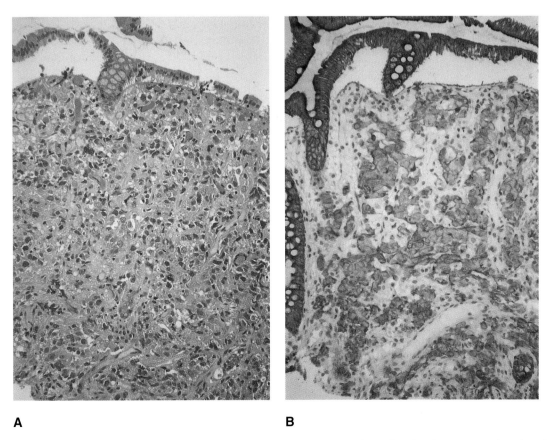

Figure 15–36. A: In comparison with Figure 15–35, the infiltrate in this lymphoma appears as large cells with moderate amounts of cytoplasm. Although no glandular differentiation is apparent, the abundant amount of eosinophilic cytoplasm favors a diagnosis of carcinoma. Also, few rare cells are suggestive of signet rings. B: The infiltrating cells are positive for keratin, proving that this is a poorly differentiated carcinoma.

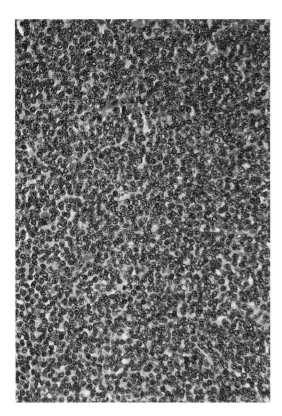

Figure 15–37. Small-lymphocytic lymphomas (SLL) can secondarily involve the stomach. Compared with the lymphoid cells in MALTomas, these lymphoid cells have relatively uniform, round nuclei with scant amounts of cytoplasm. Compared with lymphomas of MALT, SLL characteristically is positive for CD5, CD23, and CD43 antigens.

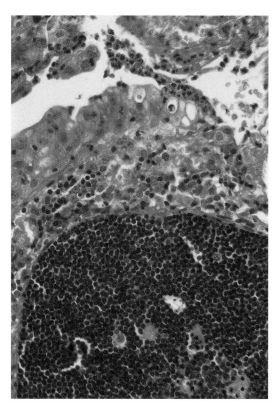

Figure 15–39. On staging, this patient was found to have small-intestinal involvement by high-grade, small, noncleaved, non-Burkitt's lymphoma (Burkitt's-like, or sporadic Burkitt's).

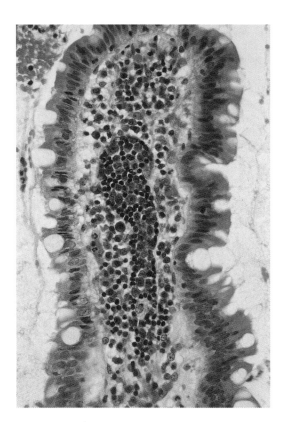

Figure 15–38. Small intestine with secondary lymphomatous involvement. The infiltrate of large atypical lymphoid cells infiltrates a lacteal and the lamina propria of a villus.

anorexia, weight loss, and diarrhea. Occasionally, a palpable mass is found on external abdominal examination.

Pathologic Features

Typical gross findings include diffuse thickening of the mucosal folds, with edema and flattening of the villi. Stage A lesions (see following section) are most likely to appear as regularly thickened or even normal mucosa. Stage B and C lesions are invariably thickened and frequently show multiple nodules or larger tumor masses.[87,88] On histologic examination, these nodules and tumor masses often represent focal areas of high-grade lymphoma.[88]

The pathologic changes involve long segments of the small intestine. The lesions can occur anywhere and can even involve the entire length of the small intestine; usually, the changes are most pronounced in the proximal duodenum.[88,89] Mesenteric lymph node involvement is common at presentation, and involvement of extraabdominal lymph nodes, such as the cervical and axillary lymph nodes, has been reported.[87] Extension to other abdominal organs, including the stomach, liver, peritoneum, the periaortic lymph nodes, and the large intestine, can also occur.

Histologically, IPSID is characterized by the presence of a diffuse band-like plasma cell infiltrate in the mucosa of the more proximal portion of the small intestine (Fig. 15–40A and

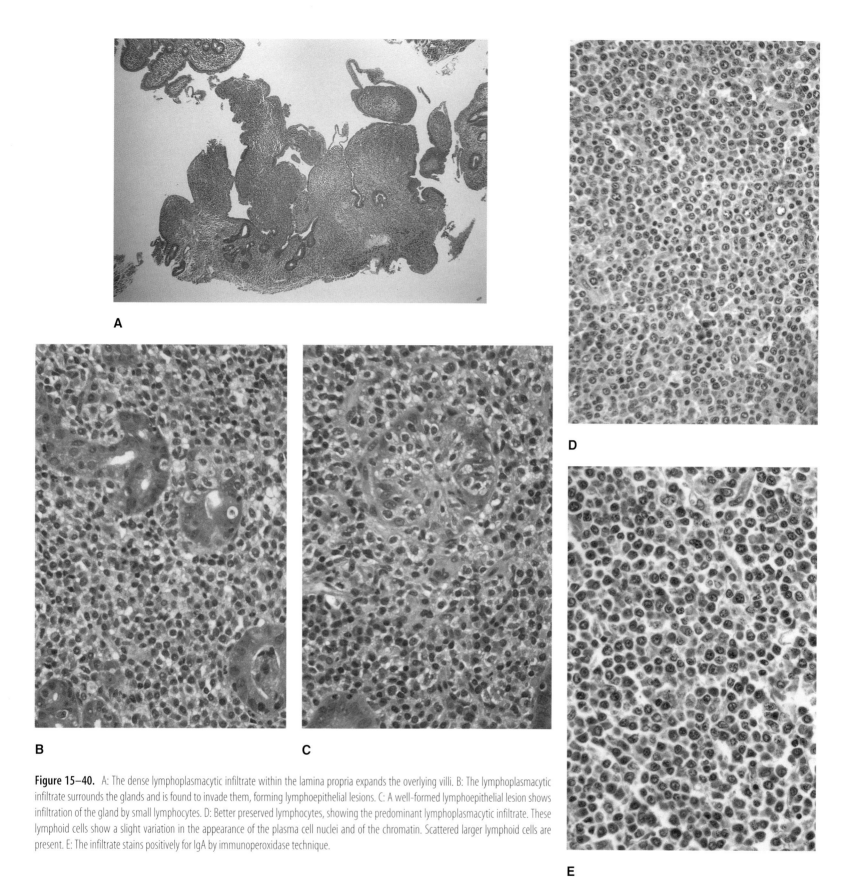

Figure 15–40. A: The dense lymphoplasmacytic infiltrate within the lamina propria expands the overlying villi. B: The lymphoplasmacytic infiltrate surrounds the glands and is found to invade them, forming lymphoepithelial lesions. C: A well-formed lymphoepithelial lesion shows infiltration of the gland by small lymphocytes. D: Better preserved lymphocytes, showing the predominant lymphoplasmacytic infiltrate. These lymphoid cells show a slight variation in the appearance of the plasma cell nuclei and of the chromatin. Scattered larger lymphoid cells are present. E: The infiltrate stains positively for IgA by immunoperoxidase technique.

B). The infiltrate leads to villous broadening and shortening, and, rarely, intraepithelial lymphocytic infiltration leads to the formation of lymphoepithelial lesions (Fig. 15–40C). Focal overlying mucosal ulcerations may be seen.

IPSID has three histologic stages:

Stage A: Characterized by a mature plasmacytic or lymphoplasmacytic infiltrate confined to the lamina propria, associated with variable villous atrophy. The mesenteric lymph nodes show mature plasmacytic infiltration with no or limited disruption of nodal architecture. This early-stage disease has been reported to regress after antibiotic therapy; long-term control with antibiotics is reported in 71% of patients.[90]

Stage B: Characterized by atypical plasmacytic or lymphoplasmacytic infiltrate; immunoblastic cells may be present. The infiltrate extends across the muscularis mucosae into the submucosa, and subtotal or total villous atrophy occurs. Distortion of the crypts occurs along with displacement of the crypts away from the muscularis mucosae. Reactive follicles are often present[87,88]; the neoplastic lymphoid cells surround and often partially destroy these reactive follicles. Colonization of the follicles by neoplastic lymphoid cells can result in nodule formation.[91] Scattered or in small aggregates among the lymphoplasmacytic infiltrate are occasional immunoblastic lymphoid cells (Fig. 15–40D). Mesenteric lymph nodes show total or partial obliteration of nodal architecture and an atypical plasmacytic infiltrate with some immunoblastic cells.

Stage C: Characterized by high-grade malignant lymphoma with features of either large-cell immunoblastic or small-, noncleaved cell lymphoma involving the entire wall.[92] Mesenteric lymph nodes are totally replaced by high-grade lymphoma.

Genetic Features

The neoplastic plasma cells synthesize the α-heavy chain of the immunoglobulin molecule without the accompanying light chain (Fig. 15–40E).[85,91] A minority of these cases do not secrete the α-heavy chain; in these nonsecretory cases, intracytoplasmic α-chain is demonstrable.[93] In the past, it was thought that the early stages of IPSID were benign and the diagnosis of malignant lymphoma could be made only when histologic evidence of high-grade lymphoma developed. Based on the fact that gene rearrangement studies show heavy- and light-chain immunoglobulin monoclonality even in the early lesions,[94] IPSID is now classified as a malignant lymphoma in all its stages.

Immunophenotypic Expression

The neoplastic plasmacytoid cells in IPSID express B-cell antigens CD20 and CD22. They do not express CD5 antigen. Reactive follicles are CD10 antigen-positive, but the neoplastic cells are CD10-negative. In some cases, infiltration of the reactive follicles can be demonstrated by a population of CD10-negative neoplastic cells, which invade and displace the native CD10-positive reactive follicular lymphocytes to the periphery of the follicle.[91]

Prognosis

IPSID in its early stages behaves as an indolent disease with long survival times and good response to antibiotic therapy. Entry of the disease into stage B is an indication for chemotherapy. Response to chemotherapy is associated with reported 5-year survival rates around 70%.[90,95] Entry into stage C, the high-grade lymphoma phase, indicates a poor prognosis with a poor response to treatment and a median survival time of 7 months.[90]

ENTEROPATHY-ASSOCIATED T-CELL LYMPHOMA

Enteropathy-associated T-cell lymphoma (EATL) is a relatively uncommon complication of celiac disease.[95,96]

Clinical Presentation

EATL typically occurs in patients who are older than 50 years. Presenting symptoms are abdominal pain, weight loss, malabsorption, and abdominal mass. Most patients have a diagnosis of celiac disease; lymphoma can appear as soon as a few months after diagnosis or after many years. Some patients have neither a history of celiac disease nor evidence of malabsorption, and present for the first time with intestinal obstruction secondary to the tumor.[97,98]

Some cases of EATL are associated with ulcerative jejunoileitis, which is characterized by multiple, inflammatory ulcers in the small intestine. Ulcerative jejunoileitis, which was originally thought to be a benign ulcerative complication in patients with celiac disease, is now recognized as being probably a manifestation of EATL. Histologic examination of ulcerative jejunoileitis does not show a recognizable lymphoma, but demonstration of T-cell receptor monoclonality in these lesions lends support to this condition being EATL.[99]

Pathologic Features

Any part of the small intestine can be involved, and multifocal involvement is usual.[97,98] Rarely, colonic and gastric involvement occurs. The lesion usually appears grossly as ulcerated nodular mass lesions (Fig. 15–41); plaques and strictures may also occur. Mesenteric and other abdominal lymph nodes are

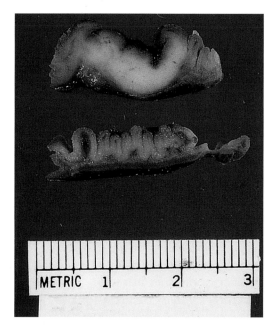

Figure 15–41. Two segments of the jejunum are presented. In the upper segment, thickening of the intestinal wall is evident. The lower segment shows relatively intact normal architecture.

commonly involved,[100] and extraabdominal dissemination to the bone marrow, liver, lung, and skin can occur.

In the involved segments of the intestine, neoplastic T cells accumulate in the lamina propria, progressively infiltrating and destroying the epithelial cells of the crypts and villi (Fig. 15–42). The histologic appearance of the neoplastic T cells varies considerably in EATL.[98] Based on morphology, the cells fall into one of several lymphoma categories within the working formula-

tion. Most commonly, the cells appear as sheets or groups of large cells with vesicular nuclei that contain multiple nucleoli, suggesting immunoblastic lymphoma. Less commonly, they show cytologic features suggestive of diffuse small cleaved, mixed, or large-cell lymphoma.[101]

The adjacent, nonlymphomatous mucosa usually shows changes typical of celiac disease. In patients who have been on a strict gluten-free diet, these changes may be minimal (see Chap-

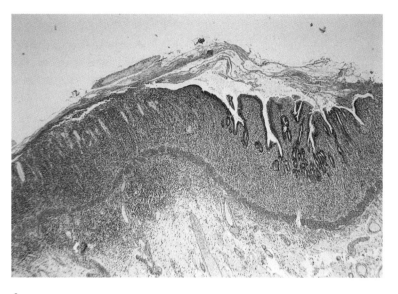

A

B

C

Figure 15–42. A: The neoplastic lymphoid cells have infiltrated the villi, causing broadening and loss of the normal architecture. Focally, the infiltrate has gone beyond the muscularis mucosae into the submucosa. B: Several glands show invasion by neoplastic T-lymphoid cells. The cells have irregular, twisted, and angulated nuclear contours and moderate amounts of pale cytoplasm. Within the lamina propria, these cells are accompanied by occasional plasma cells and eosinophils. C: The tips of the residual villi are infiltrated by atypical-appearing T lymphocytes. Plasma cells and eosinophils usually accompany the neoplastic T cells.

ter 7). Occasionally, neoplastic T cells can be identified in the atrophic, grossly normal mucosa.[98]

Immunophenotypic Expression

In celiac disease, the normal subpopulation of intraepithelial T lymphocytes increases; these are characteristically CD3-positive, and CD4- and CD8-negative. EATL shows a similar increase in this subset of intraepithelial lymphocytes.[102] Neoplastic lymphoid cells express CD45 but do not express B-cell markers or immunoglobulin light chains. Most of the neoplastic lymphoid cells stain positively for CD45RO, CD3, and CD7 antigens, but are CD4- and CD8 antigen-negative.[96-98] CD30 antigen positivity is found in cases showing large, anaplastic-appearing lymphocytes.[98]

The monoclonal antibody HML-1 has been reported to stain the neoplastic T cells in cases of EATL.[103] Care must be taken in interpreting HML-1 positivity, however, because HML-1 also recognizes almost all small-intestinal intraepithelial and some lamina propria T cells.[104] In addition, HML-1 has been found to stain some extraintestinal non-Hodgkin's lymphomas.[105]

Genetic Features

The neoplastic T cells have been shown to have T-cell receptor β-chain gene rearrangements.[95] T-cell receptor monoclonality can be detected in some celiac disease specimens without histologic evidence of lymphoma, and in uninvolved mucosa adjacent to EATL.[106,107] This finding supports the concept that the lymphoma arises from the T-cell population found in the enteropathic bowel.

The role of Epstein-Barr virus (EBV) in the development of EATL is controversial. Some authorities have found evidence of EBV genomic material in the neoplastic cells of EATL and have suggested an etiologic role for EBV in the development of EATL[108]; other studies have found no EBV genomic material.[109]

Prognosis

Due to its propensity to involve multiple segments of the intestine, local curative resection is not usually possible. Surgical resection is generally undertaken if complications like obstruction, perforation, and uncontrollable hemorrhage occur. Some cases show temporary remission with surgery and chemotherapy, but most cases relapse. EATL should be considered a highly aggressive malignant lymphoma; most patients die within a few months of diagnosis.[97,98]

MULTIPLE LYMPHOMATOUS POLYPOSIS

Multiple lymphomatous polyposis (MLP) is generally considered to be a distinct clinical presentation of mantle cell lymphoma.[110,111] Because other gastrointestinal lymphomas such as follicular center cell lymphomas[112] and T-cell lymphomas[113] can present as multiple polyps, however, some authors believe that the term "multiple lymphomatous polyposis" should be used as a clinical syndrome with multiple causes rather than as a specific diagnosis. We use the term in its restrictive sense as equivalent to mantle cell lymphoma involving the gastrointestinal tract.

Clinical Presentation

MLP is an uncommon lymphoma,[114,115] most often affecting individuals older than 50. Presentation is with diarrhea, weight loss, abdominal pain, or gastrointestinal bleeding.

Pathologic Features

The gastrointestinal tract is studded with multiple polypoid tumors, sometimes with larger dominant mass lesions.[112,115] The polyps range in size from millimeters to several centimeters. Any portion of the gastrointestinal tract can be involved, but the ileocecal region is most commonly affected. Adjacent mesenteric lymphadenopathy is usually present.

Histologically, a dense lymphoid infiltrate occurs, involving the mucosa and submucosa in a diffuse or nodular pattern (Fig. 15–43A), and filling the polypoid masses (Fig. 15–43B). Residual reactive follicular centers are often identified entrapped within the lymphomatous infiltrate. The overlying mucosa is usually intact, but lymphoepithelial lesions can be found.[111,115] The neoplastic cells are cytologically similar to mantle cells (Fig. 15–43C). They are uniformly small- to medium-size cells, with irregularly angular or cleaved nuclei, inconspicuous nucleoli, and scanty cytoplasm.[114]

When nodules become numerous, the lesion can be mistaken for a follicular center cell lymphoma, which can also present with multiple polypoid lesion.[112] The distinction is based on the fact that in MLP, the nodularity results from colonization of reactive follicles by the neoplastic mantle cells.[110]

Immunophenotypic Expression

The immunophenotypic features of the neoplastic cells in MLP are the same as for nodal-based mantle cell lymphoma.[114] The cells express mature B-cell markers (CD19, CD20, and CD22) and surface IgM or IgD. They are positive for CD5 antigen, negative for CD10 and CD23 antigens. Although not reported with specific reference to MLP, the majority of nodal-based mantle cell lymphomas express CD43 (see Table 15–4).[52,116]

Genetic Features

Molecular probe studies show rearrangement of *bcl*-1 locus or the t(11;14)(q13;q32) translocation.[117] Rearrangement of the *bcl*-1 locus leads to overexpression of the cyclin D1/PRAD1 protein.[118]

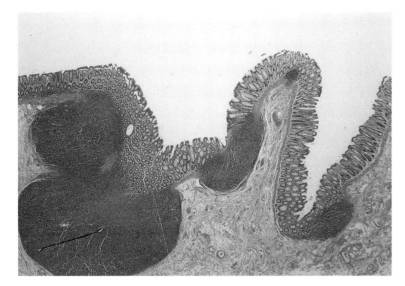

A

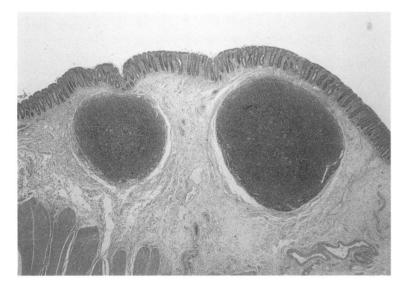

B

C

Figure 15–43. A: Several mantle cell nodules are evident in this example of multiple lymphomatous polyposis (MLP). The colon was studded with numerous such nodules. B: Multiple lymphomatous polyposis, showing two well-defined submucosal nodules. C: The nodule of mantle cells is composed of monotonous-appearing cells. The lymphocytes are small, with slightly irregularly shaped nuclear contours, inconspicuous nucleoli, and scanty cytoplasm.

Prognosis

Similar to nodal-based mantle cell lymphomas, MLP disseminates early, with involvement of extragastrointestinal organs such as liver, spleen, bone marrow, and peripheral lymph nodes. These disseminated cases cannot be differentiated from disseminated nodal-based mantle cell lymphoma with secondary GI tract involvement. The disease follows a moderately aggressive course, with a median survival time of less than 5 years,[110,119] with rare reported cases of transformation to high-grade B-cell lymphoma.[119]

HIGH-GRADE BURKITT'S LYMPHOMA

Burkitt's lymphoma is an entity of the non-Western world, occurring especially in the Middle East and Africa. It is a childhood disease, and in some countries it accounts for as much as half of all pediatric non-Hodgkin's lymphomas, with 60% of these cases presenting as primary intestinal lymphomas.[120,121] In the United States, sporadic Burkitt's lymphoma (also called Burkitt-like lymphoma) has somewhat different clinicopathologic features.[122,123] A higher frequency of Burkitt-like lymphomas is also seen in immunodeficient patients, particularly those with acquired immunodeficiency syndrome.

Clinical Presentation

Interestingly, the endemic form of Burkitt's lymphoma seen in Africa commonly presents with lesions of the jaw rather than with gastrointestinal involvement.[124] In contrast, ileocecal involvement is the common manifestation of Burkitt-like or sporadic Burkitt's lymphoma occurring in the Western world and the Middle East.[121]

Endemic African Burkitt's lymphoma is a disease that affects children in the first decade of life; males are more frequently affected.[124] Sporadic Burkitt's lymphoma tends to affect patients in the 30–60-year age group.[123,124]

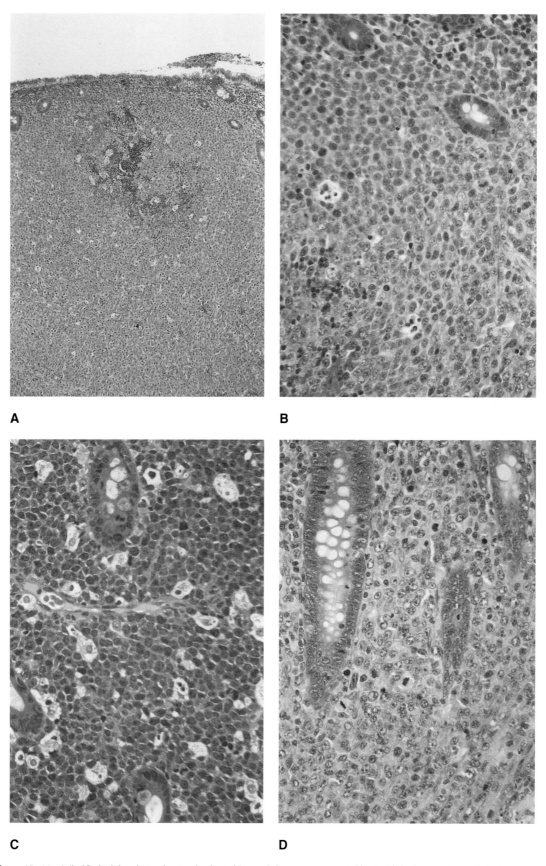

Figure 15–44. A: Ileal Burkitt's lymphoma showing the classical "starry sky" appearance imparted by tingible body macrophages. B: Higher power micrograph of part A, showing the monotonous population of medium-size lymphocytes with one to three nucleoli. C: Burkitt's lymphoma of the small intestine, showing typical small, noncleaved lymphocytes. D: Burkitt-like lymphoma has a similar appearance to Burkitt's lymphoma, except that there is more size variation of the lymphoid cells.

reveal follicular lymphoma as a subtype. *Leukemia*. 1993;7: 268–273.

56. Zamboni GM, Franzin G, Scarpa A, et al. Carcinoma-like signet-ring cells in gastric mucosa-associated lymphoid tissue (MALT) lymphoma. *Am J Surg Pathol*. 1996;20:588–598.

57. Carbone PP, Kaplan HS. Report of the committee on Hodgkin's disease staging classification. *Cancer Res*. 1971;31:1860–1861.

58. Musshoff K. Klinische stadieneinteilung der Nicht-Hodgkin lymphome. *Strahlentherapie*. 1977;153:218–221.

59. Caletti GC, Lorena Z, Bolondi L. Impact of endoscopic ultrasonography on diagnosis and treatment of primary gastric lymphoma. *Surgery*. 1988;103:315.

60. Horstmann M, Erttmann R, Winkler K. Relapse of MALT lymphoma associated with *Helicobacter pylori* after antibiotic treatment. *Lancet*. 1994;343:1098–1099.

61. Karat D, O'Hanlon DM, Hayes N, et al. Prospective study of *Helicobacter pylori* infection in primary gastric lymphoma. *Br J Surg*. 1995;82:1369–1370.

62. Ruskone-Fourmestraux A, Aegerter P, Delmer A. Primary digestive tract lymphoma: A prospective multicentric study of 91 patients. *Gastroenterology*. 1993;105:1662–1671.

63. Bartlett DL, Karpeh MS, Filippa DA, et al. Long-term follow-up after curative surgery for early gastric lymphoma. *Ann Surg*. 1996;223:53–62.

64. Radaszkiewicz T, Dragosics B, Bauer P. Gastrointestinal malignant lymphomas of the mucosa-associated lymphoid tissue: Factors relevant to prognosis. *Gastroenterology*. 1992;102: 1628–1638.

65. Shimm DS, Dosoretz DE, Anderson T et al. Primary gastric lymphoma. An analysis with emphasis on prognostic factors and radiation therapy. *Cancer*. 1983;52:2044–2048.

66. Lybeert ML, De Neve W, Vrints LW, et al. Primary gastric non-Hodgkin's lymphoma stage IE and IIE. *Eur J Cancer*. 1996;32A: 2306–2311.

67. Cogliatti SB, Schmid U, Schumacher U, et al. Primary B-cell gastric lymphoma: A clinicopathological study of 145 patients. *Gastroenterology*. 1991;101:1159–1170.

68. Nakamura S, Akazawa K, Yao T, et al. Primary gastric lymphoma: A clinicopathologic study of 233 cases with special reference to evaluation with the MIB-1 index. *Cancer*. 1995;76: 1313–1324.

69. Castrillo JM, Montalban C, Obeso G, et al. Gastric B-cell mucosa associated lymphoid tissue lymphoma: A clinico-pathological study in 56 patients. *Gut*. 1992;33:1307–1311.

70. Eidt S, Stolte M, Fischer R. Factors influencing lymph node infiltration in primary gastric malignant lymphoma of the mucosa-associated lymphoid tissue. *Pathol Res Pract*. 1994;190: 1077–1081.

71. Isaacson PG. Gastrointestinal lymphoma. *Hum Pathol*. 1994;25: 1020–1029.

72. Domizio P, Owen RA, Shepherd NA, et al. Primary lymphoma of the small intestine. A clinicopathological study of 119 cases. *Am J Surg Pathol*. 1993;17:429–442.

73. Shepherd NA, Hall PA, Coates PJ, et al. Primary malignant lymphoma of the colon and rectum. A histopathological analysis of 45 cases with clinicopathological correlations. *Histopathology*. 1988;12:235–252.

74. Greenstein AJ, Mullin GE, Strauchen JA, et al. Lymphoma in inflammatory bowel disease. *Cancer*. 1992;69:1119–1123.

75. Li G, Ouyang Q, Liu K, et al. Primary non-Hodgkin's lymphoma of the intestine: A morphological, immunohistochemical and

clinical study of 31 Chinese cases. *Histopathology*. 1994;25: 113–121.

76. Herrmann R, Panahon AM, Barcos MP, et al. Gastrointestinal involvement in non-Hodgkin's lymphoma. *Cancer*. 1980;46: 215–222.

77. Fischbach W, Kestel W, Kirchner T, et al. Malignant lymphomas of the upper gastrointestinal tract. Results of a prospective study in 103 patients. *Cancer*. 1992;70:1075–1080.

78. Solidoro A, Salazar F, de la Flor J, et al. Endoscopic tissue diagnosis of gastric involvement in the staging of non-Hodgkin's lymphoma. *Cancer*. 1981;48:1053–1057.

79. Malik IA, Shamsi Z, Shafquat A, et al. Clinicopathological features and management of immunoproliferative small intestinal disease and primary small intestinal lymphoma in Pakistan. *Med Pediatr Oncol*. 1995;25:400–406.

80. Akbulut H, Soykan I, Yakaryilmaz, et al. Five-year results of the treatment of 23 patients with immunoproliferative small intestinal disease: A Turkish experience. *Cancer*. 1997;80:8–14.

81. Shih LY, Liaw SJ, Dunn P, et al. Primary small-intestinal lymphomas in Taiwan: Immunoproliferative small-intestinal disease and nonimmunoproliferative small-intestinal disease. *J Clin Oncol*. 1994;12:1375–1382.

82. Arista-Nasr NJ, Gonzalez-Romo MA, Mantilla-Morales A, et al. Immunoproliferative small intestinal disease in Mexico. *J Clin Gastroenterol*. 1994;18:67–71.

83. Al-Bahrani ZR, Al-Mondhiry H, Bakir F, et al. Clinical and pathologic subtypes of primary intestinal lymphoma. Experience with 132 patients over a 14-year period. *Cancer*. 1983;52: 1666–1672.

84. Salem P, Nassar V, Shahid M, et al. "Mediterranean abdominal lymphoma," or immunoproliferative small intestinal disease, I: Clinical aspects. *Cancer*. 1977;40:2941–2947.

85. Price SK. Immunoproliferative small intestinal disease: A study of 13 cases with alpha heavy-chain disease. *Histopathology*. 1990;17:7–17.

86. Rogers P, Hill I, Sinclair-Smith C, et al. Clinical and pathological evolution of alpha chain disease to immunoblastic lymphoma and response to COMP chemotherapy. *Med Pediatr Oncol*. 1988;16:128–131.

87. Nassar VH, Salem PA, Shahid MJ, et al. 'Mediterranean abdominal lymphoma' or immunoproliferative small intestinal disease. Part II. Pathological aspects. *Cancer*. 1978;41:1340–1354.

88. Cammoun M, Jaafoura H, Tabbane F, et al. Immunoproliferative small intestinal disease without alpha-chain disease: A pathological study. *Gastroenterology*. 1989;96:750–763.

89. Tabbane F, Mourali N, Cammoun M, et al. Results of laparotomy in immunoproliferative small intestinal disease. *Cancer*. 1988;61:1699–1706.

90. Akbulut H, Soykan I, Yakaryilmaz, et al. Five-year results of the treatment of 23 patients with immunoproliferative small intestinal disease: A Turkish experience. *Cancer*. 1997;80:8–14.

91. Isaacson PG, Dogan A, Price SK, et al. Immunoproliferative small-intestinal disease. An immunohistochemical study. *Am J Surg Pathol*. 1989;13:1023–1233.

92. Salem P, El-Hashimi L, Anaissie E, et al. Primary small intestinal lymphoma in adults. A comparative study of IPSID versus non-IPSID in the middle east. *Cancer*. 1987;59:1670–1676.

93. Rambaud JC, Modigliani R, Phuoc BK, et al. Non-secretory alpha-chain disease in intestinal lymphoma. *N Engl J Med*. 1980;303:53.

94. Smith WJ, Price SK, Isaacson PG. Immunoglobulin gene re-

arrangement in immunoproliferative small intestinal disease (IPSID). *J Clin Pathol.* 1987;40:1291–1297.

95. Isaacson PG, O'Connor NT, Spencer J, et al. Malignant histiocytosis of the intestine: A T-cell lymphoma. *Lancet.* 1985;2:688–691.

96. Mathus-Vliegen EM, Van-Halteren H, Tytgat GN. Malignant lymphoma in coeliac disease: Various manifestations with distinct symptomatology and prognosis? *J Intern Med.* 1994;236:43–49.

97. Murray A, Cuevas EC, Jones DB, et al. Study of the immunohistochemistry and T cell clonality of enteropathy-associated T cell lymphoma. *Am J Pathol.* 1995;146:509–519.

98. Chott A, Dragosics B, Radaszkiewicz T. Peripheral T-cell lymphomas of the intestine. *Am J Pathol.* 1992;141:1361–1371.

99. Ashton KM, Diss TC, Pan L, et al. Molecular analysis of T-cell clonality in ulcerative jejunitis and enteropathy-associated T-cell lymphoma. *Am J Pathol.* 1997;151:493–498.

100. O'Farrelly C, Feighery C, O'Briain DS, et al. Humoral response to wheat protein in patients with coeliac disease and enteropathy associated T cell lymphoma. *Br Med J Clin Res.* 1986;293:908–910.

101. Chan JK, Banks PM, Cleary ML, et al. A revised European-American classification of lymphoid neoplasms proposed by the International Lymphoma Study Group. A summary version. *Am J Clin Pathol.* 1995;103:543–560.

102. Spencer J, MacDonald TT, Diss T, et al. Changes in intraepithelial lymphocyte subpopulations in coeliac disease and enteropathy associated T cell lymphoma (malignant histiocytosis of the intestine). *Gut.* 1989;30:339–346.

103. Spencer J, Cerf-Bensussan N, Jarry A, et al. Enteropathy associated T cell lymphoma (malignant histiocytosis of the intestine) is recognized by a monoclonal antibody (HML-1) that defines a membrane molecule on human mucosal lymphocytes. *Am J Pathol.* 1988;132:1–5.

104. Cerf-Bensussan N, Jarry A, Brousse N, et al. A monoclonal antibody (HML-1) defining a novel membrane molecule present on human intestinal lymphocytes. *Eur J Immunol.* 1987;17:1279–1285.

105. Falini B, Flenghi L, Fagioli M, et al. Expression of the intestinal T-lymphocyte associated molecule HML-1: Analysis of 75 non-Hodgkin's lymphomas and description of the first HML-1 positive lymphoblastic tumor. *Histopathology.* 1991;18:421–426.

106. Strickland A, Jones DB, Wright DH. T-cell clonality in neoplastic and enteropathic adjacent bowel in enteropathy-associated T-cell lymphoma. *J Pathol.* 1992;168(Suppl):95A.

107. Leung ST, Murray A, Jones DB, et al. Genotypic analysis of celiac disease and enteropathy-associated T-cell lymphomas. *J Pathol.* 1993;170(Suppl)335A.

108. Pan L, Diss TC, Peng H, et al. Epstein-Barr virus (EBV) in enteropathy-associated T-cell lymphoma (EATL). *J Pathol.* 1993;170:137–143.

109. Ilyas M, Niedobitek G, Agathanggelou A, et al. Non-Hodgkin's lymphoma, coeliac disease, and Epstein-Barr virus: A study of 13 cases of enteropathy-associated T- and B-cell lymphoma. *J Pathol.* 1995;177:115–122.

110. O'Briain DS, Kennedy MJ, Daly PA, et al. Multiple lymphomatous polyposis of the gastrointestinal tract. A clinicopathologically distinctive form of non-Hodgkin's lymphoma of B cell centrocytic type. *Am J Pathol.* 1989;13:691–699.

111. Fraga M, Lloret E, Sanchez-verde L, et al. Mucosal mantle cell (centrocytic) lymphomas. *Histopathology.* 1995;26:413–422.

112. Moynihan MJ, Bast MA, Chan WC, et al. Lymphomatous polyposis. A neoplasm of either follicular mantle or germinal center cell origin. *Am J Surg Pathol.* 1996;20:442–452.

113. Hirakawa K, Fuchigami T, Nakamura S, et al. Primary gastrointestinal T-cell lymphoma resembling multiple lymphomatous polyposis. *Gastroenterology.* 1996;111:778–782.

114. Isaacson PG, MacLennan KA, Subbuswamy SG. Multiple lymphomatous polyposis of the gastrointestinal tract. *Histopathology.* 1984;8:641–656.

115. Ruskone-Fourmestraux A, Delmer A, Levergne A, et al. Multiple lymphomatous polyposis of the gastrointestinal tract: Prospective clinicopathologic study of 31 cases. *Gastroenterology.* 1997;112:7–16.

116. Gelb AB, Rouse RV, Dorfman FR, et al. Detection of immunophenotypic abnormalities in paraffin-embedded B-lineage non-Hodgkin's lymphomas. *Am J Clin Pathol.* 1994;102:825–834.

117. Smir BN, Ramaika CA, Cho CG, et al. Molecular evidence links lymphomatous polyposis of the gastrointestinal tract with mantle cell lymphoma. *Hum Pathol.* 1995;26:1282–1285.

118. Ruskone-Fourmestraux A, Delmer A, Lavergne A, et al. Multiple lymphomatous polyposis of the gastrointestinal tract: Prospective clinicopathologic study of 31 cases. *Gastroenterology.* 1997;112:7–16.

119. Harris M, Blewitt RW, Davies VJ, et al. High grade non-Hodgkin's lymphoma complicating polypoid nodular lymphoid hyperplasia and multiple lymphomatous polyposis of the intestine. *Histopathology.* 1989;15:339–350.

120. Ladjadj Y, Philip T, Lenoir GM, et al. Abdominal Burkitt-type lymphomas in Algeria. *Br J Cancer.* 1984;49:503–512.

121. Anaissie E, Geha S, Allam C, et al. Burkitt's lymphoma in the Middle East: A study of 34 cases. *Cancer.* 1985;56:2539–2543.

122. Levine AM, Pavlova Z, Pockros AW, et al. Small noncleaved follicular center cell (FCC) lymphoma: Burkitt and non-Burkitt variants in the United States. I. Clinical features. *Cancer.* 1983;52:1073–1079.

123. Pavlova Z, Parker JW, Taylor CR, et al. Small noncleaved follicular center cell lymphoma: Burkitt's and non-Burkitt's variants in the U.S. II. Pathologic and immunologic features. *Cancer.* 1987;59:1892–1902.

124. Burkitt D, O'Connor GT. Malignant lymphoma in African children. I. A clinical syndrome. *Cancer.* 1961;14:258–269.

125. Miliauskas JR, Berard CW, Young RC, et al. Undifferentiated non-Hodgkins' lymphomas (Burkitt's and non-Burkitt's types): The relevance of making this histologic distinction. *Cancer.* 1982;50:2115–2221.

126. The Non-Hodgkin's lymphoma Pathologic Classification Project. National cancer institute sponsored study of non-Hodgkin's lymphomas: Summary and description of a working formulation for clinical usage. *Cancer.* 1982;49:2112–2135.

127. Garcia CF, Weiss LM, Warnke RA. Small noncleaved cell lymphoma: An immunophenotypic study of 18 cases and comparison with large cell lymphoma. *Hum Pathol.* 1987;17:454–461.

128. Yano T, van Krieken JH, Magrath IT, et al. Histogenetic correlations between subcategories of small noncleaved cell lymphomas. *Blood.* 1992;79:1282–1290.

129. Haluska FG, Finger LR, Kagan J, et al. Molecular genetics of chromosomal translocations in B- and T-lymphoid malignancies. *In* Cossman J (ed.): *Molecular Genetics in Cancer Diagnosis.* New York, Elsevier, 1990. pp. 143–162.

16

THE ANAL CANAL

Jennifer Cho Sartorelli and Parakrama Chandrasoma

▶ CHAPTER OUTLINE

STRUCTURE AND FUNCTION

The anal canal is that part of the distal GI tract that is distal to the rectum and proximal to perianal skin. It is defined histologically and consists of two parts:

1. The mucosa of the anal transitional zone (ATZ) is the non-columnar epithelium between the columnar, crypt-bearing, rectal mucosa and the normally maturing squamous epithelium that lines the distal anal canal. The epithelium lining the ATZ resembles transitional epithelium, being flat, stratified, and composed of small, cuboidal cells (Fig. 16–1). Small crypt-like structures are sometimes present in this transitional epithelium (Fig. 16–2); these may contain Paneth cells and, on rare occasion, gastric parietal cells.[1] The extent of the ATZ varies from less than 1 mm to 2 cm in different people.

Most of the ATZ lies above the dentate, or pectinate, line and grossly resembles rectal mucosa, with which it blends imperceptibly at endoscopy. The ATZ usually lines the columns of Morgagni, which end distally at the dentate line. In inflammatory diseases of the anal canal, reactive changes may occur in the ATZ epithelium; these can be difficult to differentiate from dysplasia (see Fig. 16–2).

2. The pecten, which is the nonkeratinizing, pigmented, squamous epithelium that lines the anal canal distal to the dentate line, merges with the ATZ proximally and with hair-containing, keratinized perianal skin at the anal verge. The pecten usually measures 2–4 cm. Melanocytes appear in the pecten and progressively increase in number as it nears the perianal skin.

The anal glands are simple mucous glands found at the level of the dentate line, commonly within the internal sphincter. The anal gland duct is lined by a transitional type of epithelium that may contain goblet cells (Fig. 16–3). The duct opens into the anal canal at the valves of the dentate line. The anal glands secrete a mixture of sulfomucins and sialomucins.[2]

The sphincteric mechanism of the anus consists of (1) the internal sphincter, which is the distal limit of the circular muscle of the GI tract, and (2) the external sphincter, the upper part of which is associated with the levator ani muscle of the pelvic floor, which attaches the rectum to the lateral pelvic wall.

The arterial supply of the upper part of the anal canal is from the superior rectal artery, which is the termination of the inferior mesenteric artery. The lower part is supplied by branches of the iliac arteries. The anal canal is a site of communication between the portal and systemic venous circulations.

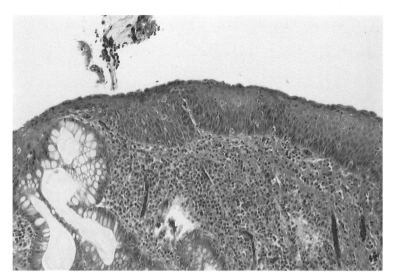

A

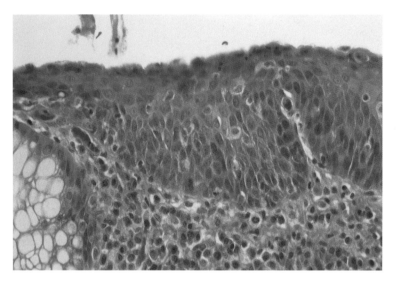

B

Figure 16–1. A: Normal anorectal transitional region. B: Anal transitional zone epithelium, which resembles transitional epithelium with vertically oriented basaloid cells and horizontally oriented surface cells.

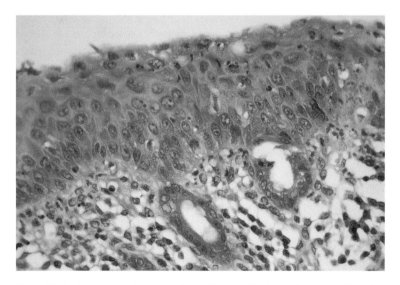

Figure 16–2. Anal transitional zone epithelium with two small, columnar-lined crypts. The epithelium shows inflammation and reactive changes that mimic dysplasia.

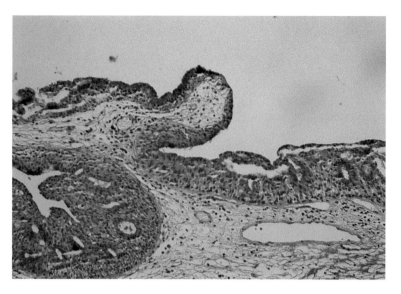

Figure 16–3. Anorectal transitional zone, stained with mucicarmine, showing scattered mucin-positive goblet cells in the surface epithelium and the anal gland duct.

The veins form submucosal plexuses; the internal hemorrhoidal plexus is above the dentate line, and the external hemorrhoidal plexus is below it. The upper part of the plexus drains via the portal venous system; the lower part drains into the systemic pelvic veins. Similarly, the lymphatic drainage of the ATZ follows the rectal lymphatics to the paraaortic nodes, whereas the lymphatics from the pecten drain to the inguinal nodes.

Physiologic studies of anal function using manometric probes that measure resting and squeeze pressures of the anal sphincter, and radiologic assessment of defecation (defecography) provide insights into anal motor function. These are used in specialized centers and are beyond the scope of the average pathologist.

BENIGN ANORECTAL LESIONS

Hemorrhoids

Hemorrhoids are among the most common specimens received by the surgical pathologist. They are the commonest cause of lower GI bleeding, which is often profuse. Rectal pain, itching, and tenesmus also occur and may be precipitated by thrombosis of the hemorrhoidal veins. The cause of hemorrhoids is unknown. Their relationship to constipation and straining is not constant; manometry shows an increased resting anal pressure in many patients, but this is believed to be a result rather than the cause of hemorrhoids.[3] Hemorrhoids are surgically resected only when they are large or complicated.

Hemorrhoids can be divided into internal hemorrhoids, which are above the dentate line and lined by rectal or transitional mucosa, and external hemorrhoids, which are below the dentate line and lined by squamous epithelium. The submucosa contains numerous dilated veins; thrombosis may be present and should be recorded in the report (Fig. 16–4). Unexpected

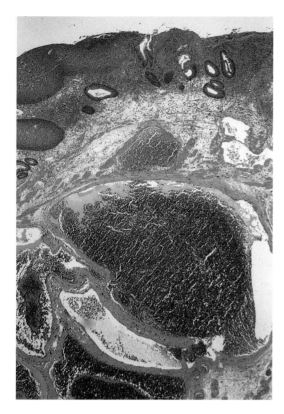

Figure 16–4. Internal hemorrhoid with thrombosis.

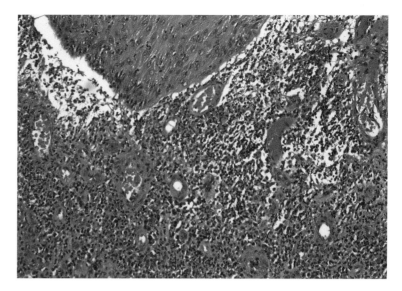

Figure 16–5. Anal fistula track, showing squamous epithelium and inflammation, including neutrophils, histiocytes, plasma cells, lymphocytes, and foreign body-type giant cells.

pathologic lesions such as squamous dysplasia are rarely seen in hemorrhoids[4]; very rarely, specimens submitted as hemorrhoids are neoplastic lesions; we have seen a polypoid anorectal melanoma submitted as a thrombosed hemorrhoid.

Anal Fissure

Anal fissure is a common cause of severe anorectal pain. Fissures are characterized by a linear ulcer, usually vertical, and usually in the posterior midline of the anal canal overlying the internal sphincter. Most anal fissures are idiopathic and are causally related to high internal sphincter pressures, which can be demonstrated electromanometrically. Surgery is necessary only for chronic intractable cases and consists of lateral sphincterotomy, which is effective in both reducing the sphincter pressure and healing the fissure.[5] Debridement of the ulcer tissue and prolapsed parts of the internal sphincter results in a pathologic specimen. This consists of epithelium with reactive changes, granulation tissue with nonspecific acute and chronic inflammation including foreign body giant cells, and smooth muscle with fibrosis. Rarely, epithelioid granulomas are found; in these cases, acid-fast staining for mycobacteria and the possibility of associated Crohn's disease must be considered.

Anal Fistula

Anal fistula is a complication of an untreated anorectal abscess formed by a suppurative inflammation of the anal glands. The organisms involved are usually a mixture of colonic luminal bacteria such as *Escherichia coli* and *Bacteroides fragilis*. The abscess usually involves the ischiorectal soft tissues between the anal sphincter and perianal skin and drains into both the anal canal and perianal skin, resulting in a fistula. Anal fistulas are classified as either high or low by their point of opening in the anal canal. Anal fistulas are usually treated by laying open the fistulous tract. The excised fistulous tract is submitted to pathology and shows inflamed granulation tissue with foreign body giant cells (Fig. 16–5). Rarely, untreated perianal infections can spread locally; in immunocompromised patients and uncontrolled diabetics, this may result in a spreading necrotizing cellulitis of the perineum, extending to the thigh and abdomen.

Infectious Diseases

The anal canal is a common site for sexually transmitted infections, particularly in anoreceptive individuals. Infections include proctitis due to *Neisseria gonorrhoeae*, Herpes simplex

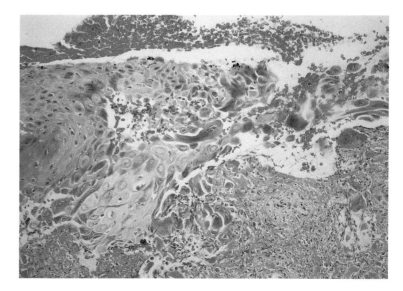

Figure 16–6. Anal canal ulcer in herpes simplex infection, showing numerous multinucleated epithelial cells, many of which have "ground glass" nuclei typical of herpes virus.

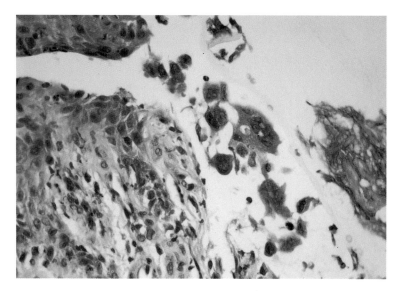

Figure 16–7. Multinucleated giant cells with glassy nuclei from the edge of an anal ulcer. These are not typical herpetic inclusions, but showed positivity for herpes simplex type II antigens on immunohistochemistry.

virus type 2 (Figs. 16–6 and 16–7), syphilis (primary chancre and condyloma latum), chlamydial infections including lymphogranuloma venereum (LGV) (Fig. 16–8), and granuloma inguinale caused by *Calymmatobacterium donovani.* LGV and granuloma inguinale have chronic disease phases, with severe ulceration and pseudo-epitheliomatous hyperplasia of the anal canal mucosa and inguinal lymphadenopathy.

The diagnosis is made clinically and by culture. Rarely, in granuloma inguinale, the organism can be identified in macrophages in a silver-stained section.

Inflammatory Cloacogenic Polyp

The term "inflammatory cloacogenic polyp" is still sometimes applied to polyps in the anal canal associated with rectal mucosal prolapse. The polyps are lined by hyperplastic rectal mu-

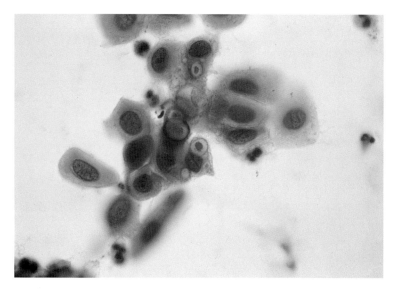

Figure 16–8. Smear from anal lesion, showing intracytoplasmic chlamydial inclusions in epithelial cells.

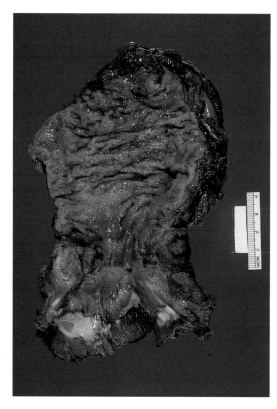

Figure 16–9. Anal involvement in Crohn's disease, showing mucosal erythema, thickening, and granularity in the anal canal and white patches in perianal skin.

cosa, which shows crypt elongation and distortion, fibromuscular replacement of the lamina propria, and relatively mild inflammation. The changes are identical to those seen in solitary rectal ulcer syndrome, and inflammatory cloacogenic polyp is now considered part of that syndrome (see Chapter 10).

Anal Lesions in Crohn's Disease

Perianal disease occurs in up to 90% of patients with Crohn's disease. Most of these patients have mild symptoms and need no treatment. Lesions include hypertrophic perianal skin tags; perianal abscess and fistula; anal fissures; and ulceration, induration, and narrowing of the anal canal (Figs. 16–9 and 16–10). Unlike the rest of the GI tract, surgical resection is not a treatment option for anal canal Crohn's disease. Patients are treated conservatively. Rarely, pathologic specimens may result from excision of anal fissures and fistulas; these usually show nonspecific inflammation and only rarely contain epithelioid granulomas (Fig. 16–11).

NEOPLASMS

Neoplasms of the anal canal arise between the rectal mucosa and the anal verge. They must be clearly distinguished from rectal neoplasms and from neoplasms of the perianal skin. Differentiation from rectal neoplasms is a problem only in the rare,

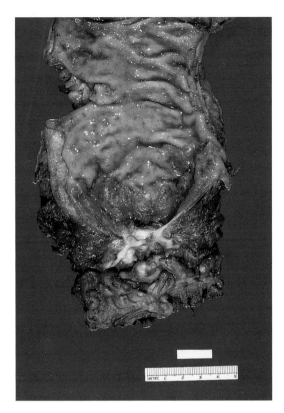

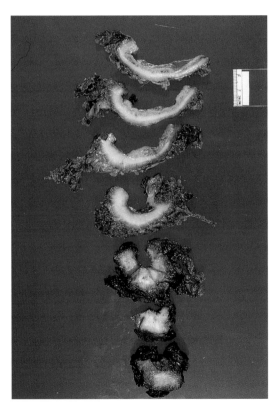

Figure 16–10. A: Crohn's disease involving the anal canal, showing a fibrous stricture in a severely abnormal anal canal. B: Cut sections from anal stricture in Crohn's disease, showing progressive thickening of the wall with luminal narrowing.

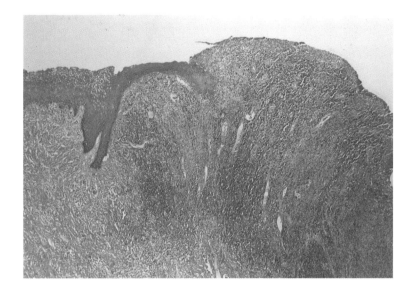

A

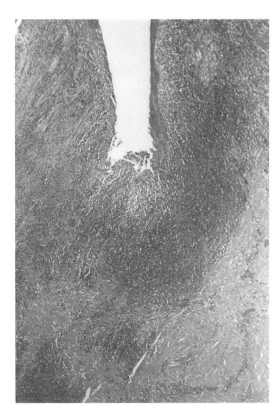

B

Figure 16–11. A: Crohn's disease of the anal canal, showing nonspecific severe acute and chronic inflammation in the base of a flat aphthoid ulcer. B: Crohn's disease of the anal canal, showing ulceration with acutely inflamed granulation tissue. The intact squamous epithelium adjacent to the ulcer shows marked subepithelial, mainly chronic, inflammation.

undifferentiated malignant neoplasm occurring in the anorectal junctional region, which could represent either a poorly differentiated rectal adenocarcinoma or a poorly differentiated carcinoma arising in the epithelium of the ATZ. Squamous carcinoma and high-grade dysplasia of the lower anal canal, however, are often difficult to differentiate from perianal squamous epithelial lesions. Although similarities exist between these, such as an association with human papillomavirus infection, differentiation is important because perianal squamous neoplasms are treated primarily by surgery, and anal canal squamous carcinoma is treated primarily by chemotherapy and radiation.[6]

Condyloma Acuminatum

Condyloma acuminatum is a sexually transmitted human papillomavirus (HPV) infection that results in the formation of viral warts in perianal skin and inside the anal canal. Warts within the anal canal occur mainly in anoreceptive individuals. A large number of different serotypes of HPV, including 6, 11, 16, 18, 31, 33, 35, and 51, have been associated. Serotypes 6 and 11 are the most commonly associated with ordinary condylomas (Fig. 16–12A); these serotypes are thought not to have malignant potential. The other serotypes, notably 16 and 18, are most frequently associated with malignancy. HPV infection is also common in the noncondylomatous epithelium adjacent to the anal canal (Fig. 16–12B), explaining the high incidence of recurrent condylomata after surgical removal. Anal canal condylomas commonly coexist with perianal, penile, and uterine cervical condylomas.

Condylomata acuminata are wart-like papillomatous lesions characterized by squamous epithelial proliferation (Fig. 16–13A). The squamous epithelium is acanthotic and commonly has a more basaloid appearance than verruca vulgaris. Cell polarity is maintained, and surface maturation takes place into keratinized cells. Many condylomas show koilocytosis in the surface region; this is characterized by cytoplasmic vacuolation and the presence of nuclei that show irregularity, increased chromatin, and cytologic characteristics of low-grade dysplasia ("raisinoid nuclei") (Fig. 16–13A–C). The presence of specific HIV serotypes can be demonstrated by immunoperoxidase techniques (see Fig. 16–12A). High-grade dysplasia and squamous carcinoma may be seen rarely in condylomas.

Condylomas treated with podophyllin show atypic cytologic features that cannot be reliably distinguished from high-grade dysplasia. When a history of podophyllin treatment is available, these changes can be ascribed cautiously to this drug, but it is advisable to keep these patients under observation for recurrent lesions and be more active in removing any new lesions.

Squamous Dysplasia

Squamous dysplasia of the anal canal is classified into low-grade anal intraepithelial neoplasia (AIN) and high-grade AIN. Low-grade AIN is commonly associated with condylomata acuminata and is usually due to HPV serotypes 6 and 11 (Fig. 16–14). High-grade AIN, which includes carcinoma in situ, may occur in a condyloma or in visually normal anal epithelium. HPV type 16 is the dominant serotype in high-grade AIN,[7] with type 18 being less commonly associated. High-grade AIN is associated with activation of c-Ha-*ras* and c-*myc* oncogenes and expression of their protein products p21ras and p62myc in the infected cells.[8]

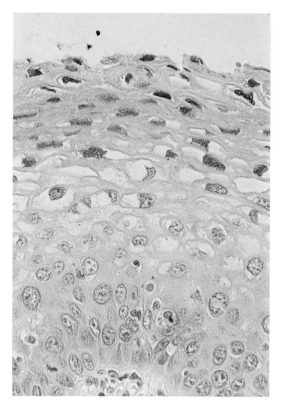

A

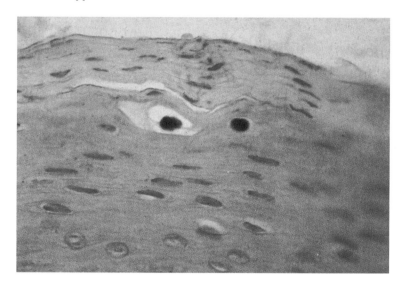

B

Figure 16–12. A: Immunoperoxidase stain for human papillomavirus serotype 6 in condyloma acuminatum, showing positive nuclear staining in infected cells. B: Immunoperoxidase stain for human papillomavirus serotype 6 in normal anal canal epithelium adjacent to a condyloma acuminatum, showing positive nuclear staining in infected cells.

High-grade AIN in a visually normal anal canal can be detected by random biopsy or cytologic preparations (Fig. 16–15; see also Chapter 18. The diagnostic criteria for dysplasia and its grade are identical to those used for the uterine cervix. In anal canal biopsies, it is important not to misinterpret transitional epithelium of the anal transitional zone for dysplasia. The epithelium of the ATZ frequently shows nuclear enlargement, hyperchromasia, and mild disorganization, particularly in the

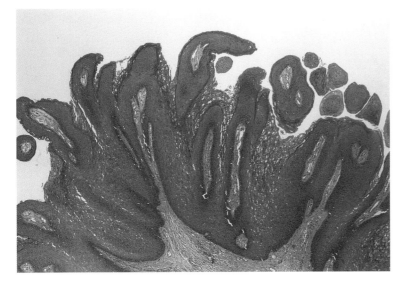

A

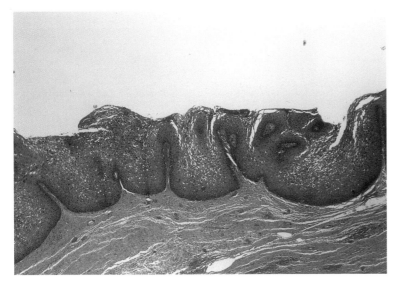

B

C

Figure 16–13. A: Condyloma acuminatum, showing squamous proliferation with acanthosis and papillomatosis. B: Condyloma acuminatum, showing acanthosis and koilocytotic change in epithelial cells in relatively flat anal canal epithelium. C: Condyloma acuminatum, showing koilocytotic change in epithelium.

basal region. Reactive changes associated with fissures and fistulas may also cause occasional difficulty in diagnosis.

The finding of high-grade AIN in a mass lesion such as a condyloma is an indication for complete surgical excision of all visible lesions. If no invasive carcinoma is found, these patients should be followed. The finding of high-grade AIN in an endoscopically normal anal canal is an indication for careful follow-up for the development of any visible lesion. The risk of progression to invasive carcinoma is high in these patients.[9] Extensive surgical resection of anal canal mucosa is not feasible, but mucosal ablative procedures are of potential value.[10]

High-grade AIN may be associated with high-grade squamous dysplasia of the perianal skin. High-grade dysplasia of the perianal skin is commonly treated by surgical resection; this may be followed by skin grafting if the area of involvement is large.[9] The term "Bowen's disease" is avoided here because to some authorities it is synonymous with high-grade dysplasia (carcinoma in situ), whereas others use it more restrictively for high-grade dysplasia of the perianal skin.

Squamous Carcinoma

Two pathologically distinct types of squamous carcinoma are recognized in the anal canal.

Verrucous Carcinoma

Verrucous carcinoma is rare in the anal canal, occurring more commonly in the penis and in perianal skin. This lesion is also called giant condyloma of Bushke and Löwenstein. Verrucous carcinoma is an exophytic, cauliflower-like, warty lesion that is larger than 2 cm. Its histologic features are identical to those of condyloma acuminatum, and it does not contain the cytologic features of high-grade dysplasia or malignancy (Fig. 16–16A). They are distinguished from condyloma acuminatum by their large size and by the fact that they show evidence of invasion at the base into the anal canal wall (Fig. 16–16B). The pattern of infiltration is as a broad, pushing margin and not as individual cells and is therefore difficult to assess accurately. Little data are available on HPV serotyping of these rare tumors; aggres-

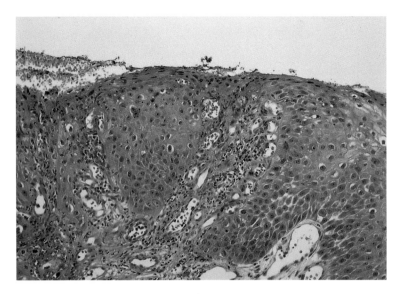

A

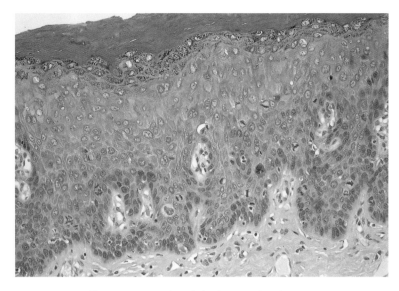

Figure 16–15. High-grade dysplasia in anal canal mucosa.

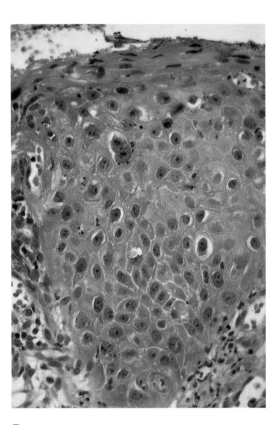

B

Figure 16–14. A: Low-grade epithelial dysplasia in the anal canal, showing mild dysplastic changes in flat epithelium with minimal koilocytosis. This specimen was positive for human papillomavirus, serotype 11, by immunohistochemistry. B: Higher power micrograph of part A.

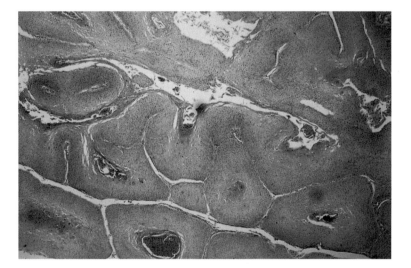

A

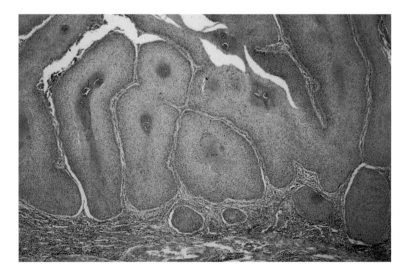

B

Figure 16–16. A: Verrucous carcinoma, tangentially cut surface of the tumor, showing papillomatosis and lack of dysplasia in the proliferating squamous epithelium. This appearance is indistinguishable from a large condyloma acuminatum. B: Base of verrucous carcinoma, showing minimal invasion at the interphase between epithelium and stroma.

sive behavior has been associated with the presence of HPV 11 and 16.[11]

All squamous papillomatous lesions clinically resembling condylomas that are larger than 2 cm should be excised with a sufficient deep surgical margin. Histologic examination of the specimen differentiates these into verrucous squamous carcinomas or large condylomata acuminata based on the presence or absence of an infiltrative base.

Verrucous carcinoma of the anorectal and perineal region

has a 66% likelihood of local recurrence. No metastases have been reported.[12] Recurrences require radical surgery. The overall mortality rate is 20%, all related to the effects of locally uncontrollable disease.[12]

Squamous Carcinoma of the ATZ and Pecten

These neoplasms were previously classified by (1) location, into tumors above and below the dentate line, (2) histologic appearance into basaloid (cloacogenic), mixed basaloid and squamous, squamous, and squamous with glandular differentiation, and (3) histologic grade. These classifications are no longer considered to be of value, mostly because all squamous carcinomas of the anal canal except verrucous carcinoma are treated in a similar manner.

Eighty-five percent of squamous carcinomas of the anal canal are associated with HPV infection. By far the most common serotype involved is HPV type 16, with type 18 being less frequent.[13] Squamous carcinomas may arise in either the flat anorectal mucosa or develop in a condyloma. The association with HPV types 16 and 18 is similar in both situations. No difference exists between HPV-positive and HPV-negative and carcinomas.[14]

Anal carcinoma presents with rectal bleeding or discharge. The majority of patients are anoreceptive male homosexuals. Grossly, the tumors are ulcerative, with typical everted edges present in most cases. Marked induration of the wall of the anal canal is usually present. Thirty-five percent of tumors arise in the ATZ and cannot be reliably differentiated from a low rectal adenocarcinoma at endoscopy (Fig. 16–17); the other 65% occur in the pecten.[6]

The diagnosis is made by adequate biopsy specimens, showing infiltrating squamous carcinoma of varying degrees of differentiation (Fig. 16–18). Basaloid features and focal glandular differentiation are commonly admixed with squamous elements in tumors arising in the ATZ (Fig. 16–19), some of which are pure basaloid carcinomas. Basaloid carcinomas resemble basal cell carcinoma of the skin, with nests of small cells with scanty cytoplasm and small ovoid nuclei that tend to show peripheral palisading. Some basaloid tumors have an adenoid pattern and may contain mucin-secreting cells (Fig. 16–19C); the presence of mucin should therefore not be taken as a criterion to negate a diagnosis of squamous carcinoma of the anal canal. Tumors of the low pecten are commonly well-differentiated, pure squamous carcinomas. These tumors diffusely infiltrate the underlying wall. Evidence of high-grade dysplasia may be present in the adjacent uninvolved anal canal mucosa.

Radiation therapy, given by external beam and brachytherapy, with or without chemotherapy, has replaced abdominoperineal resection as the primary treatment modality for anal canal squamous carcinomas of all histologic types and grades. Eighty percent of patients have a complete response to this treatment. The 5-year survival rate is 60–70%.[6,15] Survival decreases with advanced stage tumors, tumors larger than 4 cm in size, the presence of node involvement, and tumors that do not respond completely to initial external beam radiation.[15] Patients experi-

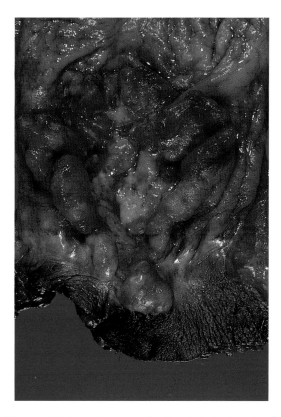

Figure 16–17. Low rectal adenocarcinoma extending down to involve the region of the pectinate line. This can be difficult to differentiate from high anal transitional zone carcinomas at endoscopy. Microscopically, the distinction is easy when the adenocarcinoma is typical, but when poorly differentiated, a basaloid carcinoma with glandular differentiation must be considered.

encing recurrence can be treated with salvage chemoradiation therapy.[16] It is extremely uncommon for patients to have surgical resections, except as palliation for advanced cases that have failed all other treatment modalities.

Biopsy samples are sometimes taken from the posttreated anal canal. Biopsy may be prompted by the presence of nodularity, unusual induration, or unusual symptoms. The presence of squamous carcinoma in these cases should be diagnosed only when cohesive groups of malignant epithelial cells are present. Single atypical cells are commonly present in postradiation tissue, representing radiation-altered stromal cells. Staining for keratin by immunoperoxidase may be helpful in these cases, but caution is necessary because stromal cells rarely show keratin positivity.

Although radiation and chemotherapy are excellent means of controlling local tumors, metastatic disease is not as well controlled. Metastases may appear in the inguinal lymph nodes, pelvic nodes, and paraaortic nodes in the region of origin of the inferior mesenteric artery.

Neoplasms of Anal Glands and Ducts

Anal Gland Adenoma

Adenomas arising in anal glands are extremely rare. They present as small, intramural nodules at the anorectal junction and are circumscribed, with the histologic features of either cystadenoma, apocrine adenoma, or hidradenoma. In small samples,

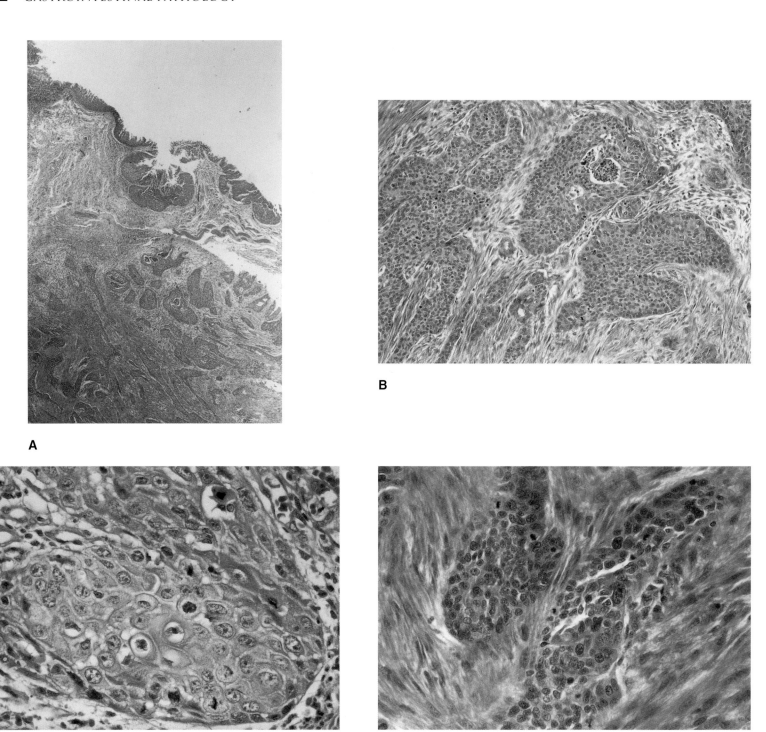

A

B

C

D

Figure 16–18. A: Squamous carcinoma of anal transitional zone arising from the epithelium of the anal transitional zone. B: Well-differentiated squamous carcinoma, showing infiltrating nests of malignant squamous epithelium. C: Squamous carcinoma, showing a nest of malignant epithelial cells with focal keratinization. D: Squamous carcinoma of the anal transitional zone, showing a lesser degree of differentiation than in part B.

distinction from well-differentiated anal gland adenocarcinoma can be difficult. Complete excision with clear margins permits accurate diagnosis by lack of infiltration and is curative.

Adenocarcinoma of Anal Glands and Ducts

These tumors are also rare; they may complicate chronic anal fistulas.[17] Anal gland adenocarcinoma should be considered when an adenocarcinoma occurs in the wall of the anal canal lined by a normal or minimally ulcerated squamous epithelium (Fig. 16–20). Most anal gland adenocarcinomas are well differentiated, with irregularly infiltrating mucin-containing spaces lined by malignant columnar epithelial cells. Desmoplasia is common. Anal gland adenocarcinomas are difficult to excise surgically, have a high likelihood of local recurrence and metastasis, and a low survival rate.[18]

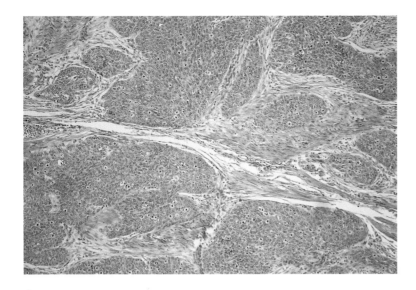

A

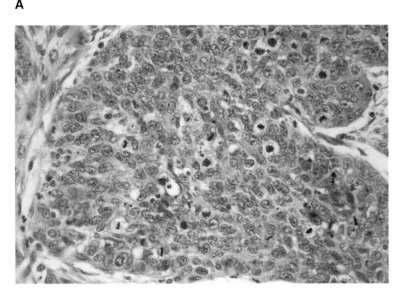

B

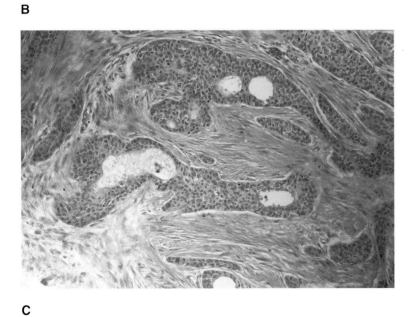

C

Figure 16–19. A: Basaloid carcinoma of the anal transitional zone, showing infiltrative nests of basaloid cells. B: Basaloid carcinoma, higher power micrograph of part A, showing small basaloid cells with high mitotic activity. C: Basaloid carcinoma of the anal transitional zone, showing glandular structures in the basaloid cell nests.

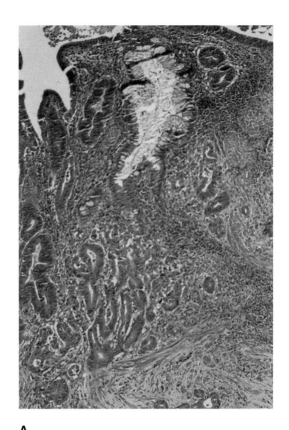

A

B

Figure 16–20. Adenocarcinoma of the anal glands. A: This is a section through the muscle wall of the anal canal, showing an infiltrating adenocarcinoma arising from an anal gland. A residual benign glandular element is present. B: Mucicarmine stain, showing malignant glands in relation to a sinus tract lined by flat glandular epithelium that shows dysplasia.

Anorectal Malignant Melanoma

Malignant melanoma of the anorectal region is very rare, accounting for 1% of all anorectal malignancies. It arises in the region of the dentate line and usually presents with rectal bleeding. Grossly, they are commonly polypoid masses, usually of large size (median size: 4 cm). Two thirds are black (Figs. 16–21 and 16–22); the rest do not appear pigmented grossly. In some patients, the anorectal melanoma is found during a search for a primary after a diagnosis of metastatic melanoma has been made in an inguinal lymph node.

Histologically, the tumors consist of sheets and nests of epithelioid melanocytes (Fig. 16–23A). The cells have round, central nuclei, which contain prominent nucleoli and intranuclear pseudo-inclusions (Fig. 16–23B). The diagnosis is usually obvious because of the presence of abundant cytoplasmic melanin pigment in the malignant cells (Fig. 16–23A). In achromatic tumors (Fig. 16–23C), the presence of the typical nuclear features and glassy eosinophilic cytoplasm, the presence of a junctional component in the adjacent epithelium (Fig. 16–23D), and immunoperoxidase staining for S100 protein and HMB45 permit diagnosis. Large, ulcerated achromatic malignant melanomas that extend up into the rectum may be difficult to differentiate from GI stromal neoplasms without immunohistochemistry (Fig. 16–24).

Anorectal malignant melanomas are treated by surgical resection, either limited resection for palliation in tumors with evidence of distant spread, or by radical surgery for localized tu-

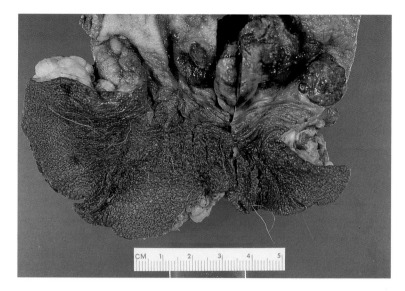

A

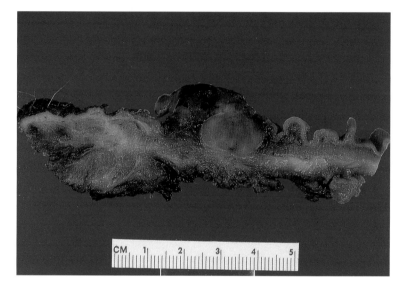

B

Figure 16–22. A: Malignant melanoma of the anal canal, showing a multinodular pigmented mass in the low anal canal near its junction with perianal skin. B. Cut section of part A, showing a nodular fleshy mass that is pigmented in one part and nonpigmented in the deeper region.

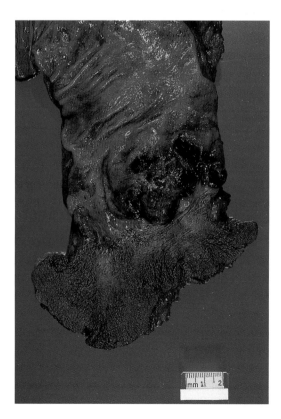

Figure 16–21. Malignant melanoma of the anal canal, showing pigmented large polypoid mass.

mors. The prognosis is uniformly bad, with a median survival time of less than 12 months and a very low survival rate.[19,20]

Other Neoplasms

Many other neoplasms have been reported in the anorectal region. Malignant lymphoma and Kaposi's sarcoma occur in immunocompromised patients, particularly those with AIDS. Small-cell, undifferentiated, neuroendocrine carcinoma can occur primarily as well as represent a metastasis from a lung primary. Other metastatic neoplasms are rare. Gastrointestinal stromal neoplasms (Chapter 14), lipomas, granular cell tumors, leukemic infiltration (granulocytic sarcomas), and hemangiomas occur very rarely.

17

GASTROINTESTINAL PATHOLOGY IN THE IMMUNOCOMPROMISED PATIENT

Pamela B. Sylvestre

Gastrointestinal disease is frequent in all types of immunocompromised patients but occurs with greatest frequency in patients with acquired immunodeficiency syndrome (AIDS). Diarrhea is an extremely common symptom in AIDS, affecting 50–90% of patients during the course of their disease.[1] Sometimes intractable diarrhea is the major symptom. Enteric infections are responsible for most cases of diarrhea in AIDS. Alterations in mucosal immunity may explain the increased susceptibility to enteric infections in AIDS; decrease in total T cells, CD4+ T cells, and IgA-producing cells have all been reported.[2,3]

Infections in immunocompromised patients include reactivation of latent infections and opportunistic infection by ubiquitous microorganisms.[4] The most important opportunistic pathogens of the GI tract are *Candida albicans* (stomatitis and esophagitis), cytomegalovirus (entire GI tract), herpes simplex virus (esophagus and anal canal), *Cryptosporidium* (small intestine), *Isospora belli* (small intestine), and *Mycobacterium avium-intracellulare* (stomach and intestine). Kaposi's sarcoma commonly involves the GI tract in patients with disseminated disease; however, it rarely causes GI symptoms. In contrast, malignant lymphomas, although less frequent, are aggressive, rapidly progressive tumors.[5] Graft-versus-host disease (GVHD) and posttransplant lymphoproliferative disorder (PTLD)[6] are conditions unique to transplant recipients.

The specific symptomatology and pathologic lesions associated with many of these diseases have been considered in relation to the respective organs. In this chapter, the factors predisposing to these diseases and their diagnosis will be considered more thoroughly.

VIRAL INFECTIONS

Cytomegalovirus

Cytomegalovirus (CMV) is a ubiquitous agent and is recognized as a pathogen in all age groups. CMV naturally persists in humans and is readily reactivated in immunocompromised states.[7] The spectrum of clinical disease due to CMV ranges from an asymptomatic carrier state to life-threatening infection. In the immunocompetent host, CMV either causes no disease or mild illnesses. Serious CMV infection occurs in AIDS, after organ transplantation, and during cancer chemotherapy and high-dosage corticosteroid therapy.

CMV in Patients with AIDS

CMV is a major cause of morbidity in patients with AIDS. It is the most common viral pathogen in this group, occurring in 40–90% of patients.[8,9] Infection usually manifests in patients at a stage of profound immunodeficiency with a CD4 cell count lower than 50 /μL.[8] The most common sites of CMV infection are the retina and the GI tract[8]; one third of AIDS patients who develop CMV infections have digestive tract involvement.[10]

CMV can cause disease throughout the GI tract from mouth to rectum; the stomach (Chapter 4) and colon (Chapter 10) are the sites of maximum involvement.[11] CMV esophagitis is a common cause of dysphagia, odynophagia, and esophageal ulceration in AIDS (Chapter 2). Symptoms of gastrointestinal involvement include epigastric pain, nausea and recurrent vomiting, diarrhea, and upper and lower GI bleeding.[12,13] Gastrointestinal complications from CMV include perforation, hemorrhage, pseudotumoral mass lesions, small-bowel obstruction, ischemic colitis secondary to CMV vasculitis, and CMV appendicitis.[14–17] Healing ulcers may cause fibrous strictures.[18]

Treatment with ganciclovir or forcarnet often heals intestinal lesions and improves the clinical situation in most AIDS patients.[14] Nevertheless, symptomatic CMV infection is associated with a poor long-term outlook because of its association with severe immunodeficiency. The median survival after a CMV infection in AIDS is 7 months, whether or not the patient receives anti-CMV maintenance treatment.[10]

CMV in Transplant Patients

Upper gastrointestinal symptoms are indicative of serious opportunistic infections such as CMV and invasive fungal infection in a significant number of transplant recipients.[19] Infection of the upper GI tract with CMV is a major cause of morbidity in cardiac transplant patients and may be life-threatening if untreated.[20] Kaplan and colleagues[21] report that GI disease was the most prominent manifestation of CMV infection in heart and heart–lung transplant patients, with an occurrence rate of 9.9%.

There are several sources of CMV infection in transplant patients: (1) immunosuppression secondary to drug therapy can result in reactivation of the latent infection present before transplantation; (2) blood transfusion required at the time of surgery can cause CMV transmission and primary infection; and (3) the transplanted organ, particularly in situations in which seropositive organs are transplanted into seronegative recipients, can serve as the vehicle for CMV transmission.

After transplantation, patients in whom CMV is identified are more likely to have been CMV-seronegative recipients of organs from CMV-seropositive donors.[21] It is generally accepted that primary infections in patients who were seronegative before transplantation are more severe than reactivated infections.[22] Involvement of multiple organ systems is common; gastrointestinal manifestations include gastritis, gastric ulceration, duodenitis, esophagitis, pyloric perforation, and colonic hemorrhage.[21] Because opportunistic infections may jeopardize allograft function and patient survival, all patients with upper GI tract symptoms require prompt endoscopy and biopsy for diagnosis of cause.

Although CMV infections continue to occur frequently after organ transplantation, a decrease in their severity has been described with the use of newer immunosuppressive regimens.[22] Patients receiving FK506 following orthotopic liver transplantation have a lower tendency to develop enteric CMV infection than those receiving cyclosporin A (CsA) treatment. Of those who do experience CMV infection, enteric CMV infection is less severe in the FK506-treated liver recipients than the CsA-treated patients.[23]

Although the tendency of CMV disease in transplant patients at risk of primary disease (seronegative recipients) is not influenced by the immunosuppressive regimen, immunosuppression has a profound effect on the reactivation of CMV disease in CMV-seropositive transplant recipients. Hibberd and colleagues[24] report a 59% prevalence of CMV disease in seropositive renal transplant patients receiving OKT3 but only 21% in those who did not receive OKT3.

In transplant patients, the presence of GI tract CMV infection is associated with a decreased T-lymphocyte helper/suppressor ratio in peripheral blood.[25] Although infection due to CMV has been a substantial cause of morbidity and mortality among transplant patients, the prognosis of the disease has improved dramatically since the introduction of ganciclovir.[26]

Diagnosis of CMV Infection

In patients at high risk for CMV, histologic evidence of infection is uncommon in normal mucosa but is frequent in lesions.[27] Histologic changes produced in CMV-infected cells are (1) cell enlargement; (2) a large, round, eosinophilic, intranuclear inclusion surrounded by a halo (Cowdry A inclusion); and (3) multiple, small, granular, basophilic intracytoplasmic inclusions (Fig.

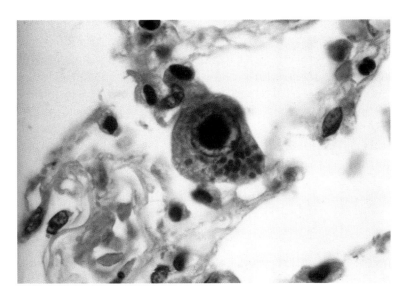

Figure 17–1. Cytomegalovirus-infected cell, showing marked cytomegaly, a large intranuclear inclusion separated from the nuclear membrane by a halo, and multiple granular intracytoplasmic inclusions.

17–1). The presence of any two of these three features in a cell is considered diagnostic for CMV by routine light microscopy. Evidence of CMV infection may be seen in glandular epithelial cells, vascular endothelial cells, and lamina propria stromal cells. CMV does not infect squamous epithelial cells in the eosphagus; deep biopsy samples containing subepithelial lamina propria are therefore essential for a diagnosis of CMV esophagitis. No correlation exists between the number of CMV-infected cells and the inflammatory response.[28]

Although the pathologic criteria for classic CMV inclusions have been well described, morphologically atypical inclusions are not well characterized (Fig. 17–2). The atypical inclusions, which are difficult to precisely identify on routine hematoxylin and eosin (H&E) sections as CMV-infected cells,

can be characterized using other diagnostic techniques. In situ hybridization for cytomegalovirus DNA is more sensitive than immunostaining (Fig. 17–3), and both are superior to routine H&E staining in terms of sensitivity.[29] Hackman and colleagues[30] report that the most sensitive method for diagnosing CMV is cell culture (sensitivity of 57%), followed by indirect fluorescent antibody staining for a late CMV antigen (53% sensitivity), in situ DNA hybridization (40% sensitivity), indirect fluorescent antibody and immunoperoxidase staining for an early CMV antigen (37% and 43% sensitivities, respectively), and routine histology (30% sensitivity). No single detection technique is completely adequate for rapid identification of CMV in small endoscopic biopsy samples. When routine H&E histology is negative, immunohistochemical staining for CMV is recommended on specimens from patients at risk for CMV or those in

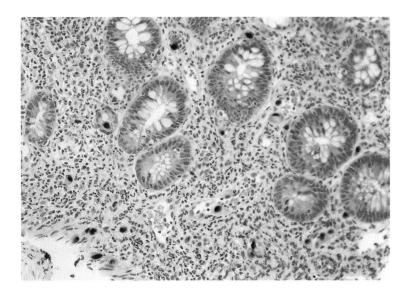

A

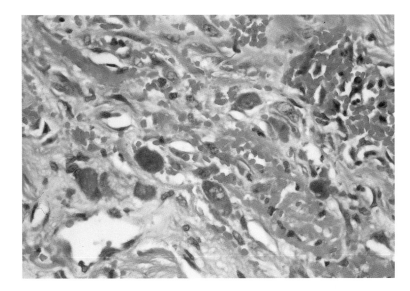

Figure 17–2. Cytomegalovirus colitis, section from a tumor-like lesion, showing multiple enlarged cells with nuclei that have smudged chromatin without definite inclusions. Some nuclei are clear with a possible inclusion, which makes them difficult to differentiate from a nucleolus. Immunoperoxidase stain for CMV was positive.

B

Figure 17–3. A: CMV gastritis, immunoperoxidase stain, showing numerous CMV-infected cells in the mucosa. B: Higher power micrograph of part A, showing predominantly nuclear staining of infected cells.

whom CMV infection is suspected by the presence of cells with atypical inclusions.

Herpes Simplex Virus

Both herpes simplex virus type I (HSV-1) and type II (HSV-2) are a cause of infections in immunocompromised patients. In the GI tract, HSV tends to infect mucosae lined by squamous epithelial cells; HSV-1 infection usually causes esophagitis, and HSV-2 infection occurs in the anal canal. Infection of the stomach, small intestine, and colon by HSV is extremely uncommon.

HSV-1 is an extremely common infection of the mouth in the normal population. After resolution of the primary infection, the virus remains latent in the nerve ganglia around the mouth, usually for the lifetime of the individual. Immunosuppression results in reactivation, causing herpetic lesions in the mouth, pharynx, and esophagus (Chapter 2). These lesions occur in all types of immunocompromised patients. Clinical features of HSV-1 infection include painful stomatitis, dysphagia, and odynophagia. Vesicular lesions, which rapidly become ulcerated, occur in the mouth, pharynx, and esophagus. The appearance of herpetic esophagitis at endoscopy is indistinguishable from CMV infection.

HSV-2, on the other hand, is a sexually transmitted infection. In anoreceptive individuals, particularly male homosexuals, HSV-2 infection occurs in the anal canal. After the primary phase, the virus remains dormant in the pelvic ganglia to become reactivated if the patient's immunity becomes compromised. Because of the common association between HSV-2 infection and AIDS, anorectal herpes occurs much more commonly in the AIDS population than in the transplant population. Herpetic proctitis causes anal pain, tenesmus, discharge, and rectal bleeding. Multiple superficial ulcers are present in the diffusely inflamed mucosa of the anal canal.

Diagnosis of HSV infection can be made by the Tzanck test (Fig. 17–4), in which a smear of the fluid from a vesicle or base of the ulcer is examined for HSV-infected cells or by biopsies

from the ulcer edge (Fig. 17–5). HSV infection of squamous epithelial cells results in multinucleation (four to eight nuclei per cell) and the presence of intranuclear inclusions. In the early stage, viral replication produces a glassy basophilic inclusion that fills the nucleus; later, the typical Cowdry A inclusion develops. The diagnosis can be confirmed in biopsy specimens by immunohistochemical staining for HSV antigens, which permits differentiation of HSV-1 and HSV-2. Viral culture is the most sensitive diagnostic test.

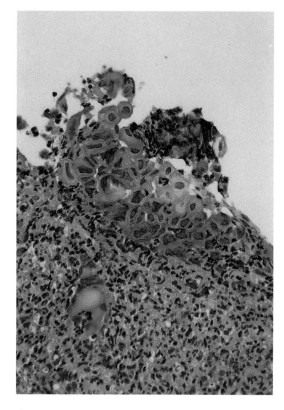

A

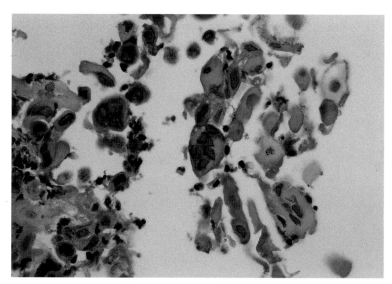

B

Figure 17–5. A: Esophageal ulcer showing herpes simplex-infected cells at the ulcer's edge. B: Higher power micrograph of part A, showing herpes simplex-infected cells, characterized by multinucleation and glassy intranuclear inclusions.

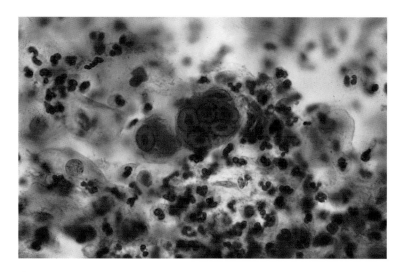

Figure 17–4. Smear from an anal canal ulcer, showing herpes simplex-infected cells. These are multinucleated and show intranuclear inclusions.

BACTERIAL INFECTIONS

Mycobacterium Avium-Intracellulare

Mycobacterium avium-intracellulare complex (MAI) is the predominant isolate in both AIDS- and non-AIDS-associated MOTT (*Mycobacterium*-other-than-*tuberculosis*) disease.[31,32] *Mycobacterium avium* and *M. intracellulare* are opportunistic pathogens that may complicate the course of AIDS and contribute significantly to morbidity and mortality in patients with AIDS.[33] MAI can colonize the intestinal mucosal surfaces of healthy individuals, becoming virtual members of the commensal gut microflora. Disease develops when the normal T-cell-mediated immunity becomes deficient, as in old age, during cancer chemotherapy, and in AIDS. As many as 50% of AIDS patients develop mycobacterial infections at some time during their disease[34]; over 50% of AIDS patients with MAI infection have a peripheral blood CD4+ lymphocyte count of less than 50/μL.[35] These patients typically have disseminated MAI infec-

tions, show little or no inflammatory tissue response, and often fail to respond to multiple-drug therapy.[36]

Clinically, patients with MAI infections present with diffuse abdominal pain, prolonged fever, weight loss, watery diarrhea, and lymphadenopathy.[37] Unusual presentations include intestinal obstruction, ileal volvulus due to matted mesenteric lymph nodes, intussusception due to engorged infected ileal mucosa, massive lower GI bleeding due to intestinal ulceration, and terminal ileitis resembling Crohn's disease.[38–40] The diagnosis of intestinal MAI infection is best made by demonstrating the acid-fast bacillus in a stool sample.

On pathologic examination, MAI infection resembles Whipple's disease.[41] On routine light microscopy, a diffuse expansion of the lamina propria by pale blue, striated histiocytes with numerous intracellular and extracellular mycobacteria takes place (Fig. 17–6).[42] The organisms appear as negative images of unstained rod-shaped structures against a blue background.[43] Well-formed granulomas with epithelioid histiocytes are seen rarely. MAI stains positively with acid-fast stains (Fig. 17–6C); periodic acid–Schiff (PAS) stain is also faintly positive.[44]

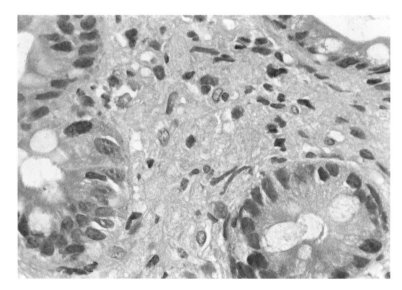

A

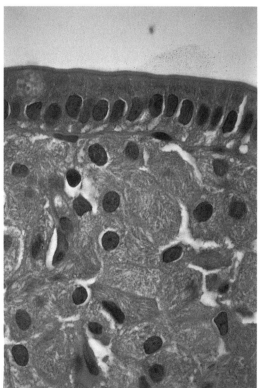

B

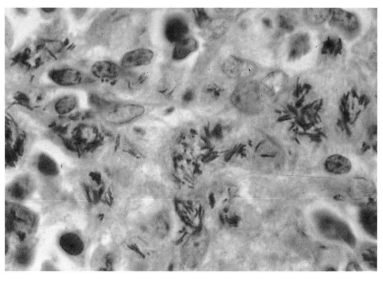

C

Figure 17–6. A: *Mycobacterium avium-intracellulare* infection of the colonic mucosa, showing expansion of the lamina propria between crypts by an accumulation of foamy histiocytes. B: *Mycobacterium avium-intracellulare* infection of the duodenum, showing more defined macrophages in the lamina propria. The macrophage cytoplasm has a fibrillary appearance due to negative staining of the bacilli. C: *Mycobacterium avium-intracellulare* infection, stained by acid-fast stain, showing numerous bacilli in infected macrophages.

Mycobacterium Tuberculosis

Tuberculosis is caused by *Mycobacterium tuberculosis*. After the primary infection, bacteria remain dormant in organs throughout the body; in the intestine, the terminal ileum and cecal region are the sites of maximal involvement. Immunodeficiency from any cause reactivates dormant mycobacteria, causing disease. Tuberculosis is prevalent in developing countries. It had been well controlled in the United States until the mid-1980s when a resurgence of the disease occurred,[45] simultaneously with the AIDS epidemic.

Tuberculosis is a common infection in HIV-positive individuals, often occurring before the common AIDS-defining infections. In sub-Saharan Africa, dual infection with HIV and *M. tuberculosis* is a major problem; many of these patients succumb to the virulent tuberculous disease before they become sufficiently immunocompromised to develop the opportunistic infections typically associated with AIDS in developed countries.[46]

Clinically, tuberculosis occurring in HIV-positive individuals are often extrapulmonary and disseminated, without cavitary lung disease.[47] Abdominal tuberculosis presents insidiously with fever, abdominal pain, ascites, diarrhea, weight loss, and rectal bleeding. Unusual presentations include intestinal obstruction, perforation, and anal fistula.[48-51] Rarely, tuberculosis involves the esophagus, causing deep ulceration, intramural inflammation with stricture formation, and tracheoesophageal fistula.[52]

The diagnosis is made by examination of stool samples by smear and culture. Biopsy specimens of affected lesions show granulomatous inflammation with necrosis; acid-fast bacilli can be demonstrated (see Chapters 8 and 10). In severely immunocompromised patients, granulomas may be poorly formed and necrosis absent; these cases usually have larger numbers of acid-fast bacilli, but diagnostic acumen is necessary to recognize the relatively nonspecific inflammatory reaction as being possibly due to tuberculosis.

Intestinal Spirochetosis

A group of phenotypically and genotypically distinct intestinal spirochetes have been associated with a mild, chronic diarrheal disease called intestinal spirochestosis.[53] Although disputed, some studies indicate that these microorganisms are capable of causing disease.[54] Intestinal spirochestosis is common in homosexual males; 36% of rectal biopsy samples show intestinal spirochetosis in homosexual men compared with 2–7% in heterosexual males.[55]

In colonic mucosal biopsy samples, intestinal spirochetosis appears as a thick, fuzzy fringe, 3–7 μm thick, on the surface.[56] This fringe appears blue in H&E sections (Fig. 17–7), purple in PAS-stained sections, and blue with Giemsa stain. Warthin-Starry stain shows positive staining and spiral structure of the organisms. Extension of the spirochetes into the crypts and invasion of the mucosal cell and lamina propria occur rarely and are associated with a conspicuous inflammatory response.[57] Under electron microscopy, the spirochetes measure 3–5 mm in length and 0.2 mm in width, contain four to eight axial fibrils, and closely resemble *Brachyspira aalborgi*.[57]

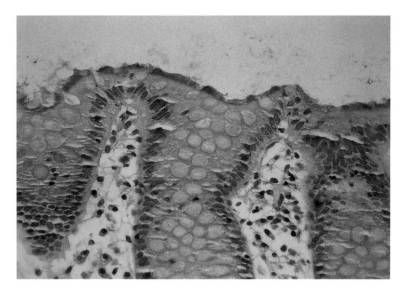

Figure 17–7. Colonic spirochetosis, showing a basophilic "fringe" of bacilli on the surface epithelial cells.

FUNGAL INFECTIONS

Candida Albicans

Candida albicans infections of the mouth and esophagus are among the commonest opportunistic infections in immunocompromised patients of all types. Candida esophagitis (see Chapter 2) is the commonest AIDS-defining infection.

Cryptococcus Neoformans

Cryptococcus neoformans is a opportunistic pathogen in immunocompromised patients. Although central nervous system involvement and disseminated disease occur in 5–10% of patients with AIDS,[58] gastrointestinal infection is rare.[59] Localized GI tract involvement affects the stomach (see Chapter 4) and intestine and can be seen in patients with AIDS as well as patients with relatively mild immunodeficiency such as that seen postsplenectomy, with steroid therapy, and with chronic liver disease.[60]

Cryptococcus neformans is a yeast with a thick mucoid capsule that stains with mucin stains. The organism is highly variable in size, from 5–20 μm, and shows narrow-based budding (Fig. 17–8). It sometimes does not evoke a strong inflammatory response, being present as a mass of yeasts in macrophages. More rarely, granulomas are produced.

Histoplasma Capsulatum

Histoplasmosis is caused by *Histoplasma capsulatum* var. *capsulatum*. The infection is common in endemic regions and is acquired by inhaling microconidia from the soil. Ninety percent of people in the Ohio and the Mississippi Valley basin show evidence of primary infection. In these patients, the organism re-

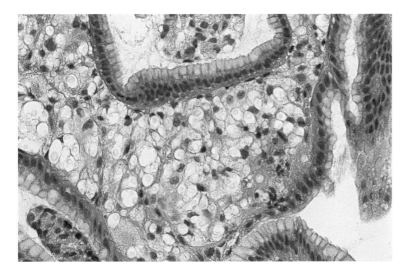

A

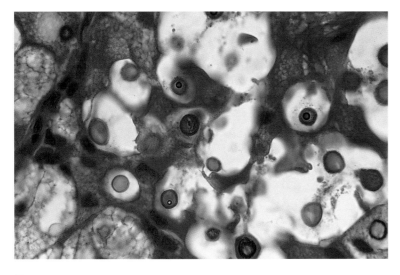

B

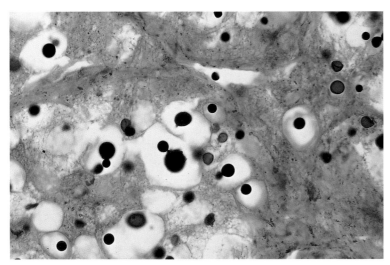

C

Figure 17–8. A: Cryptococcal gastritis, showing numerous yeast in the lamina propria. The yeasts are of varying sizes and have a halo around them, representing negative staining of the thick mucoid capsule. Note the lack of any significant inflammatory response. B: *Cryptococcus neoformans,* showing yeasts of varying size surrounded by a thick capsule. C: *Cryptococcus neoformans,* stained with methenamine silver, showing positive staining of the yeast. A budding yeast is present with the narrow-based single budding typical of *C. neoformans.*

mains dormant in the body and can be reactivated if immunodeficiency develops.

Gastrointestinal histoplasmosis is a common complication of AIDS in endemic regions.[61] The gastrointestinal tract is affected in 75% of cases of disseminated disease, but this is usually subclinical.[62] The ileocecal region is the most common area involved; although any part of the GI tract may be affected. GI tract histoplasmosis can cause small-bowel obstruction, ulceration with hemorrhage and perforation, mass lesions mimicking carcinoma and a granulomatous ileitis resembling Crohn's disease.[63–65]

In biopsy samples and resected specimens from patients with AIDS, the involved bowel shows numerous organisms in macrophages in the lamina propria (Chapters 8 and 10). Involvement can be massive, with large numbers of organisms, or limited. In the latter event, histologic diagnosis may be difficult. *Histoplasma capsulatum* is a small, round, single-budding yeast, 2–5 mm in diameter, seen as clusters in macrophages (Fig. 17–9A and B). In routine H&E sections, it has a retraction halo due to cytoplasmic retraction from the cell wall. The organisms stains positively with PAS and methenamine silver (Fig. 17–9C). The diagnosis can be confirmed in biopsy specimens by immunohistochemistry (Fig. 17–9D). Electron microscopy and immunofluorescence may also be used for diagnosis.[66]

PARASITIC INFECTIONS

Cryptosporidium

Cryptosporidiosis is an infectious disease caused by the coccidian parasite, *Cryptosporidium parvum,* which primarily infects the GI tract of humans and animals; it is prevalent in farm livestock.[67] The infection is common worldwide. It was first reported in humans in 1976[68]; during the 1980s, the number of human cases rose dramatically. Most serious infections occur in immunodeficient patients, most commonly those with AIDS.[68]

In immunocompetent persons, *C. parvum* causes a watery diarrhea that lasts several days to weeks and resolves spontaneously.[68] Water-borne outbreaks of cryptosporidiosis have occurred in the United States. The most severe of these took place in 1993, in which over 400,000 residents of the greater Milwaukee, Wisconsin, area became infected with *C. parvum* following contamination of the city's water supply by *Cryptosporidium* oocysts that passed through the filtration system of one of the city's water treatment plants.[69]

Cryptosporidiosis occurs in 5% of all HIV-positive patients and 21% of those with AIDS.[70] Severely immunocompromised patients with CD4+ lymphocyte counts less than 50/μL develop severe, prolonged, life-threatening watery diarrhea, often causing death.[70] In sub-Saharan Africa, "slim disease" (prolonged diarrhea and wasting usually due to coccidian parasites) is a common manifestation of AIDS.[71]

The diagnosis of cryptosporidiosis is generally made by the detection of oocysts in stools by means of several concentration

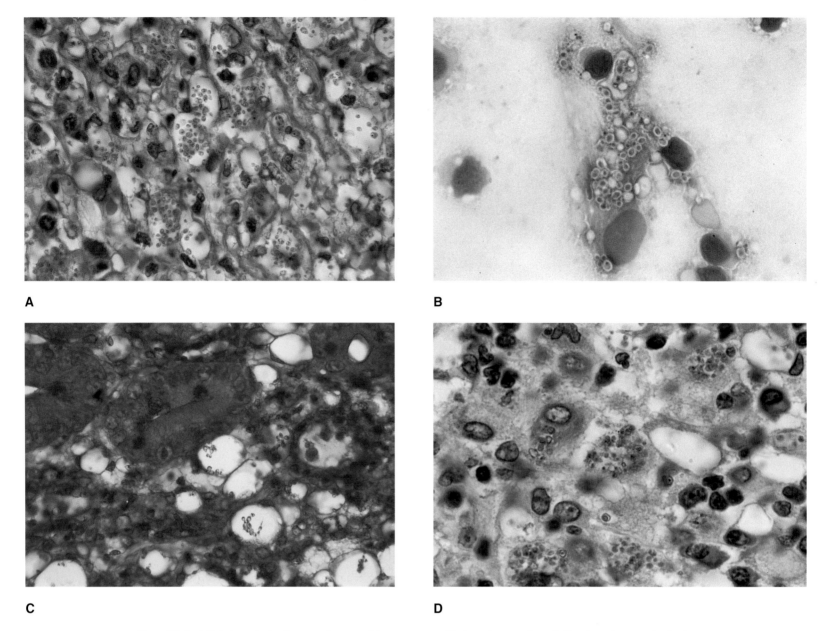

Figure 17–9. A: Histoplasmosis, showing macrophages containing numerous small 2–4-μm long yeast forms. B: Histoplasmosis, smear, showing intracellular and extracellular yeasts. These are small and round and have a halo resulting from negative staining of the capsule. This is a smear used as a negative control for immunoperoxidase staining. C: Histoplasmosis, PAS-stained section, showing positive staining of the small, round yeasts. D: Histoplasmosis, immunperoxidase stain, showing positivity of the yeasts.

and staining techniques. Common staining techniques are a modified acid-fast stain (Fig. 17–10) and fluorescent antibody stains.[72] Examination of multiple stool samples increases the diagnostic yield of *C. parvum*.[73]

The organism can also be seen in biopsy specimens of infected parts of the GI tract. *Cryptosporidium* is a small, round organism, 2–5 mm in diameter, that is seen attached to the epithelial cell surface.[74] The organisms are clearly seen on routine H&E sections (Fig. 17–11). Although it appears to be on the surface of the cell, *C. parvum* is an intracellular parasite that uses the membrane of the intestinal cell in the makeup of its cell wall. Infection is usually associated with reactive epithelial changes, such as villous atrophy in the small intestine and mixed inflammatory cell infiltration of the lamina propria. *Cryptosporidium parvum* can be found anywhere in the GI tract; biopsy speci-

mens taken from the terminal ileum are the most likely to be positive in *C. parvum* enteritis. Sensitivities of positive biopsy are 93% in terminal ileum, 60% in colon, 53% in duodenum, and 11% in stomach.[73] Electron microscopy, which shows the organism, is not usually necessary for diagnosis.

Isospora Belli

Isospora belli is an intestinal spore-forming protozoan parasite that can cause diarrhea in the immunocompetent and immunocompromised host. The organism is acquired from fecooral transmission of oocysts from human or animal sources in contaminated food or water. The oocysts excyst in the upper small intestine and invade the mucosal cell, causing destruction of the brush border.[74]

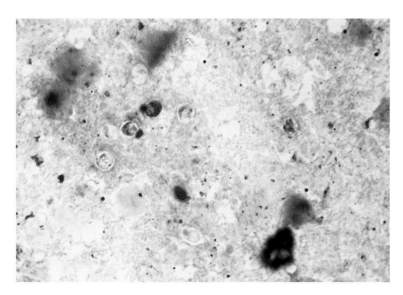

Figure 17–10. *Cryptosporidium* in a stool specimen stained with modified acid-fast stain.

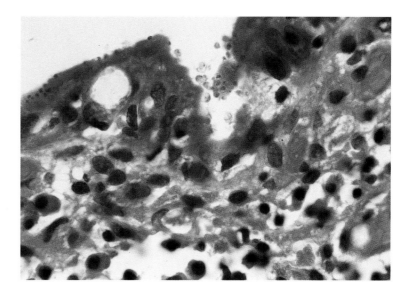

A

B

Patients infected with *I. belli* present with chronic, profuse, watery diarrhea. Other symptoms include steatorrhea, abdominal pain, vomiting, dehydration, and weight loss. Diarrhea is more prolonged and profuse in patients with AIDS,[75] in whom it may contribute significantly to death. *I. belli* accounts for approximately 2% of chronic diarrhea in patients with AIDS in the United States.[76]

The diagnosis of *Isospora belli* infection is usually made by identifying the oocysts in stool specimens, using concentration techniques (Fig. 17–12). The organism is much larger than *Cryptosporidium*, measuring 20–30 μm in diameter. Its recognition is facilitated by fluorescent antibody stains and examination of auramine-rhodamine stained smears with fluorescent microscopy (Fig. 17–13). Very rarely, the oocysts can be demonstrated as rounded structures within the surface epithelial lining of the intestine (see Chapter 6).

Microsporidia

Microsporidia are ubiquitous, obligate, intracellular protozoan parasites increasingly implicated as opportunistic pathogens in patients with AIDS enteritis and chronic diarrhea.[77] These spore-forming protozoa belong to the phylum Microspora; five genera (*Enterocytozoon, Encephalitozoon, Septata, Pleistophora,* and *Nosema*) and unclassified Microspora have been associated with human disease in immunodeficient hosts. Microsporidiosis usually infects individuals with CD4+ lymphocyte counts of less than 100/μL.[78] *Enterocytozoon bieneusi* is the commonest organism, being found as the sole pathogen in approximately 27% of AIDS patients with chronic diarrhea.[79]

The diagnosis of microsporidiosis currently depends on the morphologic demonstration of the organisms in biopsy and stool specimens. The organism is difficult to visualize because of its small size. The sensitivity of identification of Microsporida in biopsy samples by routine light microscopy is related to the parasite load and experience of the pathologist. The

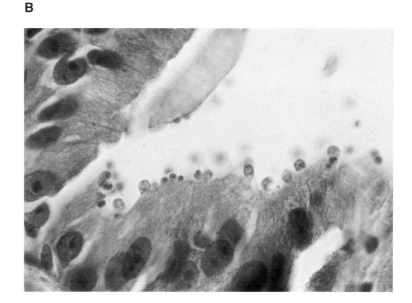

C

Figure 17–11. A: Cryptosporidiosis, involving the duodenal mucosa, showing numerous small, rounded organisms on the cell surface. B: Higher power micrograph of part A. C: Cryptosporidiosis, involving the epithelial surface of the common bile duct.

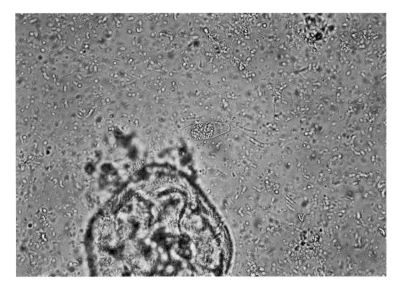

A

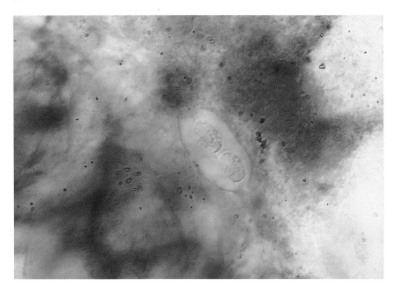

B

Figure 17–12. A: Oocyst of *Isospora belli* in wet mount of a stool sample after concentration. B: Oocyst of *Isospora belli* in stool sample.

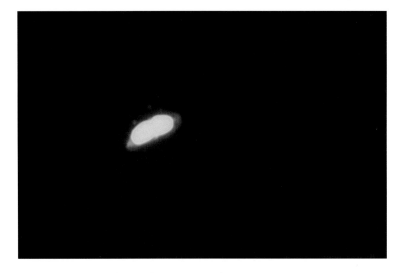

Figure 17–13. Oocyst of *Isospora belli*, as seen using fluorescent microscopy in a stool smear stained by auramine-rhodamine.

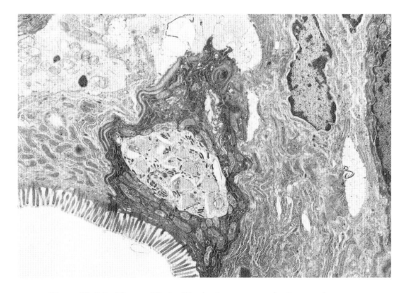

Figure 17–14. Microsporidiosis of the duodenum, as seen by electron microscopy.

organism is seen as tiny, round, intracellular structures in the supranuclear region of infected enterocytes; modified trichrome and Warthin-Starry stains facilitate identification of the organism.[80] Electron microscopy and fluorescein-tagged antibody (immunofluorescence) technique are useful in both diagnosis and definitive species characterization (Fig. 17–14).[81] In stool samples, the spores are seen by light microscopy using special staining techniques.[82] Due to erratic shedding of organisms in the feces, multiple sequential stool samples should be examined.

NEOPLASMS

Kaposi's Sarcoma

Disseminated Kaposi's sarcoma, with involvement of skin, mucous membranes, lymph nodes, and GI tract, occurs in immunocompromised patients, with the highest occurrence being in AIDS patients.[83] Gastrointestinal lesions occur in over 50% of patients with AIDS and cutaneous and lymph node involvement by Kaposi's sarcoma.[84] Kaposi's sarcoma may occur in the GI tract in the absence of cutaneous manifestations.[85] Gastrointestinal Kaposi's sarcoma is usually asymptomatic (Figs. 17–15 and 17–16); however, complications may occur and include massive hemorrhage, obstruction due to intussusception, acute appendicitis, diarrhea, and ileus.[86–89]

Specific herpesvirus-like DNA sequences have recently been found in lesions from patients with Kaposi's sarcoma and AIDS.[90] This has been characterized as a novel gamma herpesvirus, known as the Kaposi's sarcoma-associated herpesvirus/human herpesvirus-8 (KSHV/HHV-8). It is believed to be implicated in the pathogenesis of Kaposi's sarcoma. The same viral DNA sequences have also been identified in classic Kaposi's sarcoma. Testing for KSHV can be done by using the published Kaposi's sarcoma 330–233 primers by polymerase chain

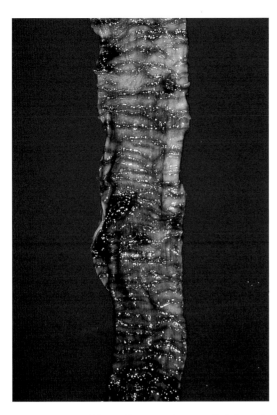

Figure 17–15. Kaposi's sarcoma of the small intestine, showing multiple hemorrhagic submucosal nodules.

reaction[91]; positively for this sequence is a specific marker for Kaposi's sarcoma and can be used to differentiate it from other vascular proliferations.[92]

Microscopically, Kaposi's sarcoma is a spindle cell proliferation (Fig. 17–17). The spindle cells show minimal atypia and moderate mitotic activity; they typically form slit-like spaces and are associated with erythrocyte extravasation and deposition of hemosiderin (see Chapters 5 and 6). In the GI tract, Kaposi's sarcoma occurs in the submucosa and lamina propria; in the latter site, the spindle cell proliferation spreads the normal glands and crypts. Electron microscopy shows cytoplasmic globules known as Weibel-Palade bodies. The histogenesis of Kaposi's sarcoma is disputed, but evidence favors an origin from lymphatic endothelium.[93]

Gastrointestinal Stromal Tumors

An increase in gastrointestinal stromal tumors has been reported in AIDS patients, in many of whom the tumors have been multiple. These neoplasms are considered in Chapter 14.

Malignant Lymphoma

Malignant lymphomas are common in immunocompromised patients, occurring in several different immunodeficiency states. They occur most commonly in AIDS, in which they are commonly high grade, aggressive neoplasms, usually with morphologic features of immunoblastic lymphoma or Burkitt-like

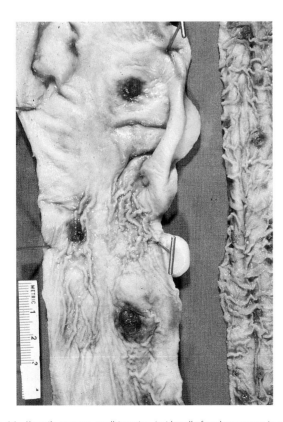

Figure 17–16. Kaposi's sarcoma, small intestine, incidentally found at autopsy in a patient with AIDS. The lesion is seen as multiple hemorrhagic nodules.

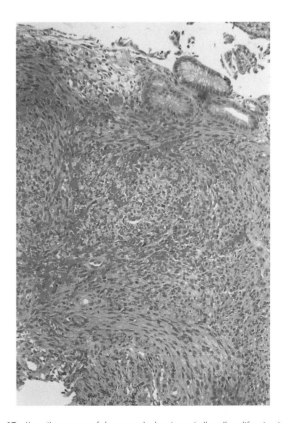

Figure 17–17. Kaposi's sarcoma of the stomach showing spindle cell proliferation in the lamina propria.

lymphoma.[94] These tumors rapidly become widely disseminated and, despite initial response to chemotherapy, have a very poor prognosis.

In AIDS, the gastrointestinal tract involvement by malignant lymphoma is second in frequency to central nervous system disease.[94] Although they are second in frequency to Kaposi's sarcoma among AIDS-associated neoplasms in the gastrointestinal tract, malignant lymphomas are much more important clinically because of their aggressive behavior. Malignant lymphomas are a common cause of death in AIDS patients.

In general, AIDS lymphomas are diagnosed and treated in a manner similar to malignant lymphomas occurring in immunocompetent hosts, which are considered in detail in Chapter 15.

Posttransplantation Lymphoproliferative Disorders

Posttransplantation lymphoproliferative disorders (PTLD) are "opportunistic neoplasms" that occur in immunosuppressed organ transplant recipients. PTLDs most commonly arise within the first posttransplant year, with a mean time of occurrence of 4.4 months.[95] They develop in 1–10% of solid organ transplant recipients and encompass a broad spectrum of lymphoid hyperplasias and "true" neoplasias, with a resultant mortality rate of up to 70%.[96,97] PTLDs are most often of the non-Hodgkin's type. Most cases are of B-lymphocyte origin and are associated with Epstein-Barr virus (EBV) infection. Less commonly, PTLDs arise from T cells or natural killer (NK) cells. The population of organ transplant recipients most at risk is that receiving potent antilymphocyte preparations in the setting of primary EBV infection.[98,99]

PTLDs may arise in lymphoid tissues such as tonsils or lymph nodes but frequently arise in extranodal sites. Major categories of clinical presentation include a mononucleosis-like syndrome, gastrointestinal disease, and solid organ disease.[95] In one series of allograft recipients with PTLDs, 17% had disease predominantly involving the GI tract. The lesions were often multiple and preferentially involved the distal small intestine.[100]

EBV infection or reactivation and intensive anti-T-lymphocyte regimens play a major role in the pathogenesis of PTLD.[101,102] EBV immortalizes B cells in vitro. It upregulates bcl-2, a protein that confers resistance to apoptosis, thus promoting cell survival and successful viral replication.[103] As demonstrated by immunohistochemistry, bcl-2 is markedly overexpressed in PTLDs.[104] Following transplantation and iatrogenic immunosuppression, the host:EBV equilibrium is shifted in favor of the virus. EBV-infected B cells proliferate in an unchecked manner due to suppression of cytotoxic T cells and elevation of B-cell-promoting cytokines.[105] Patients who develop primary EBV infection after transplantation are at greater risk of developing PTLD.[106,107] The incidence of PTLD for EBV-seronegative recipients is 24 times greater than that for EBV-seropositive recipients. The additional risk factors of anti-T-lymphocyte therapy (eg, OKT3) for rejection further amplifies this risk.[108] Most seronegative patients become infected with EBV either via the graft or through natural means. Seropositive patients begin to shed higher levels of virus and may become secondarily superinfected via the graft. A quantitative difference in circulating EBV viral load and EBV-specific antibody levels is evidence between transplant recipients with and without PTLD.[109] A "grace" period of approximately 1 month posttransplantation occurs before increased viral shedding is detected. PTLD is almost never seen during this interval.[110]

Three methods are commonly used to show EBV in tissues: (1) semiquantitative polymerase chain reaction (PCR) for EBV DNA; (2) in situ hybridization for EBV-encoded RNA (EBER), and (3) immunoperoxidase stain for EBV latent membrane protein (LMP). Cell lines containing EBV in the productive state are EBER-positive, whereas latently infected cells lines are EBER-negative.[111] EBV studies are useful in discriminating the atypical lymphoid infiltrates of early EBV-associated PTLDs from acute cellular rejection in transplanted organs. EBER and LMP studies can be done on paraffin sections, and EBER and PCR are the most sensitive techniques.[112]

The histologic spectrum of PTLD ranges from hyperplastic lesions to frank neoplasia. The appearance of the lymphoid cells ranges from nonuniform (polymorphic) to uniform (monomorphic). These lesions can be classified into polyclonal or monoclonal polymorphic tumors and monoclonal monomorphic tumors. T-cell non-Hodgkin's lymphomas are uncommon after solid organ transplantation.[113] Most PTLDs are associated with a polyclonal or monoclonal B-cell proliferation.[114] Distinctive categories of PTLDs include

1. early lesions
2. polymorphic PTLDs
3. monomorphic PTLDs (B- and T-cell lymphomas)
4. plasmacytoma-like lesions
5. T-cell-rich large B-cell lymphoma/Hodgkin's disease-like lesions[115]

Monomorphic lesions should be reported as a PTLD and classified according to a recognized classification of non-Hodgkin's lymphoma (see Chapter 15). Polymorphic lesions should be carefully evaluated for EBV genomes and for clonality by immunophenotyping or gene rearrangement studies (Fig. 17–18).

The clinical course of PTLD is unpredictable. The lesions frequently undergo regression when immunosuppression is reduced or discontinued. Nonclonal lesions with a polymorphous histology have a greater potential of regressing. Some monoclonal tumors can undergo regression; however, clonal tumors with a monomorphous histology portend a bad clinical outcome.[116,117] There is no consensus on the treatment of PTLD other than reduction of immunosuppressive therapy. Approaches to PTLD therapy may also include antiviral therapy and antilymphoma chemotherapy. In recipients of bone marrow allografts, PTLDs are often of donor origin. The majority of PTLDs in solid organ recipients are of host origin.[118] PTLDs of donor origin tend to have a better prognosis.[119]

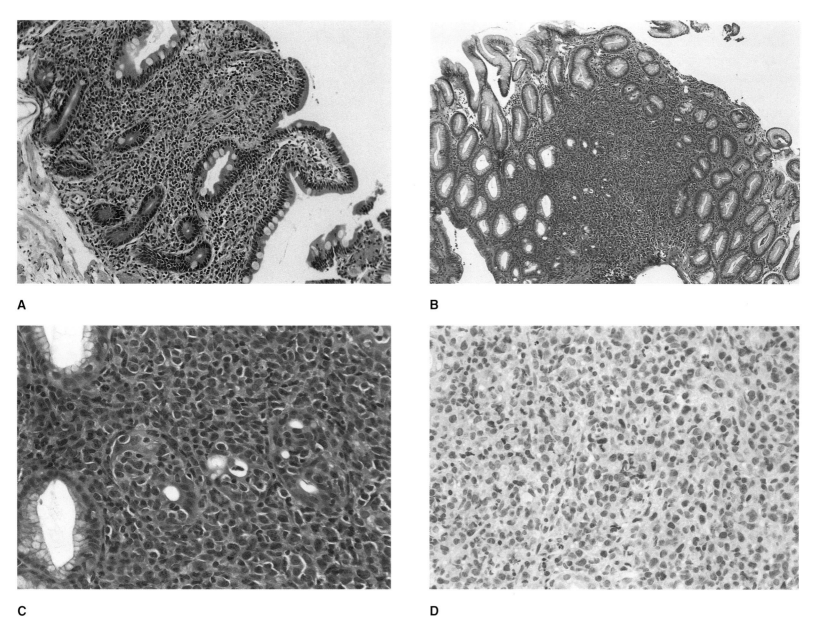

Figure 17–18. A: Posttransplantation lymphoproliferative disorder (PTLD), early stage, showing a polymorphous lymphocytic infiltrate in the lamina propria of the small intestine. (Courtesy of Dr Michael A Nalesnik, University of Pittsburgh). B: PTLD, showing intraepithelial lymphocytes and destruction of crypts in the small intestine by a polymorphous lymphocytic infiltrate. (Courtesy of Dr Randall G Lee, University of Pittsburgh). C: Higher power micrograph or part B (Courtesy of Dr Randall G Lee, University of Pittsburgh). D: PTLD, Epstein-Barr virus-encoded RNAs (EBER) in situ hybridization. Nuclear staining demonstrates EBV genome within the lymphoproliferative lesion shown in part B. (Courtesy of Dr Randall G Lee, University of Pittsburgh).

GRAFT-VERSUS-HOST DISEASE

Acute graft-versus-host disease (GVHD) remains a major complication of allogenic bone marrow transplantation (BMT), occurring in 25–70% of patients, despite GVHD prophylaxis.[120] It can also develop in immunosuppressed patients with malignancies who receive nonirradiated blood transfusions. The skin, gastrointestinal tract, and liver are the primary target organs.[120,121] GVHD may affect any portion of the GI tract. Clinical manifestations of GVHD are nausea, vomiting and upper abdominal pain, and diarrhea.[122]

The mechanism of acute GVHD is uncertain, but indications are that the primary mechanism is cell-mediated.[121] Affected sites show a prominent infiltrate of CD2+, CD8+ T lymphocytes.[123] Alloreactive donor T cells recognize foreign major and minor histocompatibility antigens of host tissues. Inflammatory cells are activated, and cytopathic molecules are secreted. Cytokines play a central role in the immunopathophysiology of acute GVHD.[124] Inflammatory cell activation and resultant secretion of cytokines may directly damage the mucosa. In the lamina propria, intercellular adhesion molecule-1 (ICAM-1) staining of endothelial cells is prominent in GVHD tissues and is significantly increased over non-GVHD specimens. Upregulation of ICAM-1 on local endothelium may lead to perpetuation of inflammation by recruitment of additional cytotoxic lymphocytes.[123]

The diagnosis of acute gastrointestinal GVHD is often based on subtle findings with considerable potential for variability in interpretation. The basic histopathologic feature of acute gastrointestinal GVHD, which occurs in the first 100 days posttransplant, is necrosis of individual cells in the regenerating compartment of the mucosa (Fig. 17–19). Severe disease may lead to loss of crypts and eventual sloughing of the mucosa.[125] Morphologic changes include the presence of ulcers and atrophy of the mucosa, nuclear atypia, inflammatory infiltrates within the lamina propria, intraepithelial lymphocytes, clusters of enterochromaffin cells, and architectural abnormalities.[126] Histologic criteria for acute GVHD involving the GI tract are apoptosis (single epithelial cell necrosis), gland destruction, inflammatory infiltrate in the lamina propria, and granular eosinophilc debris in dilated glands.[127,128] Of individual features, granular debris in glands is a specific (94% specificity) but insensitive (41% sensitivity) marker for GVHD.[127]

Distinction between GVHD and CMV infection can be difficult. The histology of acute GVHD may be simulated by cytoreductive agents and viral infections, particularly CMV. An absolute diagnosis of acute GVHD cannot therefore be made in the first 21 days posttransplant or in any mucosa-containing CMV inclusions.[125]

Chronic GVHD is a pleiotrophic syndrome with variability in the time of onset, organ systems involved, and rate of progression. The clinicopathologic features resemble an overlap of several collagen vascular diseases, with frequent involvement of the skin, liver, eyes, mouth, upper respiratory tract, and esophagus, and less frequent involvement of the serosal surfaces, lower gastrointestinal tract, and skeletal muscle.[129] The basic pathology of chronic gastrointestinal GVHD is fibrosis of the submucosa and subserosa; therefore, mucosal biopsy is of limited value in the diagnosis of chronic GVHD.[125]

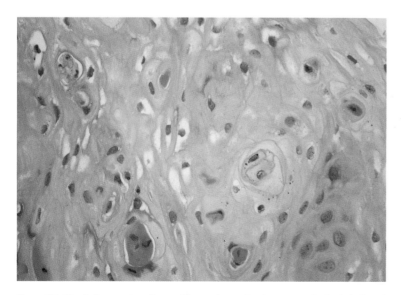

Figure 17–19. Graft-versus-host disease of the esophagus, showing necrosis of individual cells and small groups of cells.

References

1. Chui DW, Owen RL. AIDS and the gut. *J Gastroenterol Hepatol.* 1994;9(3):291–303.
2. Kotler DP, Scholes JV, Tierney AR. Intestinal plasma cell alterations in acquired immunodeficiency syndrome. *Dig Dis Sci.* 1987;32(2):129–138.
3. Frisancho Velarde O. Gastroenterologic manifestations of acquired immunodeficiency syndrome. *Rev Gastroenterol Peru.* 1991;11(2):86–96.
4. Gold JW. Overview of infection with the human immunodeficiency virus: Infectious complications. *Clin Chest Med.* 1988;9(3):377–386.
5. Hirschel B. AIDS and gastrointestinal tract: A summary for gastroenterologists and surgeons. *Schweiz Med Wochenschr.* 1990;120(14):475–484.
6. Rotterdam H, Tsang P. Gastrointestinal disease in the immunocompromised patient. *Hum Pathol.* 1994;25(11):1123–1140.
7. Tyms AS, Taylor DL, Parkin JM. Cytomegalovirus and the acquired immunodeficiency syndrome. *J Antimicrob Chemother.* 1989;23 Suppl A:89–105.
8. Raffi F. Cytomegalovirus infections in AIDS. *Rev Prat.* 1995;45(6):733–738.
9. Dayan K, Neufeld DM, Lang R, et al. Widespread gastrointestinal CMV infection as the presenting manifestation of AIDS. *Harefuah.* 1993;124(3):124–126.
10. Barbera JR, Capdevila JA, Garcia-Quintana AM, et al. Digestive cytomegalovirus disease in AIDS patients. *Engerm Infecc Microbiol Clin.* 1996;14(7):411–415.
11. Murray RN, Parker A, Kadakia SC, et al. Cytomegalovirus in upper gastrointestinal ulcers. *J Clin Gastroenterol.* 1994;19(3):198–201.
12. Nieto I, Llach J, Bordas JM, et al. Endoscopic gastrointestinal findings in patients with human immunodeficiency virus infection. *J Gastroenterol Hepatol.* 1995;18(2):57–60.
13. Hackman RC, Wolford JL, Gleaves CA, et al. Recognition and rapid diagnosis of upper gastrointestinal cytomegalovirus infection in marrow transplant recipients. A comparison of seven virologic methods. *Transplantation.* 1994;57(2):231–237.
14. Carbo J, Laguna F, Garcia-Samaniego J, et al. Gastrointestinal disease due to cytomegalovirus in patients infected with the human immunodeficiency virus. *Rev Esp Enferm Dig.* 1995;87(7):499–504.
15. Dolgin SE, Larsen JG, Shah KD, et al. CMV enteritis causing hemorrhage and obstruction in an infant with AIDS. *J Pediatr Surg.* 1990;25(6):696–698.
16. Tarng YW, Shih DF, Liu SI, et al. Cytomegalovirus appendicitis in a patient with acquired immunodeficiency syndrome: A case report. *Chung Hua I Hsueh Tsa Chih* (Taipei). 1997;60(1):48–51.
17. Muldoon J, O'Riordan K, Rao S, et al. Ischemic colitis secondary to venous thrombosis. A rare presentation of cytomegalovirus vasculitis following renal transplantation. *Transplantation.* 1996;61(11):1651–1653.
18. Goodgame RW, Ross PG, Kim HS, et al. Esophageal stricture after cytomegalovirus ulcer treated with ganciclovir. *J Clin Gastroenterol.* 1991;13(6):678–681.
19. Graham SM, Flowers JL, Schweitzer E, et al. Opportunistic upper gastrointestinal infection in transplant recipients. *Surg Endosc.* 1995;9(2):146–150.
20. Arabia FA, Rosado LJ, Huston CL, et al. Incidence and recur-

rence of gastrointestinal cytomegalovirus infection in heart transplantation. *Ann Thorac Surg.* 1993;55(1):8–11.

21. Kaplan CS, Petersen EA, Icenogle TB, et al. Gastrointestinal cytomegalovirus infection in heart and heart-lung transplant recipients. *Arch Intern Med.* 1989;149(9):2095–2100.

22. Pollard RB. Cytomegalovirus infections in renal, heart, heart-lung and liver transplantation. *Pediatr Infect Dis J.* 1988; 7(5 Suppl):S97–S102.

23. Sakr M, Hassanein T, Gavaler J, et al. Cytomegalovirus infection of the upper gastrointestinal tract following liver transplantation—incidence, location, and severity in cyclosporine—and FK506-treated patients. *Transplantation.* 1992;53(4):786–791.

24. Hibberd PL, Tolkoff-Rubin NE, Cosimi AB, et al. Symptomatic cytomegalovirus disease in the cytomegalovirus antibody seropositive renal transplant recipient treated with OKT3. *Transplantation.* 1992;53(1):68–72.

25. Alexander JA, Cuellar RE, Fadden RJ, et al. Cytomegalovirus infection of the upper gastrointestinal tract before and after liver transplantation. *Transplantation.* 1988;46(3):378–382.

26. Shrestha BM, Parton D, Gray A, et al. Cytomegalovirus involving gastrointestinal tract in renal transplant recipients. *Clin Transplant.* 1996;10(2):170–175.

27. Goodgame RW, Genta RM, Estrada R, et al. Frequency of positive tests for cytomegalovirus in AIDS patients: Endoscopic lesions compared with normal mucosa. *Am J Gastroenterol.* 1993;88(3):338–343.

28. Meybehm M, Kindermann D, Bierhoff E. Cytomegalovirus infections of the gastrointestinal tract. *Leber Magen Darm.* 1992; 22(5):185–189.

29. Wu GD, Shintaku IP, Chien K, et al. A comparison of routine light microscopy, immunohistochemistry, and in situ hybridization for the detection of cytomegalovirus in gastrointestinal biopsies. *Am J Gastroenterol.* 1989;84(12):1517–1520.

30. Hackman RC, Wolford JL, Gleaves CA, et al. Recognition and rapid diagnosis of upper gastrointestinal cytomegalovirus infection in marrow transplant recipients. A comparison of seven virologic methods. *Transplantation.* 1994;57(2):231–237.

31. Young LS, Inderlied CB, Berlin OG, et al. Mycobacterial infections in AIDS patients, with an emphasis on the *Mycobacterium avium* complex. *Rev Infect Dis.* 1986;8(6):1024–1033.

32. Dionisio D, Di Lollo S, Milo D, et al. Pseudo-Whipple disease caused by atypical mycobacteriosis in AIDS: A clinical and electron microscopic study of 2 cases. *Recenti Prog Med.* 1990; 81(9):571–575.

33. Scoular A, French P, Miller R. *Mycobacterium avium-intracellulare* infection in the acquired immunodeficiency syndrome. *Br J Hosp Med.* 1991;46(5):295–300.

34. Collins FM. Mycobacterial disease, immunosuppression, and acquired immunodeficiency syndrome. *Clin Microbiol Rev.* 1989; 2(4):360–377.

35. Dionisio D, Tortoli E, Simonetti MT, et al. Intestinal mycobacterial infections in AIDS. Clinical course and treatment of infections caused by *Mycobacterium avium, Mycobacterium kansasii, Mycobacterium genavense. Recenti Prog Med.* 1994;85(11):526–536.

36. Murray HW, Scavuzzo DA, Chaparas SD, et al. T lymphocyte responses to mycobacterial antigen in AIDS patients with disseminated *Mycobacterium avium-Mycobacterium intracellulare* infection. *Chest.* 1988;93(5):922–925.

37. Herrero Martinez JA, Sanchez Manzano MD, Palenque Mataix E, et al. *Mycobacterium avium-intracellulare* disseminated in-

fection in patients with AIDS. (Article in Spanish) *Med Clin* (Barc). 1993;100(5):171–173.

38. Cappell MS, Hassan T, Rosenthal S, et al. Gastrointestinal obstruction due to *Mycobacterium avium intracellulare* associated with the acquired immunodeficiency syndrome. *Am J Gastroenterol.* 1992;87(12):1823–1827.

39. Cappell MS, Gupta A. Gastrointestinal hemorrhage due to gastrointestinal *Mycobacterium avium intracellulare* or esophageal candidiasis in patients with the acquired immunodeficiency syndrome. *Am J Gastroenterol.* 1992;87(2):224–229.

40. Schneebaum CW, Novick DM, Chabon AB, et al. Terminal ileitis associated with *Mycobacterium avium-intracellulare* infection in a homosexual man with acquired immune deficiency syndrome. *Gastroenterology.* 1987;92(5 Pt 1):1127–1132.

41. Gillin JS, Urmacher C, West R, et al. Disseminated *Mycobacterium avium-intracellulare* infection in acquired immunodeficiency syndrome mimicking Whipple's disease. *Gastroenterology.* 1983;85(5):1187–1191.

42. Klatt EC, Jensen DF, Meyer PR. Pathology of *Mycobacterium avium-intracellulare* infection in acquired immunodeficiency syndrome. *Hum Pathol.* 1987 Jul;18(7):709–714.

43. Maygarden SJ, Flanders EL. Mycobacteria can be seen as "negative images" in cytology smears from patients with acquired immunodeficiency syndrome. *Mod Pathol.* 1989;2(3):239–243.

44. Solis OG, Belmonte AH, Ramaswamy G, et al. Pseudogaucher cells in *Mycobacterium avium intracellulare* infections in acquired immune deficiency syndrome (AIDS). *Am J Clin Pathol.* 1986;85(2):233–235.

45. Jadvar H, Mindelzun RE, Olcott EW, et al. Still the great mimicker: Abdominal tuberculosis. *AJR.* 1977;168(6):1455–1460.

46. O'Keefe EA, Wood R. AIDS in Africa. *Scand J Gastroenterol* (Suppl). 1996;220:147–152.

47. Joint Position Paper of the American Thoracic Society and the Centers for Disease Control. Mycobacterioses and the acquired immunodeficiency syndrome. *Am Rev Respir Dis.* 1987;136(2): 492–496.

48. Sircar S, Taneja VA, Kansra U. Epidemiology and clinical presentation of abdominal tuberculosis—A retrospective study. *J Indian Med Assoc.* 1996;94(9):342–344.

49. Salvati V, Fumo F, D'Armiento FP, et al. Primary intestinal tuberculosis. *Minerva Chir.* 1996;51(7–8):567–571.

50. Wong SS, Chow E. Endoscopic diagnosis of colonic tuberculosis: Unusual presentation with two colonic strictures. *Endoscopy.* 1996;28(9):783.

51. Musch E, Tunnerhoff-Mucke A. Tuberculous anal fistula in acquired immunologic deficiency syndrome. *Z Gastroenterol.* 1995;33(8):440–444.

52. de Silva R, Stoopack PM, Raufman JP. Esophageal fistulas associated with mycobacterial infection in patients at risk for AIDS. *Radiology.* 1990;175(2):449–453.

53. Muniappa N, Duhamel GE. Phenotypic and genotypic profiles of human, canine, and porcine spirochetes associated with colonic spirochetosis correlates with in vivo brush border attachment. *Adv Exp Med Biol.* 1997;412:159–166.

54. Gebbers JO, Laissue JA. Diarrhea due to rare forms of colitis: Microscopic (lymphocytic, collagenous) colitis and spirochetosis. *Schweiz Med Wochenschr.* 1994;124(42):1852–1861.

55. Surawicz CM, Roberts PL, Rompalo A, et al. Intestinal spirochetosis in homosexual men. *Am J Med.* 1987;82(3 Spec No): 587–592.

56. Dauzan YR, Merlio JP, Grelier P, et al. Colo-rectal spirochetosis: Is it an anatomo-pathologic entity? *Ann Pathol.* 1990;10(4): 258–261.

57. Guccion JG, Benator DA, Zeller J, et al. Intestinal spirochetosis and acquired immunodeficiency syndrome: Ultrastructural studies of two cases. *Ultrastruct Pathol.* 1995;19(1):15–22.

58. Levitz SM. The ecology of *Cryptococcus neoformans* and the epidemiology of cryptococcosis. *Rev Infect Dis.* 1991;13(6):1163–1169.

59. Washington K, Gottfried MR, Wilson ML. Gastrointestinal cryptococcosis. *Mod Pathol.* 1991;4(6):707–711.

60. Daly JS, Porter KA, Chong FK, et al. Disseminated, nonmeningeal gastrointestinal cryptococcal infection in an HIV-negative patient. *Am J Gastroenterol.* 1990;85(10):1421–1424.

61. Hofman P, Mainguene C, Huerre M, et al. Colonic *Histoplasma capsulatum* pseudotumor in AIDS. Morphological and immunohistochemical diagnosis of an isolated lesion. *Arch Anat Cytol Pathol.* 1995;43(3):140–146.

62. Miller DP, Everett ED. Gastrointestinal histoplasmosis. *J Clin Gastroenterol.* 1979;1(3):233–236.

63. Cappell MS, Mandell W, Grimes MM, et al. Gastrointestinal histoplasmosis. *Dig Dis Sci.* 1988;33(3):353–360.

64. Heneghan SJ, Li J, Petrossian E, et al. Intestinal perforation from gastrointestinal histoplasmosis in acquired immunodeficiency syndrome. Case report and review of the literature. *Arch Surg.* 1993;128(4):464–466.

65. Cimponeriu D, LoPresti P, Lavelanet M, et al. Gastrointestinal histoplasmosis in HIV infection: Two cases of colonic pseudocancer and review of the literature. *Am J Gastroenterol.* 1994 Jan;89(1):129–131.

66. Hofman P, Mainguene C, Huerre M, et al. Colonic *Histoplasma capsulatum* pseudotumor in AIDS. Morphological and immunohistochemical diagnosis of an isolated lesion. *Arch Anat Cytol Pathol.* 1995;43(3):140–146.

67. Tzipori S. Cryptosporidiosis in perspective. *Adv Parasitol.* 1988;27:63–129.

68. Chacin-Bonilla L. Cryptosporidiosis in humans. Review. *Invest Clin.* 1995;36(4):207–250.

69. Cicirello HG, Kehl KS, Addiss DG, et al. Cryptosporidiosis in children during a massive waterborne outbreak in Milwaukee, Wisconsin: Clinical, laboratory and epidemiologic findings. *Epidemiol Infect.* 1997;119(1):53–60.

70. Blanshard C, Jackson AM, Shanson DC, et al. Cryptosporidiosis in HIV-seropositive patients. *Q J Med.* 1992;85(307–308): 813–823.

71. O'Keefe EA, Wood R. AIDS in Africa. *Scand J Gastroenterol* (Suppl). 1996;220:147–152.

72. Chacin-Bonilla L. Cryptosporidiosis in humans. Review. *Invest Clin.* 1995;36(4):207–250.

73. Greenberg PD, Koch J, Cello JP. Diagnosis of *Cryptosporidium parvum* in patients with severe diarrhea and AIDS. *Dig Dis Sci.* 1996;41(11):2286–2290.

74. Petrella T, Bonnin A, Michiels JF, et al. Production of a monoclonal anti-*Cryptosporidium* sp. Antibody for paraffin-embedded sections. *Ann Pathol.* 1991;11(2):132–138.

75. Soave R. Cryptosporidiosis and isosporiasis in patients with AIDS. *Infect Dis Clin North Am.* 1988;2(2):485–493.

76. DeHovitz JA, Pape JW, Boncy M, et al. Clinical manifestations and therapy of *Isospora belli* infection in patients with the acquired immunodeficiency syndrome. *N Engl J Med.* 1986;315(2): 87–90.

77. Chukwuma C Sr. Microsporidium in AIDS patients: A perspective. *East Afr Med J.* 1996;73(1):72–75.

78. Eeftinck Schattenkerk JK, van Gool T, van Ketel RJ, et al. Clinical significance of small-intestinal microsporidiosis in HIV-1-infected individuals. *Lancet.* 1991;337(8746):895–898.

79. van den Bergh Weerman MA, van Gool T, Eeftinck Schattenkerk JK, Dingemans KP. Electron microscopy as an essential technique for the identification of parasites in AIDS patients. *Eur J Morphol.* 1993;31(1–2):107–110.

80. Weber R, Bryan RT, Owen RL, et al. Improved light-microscopical detection of microsporidia spores in stool and duodenal aspirates. The Enteric Opportunistic Infections Working Group. *N Engl J Med.* 1992;326(3):161–166.

81. Weber R, Bryan RT, Schwartz DA, et al. Human microsporidial infections. *Clin Microbiol Rev.* 1994;7(4):426–461.

82. Punpoowong B, Pitisuttithum P, Chindanond D, et al. Microsporidum: Modified technique for light microscopic diagnosis. *J Med Assoc Thai.* 1995;78(5):251–254.

83. Levine AM, Gill PS, Muggia F. Malignancies in the acquired immunodeficiency syndrome. *Curr Probl Cancer.* 1987;11(4): 209–255.

84. Parente F, Cernuschi M, Orlando G, et al. Kaposi's sarcoma and AIDS: Frequency of gastrointestinal involvement and its effect on survival. A prospective study in a heterogeneous population. *Scand J Gastroenterol.* 1991;26(10):1007–1012.

85. Lemlich G, Schwam L, Lebwohl M. Kaposi's sarcoma and acquired immunodeficiency syndrome. Postmortem findings in twenty-four cases. *J Am Acad Dermatol.* 1987;16(2 Pt 1):319–325.

86. Neville CR, Peddada AV, Smith D, et al. Massive gastrointestinal hemorrhage from AIDS-related Kaposi's sarcoma confined to the small bowel managed with radiation. *Med Pediatr Oncol.* 1996;26(2):135–138.

87. Hofstetter SR, Stollman N. Adult intussusception in association with the acquired immune deficiency syndrome and intestinal Kaposi's sarcoma. *Am J Gastroenterol.* 1988;83(11):1304–1305.

88. Prufer-Kramer L, Kramer A. Gastrointestinal manifestations of AIDS. 2: Bacterial and vh parasitic infections, malignant tumors. *Fortschr Med.* 1991;109(8):179–182.

89. Zebrowska G, Walsh NM. Human immunodeficiency virus-related Kaposi's sarcoma of the appendix and acute appendicitis. Report of a case and review of the literature. *Arch Pathol Lab Med.* 1991;115(11):1157–1160.

90. Moore PS, Chang Y. Detection of herpesvirus-like DNA sequences in Kaposi's sarcoma in patients with and without HIV infection. *N Engl J Med.* 1995;332(18):1181–1185.

91. Chang Y, Cesarman E, Pessin MS, et al. Identification of herpesvirus-like DNA sequences in AIDS-associated Kaposi's sarcoma. *Science.* 1994;266(5192):1865–1869.

92. Jin YT, Tsai ST, Yan JJ, et al. Detection of Kaposi's sarcoma-associated herpesvirus-like DNA sequence in vascular lesions. A reliable diagnostic marker for Kaposi's sarcoma. *Am J Clin Pathol.* 1996;105(3):360–363.

93. Dorfman RF. Kaposi's sarcoma: Evidence supporting its origin from the lymphatic system. *Lymphology.* 1988;21(1):45–52.

94. Sakurada K. AIDS-related malignancy. *Hokkaido Igaku Zasshi.* 1993;68(5):612–614.

95. Nalesnik MA, Jaffe R, Starzl TE, et al. The pathology of posttransplant lymphoproliferative disorders occurring in the setting of cyclosporine A-prednisone immunosuppression. *Am J Pathol.* 1988;133(1):173–192.

96. Badley AD, Portela DF, Patel R, et al. Development of monoclonal gammopathy precedes the development of Epstein-Barr virus-induced posttransplant lymphoproliferative disorder. *Liver Transpl Surg.* 1996;2(5):375–382.

97. Randhawa PS, Jaffe R, Demetris AJ, et al. Expression of Epstein-Barr virus-encoded small RNA (by the EBER-1 gene) in liver specimens from transplant recipients with post-transplantation lymphoproliferative disease. *N Engl J Med.* 1992;327(24): 1710–1714.

98. Boyle GJ, Michaels MG, Webber SA, et al. Posttransplantation lymphoproliferative disorders in pediatric thoracic organ recipients. *J Pediatr.* 1997;131(2):309–313.

99. Goral S, Felgar R, Shappell S. Posttransplantation lymphoproliferative disorder in a renal allograft recipient. *Am J Kidney Dis.* 1997;30(2):301–307.

100. Nalesnik MA. Involvement of the gastrointestinal tract by Epstein-Barr virus—associated posttransplant lymphoproliferative disorders. *Am J Surg Pathol.* 1990;14(Suppl)1:92–100.

101. Boubenider S, Hiesse C, Goupy C, et al. Incidence and consequences of post-transplantation lymphoproliferative disorders. *J Nephrol.* 1997;10(3):136–145.

102. Davis CL, Harrison KL, McVicar JP, et al. Antiviral prophylaxis and the Epstein Barr virus-related post-transplant lymphoproliferative disorder. *Clin Transplant.* 1995;9(1):53–59.

103. Murray PG, Swinnen LJ, Constandinou CM, et al. BCL-2 but not its Epstein-Barr virus-encoded homologue, BHRF1, is commonly expressed in posttransplantation lymphoproliferative disorders. *Blood.* 1996;87(2):706–711.

104. Chetty R, Biddolph S, Kaklamanis L, et al. bcl-2 protein is strongly expressed in post-transplant lymphoproliferative disorders. *J Pathol.* 1996;180(3):254–258.

105. O'Brien S, Bernert RA, Logan JL, et al. Remission of posttransplant lymphoproliferative disorder after interferon alfa therapy. *J Am Soc Nephrol.* 1997;8(9):1483–1489.

106. Manez R, Breinig MC, Linden P, et al. Posttransplant lymphoproliferative disease in primary Epstein-Barr virus infection after liver transplantation: The role of cytomegalovirus disease. *J Infect Dis.* 1997;176(6):1462–1467.

107. Boyle GJ, Michaels MG, Webber SA, et al. Posttransplantation lymphoproliferative disorders in pediatric thoracic organ recipients. *J Pediatr.* 1997;131(2):309–313.

108. Walker RC, Marshall WF, Strickler JG, et al. Pretransplantation assessment of the risk of lymphoproliferative disorder. *Clin Infect Dis.* 1995;20(5):1346–1353.

109. Riddler SA, Breinig MC, McKnight JL. Increased levels of circulating Epstein-Barr virus (EBV)-infected lymphocytes and decreased EBV nuclear antigen antibody responses are associated with the development of posttransplant lymphoproliferative disease in solid-organ transplant recipients. *Blood.* 1994;84(3): 972–984.

110. Nalesnik MA, Starzl TE. Epstein-Barr virus, infectious mononucleosis, and posttransplant lymphoproliferative disorders. *Transplant Sci.* 1994;4(1):61–79.

111. Montone KT, Friedman H, Hodinka RL, et al. In situ hybridization for Epstein-Barr virus NotI repeats in posttransplant lymphoproliferative disorder. *Mod Pathol.* 1992;5(3):292–302.

112. Lones MA, Shintaku UP, Weiss LM, et al. Posttransplant lymphoproliferative disorder in liver allograft biopsies: A comparison of three methods for the demonstration of Epstein-Barr virus. *Hum Pathol.* 1977;28(5):533–539.

113. Hanson MN, Morrison VA, Peterson BA, et al. Posttransplant T-cell lymphoproliferative disorders—an aggressive, late complication of solid-organ transplantation. *Blood.* 1996;88(9): 3626–3633.

114. Goral S, Felgar R, Shappell S. Posttransplantation lymphoproliferative disorder in a renal allograft recipient. *Am J Kidney Dis.* 1997;30(2):301–307.

115. Harris NL, Ferry JA, Swerdlow SH. Posttransplant lymphoproliferative disorders: Summary of Society for Hematopathology Workshop. *Semin Diagn Pathol.* 1997;14(1):8–14.

116. Delecluse HJ, Rouault JP, Ffrench M, et al. Post-transplant lymphoproliferative disorders with genetic abnormalities commonly found in malignant tumours. *Br J Haematol.* 1995;89 (1):90–97.

117. Randhawa PS, Demetris AJ, Nalesnik MA. The potential role of cytokines in the pathogenesis of Epstein-Barr virus associated post-transplant lymphoproliferative disease. *Leuk Lymphoma.* 1994;15(5–6):383–387.

118. Weissmann DJ, Ferry JA, Harris NL, et al. Posttransplantation lymphoproliferative disorders in solid organ recipients are predominantly aggressive tumors of host origin. *Am J Clin Pathol* 1995;103(6):748–755.

119. Le Frere-Belda MA, Martin N, Gaulard P, et al. Donor or recipient origin of post-transplantation lymphoproliferative disorders: evaluation by in situ hybridization. *Mod Pathol.* 1997;10(7): 701–707.

120. Woo SB, Lee SJ, Schubert MM. Graft-vs.-host disease. *Crit Rev Oral Biol Med.* 1997;8(2):201–216.

121. Matsuoka LY. Graft versus host disease. *J Am Acad Dermatol.* 1981;5(5):595–599.

122. Snover DC, Weisdorf SA, Vercellotti GM, et al. A histopathologic study of gastric and small intestinal graft-versus-host disease following allogeneic bone marrow transplantation. *Hum Pathol.* 1985;16(4):387–392.

123. Roy J, Platt JL, Weisdoft DJ. The immunopathology of upper gastrointestinal acute graft-versus-host disease. Lymphoid cells and endothelial adhesion molecules. *Transplantation.* 1993; 55(3):572–578.

124. Ferrara JL, Cooke KR, Pan L, et al. The immunopathophysiology of acute graft-versus-host-disease. *Stem Cells.* 1996;14(5): 473–489.

125. Snover DC. Graft-versus-host disease of the gastrointestinal tract. *Am J Surg Pathol.* 1990;14(Suppl)1:101–108.

126. Bombi JA, Nadal A, Carreras E, et al. Assessment of histopathologic changes in the colonic biopsy in acute graft-versus-host disease. *Am J Clin Pathol.* 1995;103(6):690–695.

127. Washington K, Bentley RC, Green A, et al. Gastric graft-versus-host disease: A blinded histologic study. *Am J Surg Pathol.* 1997;21(9):1037–1046.

128. Snover DC, Weisdorf SA, Vercellotti GM, et al. A histopathologic study of gastric and small intestinal graft-versus-host disease following allogeneic bone marrow transplantation. *Hum Pathol.* 1985;16(4):387–392.

129. Shulman HM, Sullivan KM, Weiden PL, et al. Chronic graft-versus-host syndrome in man. A long-term clinicopathologic study of 20 Seattle patients. *Am J Med.* 1980;69(2):204–217.

18

CYTOPATHOLOGY OF THE GASTROINTESTINAL TRACT

Anwar Sultana Raza and Wesley Y. Naritoku

▶ CHAPTER OUTLINE

1. The brush samples a larger surface area of the lesion, which is particularly valuable in precancerous lesions such as Barrett's esophagus and chronic ulcerative colitis in which dysplastic mucosa does not differ at endoscopy from nondysplastic mucosa.
2. The brush has a greater accessibility than a biopsy forceps in tightly stenotic lesions, particularly malignant strictures of the esophagus and colon, in which biopsy specimens have a significant false-negative rate. Accessibility is also an important advantage in sampling lesions of the ampulla of Vater, where brush samples frequently provide diagnostic material when biopsies fail to do so.
3. Brush samples are potentially cheaper than biopsies, particularly in evaluating Barrett's esophagus and ulcerative colitis, if they ever replace biopsies. At the present time, though, brush samples are an adjunct to multiple biopsies, and actually increase the cost of the procedure.
4. Cytologic preparations have a shorter turnaround time than biopsies; this is not a very relevant issue because diagnosis is rarely urgent.
5. In submucosal and intramural mass lesions, which are not accessible by biopsy, fine-needle aspiration directed by endoscopic ultrasound represents a superior diagnostic technique.[6]

Cytopathology of the gastrointestinal tract, when used as an adjunct to biopsy, increases the diagnostic yield of most inflammatory and neoplastic lesions,[1-4] and in some instances cytology is more sensitive for diagnosis than biopsy.[1,4,5] Endoscopic brush samples have the following advantages over biopsy:

Despite these advantages, cytopathologic samples are rarely obtained from gastrointestinal lesions, even in many academic centers. The reasons for this are uncertain, but may relate to the lack of specialized cytopathology expertise among pathologists trained in gastrointestinal pathology.

Cytologic preparations should be examined by scanning at low power to assess overall cellularity, degree of cellular preservation, architectural arrangements, and the smear background. This is followed by a systematic screening of the smear at high magnification for cellular abnormalities and the presence of infectious agents.

The opening line of the microscopic description in the report should indicate adequacy and preservation of the sample, similar to that required by the Revised Bethesda System of gynecologic Pap smears. Identification of a disease process should be stated in language similar to that used in surgical pathology of the gastrointestinal tract. If a specific diagnosis is not identified, the findings should be described with comments about their meaning, when relevant. It should be emphasized that cytology is a screening procedure. The absence of positivity for a malignant process does not exclude malignancy because the sensitivity of the procedure is less than 100%. More importantly, the presence of a malignancy must be confirmed by biopsy, except in rare situations such as ampullary lesions in which the lesion is inaccessible to biopsy, because false-positive diagnoses may occur.

SPECIMEN COLLECTION

Lavage Methods

Lavage of both upper and lower gastrointestinal tract with isotonic saline, with or without mucolytic agents, was the only method of obtaining cytologic samples from the gastrointestinal tract before the advent of fiberoptic endoscopy. These techniques provided samples that did little to increase diagnostic yield of biopsies and are now obsolete.[7]

Brushing Method

A small nylon brush in a thin polyethylene tube is inserted into the biopsy channel of the endoscope. Retraction of the polyethylene sheath exposes the tip of the brush, which is brushed against the entire surface of the lesion or, in the case of potentially dysplastic mucosa, over the entire area under suspicion. Best results are obtained when the brush sample is obtained prior to taking endoscopic biopsies; histologic diagnosis of biopsy specimens is not affected adversely by prior brushing. Others, however, prefer brushings to be obtained after biopsy so that the quantitative cellular yield is maximized.[8–10]

After brushing, the brush is covered by the polyethylene sheath to protect the sample and then withdrawn from the endoscope. Two or three smears are made with a rapid rolling motion of the brush covering a surface area the size of a quarter on a plain glass slide, rather than rubbing the brush over the entire slide.[11] The slides are immediately fixed in 95% ethanol for Papanicolaou staining or air-dried for Diff-Quik staining. Cell block preparations are particularly useful for clotted specimens and tissue fragments or when the need for a special stain is anticipated.

Salvage Cytology

Salvage cytology is usually performed after endoscopic biopsy samples have been taken from lesions suggestive of malignancy. The brush, biopsy forceps, or the cytology brush channel of the endoscope is rinsed with balanced salt solution. The cell suspension is then centrifuged or filtered to produce smears and cell blocks. The endoscopic brush may be immersed in CytoLyt (Cytyc) after preparing the smears, which may then be used to prepare ThinPrep slides. The average screening time per case is considerably shorter with ThinPrep slides than direct smears. The ThinPrep slides are also reported to be superior to direct smears in cellularity, quantity, and quality of diagnostic cells, with the additional advantage of reduction in the number of unsatisfactory specimens.[9,10]

Direct Smears from Biopsy Specimens

Small endoscopic biopsy specimens can be imprinted or smeared on a glass slide prior to their being placed in fixative.[12] Imprints from these samples rapidly dry out, and the imprinted slide must be placed in fixative within 4 s after preparation to prevent drying artefact if Papanicolaou staining is to be performed. The imprints can also be air-dried and stained with Diff-Quik or May-Grünwald-Giemsa stain. Imprint cytology is useful as an immediate assessment of the adequacy of a biopsy sample, providing bedside information that can influence whether additional biopsy samples should be taken from the lesion. Touch cytology is a quick, simple, and sensitive screening test, particularly for the diagnosis of mucosal infections of the gastrointestinal tract. *Candida* esophagitis, *Helicobacter pylori*, *Helicobacter heilanii* (*Gastrospirillum hominis*) gastritis, and duodenal infection with *Giardia lamblia* are the most commonly identified infections[12] using this technique.

Transmucosal Fine-Needle Aspiration Biopsy

Transmucosal fine-needle aspiration (FNA) is useful in the diagnosis of submucosal, intramural, and extrinsic mass lesions that can be either seen at endoscopy as masses covered by normal mucosa that protrude into the lumen or visualized by endoscopic ultrasonography. In the latter event, the FNA must be directed by endoscopic ultrasonography.[6] This method may also be used in preoperative staging procedures because it permits sampling of periesophageal or perigastric lymph nodes. The material obtained by FNA is processed for smears and cell block preparation. Like FNA biopsy specimens in the rest of the body, these samples can provide tissue that is adequate for immunohistochemical and ultrastructural studies.

Blind Abrasive Techniques

A balloon-like sampling device has been used predominantly in the esophagus. The balloon device, which is covered by a nylon net, is swallowed in the deflated state; in the stomach, it is inflated, and the balloon is pulled through the gastroestophageal junction and up the esophagus to the cricoid, where it is again deflated and removed. The inflated balloon surface contains cells abraded from the epithelial surface of the esophagus. The balloon surface is either smeared directly on glass slides or rinsed into a fixative solution for filtration or centrifugation to produce smears and cell block preparations.

Abrasive balloon devices are rapid, inexpensive, and easy to use. They can be used in the field by trained, nonphysician medical professionals, making their use very suited to mass screening of populations at high risk for esophageal carcinoma.[13] The cost of balloon cytology is one sixth that of endoscopy and biopsy. Efforts to use this technique in China, one of the highest risk regions in the world for esophageal squamous carcinoma, resulted in a significant rate of detection of early lesions.[14] More recently, the technique has been advocated for use in place of regular endoscopy in the United States for patients with long-segment Barrett's esophagus.[13]

Endoscopic Retrograde Cholangiopancreatography

Cannulation of the papilla of Vater during endoscopic retrograde cholangiopancreatography (ERCP) permits the aspiration of contents of the bile and pancreatic ducts, as well as brushings to be obtained. In contrast to other GI sites, cytologic preparations frequently represent the only available diagnostic material from ampullary lesions because it is rarely possible to adequately access these lesions with a biopsy forceps.

ESOPHAGEAL CYTOPATHOLOGY

Normal Cytology

Esophageal brushings in the absence of disease consist essentially of intermediate-type squamous cells, characteristized by abundant delicate cytoplasm and vesicular nuclei (Fig. 18–1), with a few superficial cells, characterized by abundant keratinized cytoplasm and pyknotic nuclei.[15] Both types of squamous cells are present in large, flat sheets; small clusters; and occasional solitary cells. Rarely, particularly in vigorously brushed specimens, smears may also contain parabasal cells that are smaller and have denser cytoplasm with vesicular nuclei. Parabasal cells are also seen if inflammation or an ulcer is present. Occasional benign squamous pearls, superficial cells with keratohyaline granules, and, rarely, melanocytes may be present.

Glandular elements may also be present in esophageal brushings from columnar cells of cardiac mucosa or due to inadvertent sampling of gastric mucosa. Glandular cells usually form clusters with cells that have finely granular cytoplasm and vesicular nuclei. Ciliated cells are present in the esophagus only during embryologic development. Their presence in esophageal brush samples usually indicates contamination from the upper respiratory tract (Fig. 18–2A). Other contaminants that may be

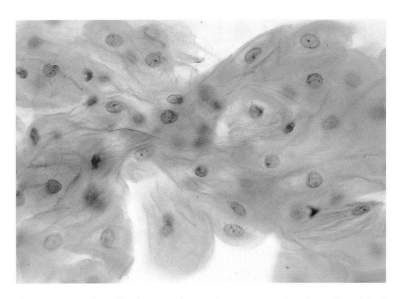

Figure 18–1. Esophageal brushing; normal intermediate squamous cells with vesicular nuclei and abundant delicate cytoplasm.

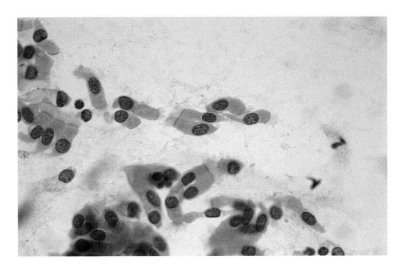

A

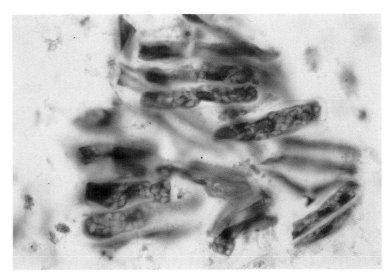

B

Figure 18–2. A: Ciliated columnar epithelial cells in an esophageal brushing; this most likely represents contamination from the upper respiratory tract. B: Plant (vegetable) cells in an esophageal brushing. These often have hyperchromatic nuclei. They should not be mistaken for dysplastic cells.

present include swallowed pigment-containing alveolar macrophages, meat fibers and plant cells (Fig. 18–2B), and bacteria and yeasts from the oral cavity.

Abnormalities in Nonneoplastic Esophageal Diseases

Certain infectious diseases of the esophagus produce characteristic abnormalities in cytologic preparations.

Candida Esophagitis

This condition shows the presence of budding yeasts and delicate pseudo-hyphae associated with neutrophils and either normal or parakeratotic squamous cells (Fig. 18–3A). Pseudo-hyphae are elongated yeast forms that are attached end-to-end. The place of attachment shows a constriction ("sausage-link" appearance). Smears stained with methenamine silver (Fig. 18–3B) are useful when the organism is not plentiful. Reactive epithelial cells and anucleate squames are commonly present (Fig. 18–3C). When atypia of the epithelial cells is marked, the possibility of secondary infection of an ulcerated tumor by *Candida* should be considered (Fig. 18–3D). Secondary *Candia* infection of an ulcer should also be a consideration when necrotic debris is present on the smear. *Candida* is a surface infection that is diagnosed with greater sensitivity by cytologic preparations than biopsies.[16–18]

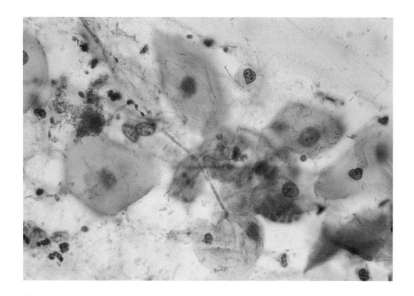

A

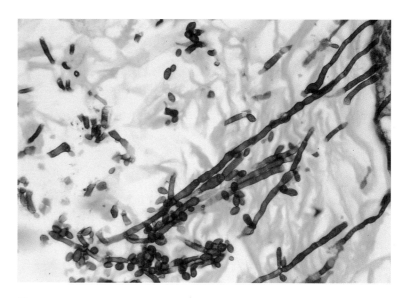

B

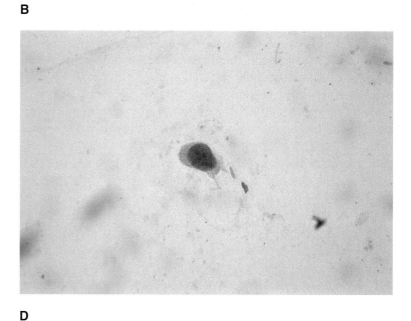

C

D

Figure 18–3. A: Esophageal brushing, showing psuedo-hyphae of *Candida* species, characterized by elongated yeast forms attached end-to-end associated with squamous cells and a few neutrophils. B: Esophageal brushing stained with methenamine silver, which highlights the pseudo-hyphae and yeasts of *Candida* species. C: Esophageal brushing, showing reactive atypia of squamous epithelial cells associated with rare *Candida* pseudo-hyphae and yeasts. D: Esophageal brushing, showing a markedly atypical cell associated with *Candida* pseudo-hypha. The degree of atypia mimics malignancy. This patient had no evidence of carcinoma.

Herpetic Esophagitis

Both herpes simplex virus and herpes varicella-zoster virus cause vesiculoulcerative lesions of the esophagus. Brushing should be done at the ulcer's base and edges. Smears show necrotic ulcer debris, inflammatory cells, reactive squamous cells, and infected cells. Aggregates of macrophages are reported to be a characteristic finding in ulcerative herpetic esophagitis; their presence warrants immunoperoxidase staining for herpesvirus when inclusions are not found. Squamous cells infected with herpesvirus show multinucleation, molding, and margination (Fig. 18–4A and B). Herpesvirus inclusions are Cowdry type A intranuclear eosinophilic inclusions surrounded by a halo and thickened nuclear membrane (Fig. 18–4C), and more diffuse nuclear inclusions with "ground glass" change in the nuclear chromatin (Fig. 18–4B).

Cytomegalovirus Esophagitis

Cytomegalovirus (CMV) does not infect squamous epithelial cells. It infects vascular endothelial cells, stromal fibroblasts, and glandular epithelial cells. Evidence of CMV infection is therefore rarely present in brushings unless ulceration is present (Fig. 18–5A); biopsies are more sensitive for diagnosis of CMV esophagitis. Cytomegalovirus-infected cells show marked cytomegaly and nucleomegaly (Fig. 18–5B). Large, ovoid, basophilic intranuclear inclusions are evident surrounded by a halo and thick nuclear chromatin marginated against the nuclear membrane (Fig. 18–5). In addition, the cytoplasm contains granular amphophilic cytoplasmic inclusions. Esophageal brushings are not a good way to exclude CMV infection, and a negative result does not permit diagnosis of idiopathic esophageal ulceration in patients with AIDS (see Chapter 3). In immunocompromised patients, infection with multiple agents is not uncommon, and careful examination of the specimen should be continued even after one agent has been found (Fig. 18–6).

Human Papillomvirus

Changes of human papillomavirus (HPV), characterized by HPV koilocytes, may rarely be seen in esophageal brushings, either in association with squamous papillomatous lesions or flat dysplastic lesions. HPV is reported to be etiologically associated with squamous carcinoma of the esophagus in some high-risk populations (see Chapter 3).

Other Infections

Aspergillus (Fig. 18–7) and bacteria are very rare causes of esophagitis. Most cases with hyphal fungi and bacteria represent contamination of the sample; these findings should be recorded in the report, but it is prudent not to ascribe an etiologic role to them without histologic confirmation in a biopsy specimen.

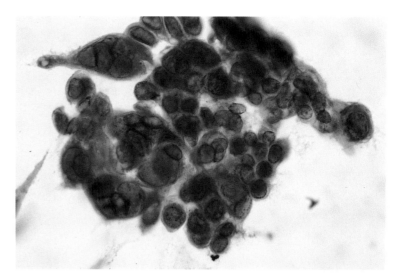

A

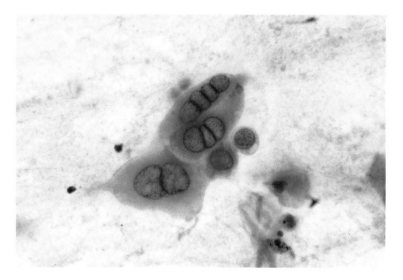

B

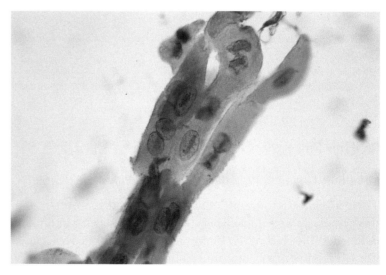

C

Figure 18–4. A: Esophageal brushing showing cytologic features of herpesvirus infection. The squamous cells show multinucleation and molding with "ground glass" intranuclear inclusions. B: Herpetic esophagitis. The squamous cells show multinucleation and molding with "ground glass" intranuclear inclusions. C: Herpetic esophagitis, showing Cowdry A intranuclear inclusions in infected squamous cells.

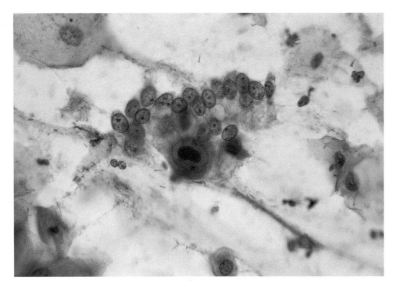

A

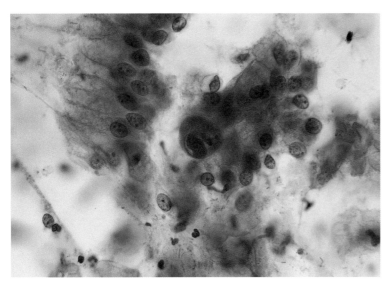

B

Figure 18–5. A: Esophageal brushing, showing cytomegalovirus-infected stromal cells demonstrating cytomegaly, nuclear enlargement, and a large intranuclear inclusion surrounded by a halo. Note the presence of parabasal cells, suggesting that this is from an area of ulceration. B: Brushing from the lower esophagus, showing cytomegalovirus-infected glandular epithelial cell, most likely from cardiac mucosa.

Reactive Processes

Radiation, Chemotherapy, and Vitamin B₁₂ and Folate Deficiency

These all cause cytomegaly, nucleomegaly, and abnormalities in the cytoplasm and nuclei (Fig. 18–8). In vitamin B_{12} and folate deficiency, the cells retain their nuclear:cytoplasmic (N:C) ratio, there is a tendency to multinucleation, and the nuclei show hyperchromasia and nuclear wrinkling. In radiation, the N:C ratio is retained, multinucleation is common, and cytoplasmic and nuclear vacuolation is evident. Chemotherapy-induced changes are similar to those seen in radiation, but there is a greater tendency to increased N:C ratios and nuclear irregularity. In all these conditions, the differential diagnosis includes squamous carcinoma. The differential diagnosis is complicated by the fact

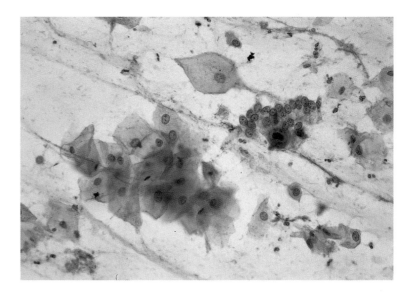

Figure 18–6. Esophageal brushing in an AIDS patient, showing infection with cytomegalovirus as well as *Candida*.

that radiation and chemotherapy changes may involve malignant cells when these treatment modalities are used for a carcinoma of the esophagus.

Pemphigus Vulgaris

This condition is characterized by abundant discohesive parabasal cells with reactive atypia and prominent bar-shaped nucleoli (Fig. 18–9). Neutrophils and eosinophils are often present (Fig. 18–9B). Differentiation from malignancy may be difficult (see Chapter 3).

Esophageal Ulcers

Ulcers occur in the esophagus in many pathologic conditions. In all of these, the presence of ulceration itself produces a constellation of cytologic changes in addition to the changes resulting from the causal factor. Changes associated with ulcers in-

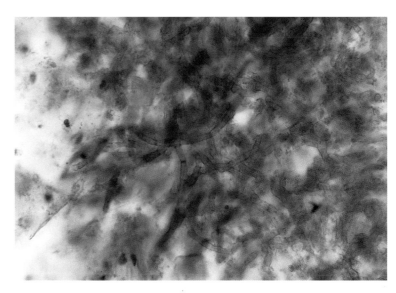

Figure 18–7. Esophageal brushing, showing hyphae of *Aspergillus* species.

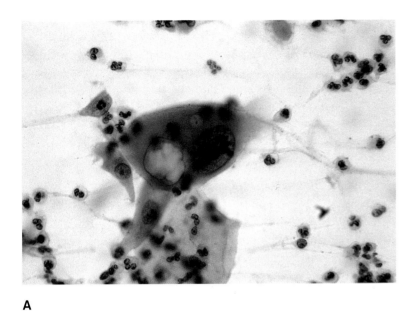

A

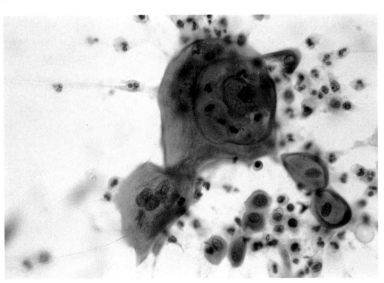

B

Figure 18–8. A: Esophageal brushing, Papanicolaou stain, showing radiation change. The affected cell shows marked nuclear enlargement associated with cytomegaly, resulting in a normal N:C ratio. The cytoplasm is vacuolated and shows varied staining. B: Radiation change, esophageal brushing, showing marked cytomegaly, vacuolated cytoplasm, and intracytoplasmic neutrophils.

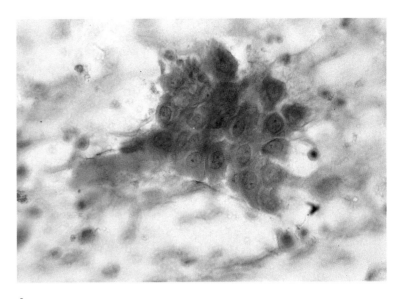

A

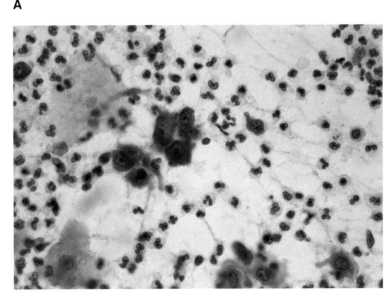

B

Figure 18–9. A: Esophageal brushing in pemphigus vulgaris, showing a group of squamous cells with early discohesive features and rounding up of superficial cells, suggestive of acantholysis. Mild nuclear atypia is evident. B: Esophageal brushing in pemphigus vulgaris, showing acantholytic single cells and loose clusters associated with neutrophils. The acantholytic cells have markedly atypical nuclei with prominent nucleoli, mimicking malignancy.

clude the presence of basal and parabasal cells, usually in cohesive groups with few single cells (see Fig. 18–5A); the cells retain their polarity with minimal overlapping and show a typical streaming effect, with the cells and nuclei appearing to flow in one direction (Fig. 18–10A). Nuclei show enlargement with smooth contours and finely granular cytoplasm. Prominent macronucleoli are typically present (Fig. 18–10B). Nuclear:nucleolar dyssynchrony is characteristic of benign repair. Only mild anisocytosis and anisonucleosis are evident. Necrotic debris and inflammatory cells are commonly present in the background.

Reactive atypia associated with ulceration can be severe enough to resemble malignancy (Fig. 18–10A and C). In extreme cases, exclusion of malignancy is difficult, and a false-

positive diagnosis is possible. The lack of discohesive single cells and the absence of pleomorphism, coarse chromatin, and irregular nuclear membranes that characterize malignant cells represent the most reliable criteria for distinguishing reactive atypia from malignancy.

Gastroesophageal Reflux Disease

No specific cytologic features help diagnose reflux disease. Brushings demonstrate acute inflammation with esoinophils and neutrophils, reactive epithelial atypia, and features of ulceration in severe cases associated with ulcers. The presence of cardiac-type mucous cells in a brushing from the esophagus is difficult to differentiate from gastric contamination.

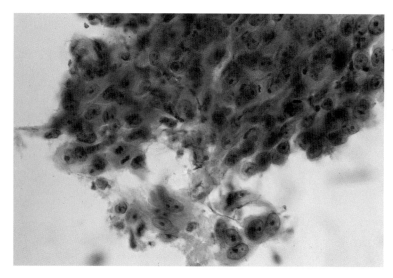

A

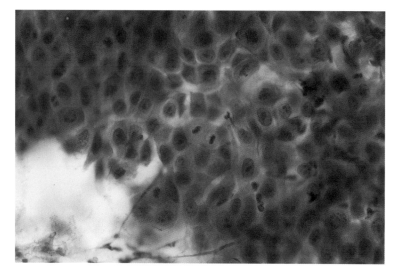

B

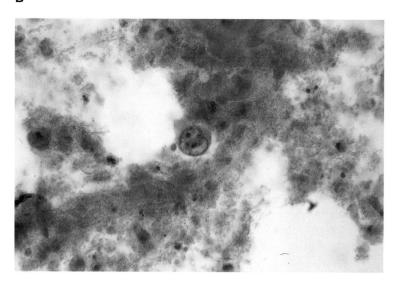

C

Figure 18–10. A: Reactive cells in ulcerative esophagitis, showing a cohesive cell group with a streaming effect. The cells have enlarged vesicular nuclei with delicate chromatin and prominent nucleoli. B: Esophageal brushing, showing atypical reactive cells that have prominent nucleoli. Note the typical mitotic figure. C: Esophageal brushing, showing necrotic cells and one large, severely atypical cell that mimics malignancy.

Barrett's Esophagus

Cells from Barrett's specialized columnar epithelium with intestinal metaplasia can be recognized in brushings (Fig. 18–11A). These appear as large, flat, sharply defined, cohesive sheets of cells with smooth edges. Goblet cells that characterize intestinal metaplasia can be been as a "swiss cheese" appearance in cell clusters that are seen en face (Fig. 18–11B).

Neoplasms of the Esophagus

Benign Neoplasms

Benign neoplasms are rare and, except for squamous papillomas, do not involve the mucosa and rarely produce abnormalities in brushings.

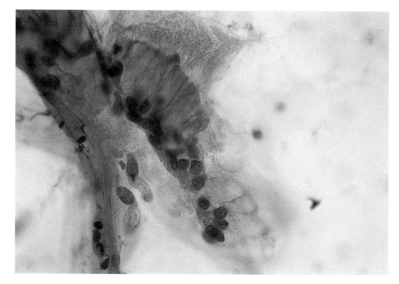

A

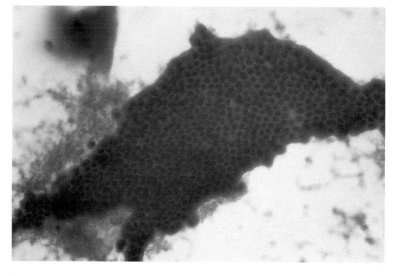

B

Figure 18–11. A: Esophageal brushing in Barrett's esophagus, showing glandular cells with goblet cells characterized by ballooning of the cytoplasm with a mucin vacuole. B: Esophageal brushing of Barrett's esophagus, showing a flat grouping of glandular epithelial cells with focal clearning ("windows") representing goblet cells.

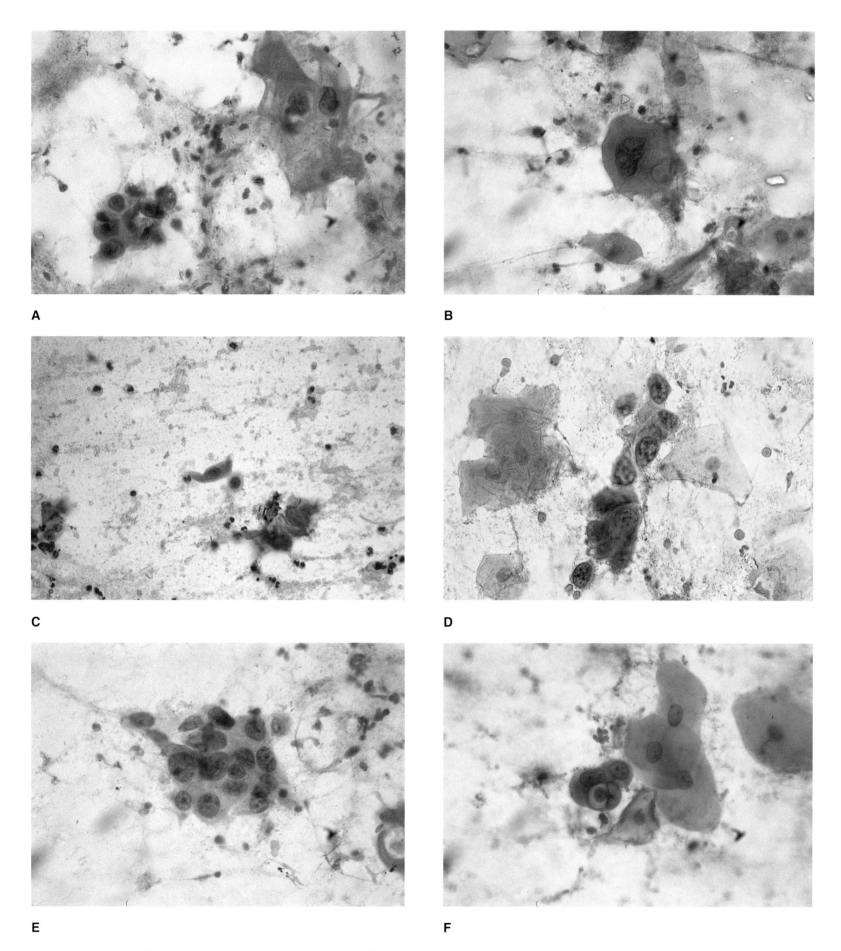

Figure 18–12. A: Esophageal brushing, showing poorly differentiated squamous carcinoma with inflammation and cells with evidence of moderate dysplasia. The dysplastic cells have abundant cytoplasm and enlarged nuclei that show an abnormal chromatin pattern. B: Esophageal brushing with well-differentiated squamous carinoma, showing a malignant cell with abundant orangeophilic cytoplasm. C: Esophageal brushing in squamous carcinoma showing a "caudate" cell with an elongated shape. D: Esophageal brushing with poorly differentiated squamous carcinoma, showing a discohesive group of malignant cells. E: Poorly differentiated squamous carcinoma. F: Poorly differentiated squamous carcinoma, showing cell-embracing and cyanophilic cytoplasm. Note the contrast with the normal intermediate cells.

Squamous Carcinoma

In the United States, most esophageal squamous carcinomas present at an advanced stage with obvious lesions, and brushings from the lesions show features of invasive carcinoma. In countries like Japan, where upper GI screening for gastric carcinoma permits simultaneous screening for esophageal carcinoma, early dysplastic changes are seen in brushings. Low-grade dysplasia is characterized by superficial or intermediate cells with slightly enlarged, hyperchromatic nuclei and a mild increase in N:C ratio (Fig. 18–12A). In high-grade dysplasia, which includes carcinoma in situ, the nuclear enlargement is greater, with higher N:C ratios, more pronounced hyperchromasia, coarser chromatin, and irregular nuclear membranes. Differentiation from invasive carcinoma is made by the absence of prominent nucleoli and a necrotic tumor diathesis.

Invasive squamous carcinomas are usually characterized by large numbers of cells, both in groups and as single cells in a background of necrosis and inflammation (Fig. 18–12A–F). Well-differentiated, keratinizing squamous carcinoma shows marked pleomorphism, with oval, spindle-shaped, elongated "tadpole" cells, and irregular bizarre cells (Fig. 18–12B). The cells have dense, opaque, orangeophilic to cyanophilic cytoplasm with refractile ringing around the necleus. Nonkeratinizing squamous carcinomas are characterized by smaller cells; with a high N:C ratio; dense cyanophilic cytoplasm; and enlarged nuclei with multiple, large, prominent nucleoli (Fig. 18–12D and E).

Dysplasia and Adenocarcinoma in Barrett's Esophagus

Brush cytology is routinely performed as part of the surveillance protocol for Barrett's esophagus in many academic centers. The use of nonendoscopic abrasive balloon cytology has also been advocated.[13] Cytologic changes of low-grade dysplasia are difficult to distinguish from reactive atypia. Cytologic changes of high-grade dysplasia are essentially similar to those in adenocarcinoma, except that the number of abnormal cells in the specimen is usually fewer, the dysplastic cell aggregates tend to be larger, and no tumor diathesis is evident (Fig. 18–13A). An even more important distinguishing feature between high grade dysplasia and adenocarcinoma is the lack of an obvious endoscopic tumor in the former.

Adenocarcinoma is characterized by loosely cohesive, small cellular aggregates with irregular borders associated with numerous, scattered, single abnormal cells in a necrotic background with inflammatory cells (Fig. 18–13B). The cell groupings show loss of polarity, crowding, and nuclear overlapping. The individual cells have high N:C ratios, and enlarged, pleomorphic, hyperchromatic, and frequently cigar-shaped nuclei with irregular nuclear membranes. One or more prominent irregular nucleoli are commonly present. The cytoplasm is delicate and finely granular without obvious vacuolation by mucin. Occasional tumor giant cells may be present. Poorly developed rudimentary cilia have been described in papillary adenocarcinomas arising in Barrett's esophagus; these are visible only under oil immersion or electron mi-

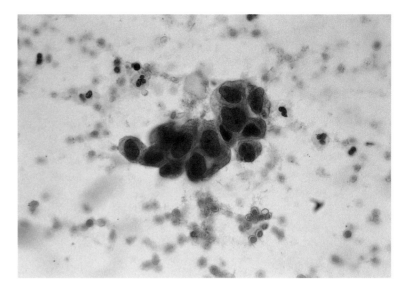

A

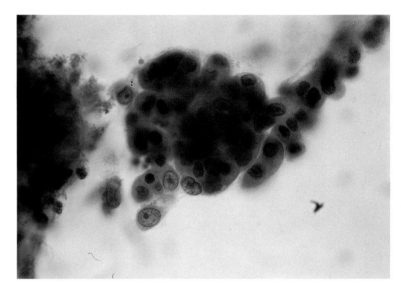

B

Figure 18–13. A: Esophageal brushing showing a group of malignant glandular epithelial cells with irregular nuclei and prominent nucleoli. This appearance can represent either high-grade dysplasia or adenocarcinoma. B: Well-differentiated adenocarcinoma, showing nuclear pleomorphism and single malignant cells.

croscopy.[19] Rare Barrett's adenocarcinomas show focal squamous differentiation.

Small-Cell Neuroendocrine Carcinoma

The esophagus is a rare site for primary extrapulmonary small cell undifferentiated neuroendocrine carcinoma. These tumors are characterized by small, round-to-ovoid cells, which may be dispersed, form small aggregates, or line up in chains. The cells have scanty cytoplasm with high N:C ratios and nuclear molding. The nuclei have dark, fine to coarsely granular, evenly distributed chromatin without nucleoli (Fig. 18–14). The differential diagnosis includes a poorly differentiated squamous carcinoma, malignant carcinoid tumor, and malignant lymphoma. Immunoperoxidase staining with punctate perinuclear

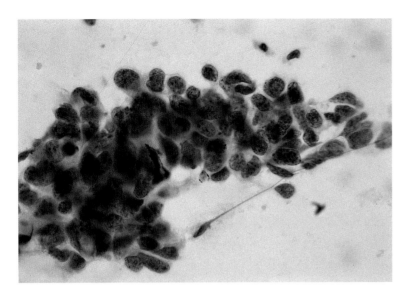

Figure 18–14. Esophageal brushing, showing a poorly differentiated carcinoma with cytologic features of small-cell undifferentiated carcinoma. The cells are cohesive, show ovoid hyperchromatic nuclei with nuclear molding and "salt and pepper" chromatin, and lack prominent nucleoili.

staining for cytokeratin and positive staining for chromogranin A and neuron specific enolase permits diagnosis.

Malignant Melanoma

The esophagus is a rare site for primary malignant melanoma. This is characterized by a cellular smear with large single cells and loosely cohesive cell clusters. The cells have distinct cell borders, cyanophilic cytoplasm, large eccentric nuclei with centrally placed macronucleoli, and nuclear pseudo-inclusions (Fig. 18–15A). When cytoplasmic melanin pigment is present, diagnosis is easy (Fig. 18–15B); in achromatic tumors, immunopositivity for S100 protein and HMB45 are of diagnostic value to differentiate melanoma from other poorly differentiated malignant neoplasms.

Other Neoplasms

Rare types of carcinoma include tumors that resemble salivary gland neoplasms such as mucoepidermoid carcinoma and adenoid cystic carcinoma (Fig. 18–16), which are believed to arise in the submucosal mucous glands of the esophagus.

Intramural mesenchymal neoplasms do not show abnormalities in brushings unless they are ulcerated; endoscopic ultrasound-directed fine-needle aspiration is an effective technique for diagnosing these neoplasms. Malignant lymphomas and carcinoid tumors rarely involve the esophagus. In immunocompromised patients, Kaposi's sarcoma rarely involves the esophagus (Fig. 18–17). Smears from ulcerated Kaposi's sarcoma may show aggregates of spindle cells that resemble mesenchymal neoplasms. In the appropriate clinical setting of a patient with acquired immunodeficiency syndrome and a red nodule seen at endoscopy, a diagnosis of Kaposi's sarcoma can be made. Biopsy is necessary for confirmation (Fig. 18–17C). Granular cell tumors of the esophagus, which are best diagnosed with Wang needle aspiration, are frequently associated

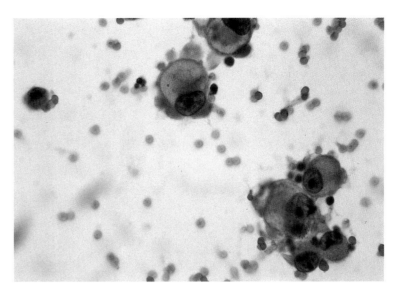

A

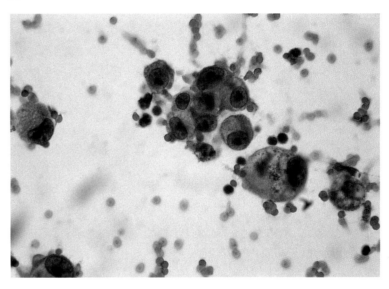

B

Figure 18–15. A: Esophageal brushing from a malignant melanoma, showing single malignant cells with large eccentric nuclei that have prominent nucleoli. The cytoplasm is clear to cyanophilic and does not contain obvious pigment. B: Malignant melanoma, showing malignant cells with scattered brown pigment granules in the cytoplasm.

with atypical hyperplasia of the squamous epithelium overlying the tumor. In an esophageal brushing of the tumor, there is a danger that the atypical squamous cells may be overinterpreted as carcinoma, particularly when the pathologist is aware of the presence of a large endoscopic mass lesion.

GASTRIC CYTOPATHOLOGY

Normal Cytology

The majority of cells from gastric brushings are derived from the surface epithelium. These appear as cohesive sheets of mucous cells with apical cytoplasm and basal nuclei (Fig. 18–18A),

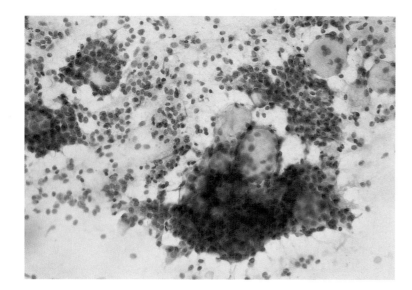

A

B

Figure 18–16. A: Adenoid cystic carcinoma, showing irregular groups of small basaloid cells with rounded basement membrane-like material. B: Adenoid cystic carcinoma, higher power micrograph of part A, showing rounded basement membrane-like material and basaloid cells with relatively bland cytologic features.

arranged in a characteristic "honeycomb," or "cartwheel" appearance (Fig. 18–18B). The deeper cells of the gastric glands, which include parietal cells, chief cells, and neuroendocrine cells, are rarely encountered in brush specimens (Fig. 18–18C).

Gastric cytologic specimens are frequently contaminated by material from the oral cavity and esophagus, and by swallowed sputum. Contaminants include squamous cells, ciliated columnar cells, alveolar macrophages, and food particles.

Benign Conditions

Chronic Gastritis

Brushings show large, cohesive aggregates of glandular epithelial cells with neutrophils and lymphocytes (Fig. 18–19A). In-

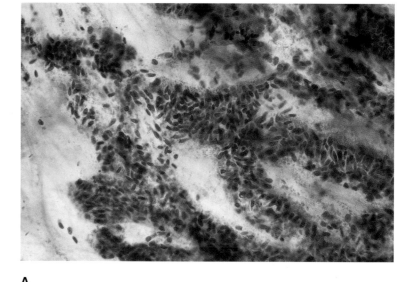

A

B

C

Figure 18–17. A: Esophageal brushing of Kaposi's sarcoma showing groupings of spindle cells. B: Kaposi's sarcoma, showing small spindle cells with discohesion. C: Esophageal biopsy specimen, showing Kaposi's sarcoma. The histologic features are difficult to differentiate from stromal tumor without clinical history and immunohistochemical stains.

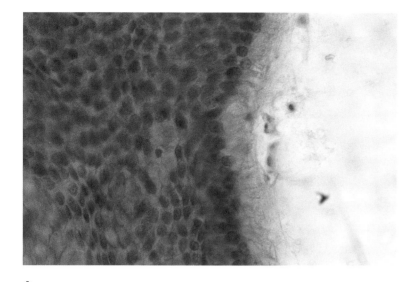

A

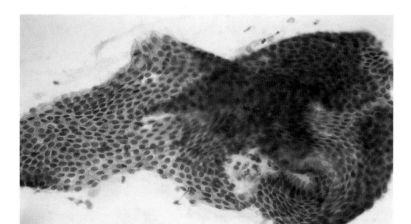

B

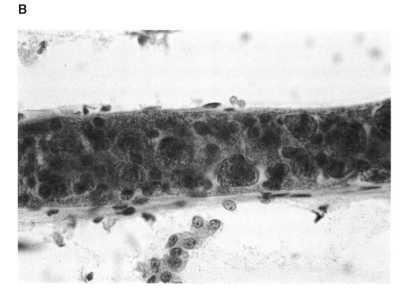

C

Figure 18–18. A: Gastric brushing, showing the edge of a grouping of benign gastric surface epithelial cells, which are columnar with basal nuclei and apical mucin that does not distend the cytoplasm. B: Gastric brushing, showing typical "honeycomb" appearance of a group of gastric surface epithelial cells. C: Normal gastric brushing, showing deep gastric glands containing parietal cells. The tubular architecture of the gland is preserved. The parietal cells have abundant granular cytoplasm.

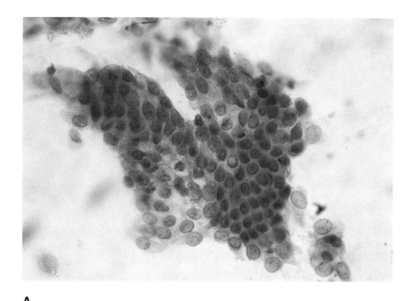

A

B

Figure 18–19. A: Gastric brushing from a patient with autoimmune chronic atrophic gastritis, showing surface epithelial cells with slight nuclear enlargement and atypia. B: Gastric brushing from a patient with autoimmune chronic atrophic gastritis, showing a greater degree of cytologic abnormality, possibly representing low-grade dysplasia.

testinal metaplasia, characterized by cells with large cytoplasmic vacuoles, may be seen. In patients with autoimmune chronic atrophic gastritis, brushing of endoscopically normal mucosa is a good method of screening for dysplasia (Fig. 18–19B). *Helicobacter pylori* is identified more easily in cytologic preparations than biopsy specimens, particularly when the density of the bacteria is low.[20] The sensitivity of *H. pylori* detection is the same for imprint cytology and brush cytology. The diagnostic sensitivity in brushings and imprints of biopsies is 97% compared with approximately 76% in biopsies. *Helicobacter pylori* is a 1–3 μm curved or spiral-shaped bacillus that is found in large numbers in the layer of mucus that covers the surface epithelial cell of the gastric mucosa (Fig. 18–20). The longitudinal axis of the organism is usually parallel to the long axis of the mucus strands.[20] *Helicobacter pylori* is seen best in

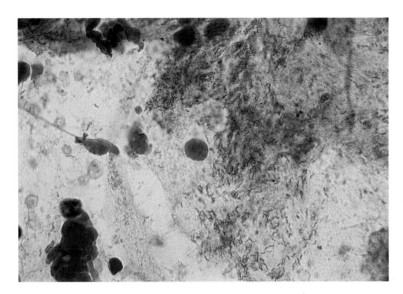

Figure 18–20. Gastric brushing showing numerous *Helicobacter pylori*, appearing as short, curved, "seagull"-shaped bacilli.

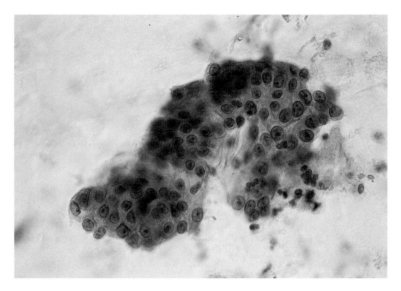

A

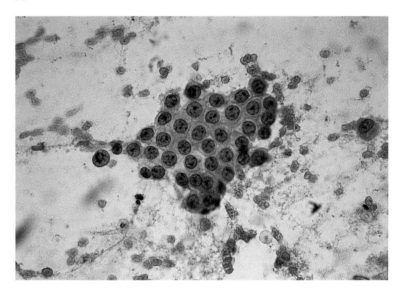

B

Figure 18–21. A: Gastric brushing, showing typical appearance of reactive epithelial cells. The cells form a cohesive grouping with normal polarity but pleomorphism is absent. B: Typical appearance of reactive atypia of gastric epithelial cells. The cells appear as a well-organized, flat sheet without pleomorphism or nuclear overlapping. The nuclei are uniformly enlarged and show delicate chromatin and prominent nucleoli. One discohesive single cell is present.

Diff Quik and Giemsa stained sections; they are less apparent in Papanicolaou stained sections. Triple stain, combining silver, hematoxylin & eosin, and alcian blue at pH 2.5, is useful in detecting *H. pylori* infection in both biopsy specimens and brushings; it also provides excellent cytologic detail in smears.[21]

Helicobacter heilanii (*Gastrospirillum hominis*) is another spiral organism that is a rare cause of chronic gastritis. The sensitivity of detection of *H. heilanii* is much greater in cytologic smears than biopsy samples.[21]

Ulcers and Erosions

Brushings should be taken from the center of the ulcer and its edges. Smears show necrotic debris and inflammatory cells along with epithelial cells that frequently show reactive atypia. Reactive gastric epithelial cells form cohesive groups of cells with enlarged nuclei and prominent large nucleoli. Cell polarity is usually maintained, and single cells are absent or very few in number (Fig. 18–21A and B). Cytologic atypia associated with reactive changes may be so marked that differentiation from malignancy can be difficult (Fig. 18–22), and there is a risk of false-positive diagnosis.[5]

Gastric Dysplasia

Low-grade gastric dysplasia cannot be reliably differentiated from reactive changes in cytologic preparations and should not be diagnosed definitively (Fig. 18–22C). High-grade dysplasia has cytologic features equivalent to adenocarcinoma.

Gastric Neoplasms

Adenocarcinoma

Intestinal-type adenocarcinoma of the stomach is characterized by multilayered disordered groups of cells associated with many single abnormal cells and a tumor diathesis (Fig.

18–23A). The cells are pleomorphic with increased N:C ratio, hyperchromasia with irregular chromatin, and nuclear borders (Fig. 18–23B and C). Prominent nucleoli are a feature. The cytoplasm is granular or, less commonly, vacuolated. Diffuse-type adenocarcinoma tends to be more infiltrative with less mucosal involvement and is associated with a higher rate of false-negative diagnosis by surface brushing techniques. Malignant cells are less numerous, and the majority are single cells (Fig. 18–24A). They are typically signet ring cells with eccentric, sharply pointed nuclei that show hyperchromasia. The cytoplasm is distended with mucin, which indents the nucleus (Fig. 18–24B and C). The background is usually clean without a tumor diathesis.

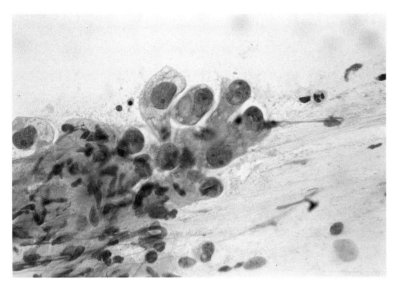

A

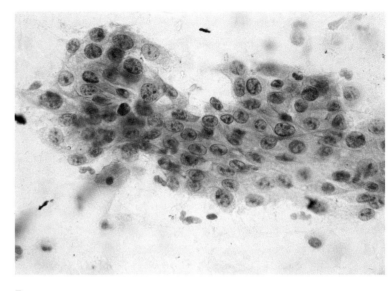

B

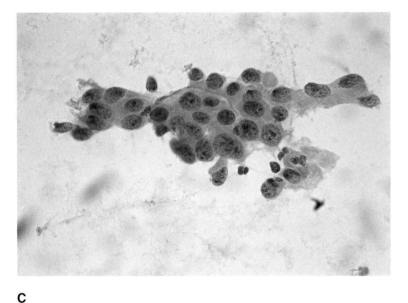

C

Figure 18–22. A: Gastric brushing from an ulcer's edge, showing spindle cells from granulation tissue and atypical reactive epithelial cells. The latter have abundant vacuolated cytoplasm and enlarged nuclei with delicate chromatin and prominent nucleoli. B: Gastric brushing, showing a group of surface epithelial cells with atypical reactive change. The cells are well organized, but show nuclear chromatin abnormality and mild pleomorphism. C: Gastric brushing, showing severe reactive atypia with cytologic features mimicking malignancy. Endoscopy and biopsy samples were negative for malignancy in this patient.

Malignant Lymphoma

Cytologic specimens are not a sensitive method for the diagnosis of malignant gastric lymphoma; brushings have a diagnostic sensitivity of 15–83%.[21] Low-grade mucosal-associated lymphoid tissue (MALT)-lymphomas cannot be diagnosed by brushings alone. High-grade lymphomas, particularly those that are associated with mucosal ulceration, appear in smears as discohesive monomorphic large round cells with high N:C ratios (Fig. 18–25). The nuclear features depend on the type of high-grade lymphoma.

Carcinoid Tumor

Carcinoid tumors usually present as polypoid structures involving the deep mucosa and are rarely encountered in brushings. They may be diagnosed by endoscopic ultrasound-directed FNA biopsy.[22] Smears of FNA specimens show cellular smears consisting of small, uniform cells appearing as small aggregates and single cells (Fig. 18–26A and B). The cells have high N:C ratios and eccentric round-to-oval uniform nuclei with evenly dispersed chromatin. Immunohistochemical positivity for chromogranin A is useful for specific diagnosis. We have encountered a case of composite, well-differentiated adenocarcinoma-carcinoid tumor of the stomach that, on brush cytology, showed only the superficial adenocarcinoma component. Resection showed the carcinoid element in the deeper regions of the tumor (see Chapter 5). The possibility of neuroendocrine carcinoma should be considered for tumors that have general features of carcinoid tumors, but have obviously malignant nuclear features (Fig. 18–26C).

Gastric GI Stromal Tumors

Fine-needle aspiration biopsy directed by endoscopic ultrasound is the most effective method of diagnosis of submucosal mass lesions such as GI stromal tumors. Smears of FNA biopsy material show cellular smears with variably sized clumps of

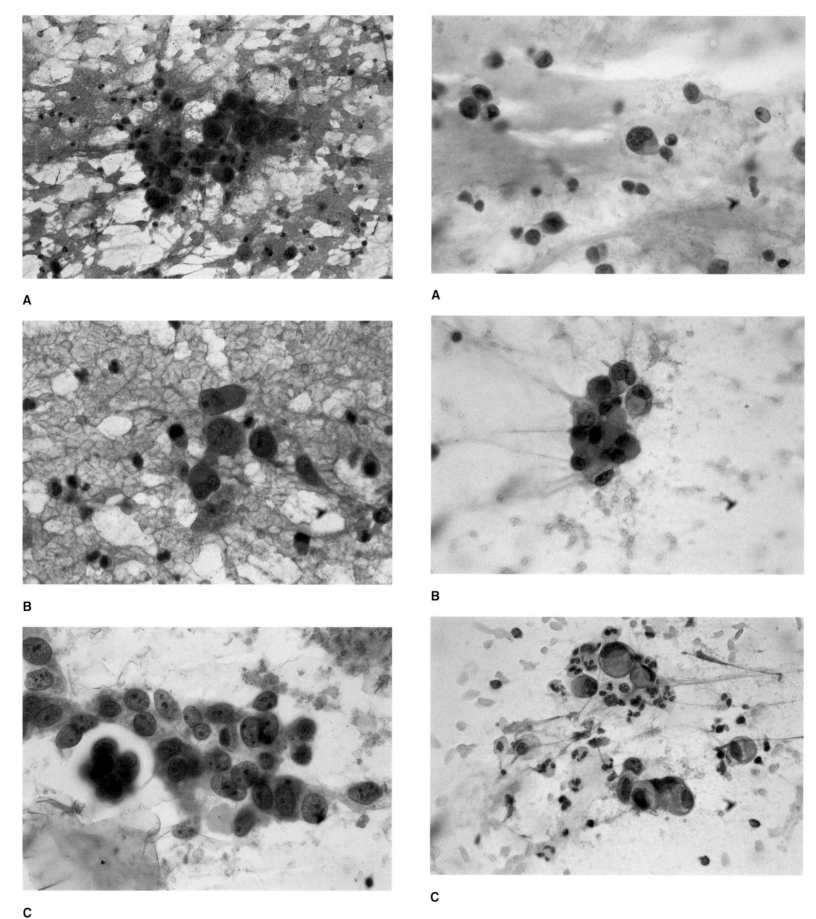

Figure 18–23. A: Gastric brushing, showing adenocarcinoma, characterized by a discohesive group of malignant epithelial cells surrounded by necrotic debris. B: Gastric adenocarcinoma, intestinal type, showing malignant glandular cells. C: Gastric adenocarcinoma, intestinal type.

Figure 18–24. A: Gastric adenocarcinoma, diffuse type with signet ring cells. The smear shows discohesive, scattered, single malignant cells. B: Gastric adenocarcinoma, signet ring cell type, showing a cohesive group of malignant cells with eccentric nuclei indented by cytoplasmic mucin. C: Signet ring cell adenocarcinoma.

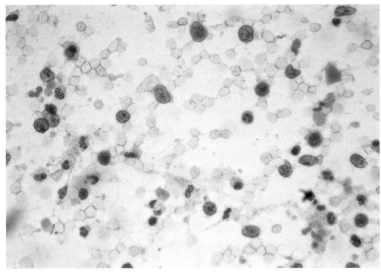

A

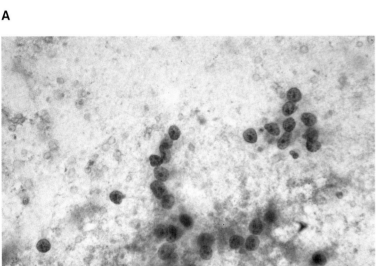

B

Figure 18–25. A: Gastric brushing in a patient with malignant lymphoma, high grade, showing discohesive round cells with round nuclei with nucleoli, resembling transformed lymphocytes. B: Malignant lymphoma of stomach, showing lymphoid cells with a tendency to grouping.

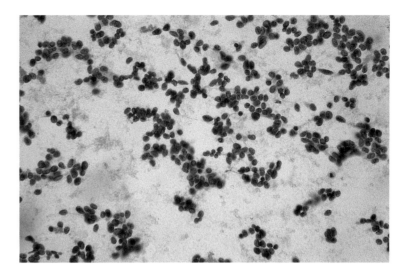

A

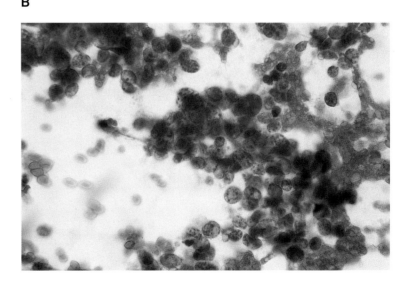

B

C

Figure 18–26. A: Carcinoid tumor of the stomach, showing irregular grouping of small round cells with round nuclei and scanty cytoplasm. B: Carcinoid tumor of the stomach showing round cells with a high N:C ratio. The cells have scanty cytoplasm and round nuclei with "salt and pepper" chromatin and nucleoli. C: Poorly differentiated malignant tumor of the stomach. The cells are round with a high N:C ratio and round nuclei. The possible diagnoses include a poorly differentiated carcinoma with neuroendocrine features.

spindle cells with a high N:C ratio (Fig. 18–27A–D). More rounded, epithelioid cells may also be present (Fig. 18–28A). The cells have cyanophilic cytoplasm and elongated blunt nuclei (spindle cell tumors) or irregular round nuclei (epithelioid tumors). Cytoplasmic vacuolation may be present in epithelioid GI stromal tumors; when pronounced, this may produce a resemblance to signet ring cell carcinoma (Fig. 18–28B and C) (see Chapter 14). In these cases, immunoperoxidase staining of smears or cell block preparations is useful. Epithelioid GI stromal tumors are usually positive for CD34 and vimentin (Fig. 18–28D); they may also show weak cytokeratin positivity, a point of importance because the differential diagnosis includes signet ring cell carcinoma. A negative mucin stain is also helpful in this differential diagnosis, because signet ring cell carcinoma is strongly positive for intracytoplasmic mucin.

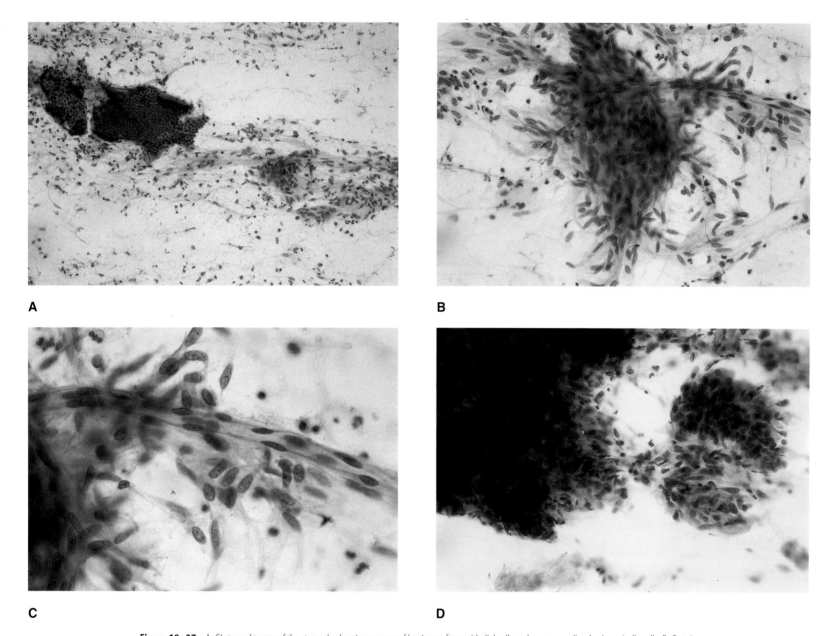

Figure 18–27. A: GI stromal tumor of the stomach, showing a group of benign surface epithelial cells and numerous discohesive spindle cells. B: Gastric GI stromal tumor, showing cellular groupings of spindle cells with numerous single cells. The nuclear features are fairly uniform. C: Higher power micrograph of part B, showing relatively uniform appearance of the spindle cells. D: Gastric GI stromal tumor, showing spindle cells with greater cellularity and more pleomorphism. Criteria for malignancy in GI stromal tumors cannot be assessed at cytology.

DUODENAL CYTOPATHOLOGY

Benign Conditions

Duodenal brushings are rarely encountered except in periampullary tumors (see following section). Normal duodenal mucosal cells are tall columnar cells seen in sheets with a "honeycomb" arrangement (Fig. 18–29). The goblet cells impart the same "swiss cheese" appearance as described in Barrett's esophagus. The cells have basal nuclei, cytoplasmic vacuolation, and apical striated borders. In erosive lesions, deeper mucous cells of the Brunner's glands and Paneth cells may be en-

countered. Erosions and ulcerations associated with acute nonspecific duodenitis and chronic peptic ulcers produce smears that are cellular, with inflammation and necrosis. The cells show reactive changes similar to those described in the stomach (Fig. 18–30). The incidence of adenocarcinoma in the duodenal bulb is so low that it is probably wise not to make a diagnosis of adenocarcinoma without having biopsy confirmation.

Infectious agents are rarely encountered in duodenal brushings. These include *Helicobacter pylori,* which is associated with gastric metaplasia, cytomegalovirus, *Cryptosporidium,* and *Giardia lamblia. Cryptosporidium* is an opportunistic parasite that occurs in normal people, but causes severe disease

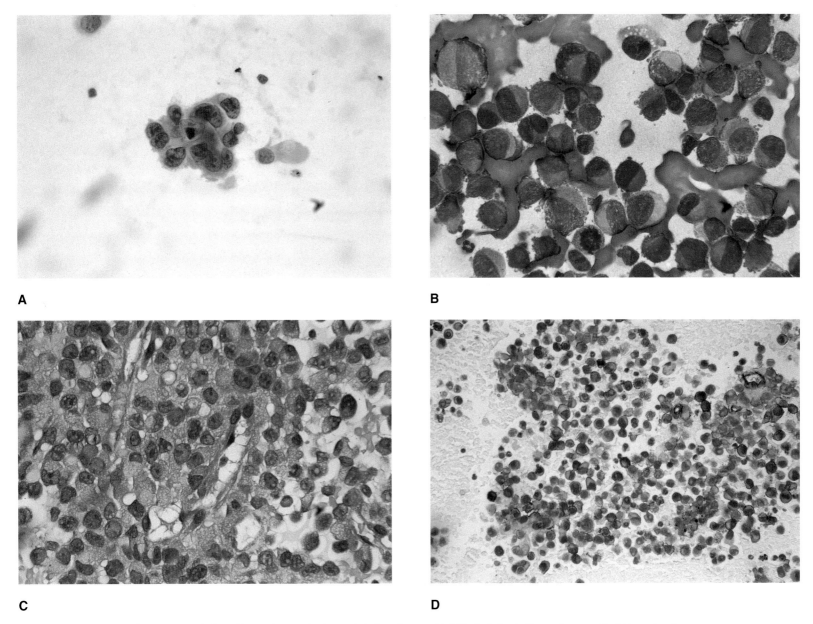

Figure 18–28. A: Gastric GI stromal tumor, showing cytologically malignant epithelioid cells. B: Gastric GI stromal tumor, epithelioid type, in a fine-needle aspiration, air-dried Diff-Quik stain, showing malignant rounded cells with eccentric nuclei and abundant cytoplasm. C: Gastric stromal tumor, epithelial type, cell block preparation, showing round cells with cytoplasmic vacuoles resembling signet ring cells. D: Gastric GI stromal tumor, immunoperoxidase stain for CD34, showing positivity in the neoplastic cells. This tumor was negative for cytokeratin and lymphoid and plasma cell markers.

only in immunocompromised hosts, appearing in smears as a round 2–4-μm basophilic protozoan, seen best in Diff-Quik stained sections. Duodenal aspiration specimens represent the most sensitive method of diagnosis of *Giardia lamblia*. In smears, the organisms resemble degenerated pale-staining nuclei; they are 12–15-μm, pear-shaped trophozoites with two nuclei and a flagellum (Fig. 18–31). When seen from the side, the organisms appear sickle-shaped.

Brush cytology of the duodenum has proven a useful adjunct to biopsy in patients who have had bone marrow transplantation for the evaluation of posttransplantation lymphoproliferative disorder and graft-versus-host disease[23] (see Chapter 17).

Neoplasms

Periampullary Tumors

Cytologic preparations, including brushings and washings, and aspirations from the terminal common duct, extrahepatic biliary system, and cannulated pancreatic duct are being increasingly used in the diagnosis of periampullary tumors. These diagnostic techniques have greater access to these structures than biopsy forceps at endoscopic retrograde cholangiopancreatography (ERCP). Bile, pancreatic, and duodenal aspirates should be processed rapidly to prevent digestion of cells by the high enzyme content of these fluids. Transporting these specimens on ice and using a refrigerated centrifuge have been recom-

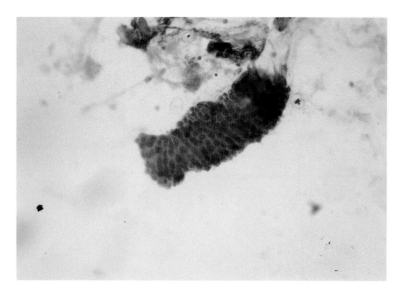

Figure 18–29. Duodenal brushing, showing normal epithelial grouping.

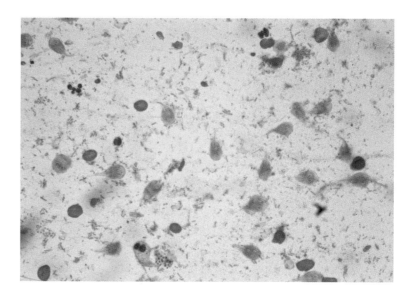

Figure 18–31. Duodenal aspirate, showing numerous trophozoites of *Giardia lamblia.*

mended.[24,25,26] Larger mass lesions of the periampullary region are frequently assessed by percutaneous FNA biopsy or intraoperative FNA by direct visualization.

Smears and cell block preparations from this region normally show cells from duodenal mucosa (see previous section) and cells from bile and pancreatic ducts (Fig. 18–32). The latter are usually few in number, appearing as cohesive, flat monolayers of medium-size columnar cells. These cell groups have a "honeycomb," or palisaded, pattern and distinct borders. The cells have a low N:C ratio; nuclei with delicate chromatin and smooth nuclear membranes; and cytoplasm that is abundant, delicate, and pale. Degenerative changes in biliary and pancreatic cells are common and consist of cytoplasmic eosinophilia, loss of nuclear detail with pyknosis and karyorrhexis, and nuclear irregularity. Long and thin "pencil" cells, or "matchstick" cells, which are elongated with a bulging polar nucleus, may be present. Rarely, infectious agents are encountered; these include *Cryptosporidium* in immunocompromised patients (see

Chapter 17), ova of *Ascaris lumbricoides,* and *Clonorchis sinensis* (Fig. 18–33).

Reactive changes in these cells may be seen in inflammatory disease, calculous disease, and benign tumors. Reactive cells are orderly, cohesive sheets of cells with absent or rare single cells, which show nuclear enlargement, but generally the N:C ratio is maintained. Polarity of the cells within aggregates is normal without nuclear crowding or overlapping. Nucleoli are commonly seen, and typical mitotic figures may be present. In inflammatory lesions, numerous neutrophils may be present. We have encountered a granular cell tumor of the terminal bile duct in a patient who presented with obstructive jaundice and a clinically and radiologically malignant stricture of the terminal bile duct.[27] Smears from this lesion showed large, discohesive cells with small, bland, central nuclei and abundant granular eosinophilic cytoplasm (Fig. 18–34). Hyperplasia and reactive change in the overlying epithelium may mimic carcinoma in smears from granular cell tumors and is a potential trap for false-positive diagnosis of cancer.

Pancreaticobiliary carcinomas are usually well-differentiated adenocarcinomas. Differentiating between papillary noninvasive tumors and well-differentiated adenocarcinomas may be impossible (Fig. 18–35). Less commonly, they are poorly differentiated and may show squamous, spindle cell, and pleomorphic features with tumor giant cells. Smears from brushings or aspirates show poorly cohesive sheets of cells with numerous single epithelial cells. Three-dimensional cell clusters with nuclear crowding and overlapping are present. The cells are larger than normal, have enlarged nuclei, a high N:C ratio, coarse chromatin, irregular nuclear membranes ("tulip," "popcorn" cells, and nuclear grooves and nipple-like protrusions of the nuclear membranes), prominent nucleoli, and pleomorphism (Fig. 18–36). Nuclear molding and atypical mitotic figures may be seen. Papillary groups are seen in both benign neoplasms (villous adenoma of papilla of Vater) and adenocarcinomas.

The difficulties with separating well-differentiated adenocarcinoma, which accounts for the majority of pancreaticobil-

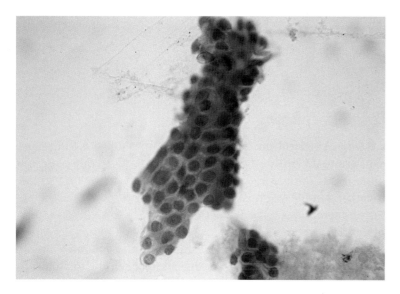

Figure 18–30. Duodenal brushing, showing benign epithelial grouping with mild reactive atypia.

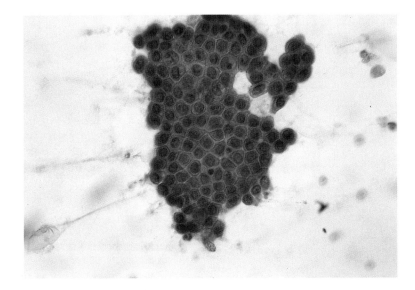

A

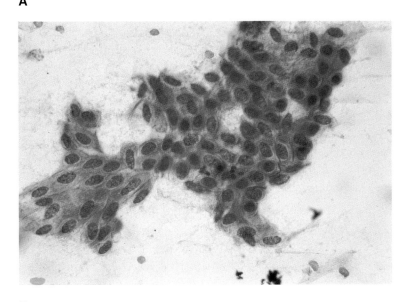

B

Figure 18–32. A: Brushing from the ampulla of Vater, showing a benign, cohesive, epithelial grouping from the terminal bile duct. Note the green-staining bile. B: Ampulla of Vater brushing, showing benign biliary epithelial cell grouping.

iary malignancies, from reactive changes in these cells makes the sensitivity of diagnosis relatively low and false-negatives frequent. False-positive diagnosis is rare in experienced hands.[28] Fine-needle aspiration biopsy has a higher sensitivity in the diagnosis of pancreatic tumors.

Neoplastic Lesions Outside the Periampullary Region

These lesions are rarely encountered in brushings. Benign duodenal tumors such as Brunner's gland hamartoma and gangliocytic paraganglioma are submucosal; they do not appear in brushings, but may be diagnosed by endoscopic ultrasound-directed FNA biopsy. Adenocarcinoma, malignant lymphoma, GI stromal tumor, and carcinoid tumors may be encountered; they have features identical to these tumors in the stomach.

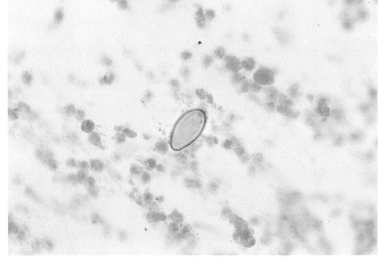

Figure 18–33. *Clonorchis sinensis.*

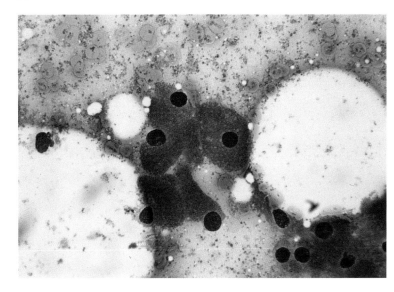

A

B

Figure 18–34. A: Granular cell tumor. B: Granular cell tumor, Diff-Quik stain, showing enlarged cells with small uniform nuclei and abundant granular cytoplasm.

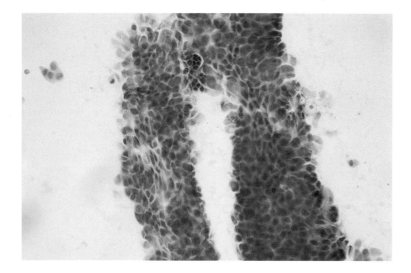

A

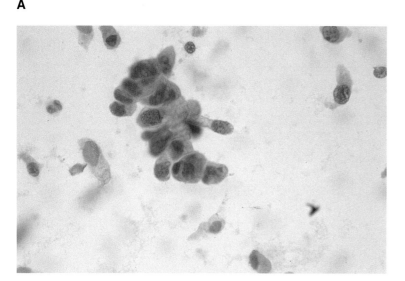

B

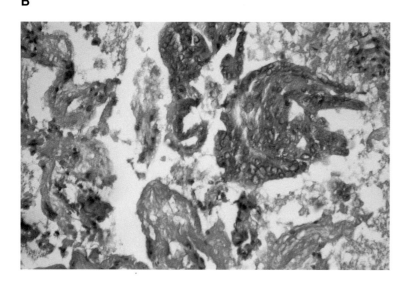

C

Figure 18–35. A: Brushing from a well-differentiated ampullary carcinoma, showing cohesive grouping of cells with cell crowding and mild pleomophism. The degree of cytologic abnormality is not marked. It is difficult to diagnose malignancy on the strength of this smear; this could be from a papillary adenoma. B: Duodenal adenocarcinoma, showing a smaller, more discohesive group of malignant cells with single malignant cells. C: Duodenal brushing, cell block, showing a well-differentiated papillary adenocarcinoma. Again, this is difficult to differentiate from a papillary adenoma.

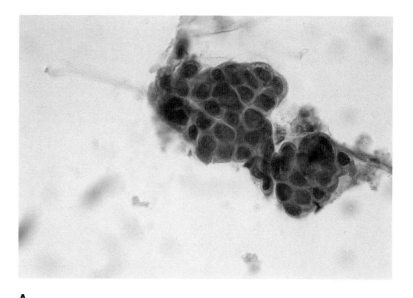

A

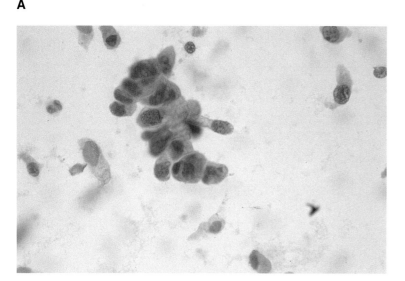

B

Figure 18–36. A: Adenocarcinoma of the ampulla of Vater, showing a cohesive grouping of cells with an increased N:C ratio, marked nuclear atypia, and pleomorphism. B: Cell block from ampullary brushing, showing malignant glandular cells in papillary clusters.

COLONIC CYTOPATHOLOGY

Benign Conditions

Colonic cytopathology specimens are rare, consisting of brushings obtained during endoscopy from visible lesions. Their rarity is due to the fact that colonoscopic biopsy has such a high rate of accuracy of diagnosis, making the addition of a cytologic specimen difficult to justify in most cases. Although cytology theoretically has a useful role in surveillance of patients with chronic ulcerative colitis, the colonic mucosal surface is so vast that endoscopic brushing is cumbersome, time-consuming, and rarely done in practice. Enemas and blind colonic lavages have been suggested, but have never achieved significant usage because they are cumbersome, cause patient discomfort, and have no proven value.

Brushings of normal colonic mucosa show sheets of cohesive cells with a honeycomb, or palisade, arrangement. The cells are tall columnar cells with many interspersed pale goblet cells with mucin vacuoles (Fig. 18–37).

Rarely, brush specimens show features of a hyperplastic polyp, characterized by mucin-distended cells (Fig. 18–38), atypia of epithelial cells associated with radiation (Fig. 18–39), and infectious agents, most commonly trophozoites of *Entamoeba histolytica* (Fig. 18–40A and B). It should be noted that the finding of infectious agents may represent commensal luminal growth rather than infection (Fig. 18–40C).

Cytology brush specimens from patients with idiopathic inflammatory bowel disease are best for the purpose of diagnosing epithelial dysplasia during the inactive phase of the disease in a

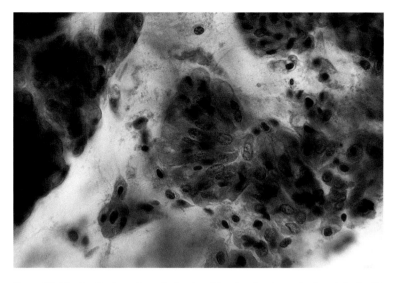

Figure 18–38. Brushing from a hyperplastic polyp of the colon, showing mucin-distended cells with small basal nuclei.

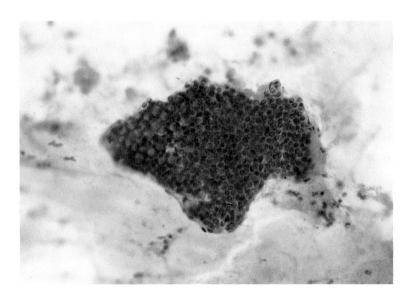

A

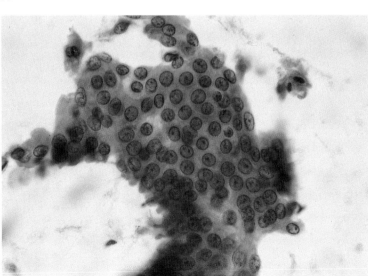

B

Figure 18–37. A: Brushing from the colon, showing normal colonic epithelial cells. These form a tightly cohesive cluster with scattered clear goblet cells. B: Colonic brushing, showing normal epithelial cell grouping. Note the scattered cells with clear cytoplasm, representing goblet cells.

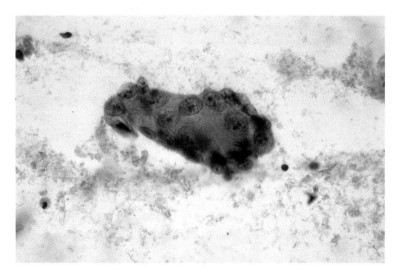

A

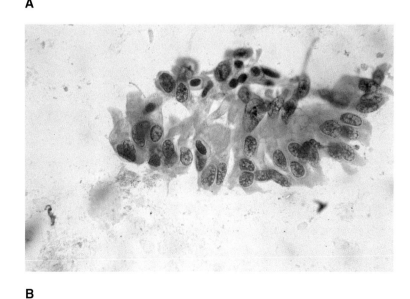

B

Figure 18–39. A: Brushing from colonic mucosa in a patient with radiation proctitis, showing markedly atypical cells in a tight cluster. B: Brushing in radiation proctitis, showing pleomorphism and atypia in columnar cells.

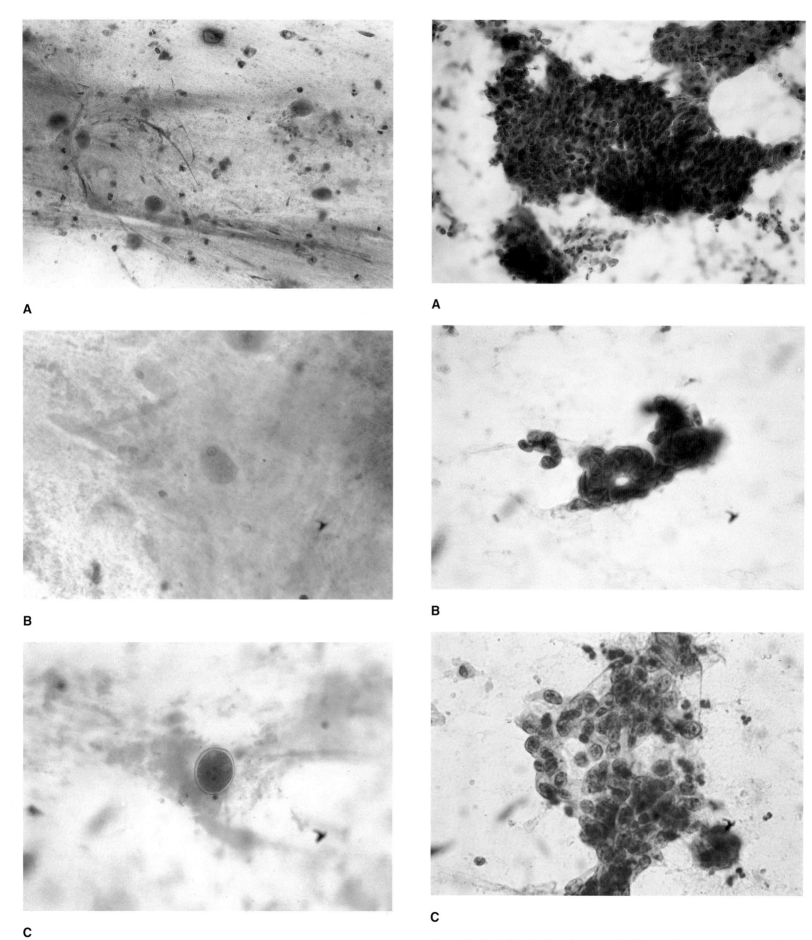

Figure 18–40. A: Colonic brushing in amebic colitis, showing trophozoites of *Entamoeba histolytica*. B: Trophozoite of *Entamoeba histolytica*. C: Cyst of *Entamoeba histolytica* in a colonic brushing.

Figure 18–41. A: Colon brushing, showing a well-differentiated adenocarcinoma, with a cohesive grouping of cells with cytologic features of malignancy. B: Colonic brushing, showing moderately differentiated adenocarcinoma. C: Colonic brushing, showing moderately differentiated adenocarcinoma.

surveillance setting. Specimens taken during the active phase of the disease show necrotic and inflammatory material from ulcers and marked reactive changes in the epithelial cells that are difficult to interpret accurately. In the nonulcerated inactive phase, epithelial cells can be evaluated for the presence of high-grade dysplasia, which has features similar to those of adenocarcinoma, but occur without a visible colonic endoscopic lesion.

Malignant Neoplasms

Most colonic brushings are from adenocarcinomas. The most valuable role for brushings is in tight malignant strictures that impede the passage of the colonoscope and biopsy forceps, and in which there is a significant false-negative rate of diagnosis. In these cases, the brush can frequently be passed through the narrowed area for accessing the tumor surface. In some instances, endoscopic transmural FNA biopsy can increase the diagnostic yield.[29]

Brushings from adenocarcinoma show cellular smears with crowded, overlapping groups of loosely cohesive cells with loss of polarity (Fig. 18–41). There are increased numbers of single cells (Fig. 18–41C). The cell groups have glandular and microacinar patterns. In well-differentiated adenocarcinoma, the cells are columnar with cigar-shaped nuclei; in less differentiated tumors, the cells tend to be rounded with round nuclei. The nuclei are enlarged, with an increased N:C ratio, pleomorphism, coarse chromatin, and prominent nucleoli.

The cytologic diagnosis of other malignant neoplasms, such as malignant lymphoma, carcinoid tumor, and GI stromal tumors, are as described for the stomach and duodenum.

THE ANAL CANAL

Benign Conditions

The anal canal is a site of high risk in anoreceptive male homosexuals, being the site of many types of sexually transmitted diseases. One of these, human papillomavirus infection, is associated with progressive dysplastic changes in the squamous epithelium, leading to squamous carcinoma. In many ways, the anal canal of anoreceptive male homosexuals is similar in its risk status to the uterine cervix of females. As such, cytologic surveillance protocols similar to Pap smears in females have been recommended in this population. Women who are HIV-positive and women with cervical intraepithelial lesions (CIN) also have a threefold increased risk of HPV infection of the anal canal and anal intraepithelial lesions; this is a second population group in whom routine anal cytology is indicated. Cytologic specimens may be obtained by the gloved finger during rectal examination or by direct scraping/brushing using an endocervical brush, wooden spatula, or moistened cotton or Dacron swabs.

Samples from the normal anal canal consist predominantly of intermediate squamous cells (Fig. 18–42A and B).

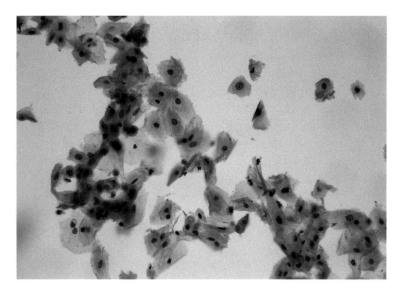

A

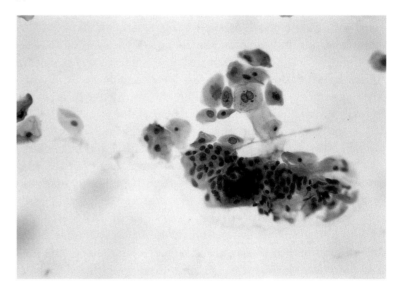

B

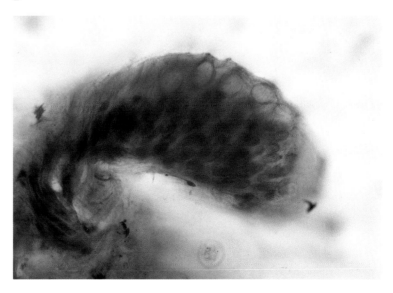

C

Figure 18–42. Normal anal smear. A: Thin-Prep, showing intermediate squamous cells. B: Thin-Prep, showing intermediate squamous cells and a group of transitional cells from the anal transitional zone. C: Smear, showing a group of benign columnar cells.

Some columnar cells (Fig. 18–42C) and "umbrella" cells from the anal transitional epithelium are often present (Fig. 18–42B). Their presence is an indication of adequacy of the specimen, because sampling must extend up to the rectum; many anal canal squamous carcinomas arise in the anal transitional zone. At present, a high proportion of cytology specimens from the anal canal are inadequate and do not contain transitional or glandular epithelium. This inadequacy results from a lack of experience and enthusiasm on the part of the person obtaining the specimen. Increased recognition of the value of this procedure in patient care and increased operator experience will improve the quality of smears. The use of automated monolayer preparations have been shown to yield more than twice as many satisfactory specimens.[30]

The main value of anal cytologic preparations is in patients in the high-risk male homosexual group who do not have a visible abnormality at proctoscopic examination. Samples are best taken when no active inflammatory or ulcerative disease is evident, with the objective of identifying subclinical flat condylomatous lesions and squamous intraepithelial lesions of increasing grade.[31,32] The evaluation of these smears uses a system similar to evaluation of Pap smears in the female. As experience with Pap smears is readily available, the knowledge base for interpretation of anal cytology is widely available.

Condyloma acuminatum is characterized by pathognomonic koilocytes with nuclear hyperchromasia and irregularity and well-defined cytolplasmic cavities (Fig. 18–43). In the anal canal, flat condylomas frequently do not have pathognomonic koilocytes; rather, less specific dyskeratotic cells occur with HPV infection.[33] The use of Thin-Prep smears (Fig. 18–42A and B) with simultaneous evaluation for human papillomavirus is the optimal method of evaluating anal cytologic specimens.

Cytologic features of squamous intraepithelial lesions (anal intraepithelial neoplasia, or AIN; also called anal squamous intraepithelial lesion, or ASIL) are cells with an increased N:C ratio, nuclear enlargement and hyperchromasia with coarse

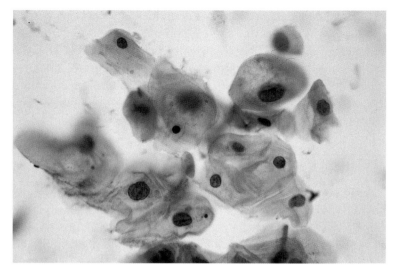

A

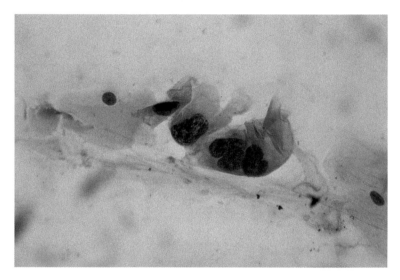

B

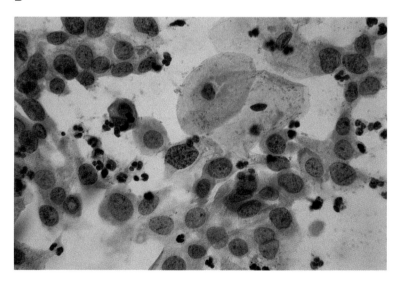

C

Figure 18–44. A: Low-grade intraepithelial neoplasia, showing squamous epithelial cells with slightly enlarged, hyperchromatic, and irregular nuclei. B: High-grade anal intraepithelial neoplasia, showing squamous cells with enlarged, irregular, hyperchromatic nuclei and an increased N:C ratio. C: High-grade anal intraepithelial neoplasia, showing enlarged irregular nuclei with hyperchromasia. The degree of cytologic abnormality is less than that shown in part B.

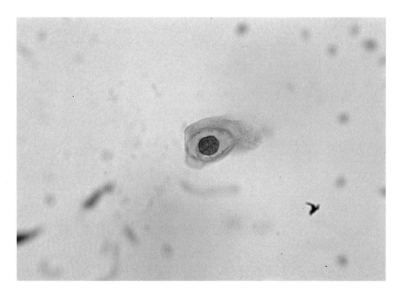

Figure 18–43. Anal canal brushing, showing a cell infected by human papillomavirus with a typical koilocyte with nuclear hyperchromasia and irregularity with a well-defined cytoplasmic cavity.

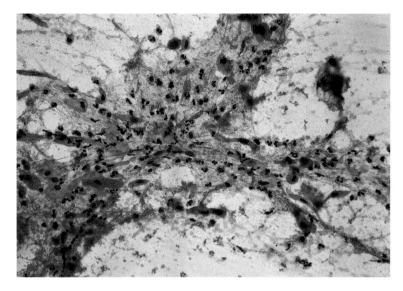

A

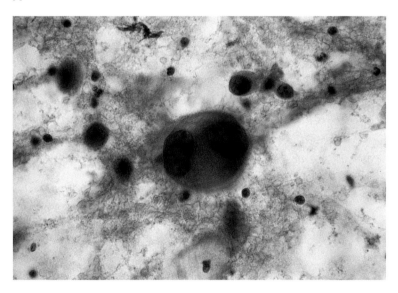

B

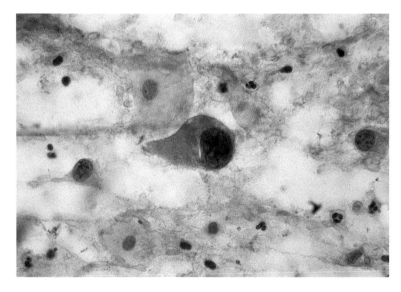

C

Figure 18–45. A: Anal smear, showing keratinizing squamous carcinoma with atypical, pyknotic nuclei. B: Squamous carcinoma of the anal canal, showing malignant, binucleated, squamous epithelial cell. C: Anal squamous carcinoma, showing a single, malignant squamous epithelial cell.

chromatin distribution, and irregular nuclear membranes (Fig. 18–44). AIN is divided into low and high grade by criteria similar to those used for cervical squamous intraepithelial neoplasia (Fig. 18–44A–C).

Malignant Neoplasms

Brush cytology from visible anal mass lesions complements biopsies, but is rarely obtained in practice because of the very high rate of accuracy of biopsy diagnosis. Most anal canal masses are squamous carcinomas with cytologic features as described previously for squamous carcinomas elsewhere (Fig. 18–45A–C). Basaloid carcinomas also occur, particularly high in the anal transitional zone. These are characterized by more basaloid-appearing squamous cells with a higher N:C ratio and scanty cyanophilic cytoplasm. They may also contain glandular elements. Small-cell undifferentiated neuroendocrine carcinoma, malignant lymphoma, malignant melanoma, and GI stromal tumors are rarely encountered (see Chapter 16).

References

1. Behmard S, Sadeghi A, Bagheri SA. Diagnostic accuracy of endoscopy with brushing cytology and biopsy in upper gastrointestinal lesions. *Acta Cytol.* 1978;22:153–154.
2. Geisinger KR, Teot LA, Richter JE. A comparative cytopathologic and histologic study of atypia, dysplasia, and adenocarcinoma in Barrett's esophagus. *Cancer.* 1992;69:8–16.
3. Lan C. Critical evaluation of the cytodiagnosis of fibrogastroendoscopic samples obtained under direct vision. *Acta Cytol.* 1990; 34:217–220.
4. Wang HH, Jonasson JG, Ducatman BS. Brushing cytology of the upper gastrointestinal tract: Obsolete or not? *Acta Cytol.* 1991;35: 195–198.
5. Moreno-Otero R, Martinez-Raposo A, Cantero J, et al. Exfoliative cytodiagnosis of gastric adenocarcinoma: Comparison with biopsy and endoscopy. *Acta Cytol.* 1983;27:485–488.
6. Wiersema MJ, Wiersema LM, Khusro Q, et al. Combined endosonography and fine needle aspiration cytology in the evaluation of gastrointestinal lesions. *Gastrointest Endosc.* 1994;40: 199–206.
7. Bardawil RG, D'Ambrosio FG, Hajdu SI. Colonic cytology: A retrospective study with histopathologic correlation. *Acta Cytol.* 1990;34:620–626.
8. Thompson H, Hoare AM, Dykes PW, et al. A prospective randomised trial to compare brush cytology before or after punch biopsy for endoscopic diagnosis of gastric cancer. *Gut.* 1977;18: 398–428.
9. Zargar SA, Khuroo MS, Jan GM, et al. Prospective comparison of the value of brushings before and after biopsy in the endoscopic diagnosis of gastroesophageal malignancy. *Acta Cytol.* 1991;35: 549–552.
10. Keighley MRB, Thompson H, Moore J, et al. Comparison of brush cytology before or after biopsy for diagnosis for gastric carcinoma. *Br J Surg.* 1979;66:246–247.
11. Ogden GR, Nairn A, Franks J, et al. Do gelatin-coated slides increase cellular retention in oral exfoliative cytology? *Acta Cytol.* 1991;35:186–188.

12. Sharma P, Misra V, Singh PA, et al. A correlative study of histology and imprint cytology in the diagnosis of gastrointestinal tract malignancies. *Indian Path Microbiol.* 1977;40:139–146.

13. Falk GW, Chittajallu R, Goldblum JR, et al. Surveillance of patients with Barrett's esophagus for dysplasia and cancer with balloon cytology. *Gastroenterology.* 1997;112:1787–1797.

14. Koss LG. Cytologic diagnosis of oral, esophageal, and peripheral lung cancer. *J Cell Biochem. (Suppl)* 1993;17:66–81.

15. Shu YJ. Cytopathology of the esophagus: An overview of esophageal cytopathology in China. *Acta Cytol.* 1983;27:7–16.

16. Geisinger KR. Endoscopic biopsies and cytologic brushings of the esophagus are diagnostically complementary. *Am J Clin Pathol.* 1995;103:295–299.

17. Wright RG, Augustine B, Whitfield A. Candida in gastroesophageal cytological and histological preparations: A comparative study. *Labmedica.* 1987;4:29–30.

18. Young JA, Elias E. Gastro-esophageal candidiasis: Diagnosis by brush cytology. *J Clin Pathol.* 1985;38:293–296.

19. Rubio CA, Jessurum J, de Ruiz PA. Geographic variations in the histologic characteristics of the gastric mucosa. *Am J Clin Pathol.* 1991;96:330–333.

20. Schnadig VJ, Bigio EH, Gourley WK, et al. Identification of *Campylobacter pylori* by endoscopic brush cytology. *Diagn Cytopathol.* 1990;6:227–234.

21. Sherman ME, Anderson C, Herman LM, et al. Utility of gastric brushing in the diagnosis of malignant lymphoma. *Acta Cytol.* 1994;38:169–174.

22. Benya RV, Metz DC, Hijazi YJ, et al. Fine needle aspiration cytology of submucosal nodules in patient with Zollinger-Ellison syndrome. *Am J Gastroenterol.* 1993;88:258–265.

23. Kuusanmaki P, Paavonen T, Pakkala S, et al. Brush cytology in the course of acute small bowel allograft rejection. *Acta Cytol.* 1997;41:1500–1509.

24. Kline TS, Joshi LP, Goldstein F. Preoperative diagnosis of pancreatic malignancy by the cytologic examination of duodenal secretions. *Am J Clin Pathol.* 1978;70:851–854.

25. Wertlake PT, Del Guercio LRM. Cytopathology of intrahepatic bile as component of integrated procedure ("minilap") for hepatobiliary disorders. *Acta Cytol.* 1976;20:42–45.

26. Yamada T, Murohisa B, Muto Y, et al. Cytologic detection of small pancreaticoduodenal and biliary cancers in the early development stage. *Acta Cytol.* 1984;28:435–442.

27. Chandrasoma P, Fitzgibbons P. Granular cell tumor of the intrapancreatic common bile duct. *Cancer* 1984;53:2178–2182.

28. Nakajima T, Tajima Y, Sugano I, et al. Multivariate statistical analysis of bile cytology. *Acta Cytol.* 1994;38:51–55.

29. Zargar SA, Khuroo MS, Mahajan R, et al. Endoscopic fine needle aspiration cytology in the diagnosis of gastro-esophageal and colorectal malignancies. *Gut.* 1991;32:745–748.

30. Sherman ME, Friedman HB, Busseniers AE, et al. Cytologic diagnosis of anal intraepithelial neoplasia using smears and Cytyc Thin-Preps. *Mod Pathol.* 1995;8:270–274.

31. Haye KR, Maiti H, Stanbridge CM. Cytological screening to detect subclinical anal human papillomavirus (HPV) infection in homosexual men attending genitourinary medicine clinic. *Genitourin Med.* 1988;64:378–382.

32. Surawicz CM, Critchlow C, Sayer J, et al. High grade anal dysplasia in visually normal mucosa in homosexual men: Seven cases. *Am J Gastroenterol.* 1995;90:1776–1778.

33. Sonnex C, Scholefield JH, Kocjan G, et al. Anal human papillomavirus infection: A comparative study of cytology, colposcopy and DNA hybridisation as methods of detection. *Genitourin Med.* 1991;67:21–25.

INDEX

Page numbers in *italics* denote figures; those followed by "t" denote tables.